Diagnostic Dermoscopy

JB
To my father.

JP
To my wife Ana for all her support.

AC
To my wife Helen, my children Henry,
Imogen and Thomas, and my parents John and Christine.

Diagnostic Dermoscopy
The Illustrated Guide

Second Edition

Jonathan Bowling MBChB FRCP
Consultant Dermatologist
Oxford, UK

Consultant Editors

John Paoli PhD
Professor, Department of Dermatology and Venereology, Institute of Clinical Sciences, Sahlgrenska Academy, University of Gothenburg; and
Consultant Dermatologist,
Sahlgrenska University Hospital, Gothenburg, Sweden

Alex Chamberlain MBBS (Hons) FACD
Adjunct Senior Lecturer, Central Clinical School, Monash University; and
Specialist Dermatologist,
Victorian Melanoma Service, Alfred Health,
Prahran, Victoria, Australia

WILEY Blackwell

This edition first published 2022

Edition History
1e © 2012 by Jonathan Bowling

Registered Offices
John Wiley & Sons, Inc., 111 River Street, Hoboken, NJ 07030, USA
John Wiley & Sons Ltd, The Atrium, Southern Gate, Chichester, West Sussex, PO19 8SQ, UK

Editorial Offices
101 Station Landing, Medford, MA 02155, USA
9600 Garsington Road, Oxford, OX4 2DQ, UK

For details of our global editorial offices, customer services, and more information about Wiley products visit us at www.wiley.com.

Wiley also publishes its books in a variety of electronic formats and by print-on-demand. Some content that appears in standard print versions of this book may not be available in other formats.

Library of Congress Cataloging-in-Publication Data

Names: Bowling, Jonathan, author.
Title: Diagnostic dermoscopy : the illustrated guide / Jonathan Bowling.
Description: Second edition. | Hoboken, NJ : Wiley-Blackwell, 2022. |
Includes bibliographical references and index.
Identifiers: LCCN 2021027285 (print) | LCCN 2021027286 (ebook) | ISBN
9781118930489 (paperback) | ISBN 9781118932056 (adobe pdf) | ISBN
9781118931622 (epub)
Subjects: MESH: Dermoscopy | Skin Diseases–diagnosis | Atlas
Classification: LCC RL105 (print) | LCC RL105 (ebook) | NLM WR 17 | DDC
616.5/075–dc23
LC record available at https://lccn.loc.gov/2021027285
LC ebook record available at https://lccn.loc.gov/2021027286

Cover Design: Wiley
Cover Images: © John Lamb/Getty, Courtesy of Jonathan Bowling

Set in 9/12pt Frutiger by Straive, Chennai, India

Printed in Great Britain by Bell and Bain Ltd, Glasgow
B000924_290824

Contents

Preface, xi

Chapter 1 Introduction, 1
Introduction, 2
Dermoscopy and diagnosis, 3
Dermoscopy principle I – illumination, 4
Dermoscopy principle II – magnification, 5
Dermoscopy colours I – eumelanin, 6
Dermoscopy colours II – non-eumelanin, 7
Imaging modes I – colours, 8
Imaging modes II – structures, 9
Dermoscopy of normal skin, 10
Dermoscopy of photodamaged skin, 11
Vascular morphologies, 12
Characteristic vascular patterns, 13
Polarised dermoscopy – shiny white structures, 14

Chapter 2 Melanocytic naevi, 15
Early naevi – globular, 16
Acquired naevi – reticular, 17
Acquired naevi – homogeneous, 18
Acquired naevi – evolving, 19
Acquired naevi in light skin, 20
Acquired naevi in medium-toned skin, 21
Atypical melanocytic lesions, 22
Atypical melanocytic lesions cases, 23
Dermal naevus – pigmented, 24
Dermal naevus – hyperpigmented, 25
Dermal naevus in dark skin, 26
Combined naevus, 27
Blue naevus, 28
Blue naevus – sclerotic/hypochromic, 29
Recurrent naevus, 30
Halo naevus, 31
Congenital naevus, 32
Agminated naevus and naevus spilus, 33
Reed naevus I, 34
Reed naevus II, 35
Pigmented Spitz naevus, 36
Hypomelanotic Spitz naevus I, 37
Hypomelanotic Spitz naevus II, 38

Chapter 3 Melanoma

Chapter 3.1 Melanoma – clinical variants, 39
Small diameter, 40
Small diameter cases, 41
Geometric border, 42
Geometric border cases, 43
Geographic border, 44
Geographic border cases, 45
Disordered polarity, 46
Disordered polarity cases, 47
Naevus-associated, 48
Naevus-associated cases, 49
Congenital melanocytic naevus-associated, 50

Chapter 3.2 Melanoma – pigment variants, 51
Multicoloured, 52
Multicoloured cases, 53
Multicomponent, 54
Multicomponent cases, 55
Hypermelanotic/hyperpigmented, 56
Hypermelanotic/hyperpigmented cases, 57
Amelanotic macules, 58
Amelanotic macules – cases, 59
Amelanotic papules, 60
Amelanotic papules – cases, 61
Hypomelanotic macules, 62
Hypomelanotic macules – cases, 63
Hypomelanotic tan plaques, 64
Hypomelanotic tan plaques cases, 65

Chapter 3.3 Melanoma – dermoscopic features, 66

Features of early melanoma, 67
Atypical network – focal, 68
Atypical network – focal cases, 69
Atypical network – multifocal, 70
Atypical network – multifocal cases, 71
Atypical beaded network, 72
Atypical beaded network cases, 73
Black dots and globules, 74
Black dots and globules cases, 75
Eccentric brown blotch, 76
Eccentric brown blotch – cases, 77
Eccentric black blotch, 78
Eccentric black blotch – cases, 79
Eccentric grey blotch, 80
Eccentric grey blotch – cases, 81
Angulated lines, 82
Angulated lines cases, 83
Negative network, 84
Negative network cases, 85
Extensive regression, 86
Extensive regression cases, 87
Focal regression, 88
Focal regression cases, 89
Blue-whitish veil, 90
Blue-whitish veil cases, 91
Dermal pigmentation, 92
Dermal pigmentation cases, 93
Polymorphous vessels, 94
Polymorphous vessels cases, 95
Skin surface markings, 96
Skin surface markings cases, 97

Chapter 3.4 Melanoma – high-risk scenarios, 98

Late features of melanoma, 99
Feature-poor melanoma, 100
Feature-poor melanoma cases, 101
Nodular melanoma, 102
Nodular melanoma cases, 103
Amelanotic nodular melanoma, 104
Amelanotic nodular melanoma cases, 105
Metastatic melanoma, 106
Metastatic melanoma cases, 107
Rare melanoma subtypes, 108
Synchronous melanoma, 109

Chapter 4 Non-melanocytic lesions, 110

Macrocomedone, 111
Solar lentigo – fingerprint pattern, 112
Solar lentigo – homogeneous pattern, 113
Solar lentigo – reticular pattern, 114
Solar lentigo – hyperpigmented 'ink spot', 115
Solar lentigo – evolving seborrhoeic keratosis, 116
Seborrhoeic keratosis – cerebriform pattern, 117
Seborrhoeic keratosis – homogeneous pattern, 118
Seborrhoeic keratosis – keratotic pattern, 119
Seborrhoeic keratosis – hyperpigmented, 120
Seborrhoeic keratosis – hypopigmented, 121
Seborrhoeic keratosis – irritated, 122
Seborrhoeic keratosis – traumatised, 123
Seborrhoeic keratosis – clonal, 124
Clear cell acanthoma, 125
Benign lichenoid keratosis – inflammatory phase, 126
Benign lichenoid keratosis – post-inflammatory phase, 127
Dermatofibroma, 128
Dermatofibroma – hypopigmented, 129
Dermatofibroma – hyperpigmented, 130
Dermatofibroma – atypical, 131
Dermatofibrosarcoma protuberans, 132
Neurofibromas, 133
Porokeratosis, 134
Porokeratosis cases, 135
Epidermal naevus, 136
Epidermal naevus cases, 137
Cutaneous T-cell lymphoma, 138
Pseudolymphoma, 139
Eccrine poroma, 140

Chapter 5 Basal cell carcinoma, 141

Superficial basal cell carcinoma – pink, 142
Superficial basal cell carcinoma – pink cases, 143
Superficial basal cell carcinoma – pigmented, 144
Superficial basal cell carcinoma – pigmented cases, 145
Nodular basal cell carcinoma – pink and small, 146
Nodular basal cell carcinoma – pink and small cases, 147
Nodular basal cell carcinoma – pigmented and small, 148
Nodular basal cell carcinoma – pigmented and small cases, 149
Nodular basal cell carcinoma – pink and large, 150
Nodular basal cell carcinoma – pink and large cases, 151
Morphoeic/infiltrative basal cell carcinoma, 152
Morphoeic/infiltrative basal cell carcinoma cases, 153

Hypopigmented basal cell carcinoma, 154
Hyperpigmented basal cell carcinoma, 155
Seborrhoeic keratosis-like basal cell carcinoma, 156
Fibroepithelioma of Pinkus, 157

Chapter 6 Keratinocyte dysplasia, 158
Actinic keratosis grade I, 159
Actinic keratosis grade II, 160
Actinic keratosis grade III, 161
Actinic keratosis – follicular hyperkeratosis, 162
Bowen's disease – classical, 163
Bowen's disease – hypertrophic, 164
Bowen's disease – pigmented, 165
Bowen's disease – digital, 166
Squamous cell carcinoma – white circles, 167
Squamous cell carcinoma – keratoacanthoma, 168
Squamous cell carcinoma – moderately differentiated, 169
Squamous cell carcinoma – ulcerated, 170
Squamous cell carcinoma – poorly differentiated, 171

Chapter 7 Special sites

Chapter 7.1 Acral melanocytic lesions, 172
Acquired acral naevi, 173
Acral parallel furrow pattern, 174
Acral lattice pattern, 175
Acral fibrillar pattern, 176
Congenital acral naevus, 177
Acral lentiginous melanoma, 178
Acral lentiginous melanoma cases, 179
ALM – brown-grey pigmentation, 180
ALM – brown-grey pigmentation cases, 181
Advanced acral lentiginous melanoma, 182

Chapter 7.2 Onychoscopy, 183
Nail matrix naevi, 184
Nail apparatus melanoma in situ, 185
Early invasive nail apparatus melanoma, 186
Advanced nail apparatus melanoma – pigmented, 187
Advanced nail apparatus melanoma – non-pigmented, 188
Nail apparatus squamous cell carcinoma, 189
Erythronychia, 190
Onychopapilloma, 191
Subungual haematoma, 192
Subungual haematoma cases, 193
Periungual warts, 194
Onychomycosis, 195
Chloronychia – green nails, 196
Nail pigmentation – exogenous, 197
Capillaroscopy, 198

Chapter 7.3 Facial lesions, 199
Venous lake, 200
Mucosal melanosis, 201
Milium/keratin cyst, 202
Hidrocystoma, 203
Epidermoid cysts, 204
Pilomatricoma, 205
Sebaceous hyperplasia, 206
Sebaceous adenoma, 207
Sebaceous naevus, 208
Malignant adnexal carcinomas, 209
Juvenile xanthogranuloma, 210
Granulomatous folliculitis, 211
Fibrous papule, 212
Trichilemmoma, 213
Dermal naevus, 214
Dermal naevus cases, 215
Solar lentigo – fingerprinting, 216
Solar lentigo – homogeneous pigmentation, 217
Solar lentigo – moth-eaten border, 218
Ink spot lentigo, 219
Benign lichenoid keratosis, 220
Benign lichenoid keratosis – post-inflammation phase, 221
Lentigo maligna, 222
Lentigo maligna – annular granular pigmentation, 223
Lentigo maligna – circles, 224
Lentigo maligna – perifollicular pigmentation, 225
Lentigo maligna – young adults, 226
Lentigo maligna melanoma – I, 227
Lentigo maligna melanoma – II, 228

Chapter 7.4 Scalp lesions, 229
Scalp naevus – dermal, 230
Scalp naevus – junctional, 231
Scalp naevus – blue, 232
Scalp naevus – reticular homogeneous, 233
Scalp seborrhoeic keratosis, 234
Scalp seborrhoeic keratosis cases, 235

Scalp melanoma – thin, 236
Scalp melanoma – thin cases, 237
Scalp melanoma – thick, 238
Scalp metastases, 239
Scalp basal cell carcinoma, 240
Scalp basal cell carcinoma cases, 241
Scalp B-cell lymphoma, 242
Scalp cylindromas/spiradenomas, 243
Scalp sarcoidosis, 244

Chapter 7.5 Trichoscopy, 245
Alopecia areata, 246
Androgenetic alopecia, 247
Frontal fibrosing alopecia, 248
Lichen planopilaris, 249
Discoid lupus erythematosus, 250
Tufted folliculitis, 251
Steroid-induced telangiectasia, 252
Pseudopelade, 253
Circle hairs, 254
Trichostasis spinulosa, 255
Picker's nodule, 256
Traction/frictional alopecia, 257
Pseudonits, 258

Chapter 8 Vascular lesions, 259
Telangiectasia, 260
Spider telangiectasia, 261
Subcorneal haematoma – parallel pattern, 262
Subcorneal haematoma – parallel pattern cases, 263
Subcorneal haematoma – homogeneous pattern, 264
Subcorneal haematoma – homogeneous pattern cases, 265
Haemangiomas – red, 266
Haemangiomas – purple, 267
Angiokeratomas, 268
Lymphangiomas, 269
Pyogenic granulomas, 270
Pyogenic granulomas – acral cases, 271
Vascular tumours, 272
Purpura – traumatic, 273

Chapter 9 Inflammoscopy, 274
Mastocytosis, 275
Acne, 276
Rosacea, 277
Eczema, 278
Psoriasis, 279
Lichen planus, 280
Lichen planus pigmentosus, 281
Capillaritis, 282
Vasculitis, 283
Granulomatous conditions, 284
Granuloma annulare, 285
Tinea corporis, 286
Pityriasis rosea, 287
Cutaneous lupus erythematosus, 288

Chapter 10 Genodermatoses, 289
Gorlin syndrome, 290
Cowden syndrome, 291
Birt-Hogg-Dubé syndrome, 292
Familial cylindromatosis syndrome, 293
Muir-Torre syndrome, 294
Reed syndrome, 295
Familial melanoma, 296
Carney complex, 297

Chapter 11 Entomodermoscopy, 298
Delusional parasitosis, 299
Scabies – *Sarcoptes scabiei*, 300
Scabies cases, 301
Head lice – *Pediculosis capitis, 302*
Bed bugs – *Cimex lectularius*, 303
Tick bites – Ixodidae, 304
Leishmaniasis, 305
Molluscum contagiosum, 306
Viral warts – Verrucae vulgaris, 307
Sea urchin – Echinoidea, 308
Jellyfish – Cnidaria, 309
Tungiasis – *Tunga penetrans*, 310
Myiasis – *Dermatobia hominis,* 311

Chapter 12 Miscellaneous, 312
Keloids and hypertrophic scars, 313
Foreign body, 314
Foreign body cases, 315
Exogenous pigmentation, 316
Exogenous pigmentation cases, 317
Laser, 318
Cryotherapy, 319
Radiotherapy, 320

Index, 321

Preface

Since the first edition of this textbook, 10 years ago, the utilisation of dermoscopy has steadily evolved. Although the principles and technology remain relatively unchanged, the main development is in relation to the language and terminology used and the widespread adoption of dermoscopy across clinical practice, beyond skin lesion diagnosis alone.

An evolving trend has now been to describe dermoscopic structures in a language or terminology which translate easily worldwide. This means that the dermoscopic future, and this textbook, will have less 'xanthomatous clouds' and 'cherry blossom vessels' and more dots, globules, blotches, circles and lines.

Having a reproducible language is clearly an advantage for education and learning, reducing uncertainty and the potential for miscommunication. Additionally, this minimalistic language lends itself to wider applications from teledermoscopy to artificial intelligence.

This book has therefore evolved and adapted its terminology wherever possible to embrace this new standardisation of the dermoscopic language. However, there will be scenarios and examples where historical descriptions remain; please accept that it is done to give more colour to the depth to the diagnostic, descriptive palette, and hopefully not to cause confusion.

Learning is a complex process which is influenced by many factors. How we learn is unique to the individual. The historical medical mantra of 'see one, do one, teach one' has been repeated for generations, particularly when learning procedural based tasks. However, this mantra is not relevant for the diagnostic arena, as you would clearly need to see more than two melanomas before being competent in melanoma diagnosis. Moreover, for improving clinical diagnosis we rely on experience, based upon repeated clinical exposure, clinical teaching, in addition to learning from an arrangement of medical media.

In this edition of this textbook we aim to increase learning for skin cancers and particularly melanoma by highlighting the many ways in which melanoma presents. But, rather than attributing melanoma diagnosis as mercurial, unpredictable and random, we have illustrated reproducible distinct morphological patterns of melanoma. These repeatable patterns of presentation create a morphological map of melanoma. Additionally, by illustrating many examples of each feature we aim to influence perceptual learning and thereby increase the readers' confidence and diagnostic ability for melanoma detection.

Understanding the presentations of this most malign medical diagnosis is the primary aim of this book. For early diagnosis is the most important factor in influencing survival from melanoma.

These changes would not have been possible without the valuable contributions of my co-editors Alex Chamberlain and John Paoli. Both are internationally known for their enthusiasm for dermoscopy education and their dermatological expertise. I have learnt numerous pearls of wisdom from these passionate diagnosticians over the course of this project. Alex has a natural flare for editing and when combined with John's multilingual approach to the dermoscopic literature the result is a comprehensive, focused and enhanced text. Their dermoscopic expertise has enriched this book with expert tips, accurate references and standardisation of terminology.

Together, this dermoscopic triumvirate has spent many months creating and editing content, and distilling the message of diagnosis in to a succinct and readable text. We hope you agree, and that you will find it a valuable addition to your clinical practice.

Jonathan Bowling

It has been a great pleasure to join with my colleagues John Paoli and Jonathan Bowling in co-editing the 2nd edition of Diagnostic Dermoscopy: The Illustrated Guide. I feel fortunate to have started my dermatology journey just as dermoscopy was taking off as a new discipline, hence my fascination and interest. This text brings together over 60 years of collective dermoscopy experience and the distance between our hometowns on opposite poles of the world has not dampened the collaborative process one bit. I owe plenty to mentors both in Australia and abroad, along with world experts I've been privileged to connect with at meetings and congresses. There has been no doubt that dermoscopy has absolutely changed the way we all approach diagnosis of skin lesions and with the concerted research efforts of many, the field has continued to evolve just when you thought everything had been described! I would urge those early in their journey to continue your professional development through reading, reflection and audit as we never truly stop learning.

I very much enjoyed the first edition of the 'Bowling textbook'. It was very readable, the images were excellent and the pearls were non-algorithm aligned. I happily recommended it to trainees and indeed endorsed it for the required reading list for the Australasian College of Dermatologists. My brief time working with Jonathan in 2007 in Oxford was a fruitful period and I'm thrilled that we've been able to collaborate again many years down the track. This text is aimed at all health practitioners willing to pick up a dermoscope. It has expanded since the 1st Edition naturally. Hopefully it will garner greater enthusiasm amongst readers to share the passion, to teach, to publish and continue to push the limits of non-invasive diagnosis.

Alex Chamberlain

Ever since I started teaching dermoscopy, I have recommended Jonathan Bowling's 1st edition of *Diagnostic Dermoscopy: The Illustrated Guide* to my students. The combination of concise and simple descriptions of dermoscopic findings, the vast collection of cases and the practical color-coding of the chapters for quick access to the chapter of interest make it a fantastic reference work for everyone learning dermoscopy. Thus, it was an enormous honour to be invited to contribute as a consultant editor together with Alex Chamberlain to this new edition you are holding in your hands.

The 2nd edition offers even more cases to be enjoyed and learned from while sticking to Jonathan's winning concept of brief but comprehensive texts presented in an orderly fashion. The chapters on melanocytic lesions and melanoma have grown substantially. The melanoma chapter has been divided into four separate sections and the previous chapter on special sites has now become five for even easier reading and comprehension. Furthermore, new diagnoses have been added to the general dermatology chapter and completely new chapters on vascular structures, genetic conditions, entomodermoscopy and miscellaneous clinical scenarios have been added. Beyond new images and more practical chapter categorisation, we have also increased the number of valuable clinical tips and references, which can now be found at the bottom of almost every page. Finally, the dermoscopic terminology has been modernised and standardised as much as possible to avoid confusion when comparing our book with other relevant modern literature on dermoscopy.

It has been a true privilege and a very rewarding experience to collaborate with Jonathan and Alex on this book. I thoroughly enjoyed our weekly Zoom meetings, email conversations and WhatsApp discussions, which helped us overcome ten-hour time zone differences and made the journey leading to the final product a real joyride. The changes and optimisations were a result of fruitful teamwork and our shared passion for dermoscopy and teaching. All in all, I feel very confident that this book will be enjoyed by you the reader.

John Paoli

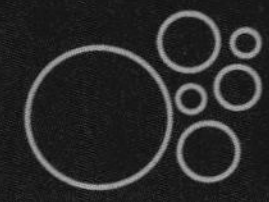

1 Introduction

Introduction 2
Dermoscopy and diagnosis 3
Dermoscopy principle I – illumination 4
Dermoscopy principle II – magnification 5
Dermoscopy colours I – eumelanin 6
Dermoscopy colours II – non-eumelanin 7
Imaging modes I – colours 8
Imaging modes II – structures 9
Dermoscopy of normal skin 10
Dermoscopy of photodamaged skin 11
Vascular morphologies 12
Characteristic vascular patterns 13
Polarised dermoscopy – shiny white structures 14

Diagnostic Dermoscopy: The Illustrated Guide, Second Edition. Jonathan Bowling.

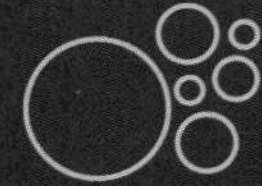

Introduction

Dermoscopy has been fully embraced by dermatologists and all those involved in skin cancer diagnosis as the gold standard tool used for clinical examination and diagnosis. It is simple to utilise, quick to apply and requires very little additional resource apart from the dermoscopy device/dermoscope itself.

However, without understanding the utility of dermoscopy, in wider clinical practice, the full diagnostic potential for the clinician may not be reached.

Format and imaging

This book is specifically a textbook with an emphasis on diagnosis, and diagnosis alone. In this way we are able to provide a comprehensive guide to the common presentations of skin lesions seen in clinics in addition to some of the more uncommon. From this starting point of diagnosis the rest of medical management flows. With greater confidence in diagnosis, a reduction in unnecessary biopsies can be achieved which frees resources to meet the increasing demand from rising skin cancer rates. Additionally, finding skin cancers at an earlier point in their evolution consumes less resources in surgical and medical management, and reduces patient morbidity and mortality.

For each topic covered, the clinical images are aimed to be standardised for illumination and orientation to aid recognition whilst illustrating the main clinical features. The adjoining dermoscopy image focuses upon key diagnostic features, which in combination with the clinical information should be all that is required for a specific diagnosis or at least a narrow differential diagnosis to be made.

Whenever possible, images of conditions have been taken across skin tones and with different dermoscope devices in different imaging modes to Illustrate the broad variety of presentations to the clinician.

Therefore, we anticipate that this book becomes a user-friendly guide, to be used in clinic by not only clinicians and nurses but also by any allied paramedical staff involved in skin lesion diagnosis.

Teledermoscopy

This format also lends itself to the growing field of teledermoscopy.

With teledermoscopy becoming an integral part of clinical practice it is helpful to have a collection of illustrated cases for reference. Therefore, throughout this book, for each topic covered, a minimal dataset, is included. This dataset includes a brief clinical description of the lesion, anatomical site and age and sex of the patient, a clear clinical image and a corresponding dermoscopic image highlighting a diagnostic feature. This textbook therefore becomes a useful reference manual, of over 500 cases, for anyone involved in teledermoscopy consultations.

Dermoscopy devices

Over the last 10 years, the greatest change in dermoscopes has been the standardisation and incorporation of both polarising and non-polarising imaging modes into the majority of dermoscopes. This leads to an increase in dermoscopic diagnostic information available for interpretation, with a simple toggle/push of a button to change between the two imaging modes. By switching between imaging modes, a composite 'occipital cortex' image can be created for interpretation and diagnosis.

There are multiple devices available for the clinician to choose. This book does not aim to advise on which device is best suited for the clinician. All we would advise is that the device sought is of a quality that allows the user to see a clear, bright, image for interpretation. The device must be robust enough for regular daily use and ergonomically designed so that it feels good in the clinician's hand. High-quality optics will ensure a crisp focused image for interpretation or image capture with a camera. The field of view needs to be of a size to provide a clear image but not too large to compromise optics or utility.

With all devices the ability to keep the dermoscope fully charged during clinical use is also an important consideration.

Therefore, for the variables mentioned above it would not be unusual for the dermoscopy enthusiast to have more than one dermoscope in regular clinical use.

Which dermoscope is best suited to your own practice is a personal choice for the clinician. Most importantly, the clinician should find a dermoscope that you want to pick up and use, feels good in your hand and fits in with your scope of clinical practice.

Clinical and histopathological correlation

We would like to emphasise that clinical diagnosis is a complex process and is based upon the summation of all relevant clinical information from the clinical history, clinical examination and dermoscopic examination.

Additionally, the importance of close clinico-pathological correlation cannot be underestimated. As dermoscopy provides a horizontal aerial view of skin microstructures, these dermoscopic findings should always be provided (in addition to the detailed clinical history and findings from clinical examination) in all samples sent for histopathology. Simple refinements such as marking the specimen for orientation, adding a map of the area of pathological interest, can help diagnosis and improve the quality of the report.

If clinical concern remains despite histopathology reporting, we would advise seeking engagement with your histopathology colleagues, for a case review, to ensure that the correct diagnosis is reached ultimately to the benefit of the patient.

As clinicians, we are accountable for our decision making, which should be based on the best possible evidence. Hopefully this book will help in that decision-making process.

The diagnosis is in the detail.

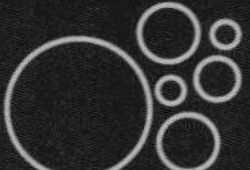

Dermoscopy and diagnosis

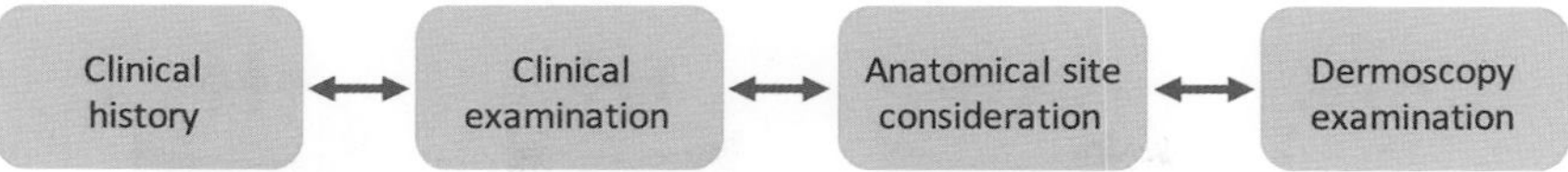

A clinical diagnosis is based upon the summation of components available for interpretation. It is not a linear progressive thread but a dynamic multiwoven fabric. Information from each progressive stage, clinical history, examination, site specifics and dermoscopy should be relayed back to the previous stages to guide analysis and refine the diagnostic process. In this way, features that were initially only thought visible on dermoscopy may also now be seen on clinical examination.

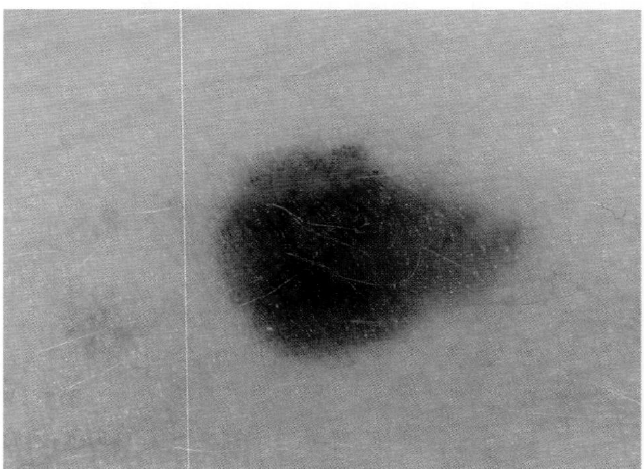

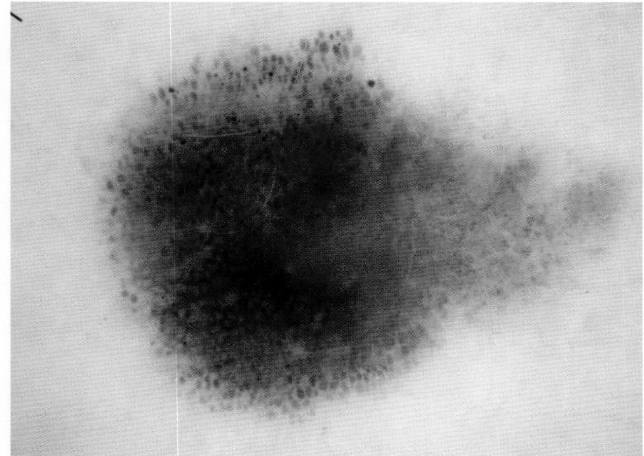

A pigmented macule on the arm of a 40-year-old woman confirmed as a 0.3 mm thick superficial spreading melanoma (SSM): dermoscopy shows eccentric irregular globules that can now also be seen on review of the clinical image.

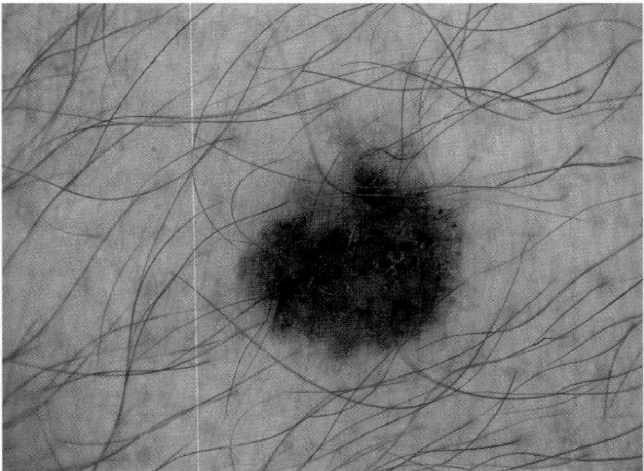

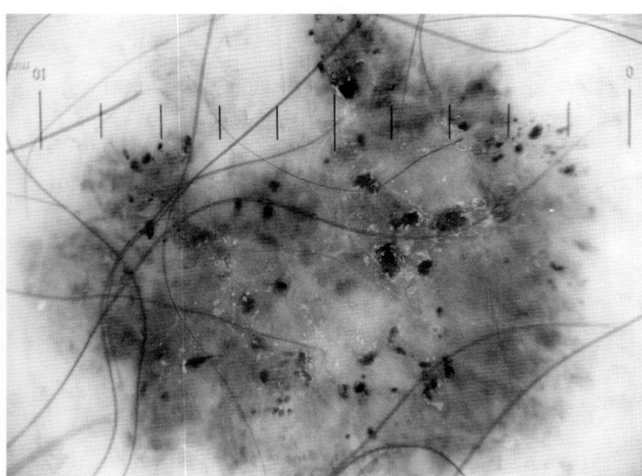

A variably pigmented macule on the arm of a 60-year-old woman confirmed as a 0.8 mm thick SSM: dermoscopy shows eccentric regression and atypical pigmented globules that can now also be seen on review of the clinical image.

Aim to constantly improve and refine clinical examination by re-assessing clinically for morphological structures once identified on dermoscopy.

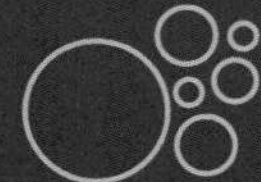

Dermoscopy principle I – illumination

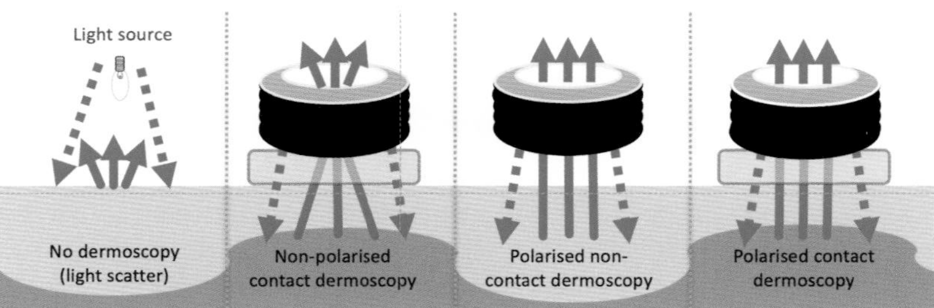

Skin is not smooth, but a layer of overlapping skin scales which scatter light when illuminated compromising visualisation of structures within the skin. This light scatter can be overcome through application of a surface interface medium, such as alcohol gel, or by using polarised light. Dermoscopes, with an internal light source and × 10 magnification, have become the standard diagnostic device for skin lesion examination. By combining contact polarised and non-polarised dermoscopy, the greatest diagnostic detail can be seen.

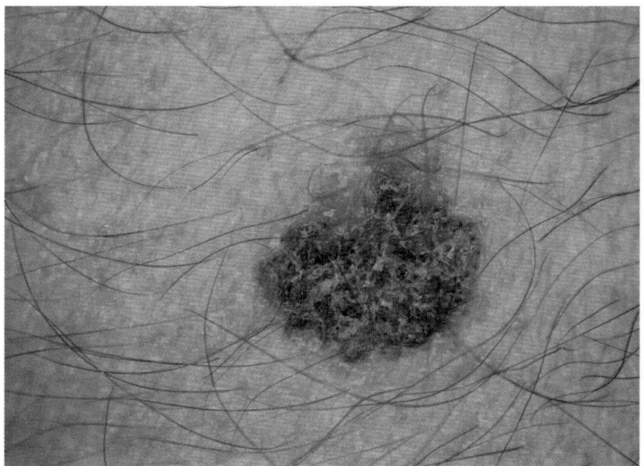

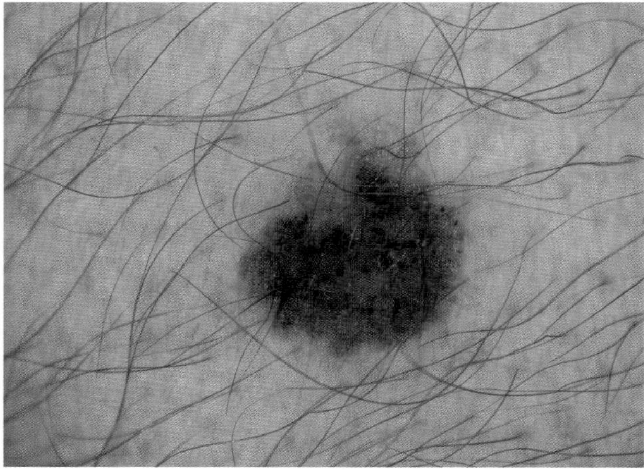

The details seen in this 0.8 mm thick SSM are more clearly seen on clinical examination following elimination of light scatter by application of alcohol gel.

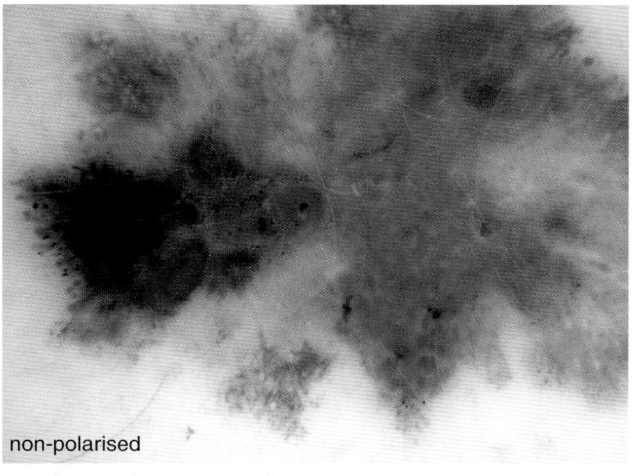

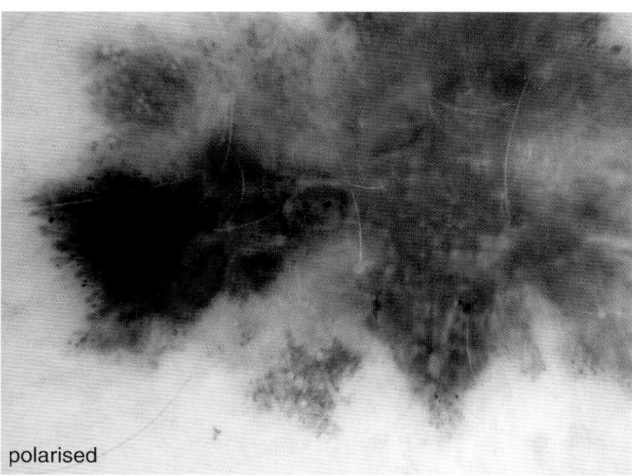

Combining dermoscopic features from both non-polarised and polarised imaging modes provides the maximum information for diagnosis in this 0.8 mm thick SSM.

Alcohol gel applied to the skin lesion prior to clinical and dermoscopic examination will aid diagnosis by reducing light scatter.

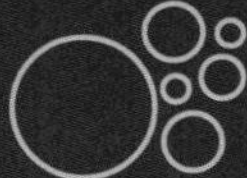

Dermoscopy principle II – magnification

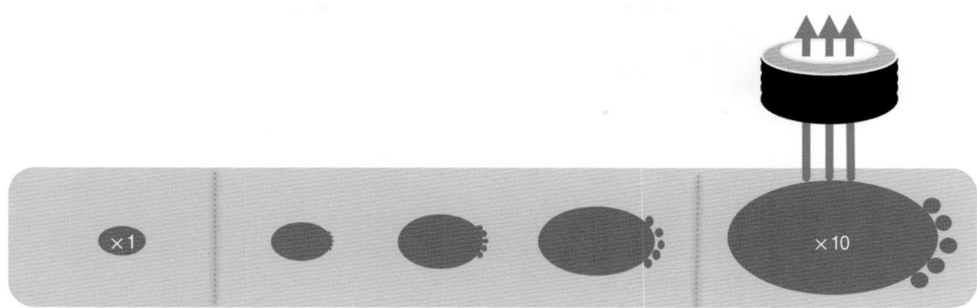

Magnification devices have been used in clinical practice for centuries. With increasing magnification, microstructures in the skin, which are invisible to the naked eye, suddenly become visible. These subtle features may be the only feature to provide early diagnosis of melanoma and hence as many lesions as possible should be examined with dermoscopy rather than naked eye preselection of a select few. Dermoscopy devices range in magnification although ×10 has become the standard.

International bank notes showing the microprint that is only visible on dermoscopy, illustrating the limitations of diagnostic detail seen on naked eye examination alone.

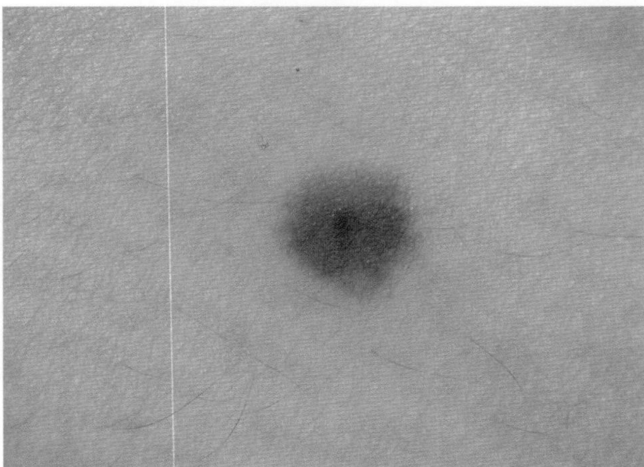

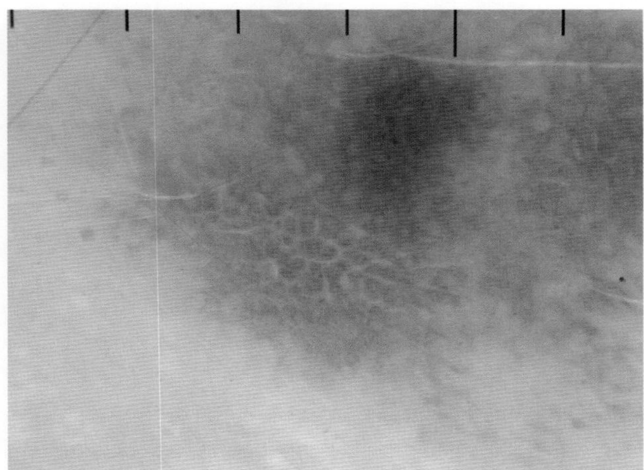

A melanocytic lesion on the knee of a 25-year-old woman: dermoscopy shows eccentric pigment globules and a focus of negative network in this case of melanoma in situ, which are only evident on dermoscopy.

Dinnes, J. et al. Dermoscopy, with and without visual inspection, for diagnosing melanoma in adults. *Cochrane Database Syst Rev*. 2018;12(12):CD011902.

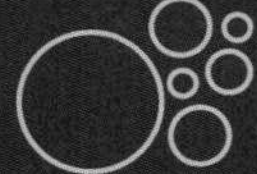

Dermoscopy colours I – eumelanin

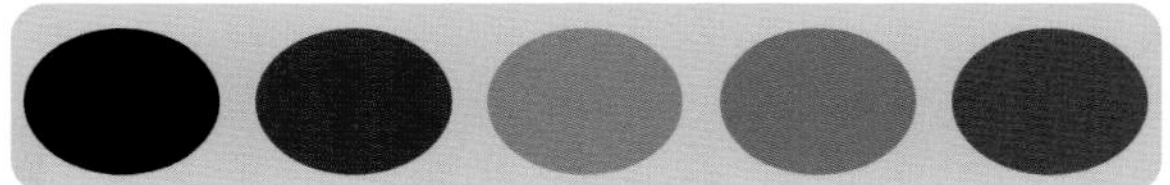

Melanin is the dominant pigment chromophore in the skin and exists in two forms, eumelanin (brown and black) and phaeomelanin (red and yellow). The colours within melanocytic skin lesions depend not only upon the ratio of eumelanin to phaeomelanin but also the pigment depth in the skin. The colour black is seen when eumelanin is present in the upper epidermis, browns in the epidermis, grey in the papillary dermis and slate blue in the deeper dermis.

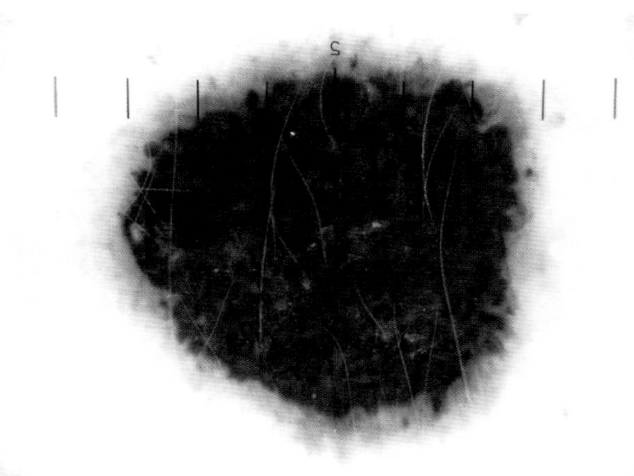

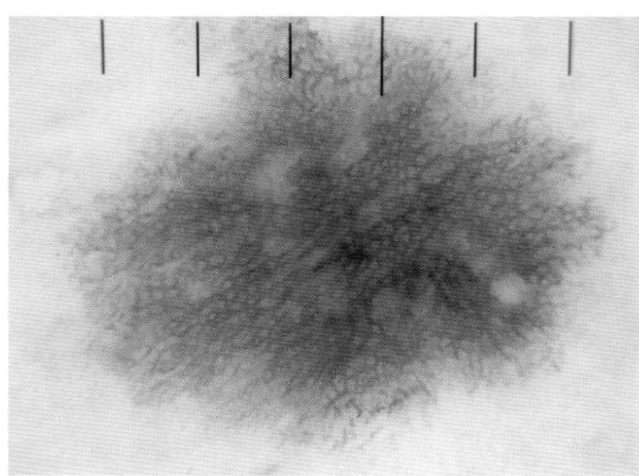

Black is a feature of eumelanin located high in the epidermis and can be seen in ink spot lentigines, Spitz naevi and melanoma; brown is the most commonly observed colour of melanocytic lesions and is due to melanin in the epidermis.

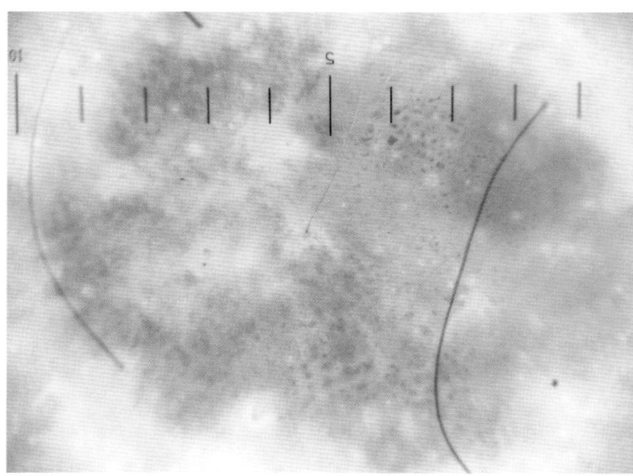

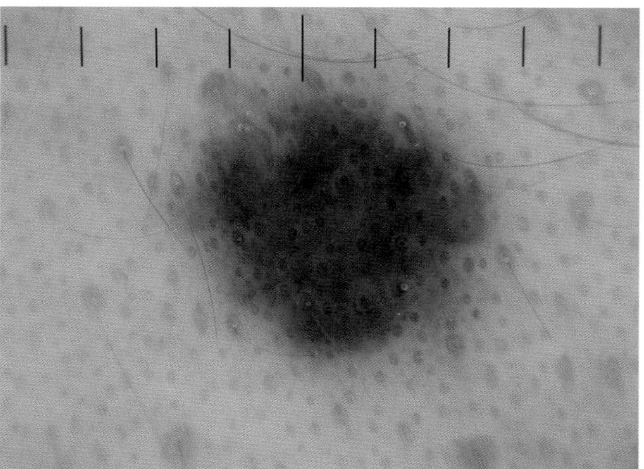

Grey pigmentation is seen when eumelanin is located in the papillary dermis (e.g. regression); slate blue is seen when eumelanin is located in the deeper dermis (e.g. blue naevi).

Note: Melanin pigmentation can be a dominant feature of non-melanocytic tumours, where tumour aggregates accumulate melanin from neighbouring melanocytes, such as seborrhoeic keratoses and pigmented basal cell carcinomas (BCC).

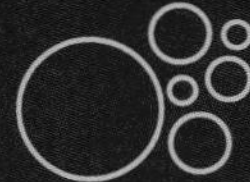

Dermoscopy colours II – non-eumelanin

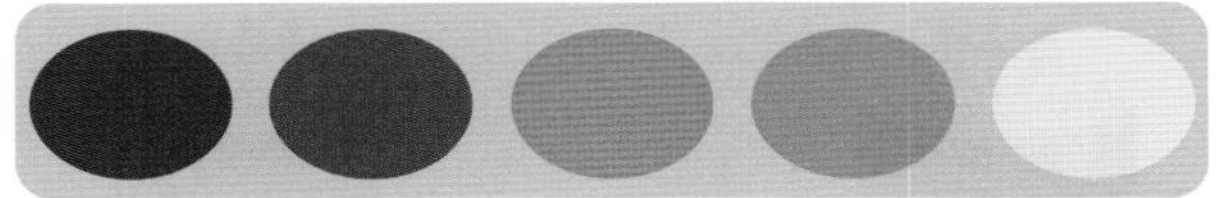

Non-eumelanin chromophores in the skin include phaeomelanin (red and yellow), haemoglobin (red and purple), keratin (white and yellow), lipids (yellow) and collagen (white). Lesions with these chromophores may show a range of colours from red, pink, orange, yellow, cream and white. If these colours predominate in the skin lesion the differential diagnosis should be extended to include not only melanocytic but non-melanocytic, inflammatory and infective skin lesions.

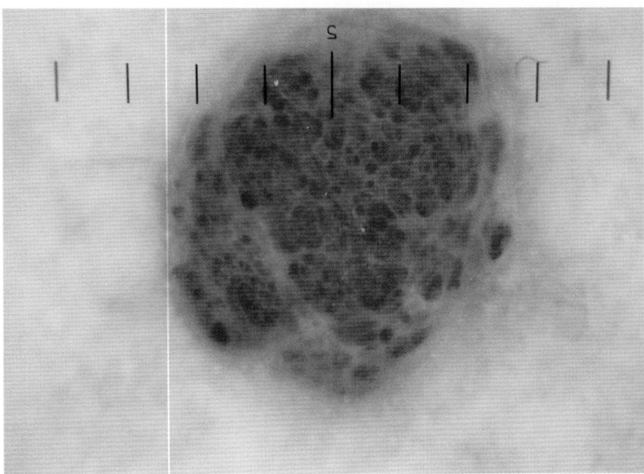

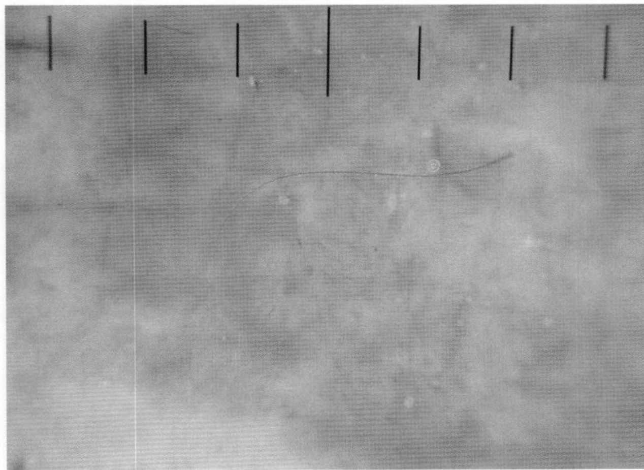

Purple and red colours are a typical feature of vascular lesions: pink colour is very non-specific and can be seen in melanocytic, non-melanocytic, infective or inflammatory lesions.

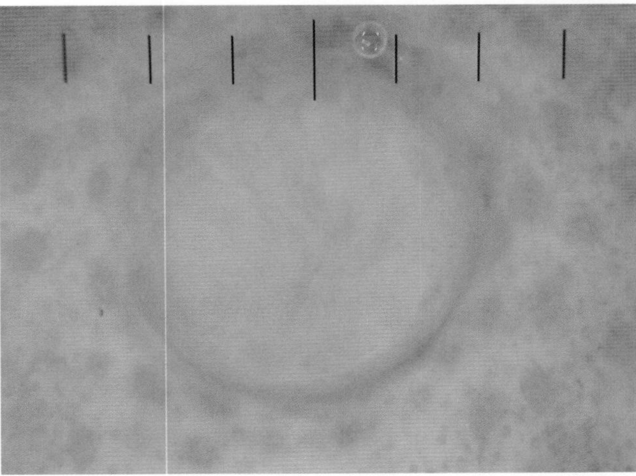

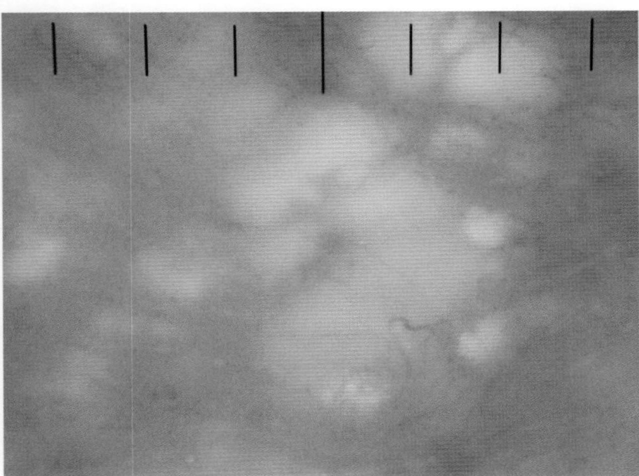

Orange is a colour that is commonly seen in melanocytic (phaeomelanin), lymphatic, granulomatous and xanthogranulomatous conditions; creamy yellow colour is seen in keratinising lesions, xanthomas, gouty tophi and sebaceous lesions.

Beware of the solitary pink lesion. Pink skin lesions can be melanocytic, non-melanocytic, infective or inflammatory. Diagnosis should be based upon clinical history and examination, dermoscopy and, where indicated, histopathology.

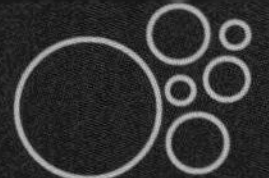

Imaging modes I – colours

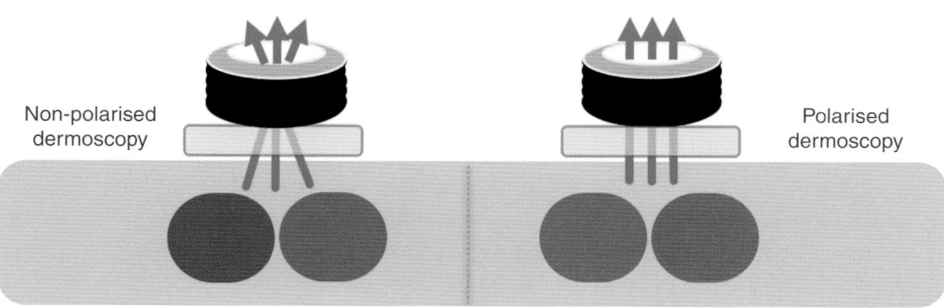

Subtle differences in colour perception are evident between polarised and non-polarised imaging modes. The most noticeable colour changes are seen in red and brown lesions. On polarised dermoscopy, reds and browns appear richer and brighter. On non-polarised dermoscopy, reds have a more purple hue and browns a duller hue. These subtle colour changes rarely cause diagnostic concern but should be considered if trying to standardise imaging for documentation or follow-up.

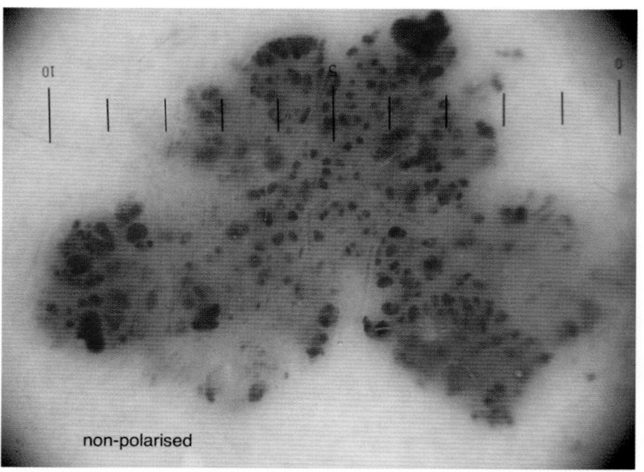

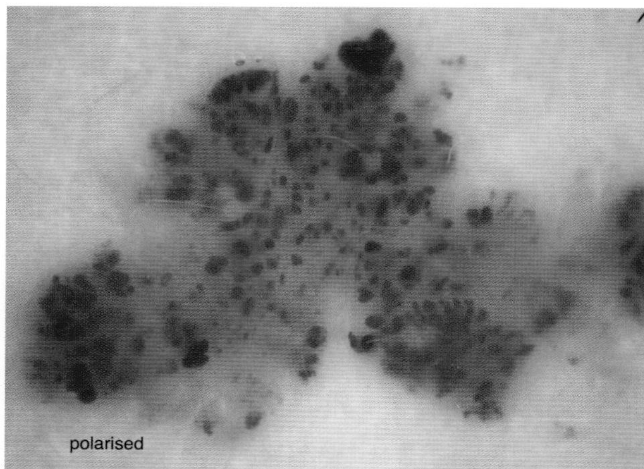

Two dermoscopic images of a benign haemangioma showing the subtle changes in red/purple colour from non-polarised to polarised imaging.

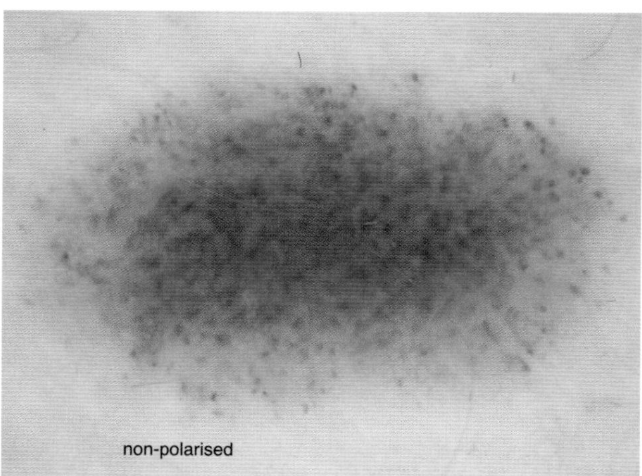

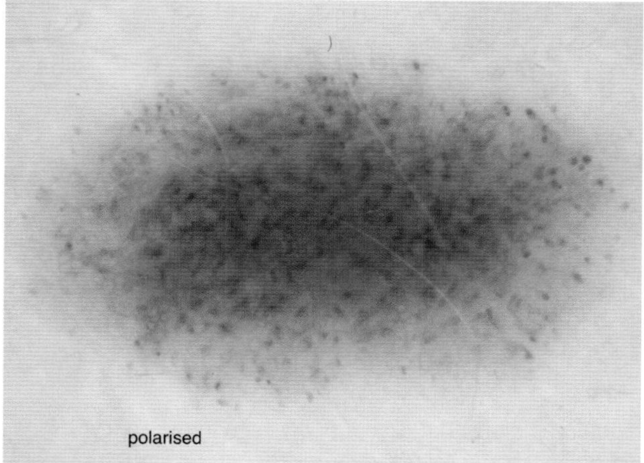

Two dermoscopic images of a melanocytic naevus showing the subtle changes in brown colour from non-polarised to polarised imaging.

Ensure the same imaging modes, same device and camera systems, whenever possible, are used if images are being taken for comparison between baseline and follow-up.

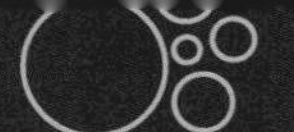

Imaging modes II – structures

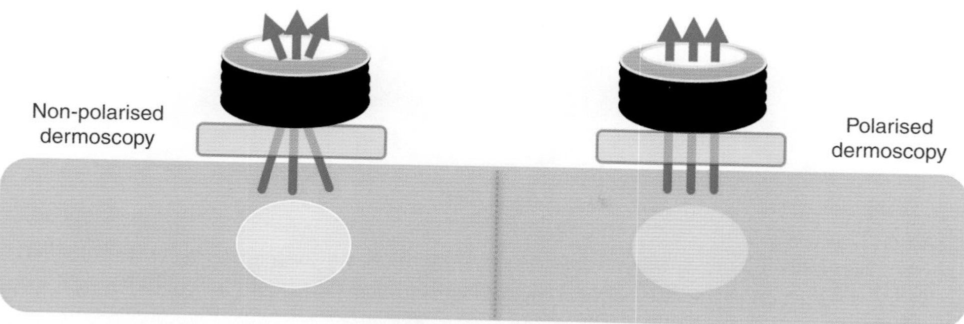

Modern dermoscopy devices allows the opportunity to examine skin lesions in both polarised and non-polarised modes. In this way, subtle changes can be seen between the two imaging modes. Foci of intraepidermal keratin can be seen commonly in seborrhoeic keratoses but also in a range of skin lesions including melanocytic lesions. On non-polarised dermoscopy, they appear as bright yellow-white globules, which are less visible on polarised dermoscopy.

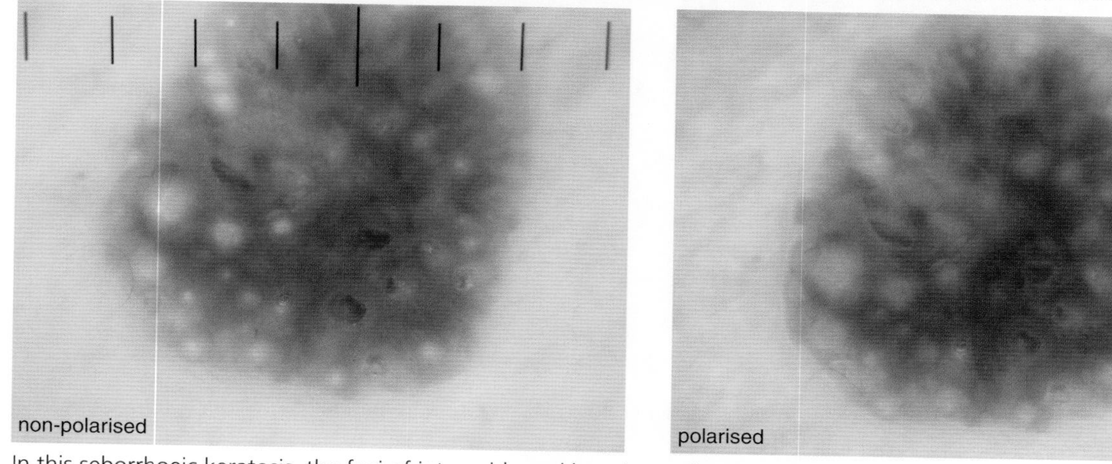

In this seborrhoeic keratosis, the foci of intraepidermal keratin can be seen on non-polarised dermoscopy as bright well-defined yellow globules; however, on polarised dermoscopy they appear as pale blurred areas.

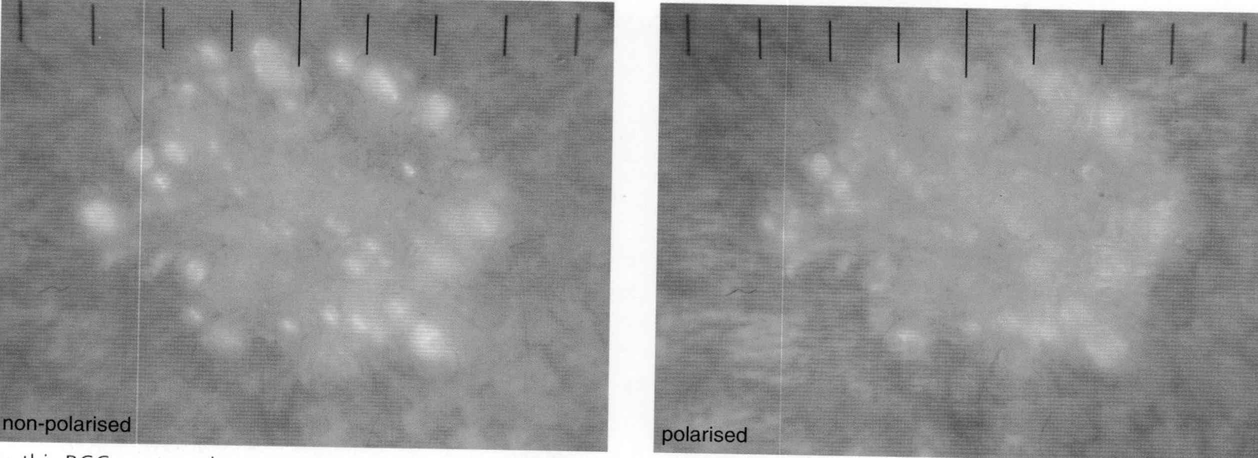

In this BCC contact dermoscopy shows bright well-defined yellow-white globules; however, on polarised dermoscopy they are less apparent.

Switching between polarising and non-polarising imaging modes can help illustrate features for diagnosis.

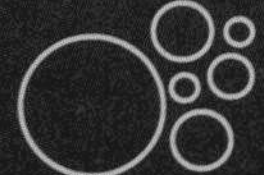

Dermoscopy of normal skin

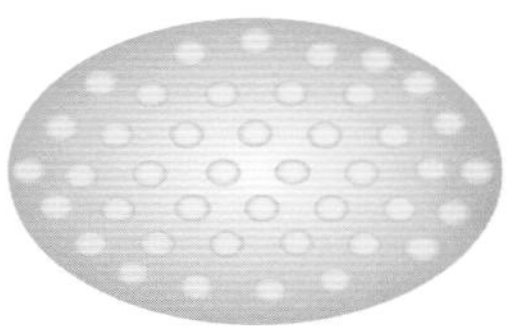
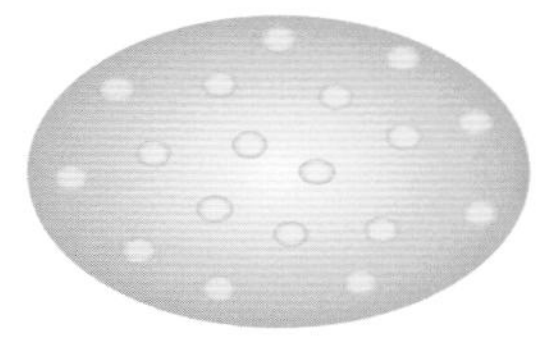
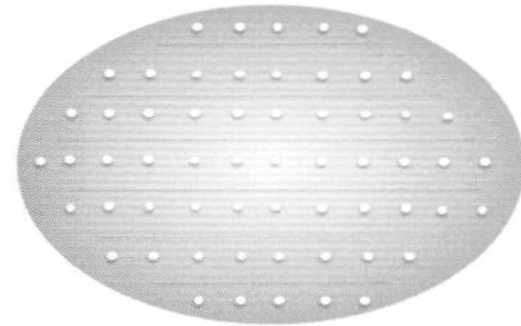

Skin lesions on different sites have features modified due to local anatomical site-specific structures. Facial skin has a higher density of follicular units and a reduction in the rete ridges compared with truncal skin where follicular density is less and rete ridges are more pronounced. Acral skin is devoid of hair follicles but shows an increase in sweat ducts visible on dermoscopy as white dots along the ridges of the dermatoglyphics. Darker skin tones highlight these background features of normal skin.

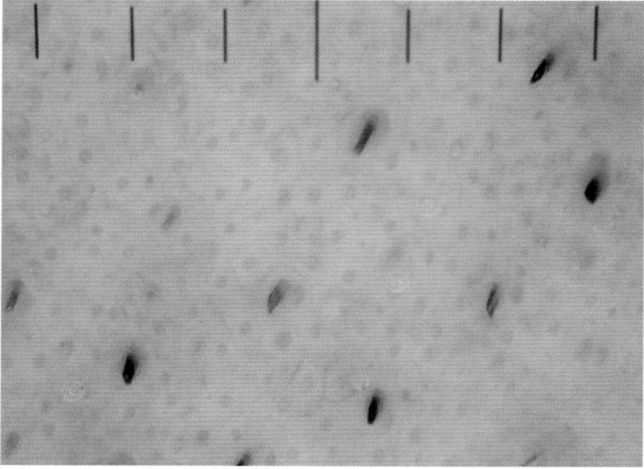
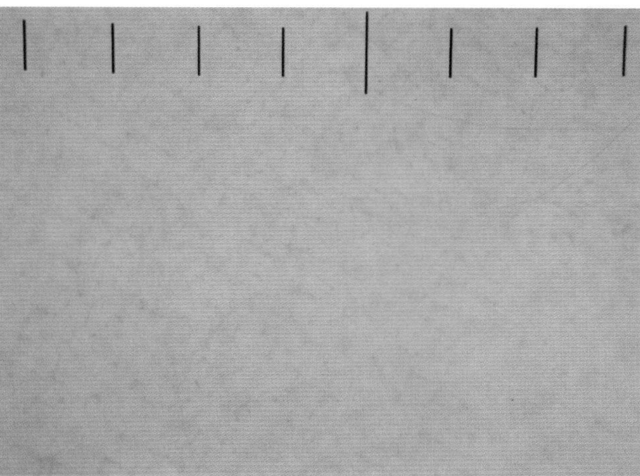

Dermoscopy of facial skin in a man with light skin showing increased follicular density with mature hair follicles. Dermoscopy of truncal skin in the same man showing fewer follicles.

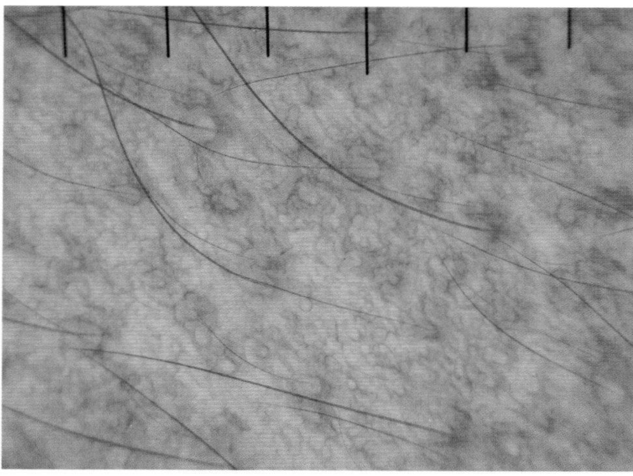
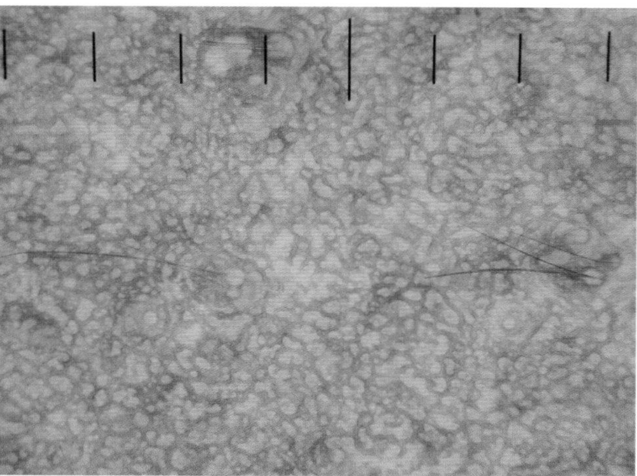

Dermoscopy of facial skin in a woman with dark skin showing background reticular pigmentation and increased follicular density. Dermoscopy of truncal skin in the same woman showing reduction in density of hair follicles.

Consider site-specific features when interpreting skin lesions.

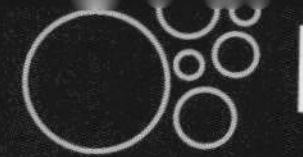

Dermoscopy of photodamaged skin

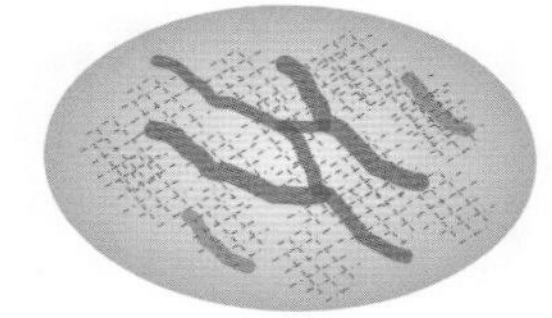

Chronic photodamage in the skin typically presents with pigmentation, vascular and atrophic changes. Dermoscopy shows widespread reticular pigmentation. The vessels are poorly focused and broad and may have increased visibility due to overlying skin atrophy.

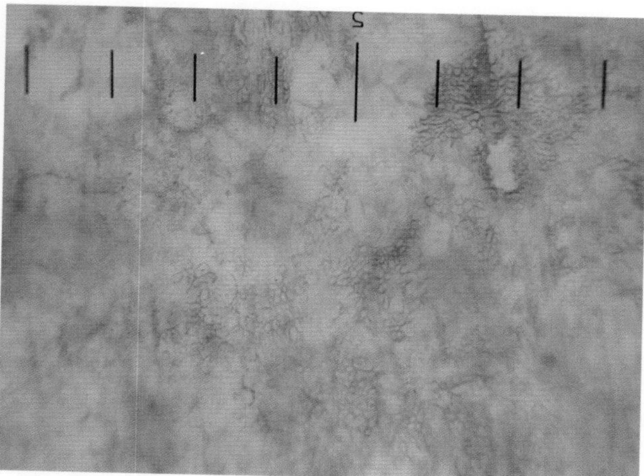

Widespread reticular pigmentation on the back of a 60-year-old man: dermoscopy shows patchy fine reticular pigmentation and ill-defined broad vessels in this non-lesional area of photodamaged skin.

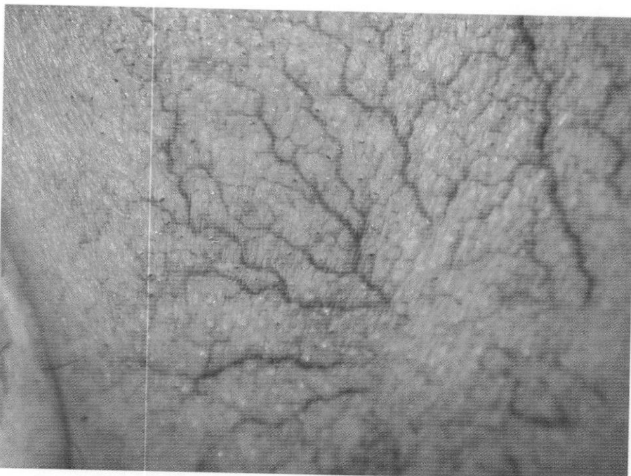

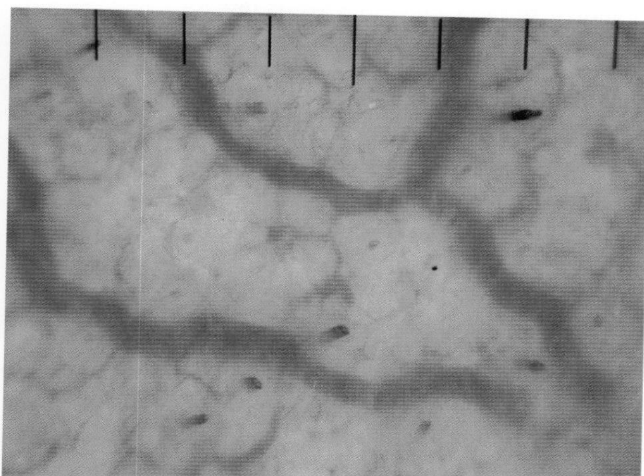

Prominent facial telangiectasia on the cheeks of a 70-year-old man: dermoscopy shows prominent broad poorly focused vessels in keeping with chronic background photodamage.

Recognising dermoscopic features found in background photodamaged skin will aid defining the margins of skin lesions found on these sites.

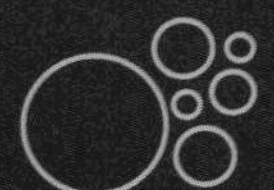

Vascular morphologies

When we see the complete spectrum of vessel types they can be seen as a vascular continuum, which explains why the same vessel types can be seen in multiple diagnoses and the same diagnosis can exhibit multiple vessel types. Although four main types are reported (dotted, coiled, linear and curved) we can describe intermediate patterns such as helical, serpentine, branching and curvilinear, to name a few. Proliferating tumours (benign or malignant) with an active growth phase tend to have more variation in vessel types whereas non-proliferating lesions tend to have a more uniform pattern.

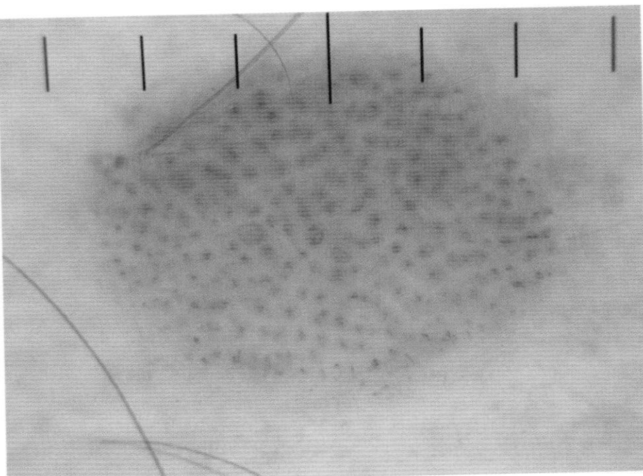

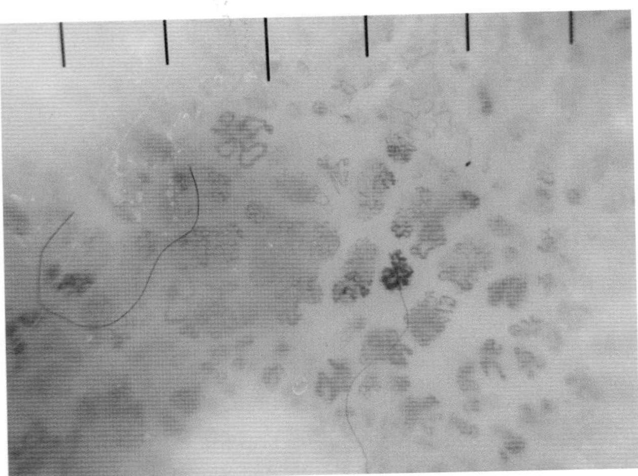

Dotted vessels are common in melanocytic lesions, dermatofibromas and inflammatory conditions. Coiled vessels are common vascular features in Bowen's disease.

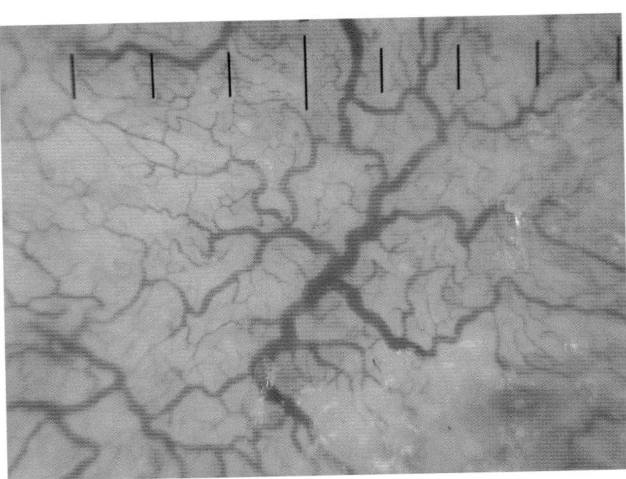

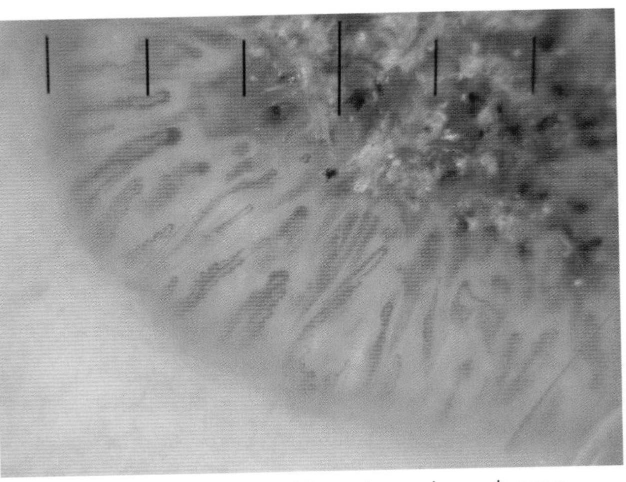

Sharply focused linear branching vessels are a common vascular feature of BCC. Radially arranged linear looped vessels are a common feature of squamoproliferative lesions.

Okkels F. Dynamic adaption of vascular morphology. *Front Physiol*. 2012;3:390.

Characteristic vascular patterns

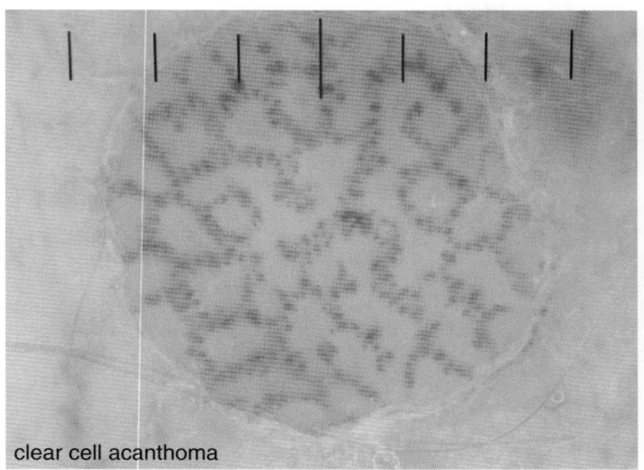
clear cell acanthoma

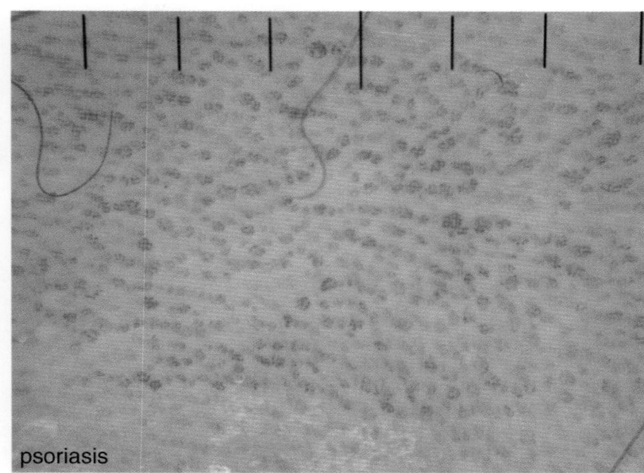
psoriasis

Uniform vascular patterns are more commonly seen in benign conditions.

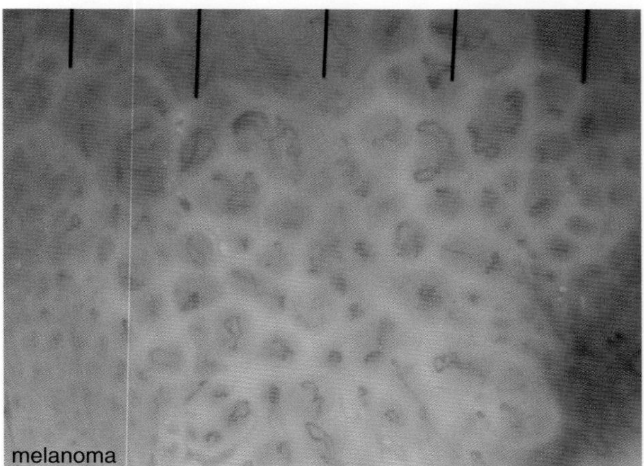
melanoma

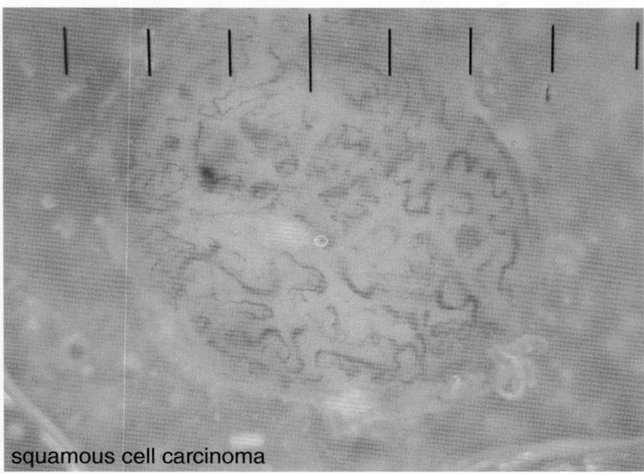
squamous cell carcinoma

Non-uniform vascular patterns are more commonly seen in malignant conditions.

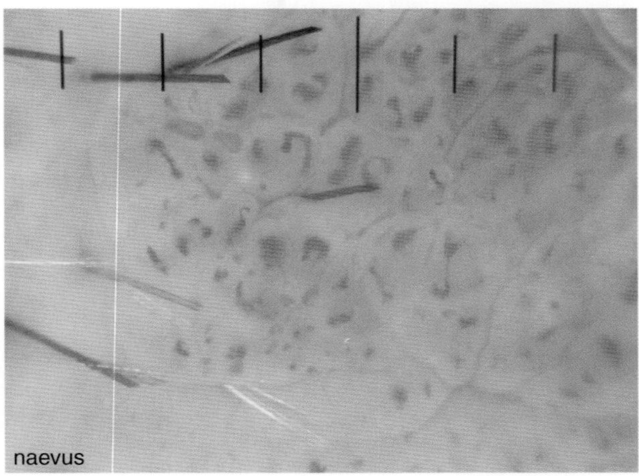
naevus

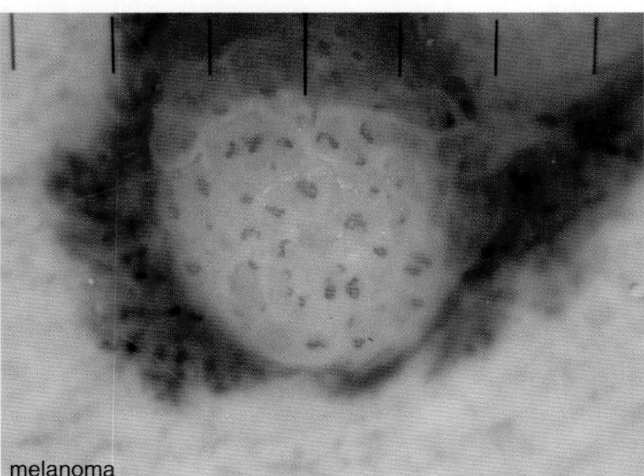
melanoma

Vascular patterns can be similar in both benign and malignant conditions.

Dermoscopic vascular patterns are useful in the diagnostic process but should not be interpreted in isolation, rather in the context of the whole lesion.

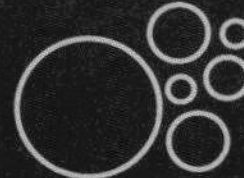

Polarised dermoscopy – shiny white structures

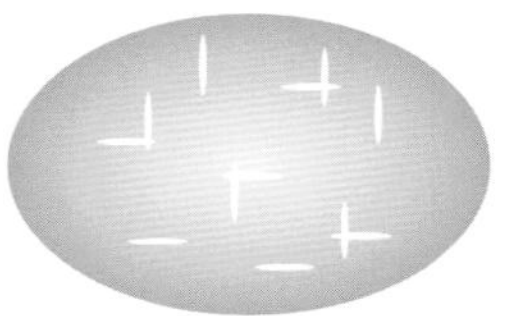
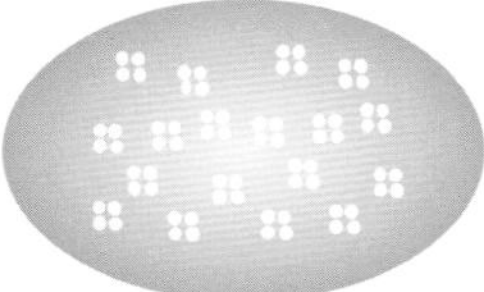
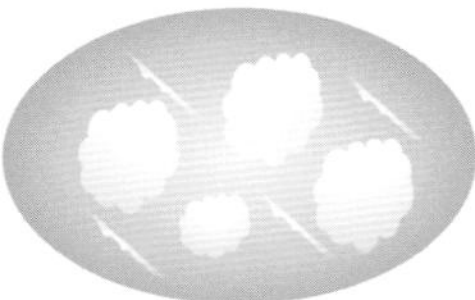

Polarised dermoscopy may show additional features that are not present on contact non-polarised dermoscopy. These shiny white structures have been described as orthogonal lines, rosettes and blotches and strands. Orthogonal lines (white lines that run perpendicular to each other) and whitish blotches and strands are caused by collagen disruption, while rosettes are a result of light reflecting off dyskeratosis at the follicular apertures.

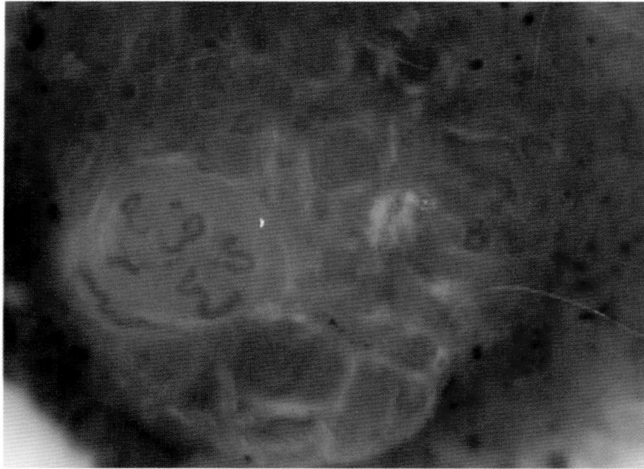

Orthogonal white lines indicating collagen disruption in this invasive melanoma.

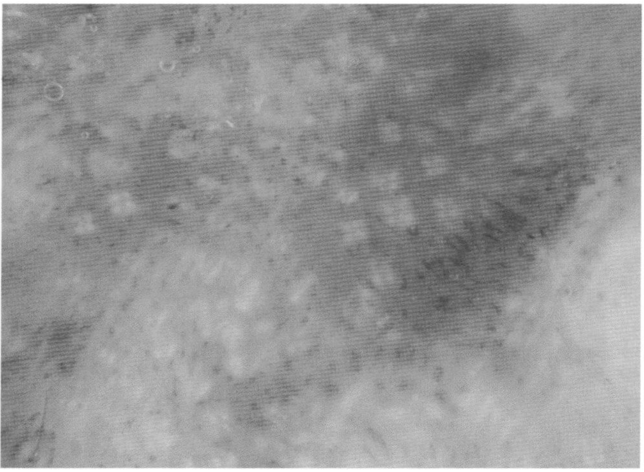

Multiple rosettes in this actinic keratosis.

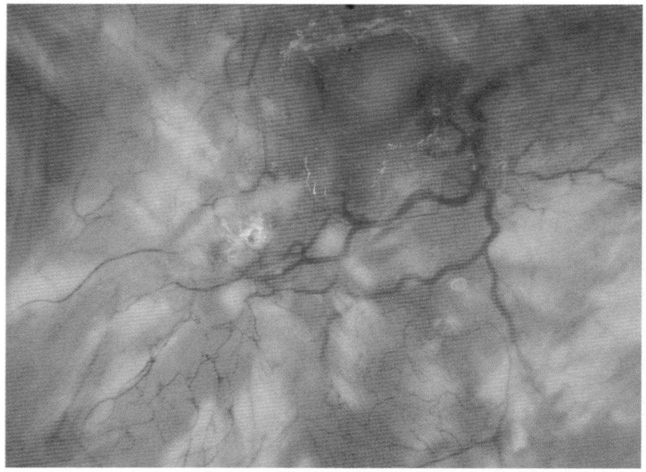

Multiple shiny white blotches and strands in this nodular BCC.

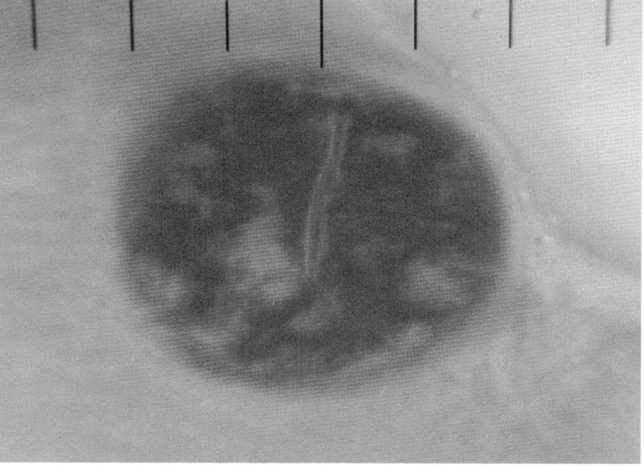

Shiny white blotches and strands in this pyogenic granuloma.

Haspeglagh M et al. Rosettes and other white shiny structures in polarised dermoscopy: histological correlate and optical explanation. *J Eur Acad Dermatol Venereol.* 2016;30(2):311–3.

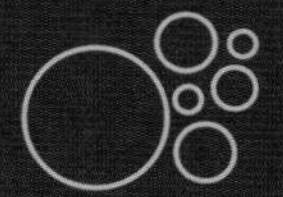

2 Melanocytic naevi

Early naevi – globular 16
Acquired naevi – reticular 17
Acquired naevi – homogeneous 18
Acquired naevi – evolving 19
Acquired naevi in light skin 20
Acquired naevi in medium-toned skin 21
Atypical melanocytic lesions 22
Atypical melanocytic lesions cases 23
Dermal naevus – pigmented 24
Dermal naevus – hyperpigmented 25
Dermal naevus in dark skin 26
Combined naevus 27
Blue naevus 28
Blue naevus – sclerotic/hypochromic 29
Recurrent naevus 30
Halo naevus 31
Congenital naevus 32
Agminated naevus and naevus spilus 33
Reed naevus I 34
Reed naevus II 35
Pigmented Spitz naevus 36
Hypomelanotic Spitz naevus I 37
Hypomelanotic Spitz naevus II 38

Diagnostic Dermoscopy: The Illustrated Guide, Second Edition. Jonathan Bowling.

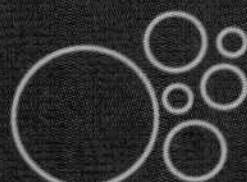

Early naevi – globular

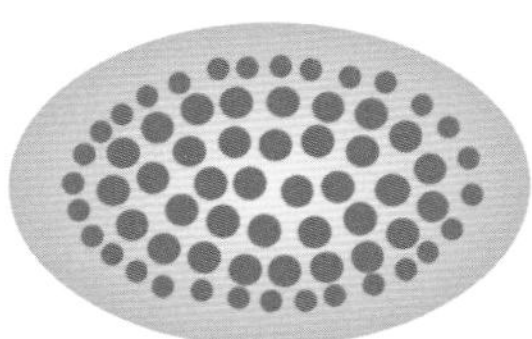

Benign naevi are typically round or oval with multiple axes of symmetry clinically. Dermoscopic features give clues as to how long a naevus has been present for. Globular morphology in children and young adults is associated with a new evolving melanocytic lesion, either junctional or early congenital dermal naevi, corresponding to a junctional nest of melanocytes on histopathology or dermal melanocytic aggregates.

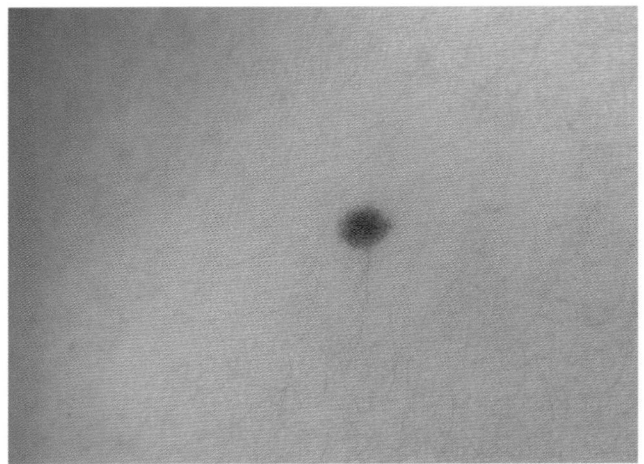

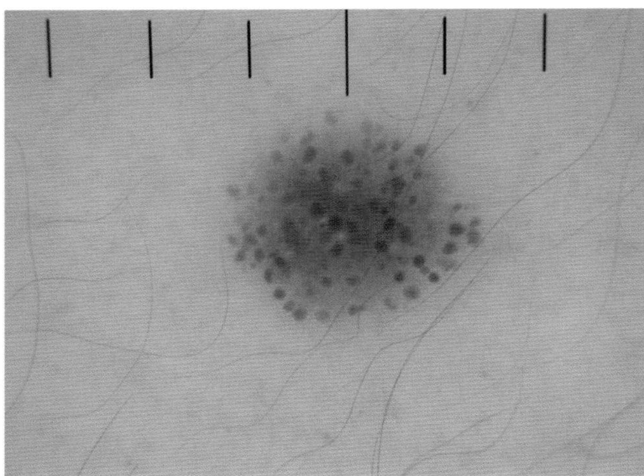

A pigmented macule on the chest of a 16-year-old boy: dermoscopy shows a predominantly globular morphology in this naevus.

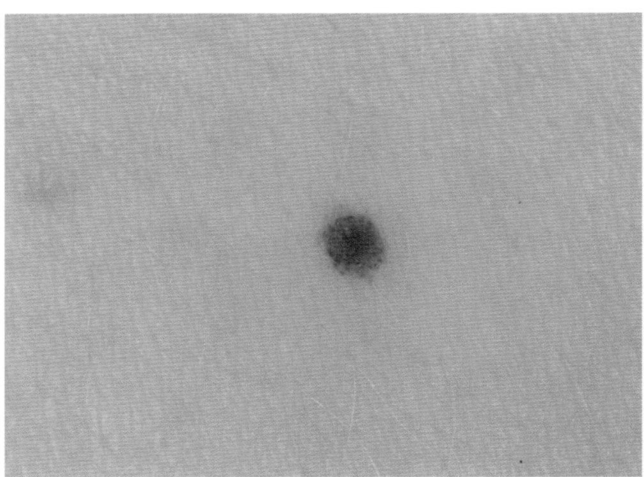

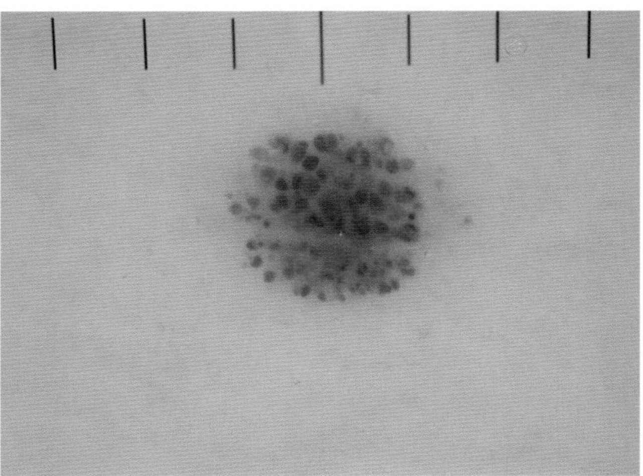

A pigmented macule on the lower back of a 13-year-old boy: dermoscopy shows a predominantly globular morphology in this naevus.

Zalaudek, I. et al. Age-related prevalence of dermoscopy patterns in acquired melanocytic naevi. *Br J Dermatol*. 2006;154(2):299–304.

Acquired naevi – reticular

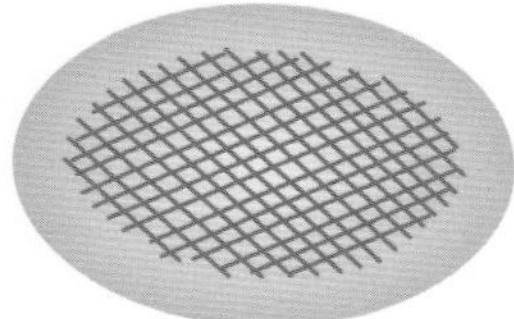

Reticular morphology formed by a pigment network is a typical feature of acquired junctional naevi, more commonly found on the sun-exposed sites of the trunk and limbs. Reticular morphology is typically seen in either new or established junctional naevi reflecting populations of melanocytes illustrating the contours of the dermoepidermal junction. The reticular pattern is more commonly seen in adults.

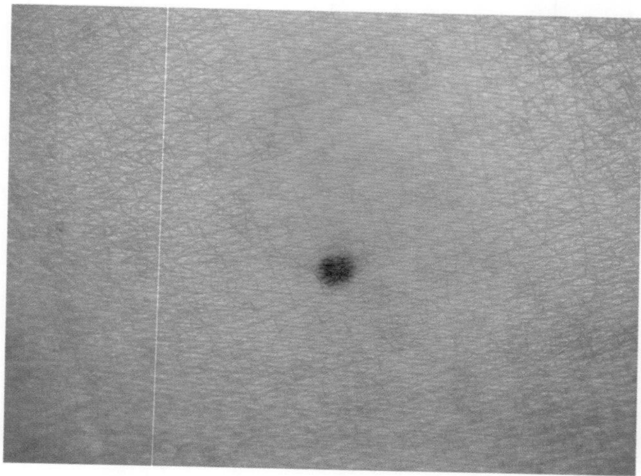

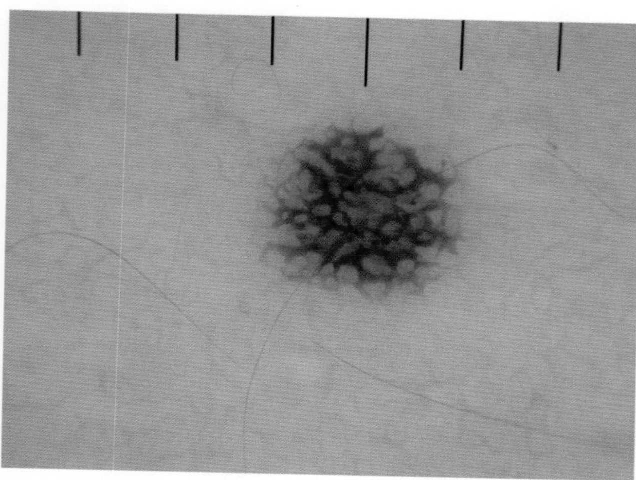

A pigmented macule on the upper arm of a 25-year-old woman: dermoscopy shows uniform reticular morphology which steadily fades out in this junctional naevus.

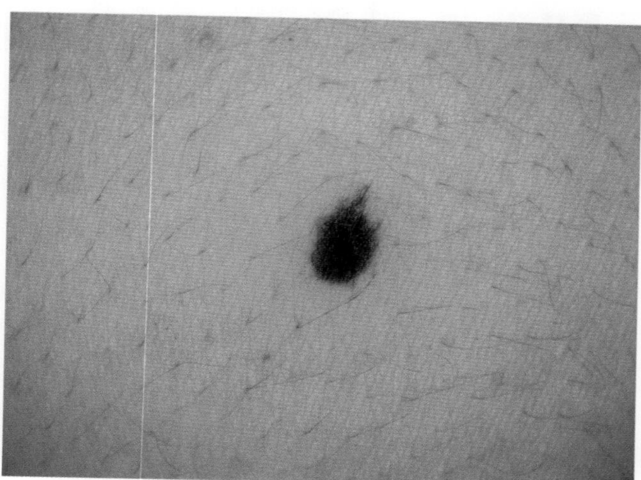

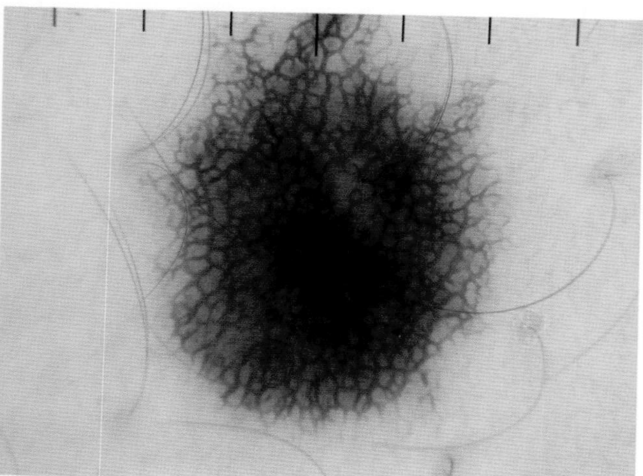

A pigmented macule on the thigh of a 30-year-old man: dermoscopy shows uniform reticular morphology in this junctional naevus.

Changchien, L. et al. Age- and site-specific variation in the dermoscopic patterns of congenital melanocytic naevi: an aid to accurate classification and assessment of melanocytic naevi. *Arch Dermatol.* 2007;143(8):1007–1014.

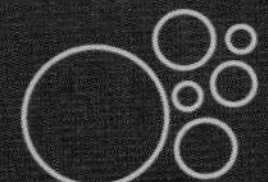

Acquired naevi – homogeneous

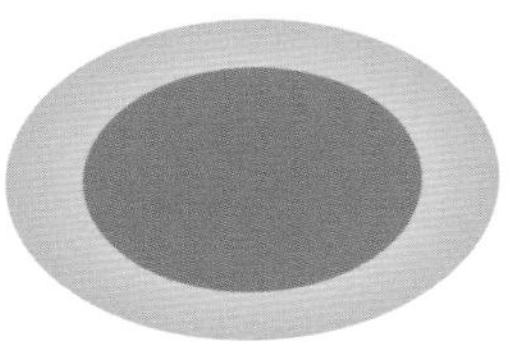

Homogeneous morphology is a typical feature of established acquired naevi. Homogeneous morphology reflects the populations of melanocytes along the dermoepidermal junction, obscuring the finer details of the rete ridge profile. A homogeneous pattern is more commonly seen in naevi in older adults.

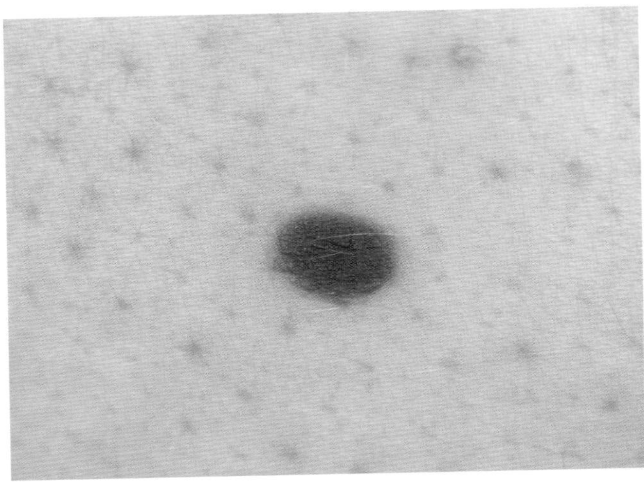

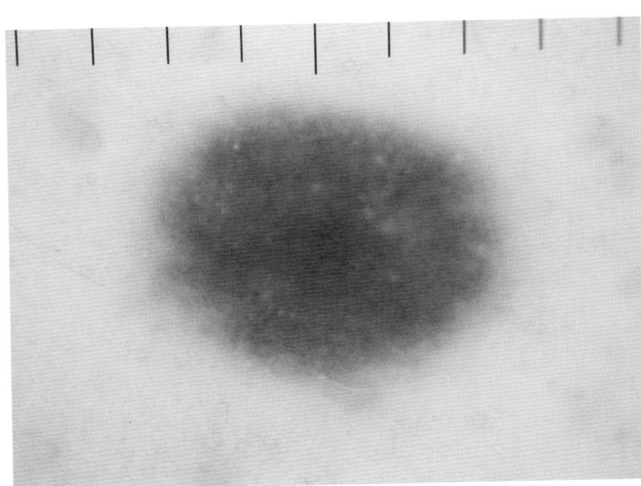

A pigmented macule on the upper back of a 55-year-old woman: dermoscopy shows uniform homogeneous morphology in this acquired naevus.

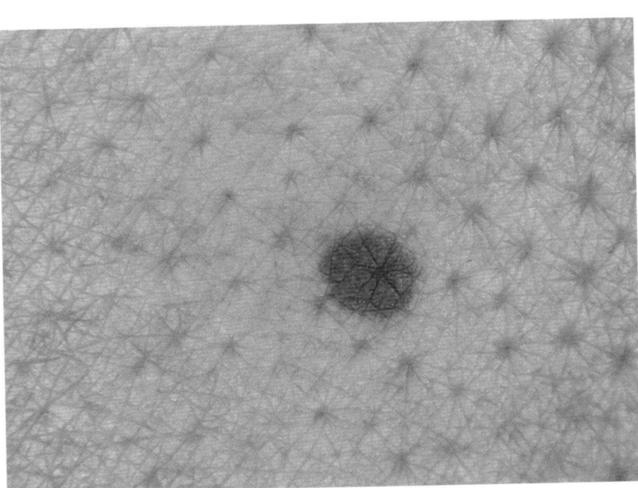

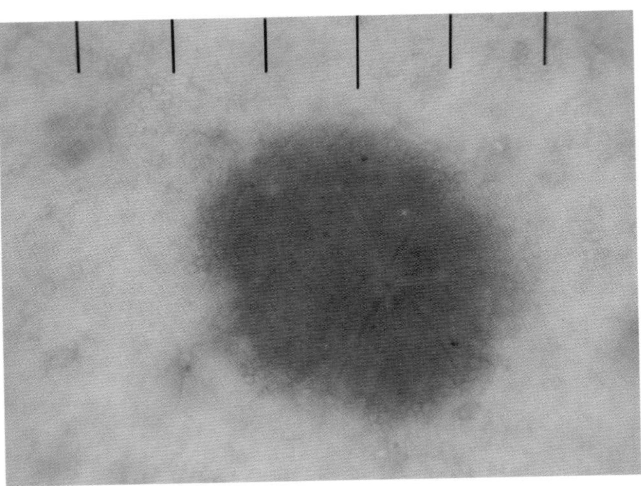

A pigmented macule on the arm of a 40-year-old woman: dermoscopy shows predominant homogeneous morphology in this acquired naevus.

Acquired melanocytic naevi change with increasing age from globular, to reticular and finally homogeneous morphology. Therefore, be suspicious if a new melanocytic lesion exhibits globular morphology in an older adult.

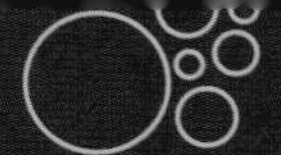

Acquired naevi – evolving

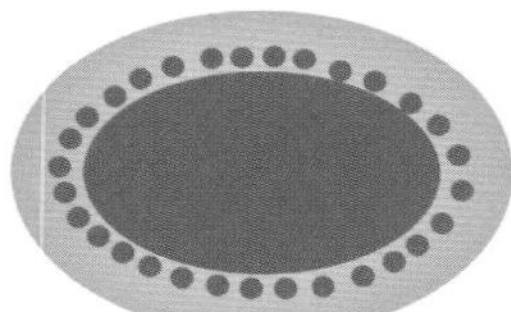

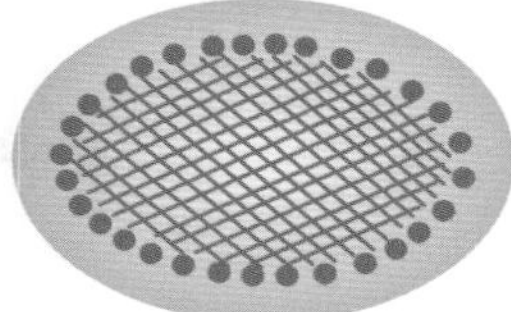

Acquired melanocytic naevi do not appear overnight but grow and evolve until they reach maturity. If they are detected at this evolving stage, a combination of dermoscopic features may be present. A symmetrical rim of uniform globules with a central uniform reticular or homogeneous pattern is typical for an evolving naevus.

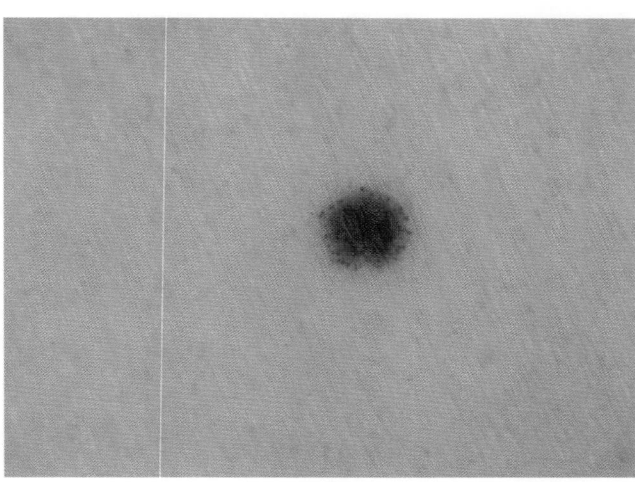

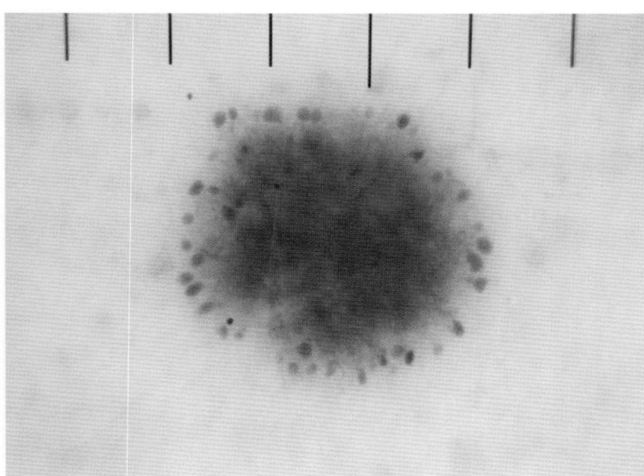

A 3 mm pigmented macule on the upper arm of a 30-year-old woman: dermoscopy shows globular homogeneous morphology with symmetrical peripheral globules in this benign evolving junctional naevus.

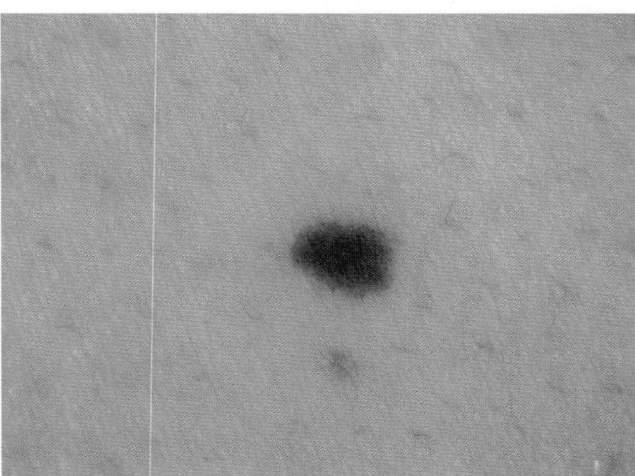

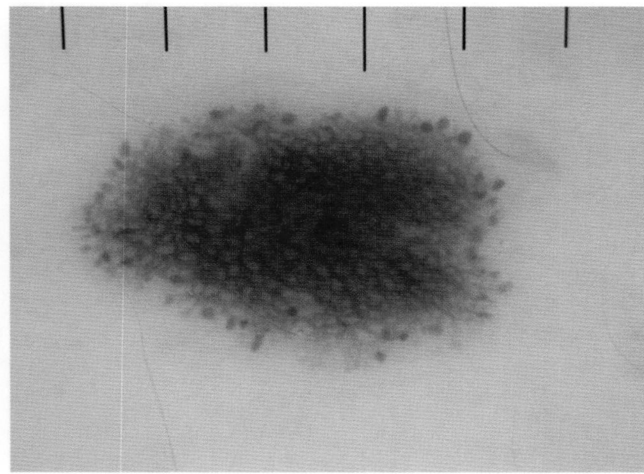

A 4 mm pigmented macule on the thigh of a 30-year-old woman: dermoscopy shows both globular and reticular morphology with symmetrical peripheral globules and central uniform reticular pigmentation in this evolving naevus.

Be suspicious of an evolving melanocytic lesion in those patients over 50 years of age or if the central component shows any non-uniform features.

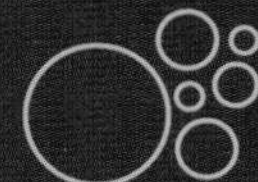

Acquired naevi in light skin

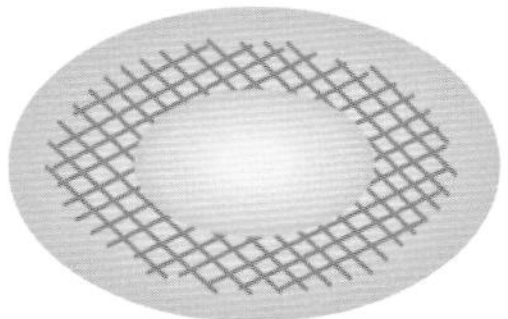

Acquired melanocytic naevi typically show a predominant pattern dependent upon skin phototype. Individuals with light skin typically have naevi with peripheral reticular pigmentation and central hypopigmentation.

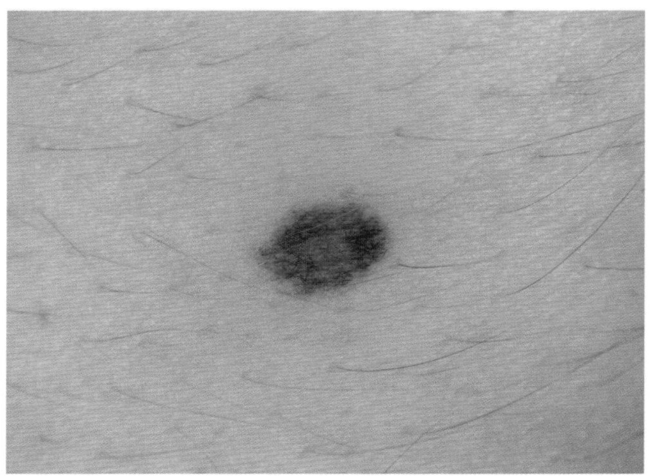

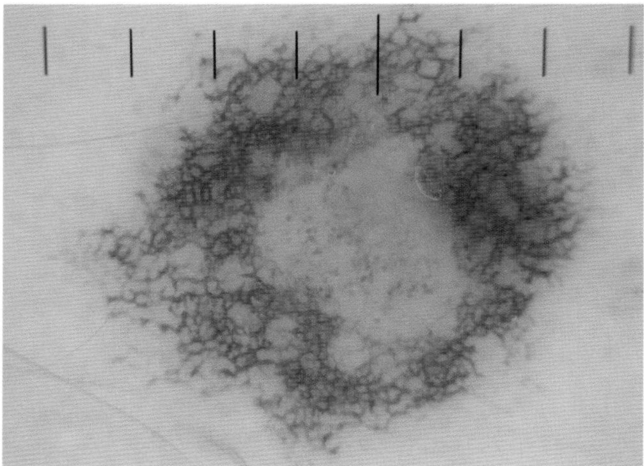

A pigmented macule on the lower abdomen of a 20-year-old man: dermoscopy shows peripheral reticular and central homogenous pigmentation in this acquired naevus.

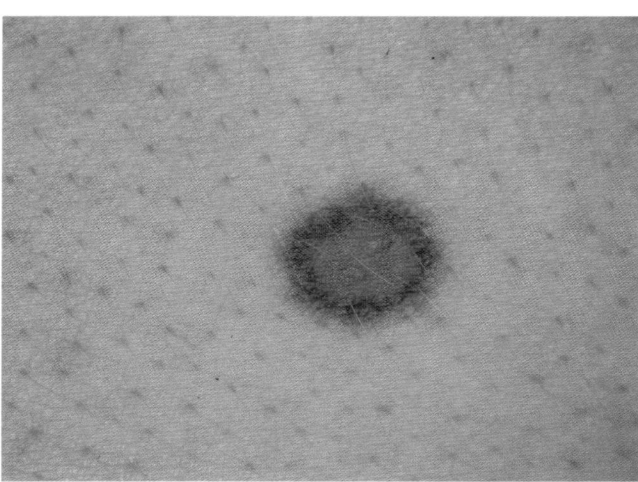

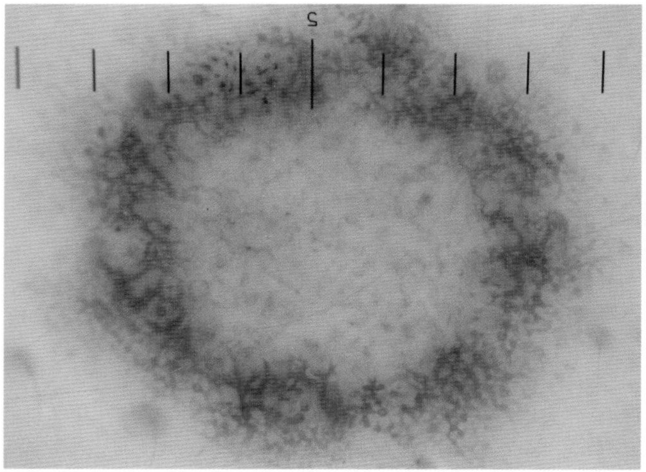

A pigmented macule on the upper back of a 30-year-old woman with a history of melanoma: dermoscopy shows peripheral reticular and central homogenous pigmentation in this acquired naevus.

Zalaudek, et al. Nevus type in dermoscopy is related to skin type. *Arch Dermatol.* 2007;143(3):351–356.

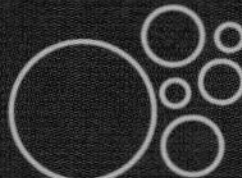

Acquired naevi in medium-toned skin

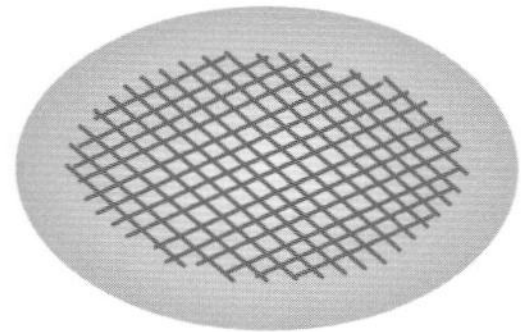

Acquired melanocytic naevi typically show a predominant pattern dependent upon skin phototype. Individuals with medium or darker toned skin typically have naevi with uniform reticular pigmentation on dermoscopy.

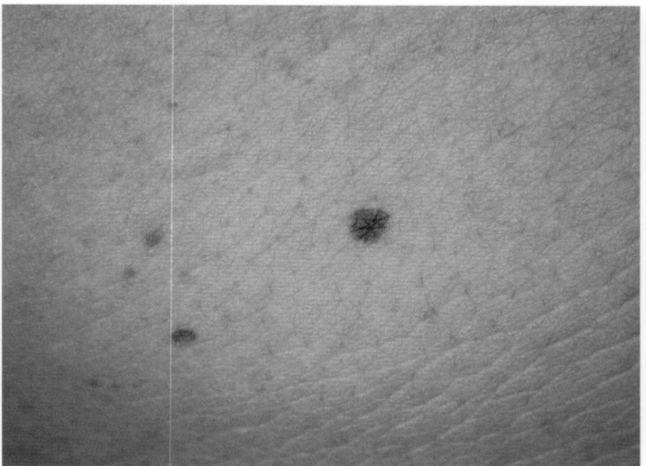

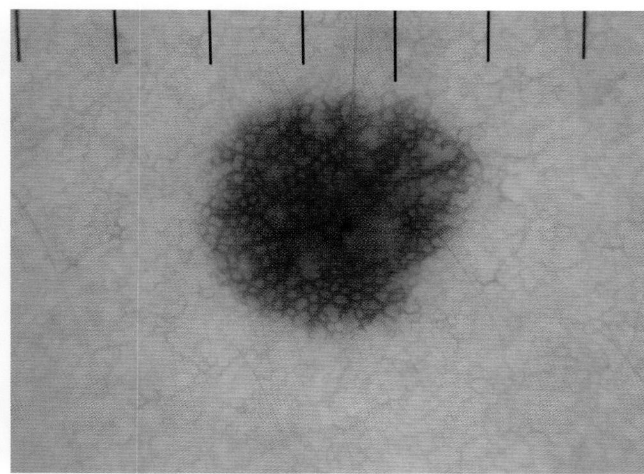

A pigmented macule on the thigh of a 40-year-old woman: dermoscopy shows uniform reticular pigmentation and perifollicular hypopigmentation in this acquired naevus.

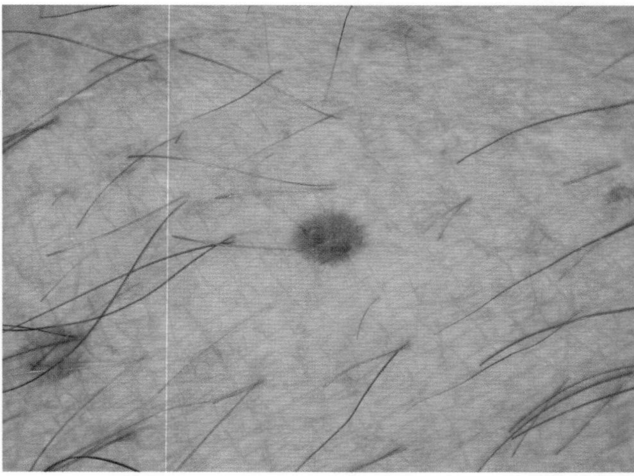

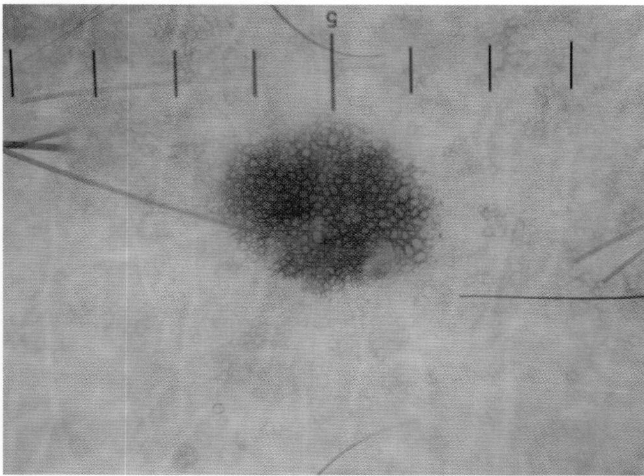

A pigmented macule on the upper back of a 30-year-old man: dermoscopy shows uniform reticular pigmentation in this acquired junctional naevus.

Be suspicious of any solitary melanocytic lesion that is out of keeping with expected morphology based on skin tone. A melanocytic lesion that is deeply pigmented despite lighter skin or pink in darker skin should be viewed with suspicion.

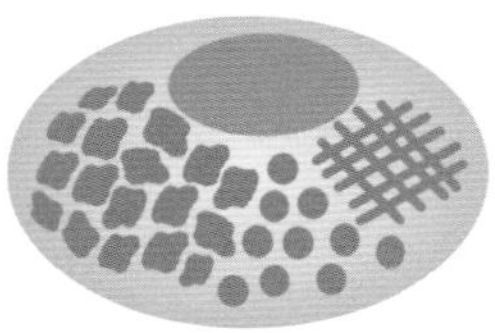

Atypical melanocytic lesions may be solitary or multiple. When features of a solitary atypical melanocytic lesion overlap with melanoma in situ, excision should be undertaken. A broad pigment network correlates histopathologically with fusion of the rete ridges. Patients with multiple naevi with atypical features require more detailed surveillance and would benefit from long-term follow-up augmented with total body photography and digital dermoscopy.

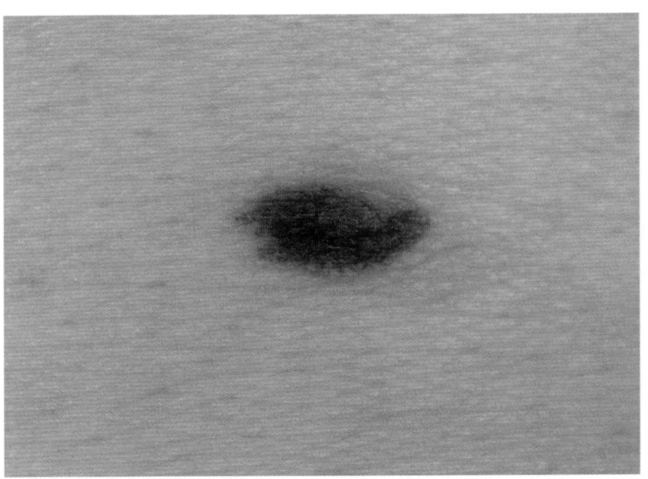

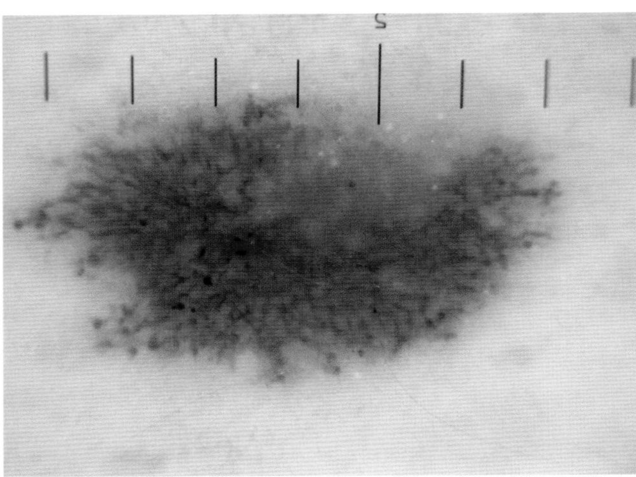

An 'ugly duckling' pigmented macule on the abdomen of a 30-year-old woman: dermoscopy shows irregularly distributed globules, irregular pigment network and homogeneous areas confirmed as a low-grade dysplastic naevus on histopathology.

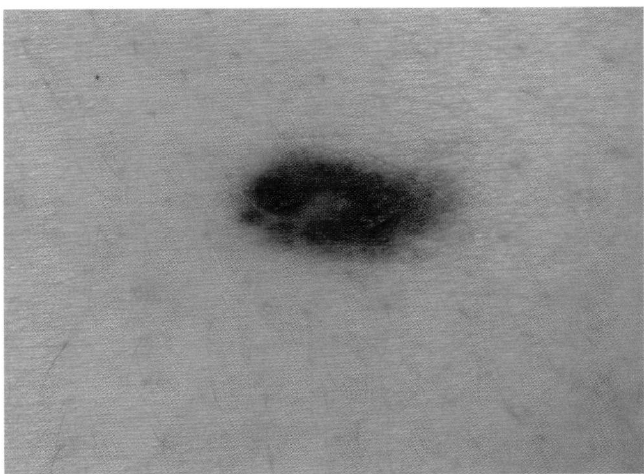

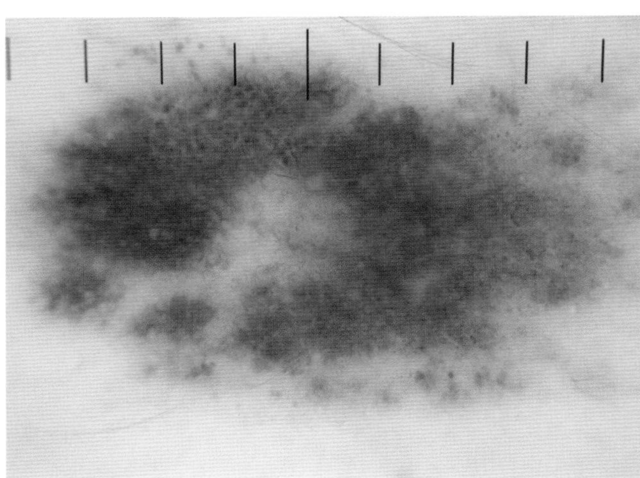

An 'ugly duckling' pigmented macule on the back of a 25-year-old woman: dermoscopy shows irregularly distributed pigment network, globules and atypically distributed cobblestone aggregates (negative network) in this dysplastic naevus.

Thomas, L. and Puig, S. Dermoscopy, digital dermoscopy and other diagnostic tools in early detection of melanoma and follow up of high-risk skin cancer patients. *Acta Dermatol Venereol*. 2017;Suppl.218:14–21.

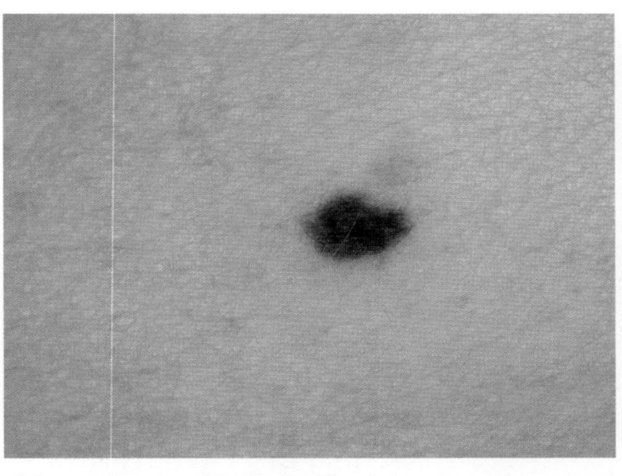
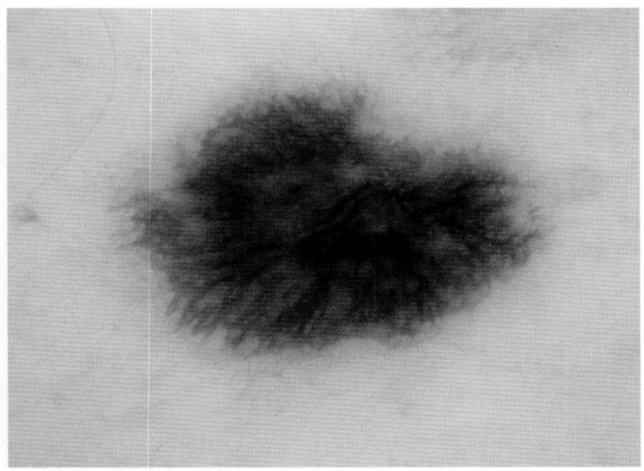

A hyperpigmented 'ugly duckling' macule on the upper back of a 45-year-old man: dermoscopy shows an atypical pigment network in this histopathologically confirmed high-grade dysplastic naevus.

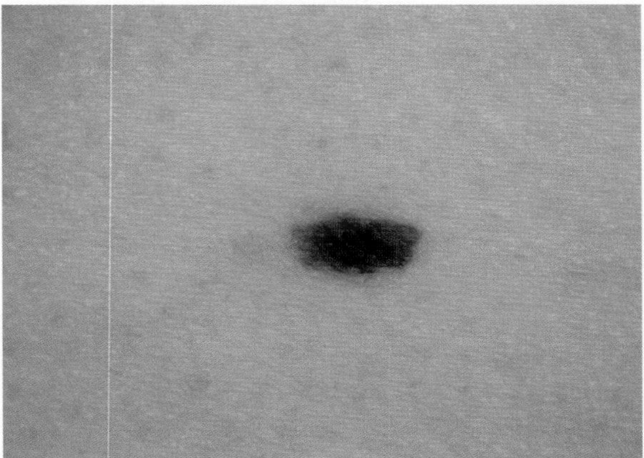
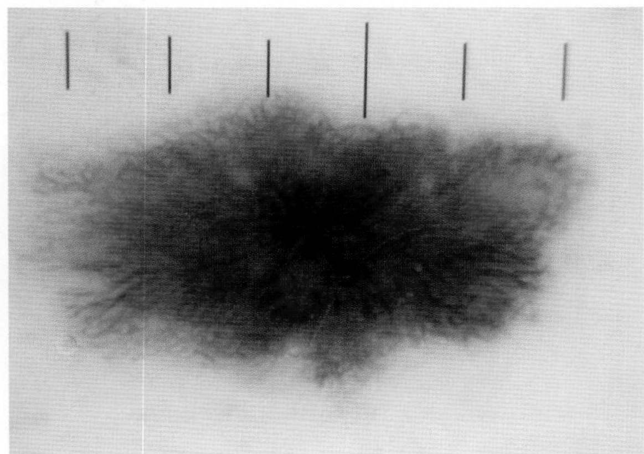

A hyperpigmented 'ugly duckling' macule on the thigh of a 55-year-old woman: dermoscopy shows an atypical pigment network and atypical peripheral pigmented streaks in this histopathologically confirmed high-grade dysplastic naevus.

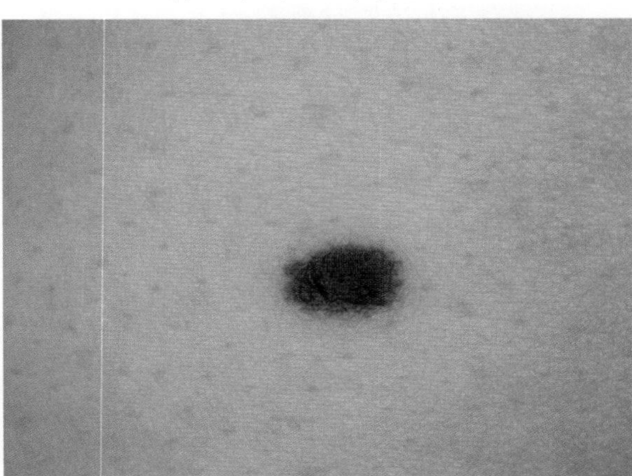
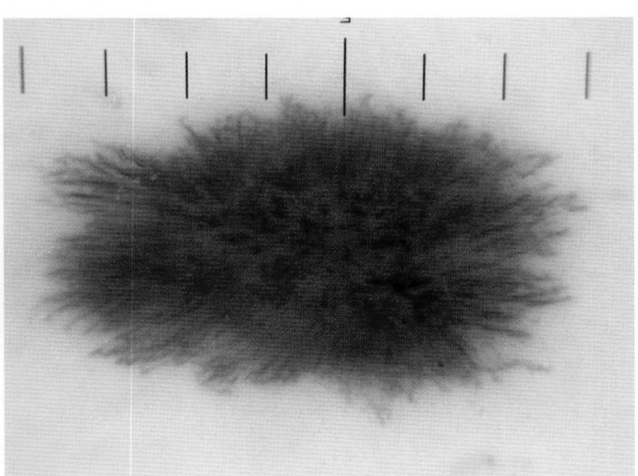

An 'ugly duckling' plaque on the abdomen of a 40-year-old woman: dermoscopy shows an atypical network, peripheral pigmented streaks, central blue-whitish structures and globules in this low-grade dysplastic naevus.

The degree of correlation between dermoscopic atypia and histopathological dysplasia is difficult to predict in solitary hyperpigmented melanocytic lesions. Therefore, excision or sequential imaging should be considered.

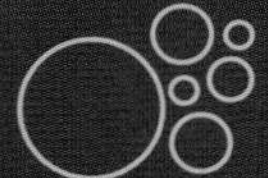

Dermal naevus – pigmented

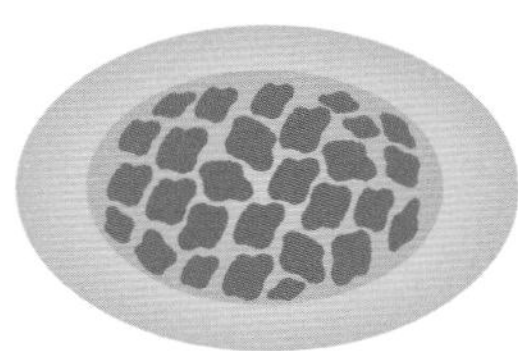

Cobblestone pigmentation is the predominant feature of congenital type naevi. The pigmented globules are round, oval or angulated, variably sized, uniformly pigmented and smooth-cornered. The histopathological correlate is dermal, dense aggregates of melanocytes. Dermal naevi develop from a genetic predisposition, rather than acquired from UV exposure, and hence are more commonly found on the trunk, head and neck rather than the limbs.

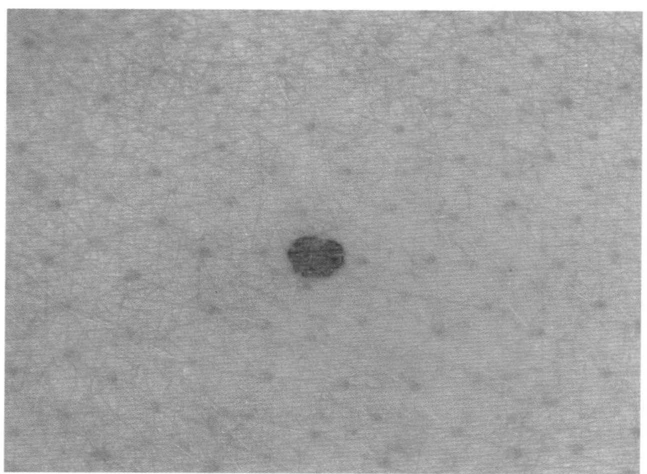

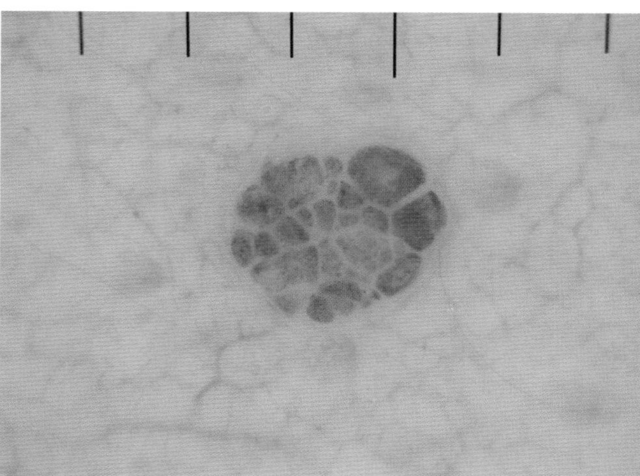

A pigmented papule on the upper back of a 20-year-old woman: dermoscopy shows a uniform cobblestone morphology with angulated, smooth-cornered globules in this dermal naevus.

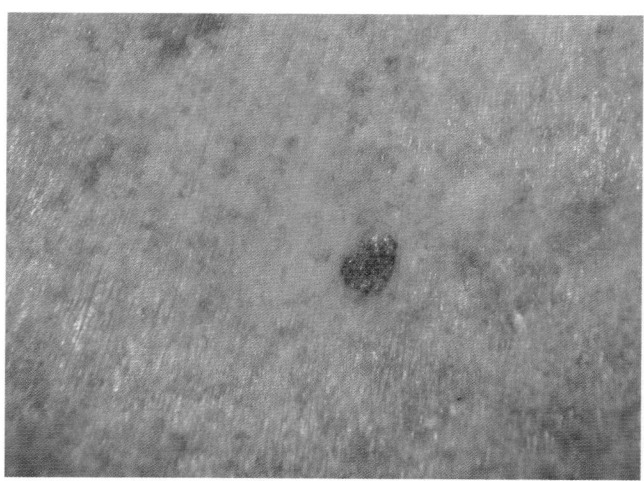

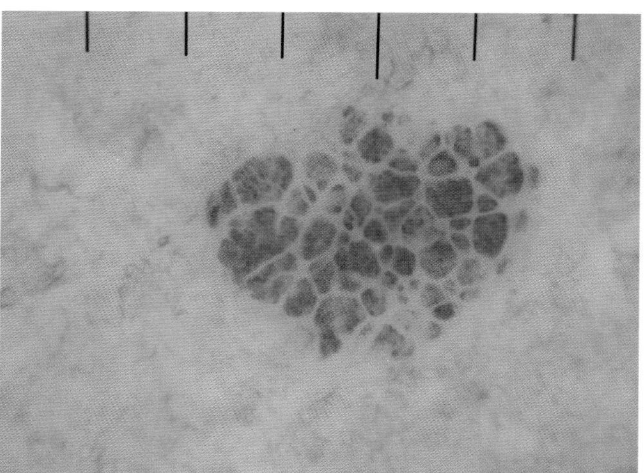

A long-standing pigmented plaque on the triceps of a 60-year-old woman with a history of melanoma: dermoscopy shows cobblestone morphology with variably sized, angulated, smooth-cornered globules in this dermal naevus.

Greco, V. et al. Dermoscopic patterns of intradermal naevi. *Australas J Dermatol*. 2020;61(4):337–341.

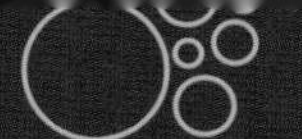

Dermal naevus – hyperpigmented

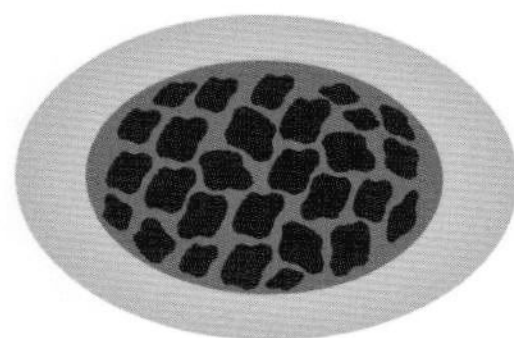

In hyperpigmented dermal naevi the dominant feature is pigmented cobblestone aggregates. With thicker naevi, keratin may build up in the surface clefts of the naevus. The vascular components may be obscured due to the increase in pigmentation. The most important differential diagnosis is a thick melanoma; hence, if any diagnostic doubt remains then consider excision.

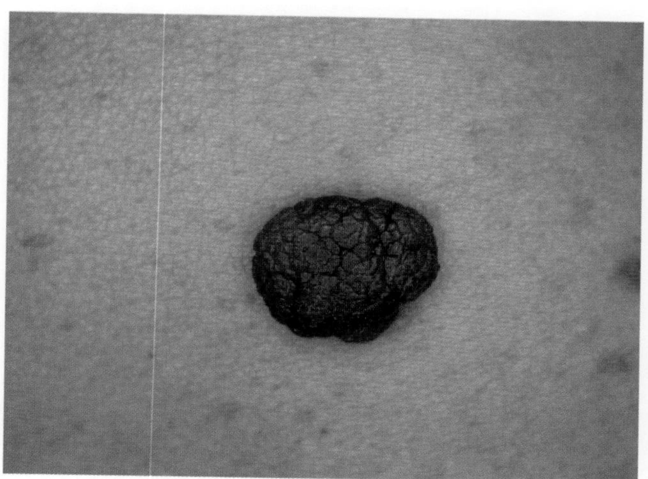

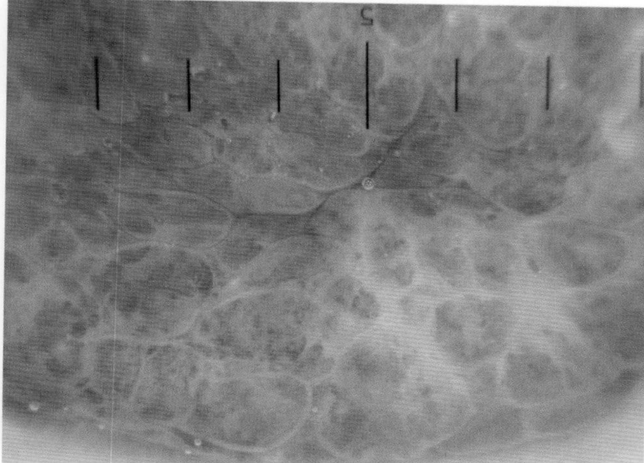

A long-standing hyperpigmented papillated exophytic lesion on the abdomen of a 40-year-old woman: dermoscopy shows hyperpigmented cobblestone pigment aggregates and poorly focused comma vessels in this dermal naevus.

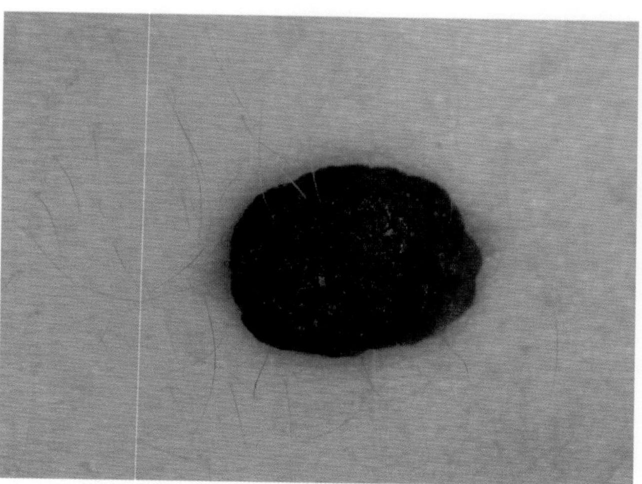

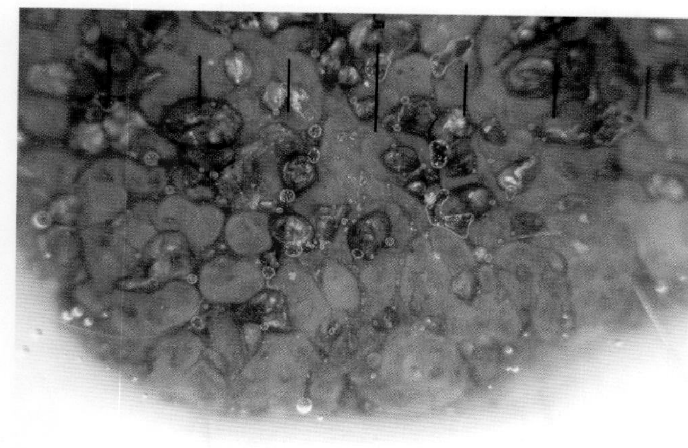

A long-standing exophytic hyperpigmented nodule on the back of a 60-year-old man: dermoscopy shows keratin-filled crypts, hyperpigmented cobblestone pigment aggregates and minimal poorly focused comma vessels in this dermal naevus.

Individuals often have more than one hyperpigmented dermal naevus – examine all naevi to look for reassuringly similar clinical and dermoscopic features. Dermal naevi will usually be soft, compressible and wobble under the dermoscope.

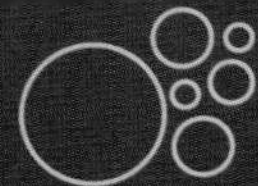

Dermal naevus in dark skin

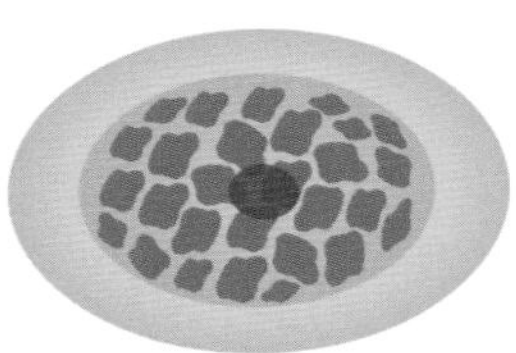

Dermal naevi in individuals with dark skin tones may show a cobblestone pattern with additional features of central perifollicular hyperpigmentation. Additional variability in pigmentation may make these naevi look more suspicious dermoscopically than clinically.

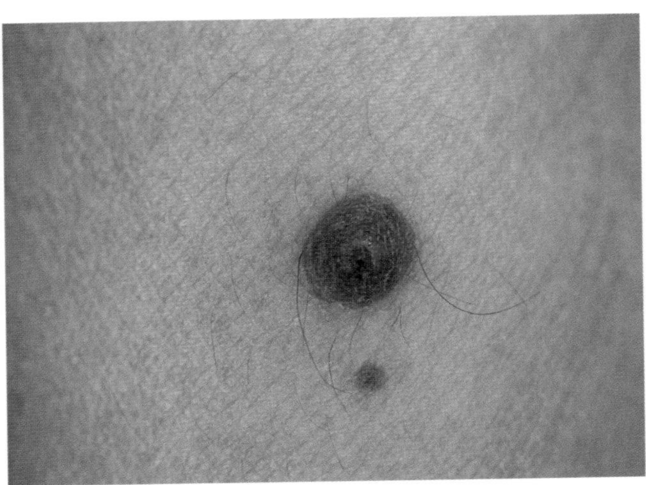

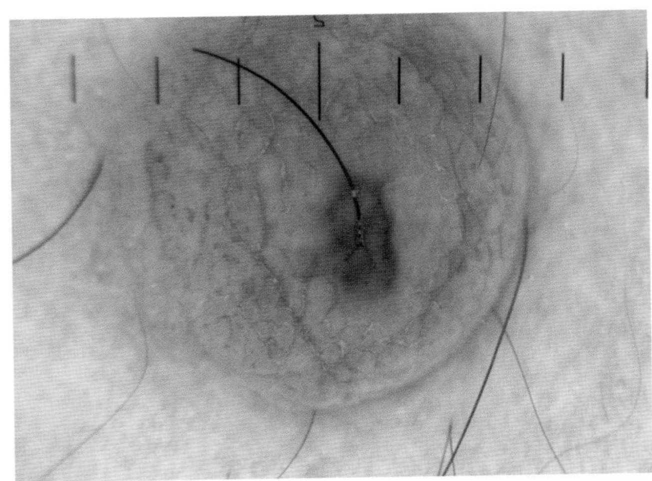

A long-standing hyperpigmented papule on the upper arm of a 40-year-old woman: dermoscopy shows a cobblestone morphology with central perifollicular hyperpigmentation in this dermal naevus.

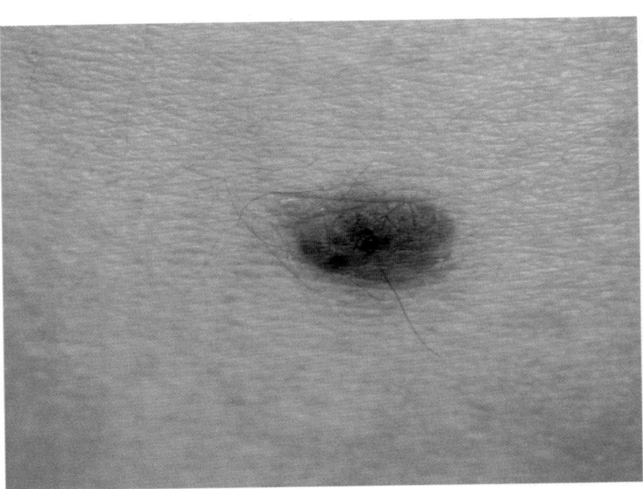

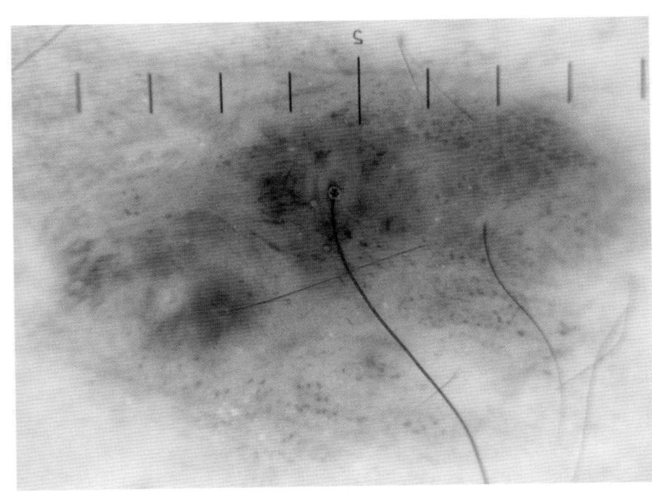

A long-standing pigmented plaque on the lower back of a 50-year-old woman: dermoscopy shows a peripheral network and central globules with slate blue areas with perifollicular hyperpigmentation in this dermal naevus.

Individuals often have more than one hyperpigmented dermal naevus – examine all naevi to look for reassuringly similar clinical and dermoscopic features. Consider a biopsy if any diagnostic doubt remains.

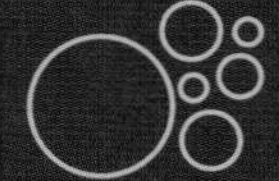

Combined naevus

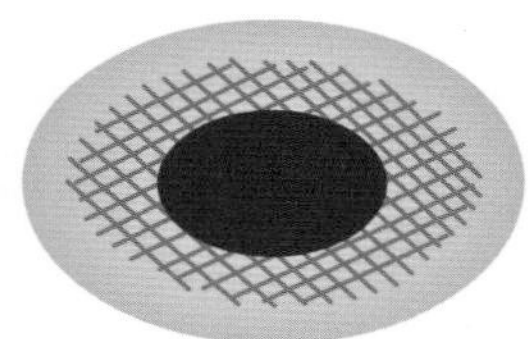

A combined naevus comprises two distinct histopathological melanocytic populations. The most common presentation is a blue naevus combined with a junctional or dermal naevus. Dermoscopy may allow visualization of the two distinct melanocytic populations. However, as this is a melanocytic lesion with a dermal component, consider excision if any diagnostic concern remains following history, clinical and dermoscopic examination.

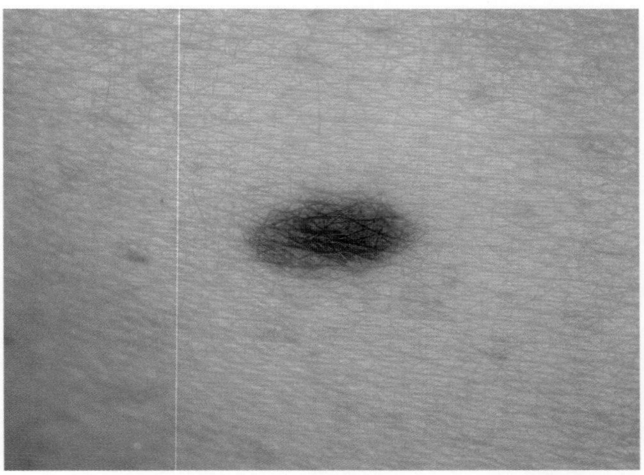

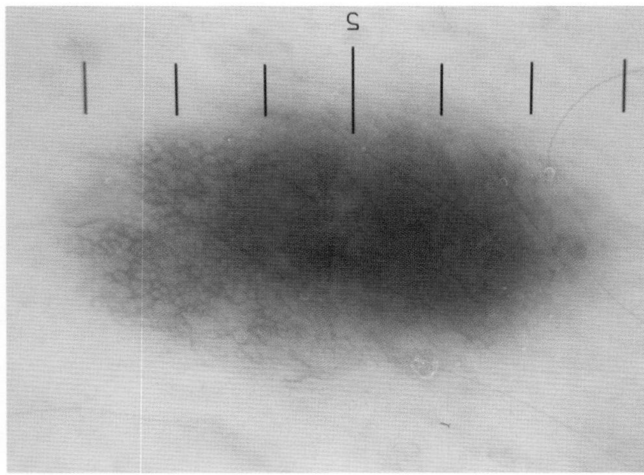

A pigmented lesion on the arm of a 50-year-old woman: dermoscopy shows one pole with reticular brown pigmentation and slate blue pigmentation at the opposite pole in this histopathologically confirmed combined junctional and blue naevus.

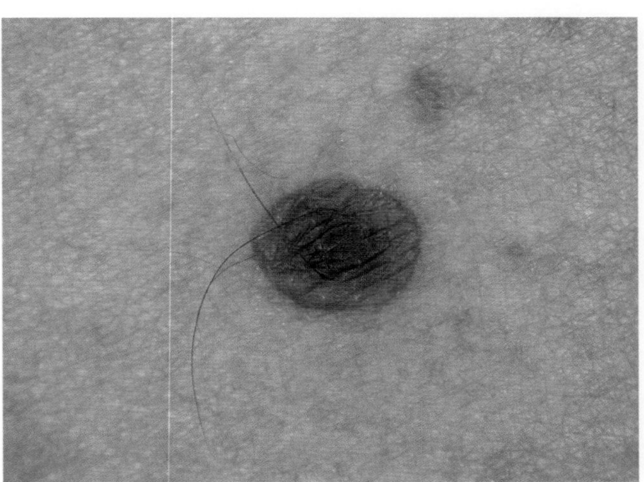

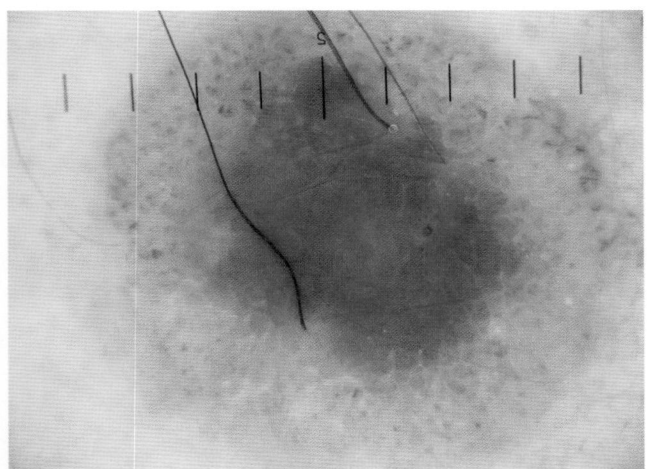

A long-standing plaque with central hyperpigmentation on the chest of a 40-year-old man: dermoscopy shows central slate blue pigmentation and peripheral cobblestone remnants in this combined blue and dermal naevus.

Combined blue naevi mimic melanoma especially where there is asymmetry. Stojkovic-Filipovic, J. et al. Dermatoscopy of combined blue naevi: A multicentre study of the International Dermoscopy Society. *JEADV* 2021;35:900–905.

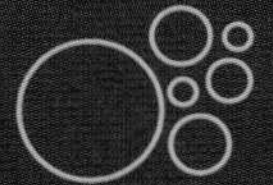

Blue naevus

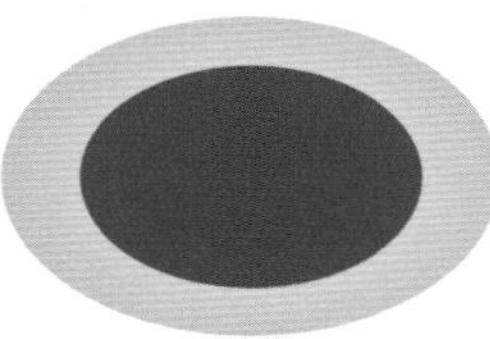

Blue naevi present as a papule or macule, with a uniform slate blue colour and typically an absence of pigment network on dermoscopy. Their blue colour is an optical effect caused by densely pigmented melanocytes located deep in the dermis. They frequently occur in childhood but may also occur in older adults where they may cause diagnostic concern, particularly if they arise in a patient with a previous melanoma.

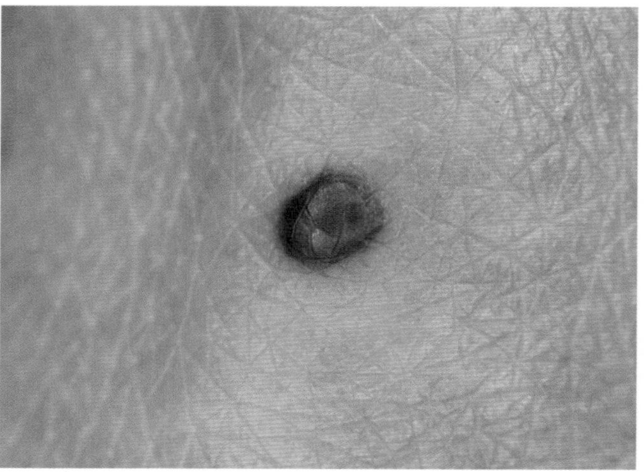

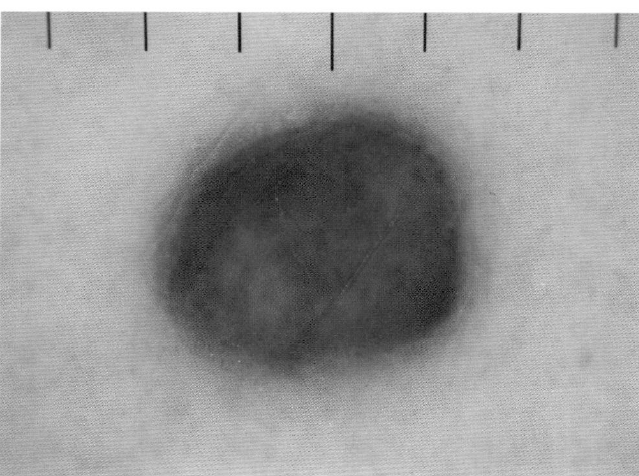

A long-standing hyperpigmented papule on the ankle of a 40-year-old woman: dermoscopy shows a uniform slate blue colour, without vascular features or pigment network in this blue naevus.

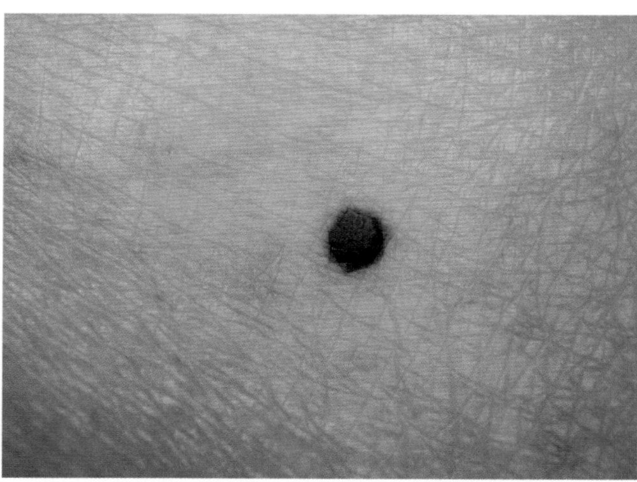

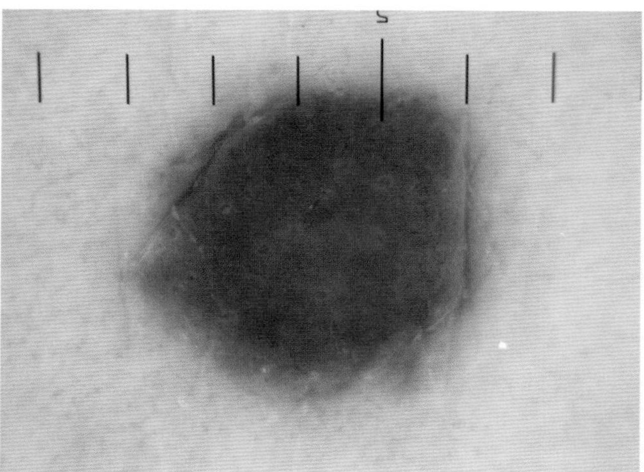

A long-standing hyperpigmented papule on the dorsum of the hand in a 50-year-old woman: dermoscopy shows a uniform slate blue colour, and an absence of vascular features or pigment network in this blue naevus.

Di Cesare, A. et al. The spectrum of dermatoscopic patterns in blue nevi. *J Am Acad Dermatol*. 2012;67(2):199–205.

Blue naevus – sclerotic/hypochromic

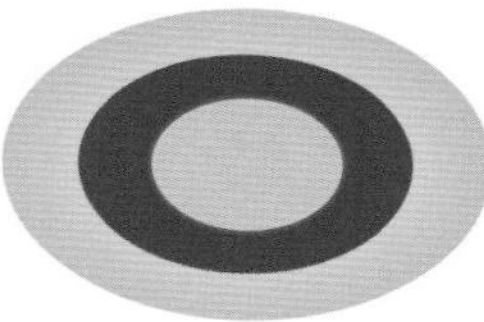

Blue naevi often have sclerotic connective tissue surrounding the melanocytes. If this sclerotic connective tissue increases then a sclerotic blue naevus becomes evident. Distinct from conventional blue naevi, the slate blue colour is typically located at the edge of the lesion with the sclerotic hypopigmented area(s) located centrally. As this is a dermal melanocytic lesion, consider excision if there is any diagnostic concern.

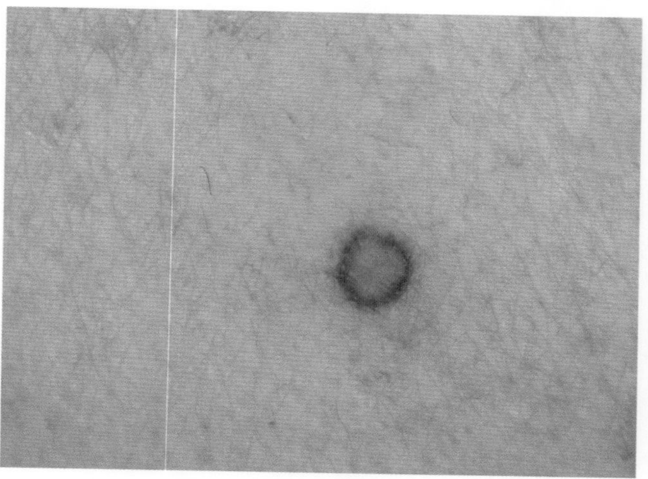

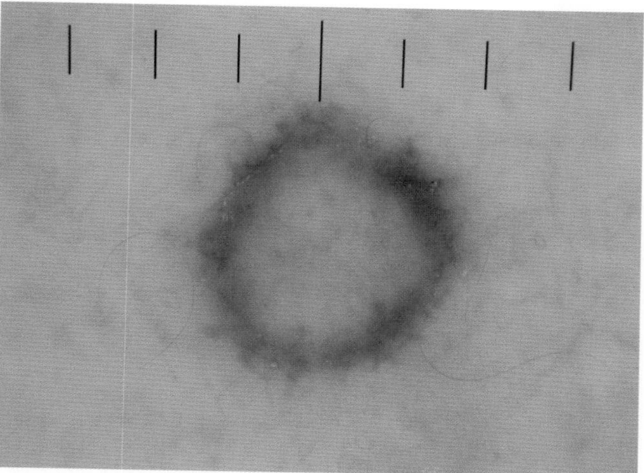

A long-standing annular blue/grey macule on the forearm of a 70-year-old woman: dermoscopy shows a uniform peripheral slate blue colour with hazy dendritic processes and central pale grey hypopigmentation in this sclerotic blue naevus.

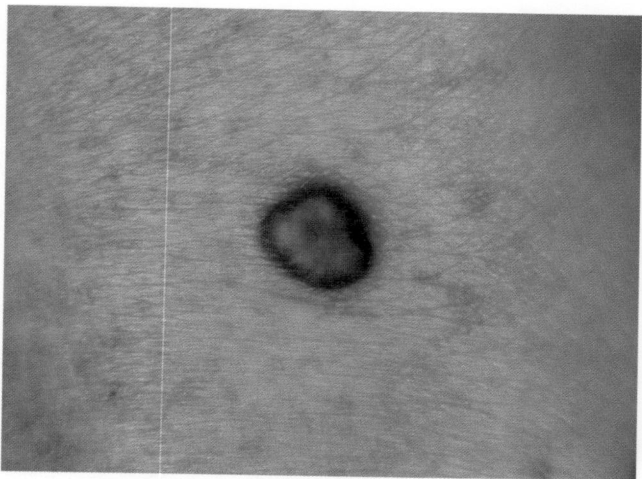

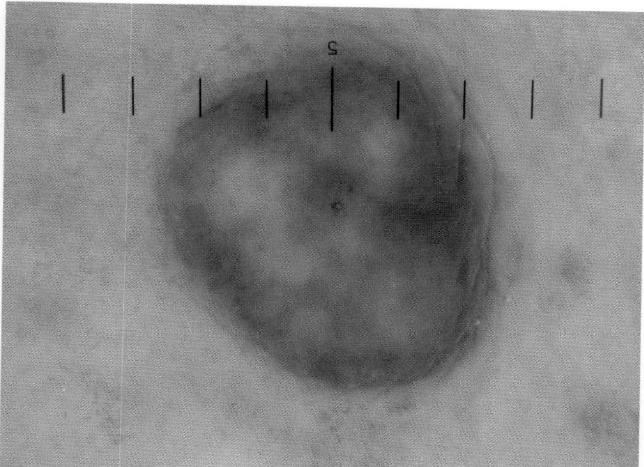

A long-standing blue/grey nodule on the ankle of a 50-year old man: dermoscopy shows peripheral slate blue colour with central coalescing grey-white pigmentation in this histopathologically confirmed sclerotic blue naevus.

Blue naevi may show hazy ill-defined dendritic processes at their periphery (which correlates well with their histopathology) Ferrara, G. et al. The many faces of blue naevus: a clinicopathologic study. *J Cutan Pathol*. 2007;34(7):543–551.

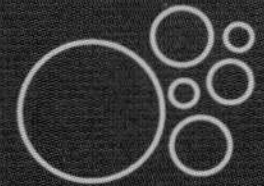

Recurrent naevus

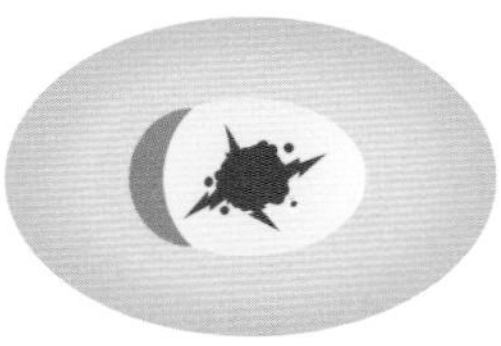

A recurrent naevus arises from residual melanocytes producing pigmentation following a traumatic episode, typically incomplete removal of a pre-existing naevus. The variable pigmentation and atypical structures may increase the index of suspicion, particularly if pigmentation is eccentric and extends beyond the scar's edge. If removed, the pathologist should be informed of the previous surgical intervention so that the original histopathology can also be reviewed.

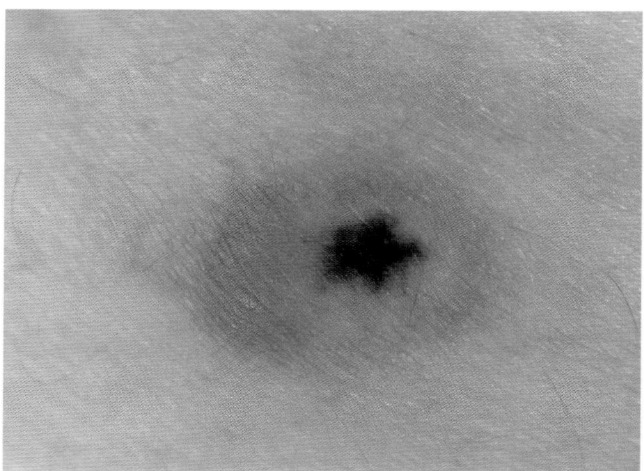

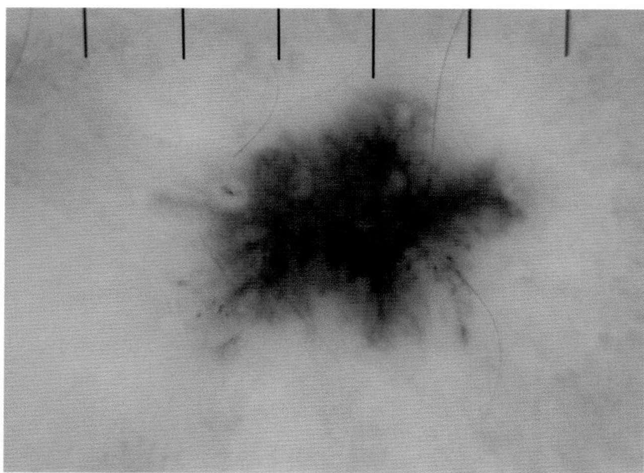

A pigmented macule on the back of a 20-year-old woman with a history of a shave biopsy: dermoscopy shows irregular pigment network and radial streaks, globules and scar-like areas in this histopathologically confirmed recurrent naevus.

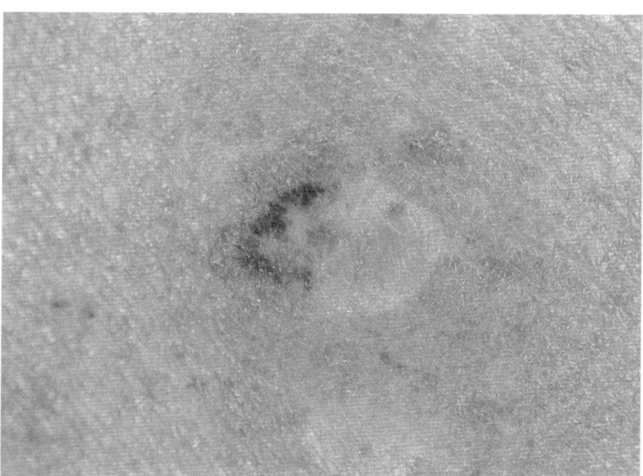

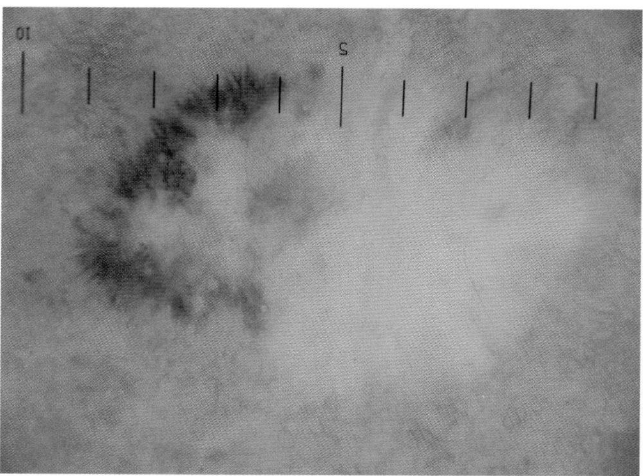

A partially pigmented lesion following a previous shave biopsy on the back of a 50-year-old man: dermoscopy shows peripheral radial streaks, granular pigmentation and scar-like areas in this histopathologically confirmed recurrent naevus.

Blum, A. et al. Recurrent melanocytic nevi and melanomas in dermoscopy: results of a multicenter study of the International Dermoscopy Society. *JAMA Dermatol*. 2014;150(2):138–145.

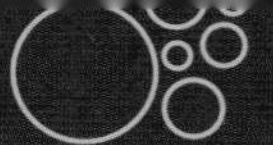

Halo naevus

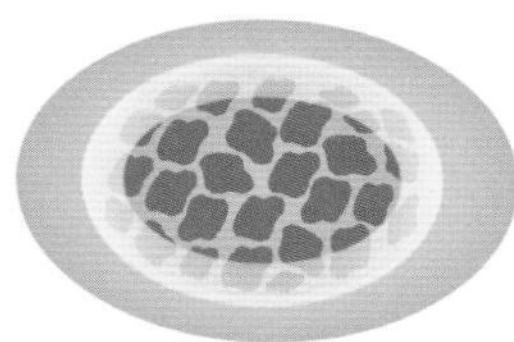

A halo naevus is a melanocytic naevus with a peripheral rim of depigmentation. The loss of pigment is due to an immune-mediated response targeted at the melanocytes. They occur commonly in children and young adults and multiple naevi are often affected. Halo naevi can take several years to fully regress. The central residual melanocytic population should show a typical pigment pattern. If not or if it occurs in an older individual, excision should be considered.

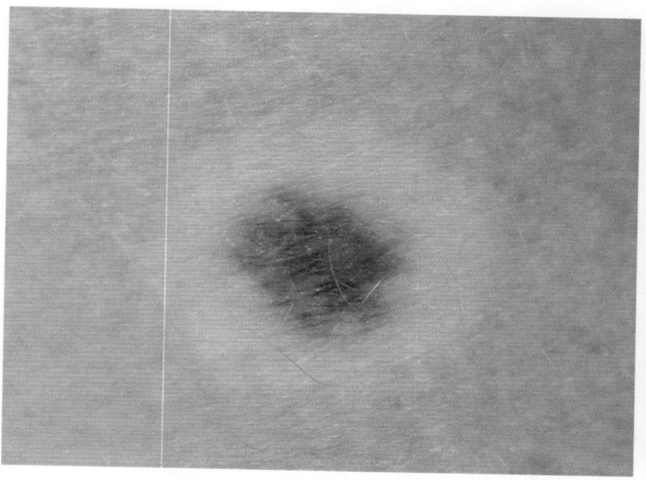
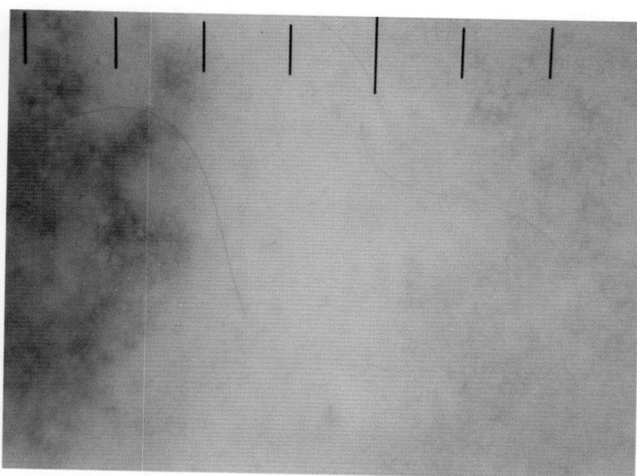

A typical halo naevus on the back of a teenage boy: dermoscopy shows peripheral depigmentation and residual reticular pigmentation centrally in this halo naevus.

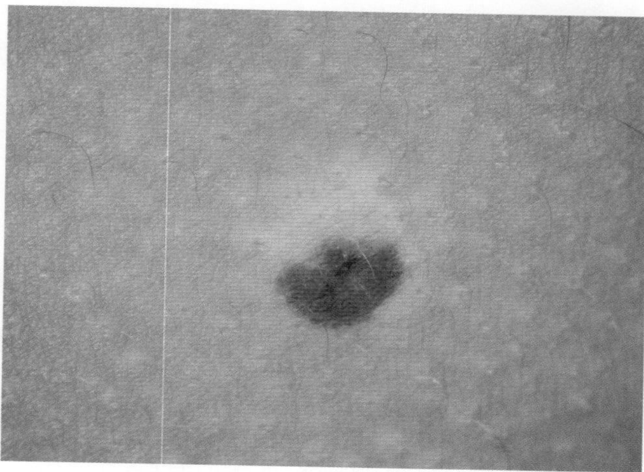
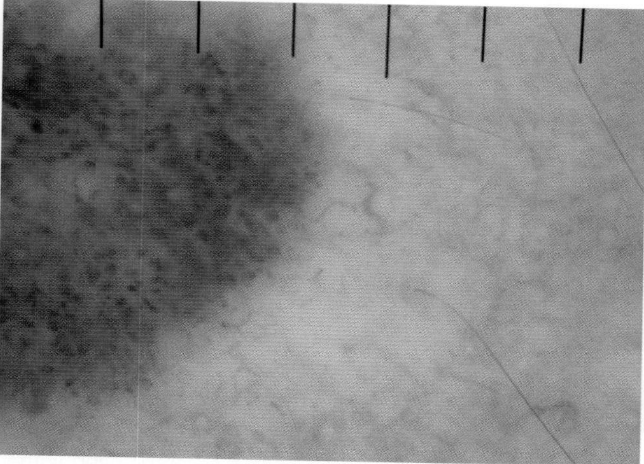

A halo naevus on the back of a 20-year-old man with an eccentric ring of depigmentation: dermoscopy shows a central residual cobblestone pattern and peripheral depigmentation in this histopathologically confirmed halo naevus.

Aouthmany, M. et al. The natural history of halo naevi: A retrospective case series. *J Am Acad Dermatol.* 2012;67(4):582–586.

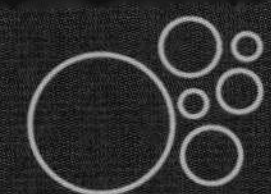

Congenital naevus

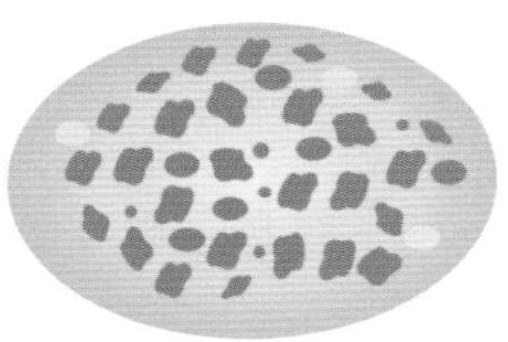

Congenital naevi typically present with a globular and/or cobblestone pattern on dermoscopy with additional clinical features of coalescing pigmented and non-pigmented papules. Small nodules and/or hypertrichosis are also commonly seen. As the child grows, congenital naevi grow proportionally.

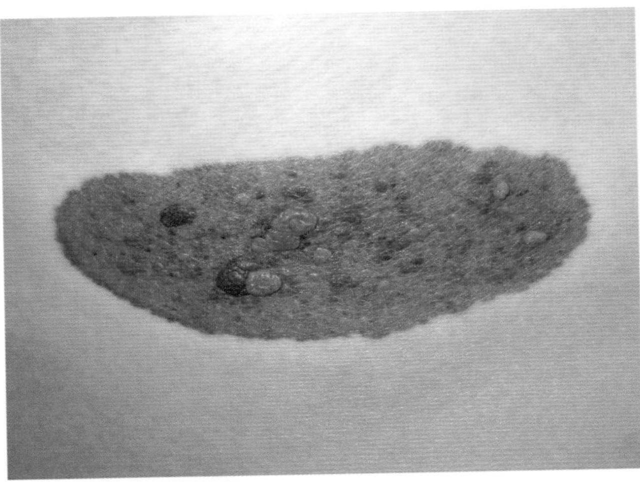

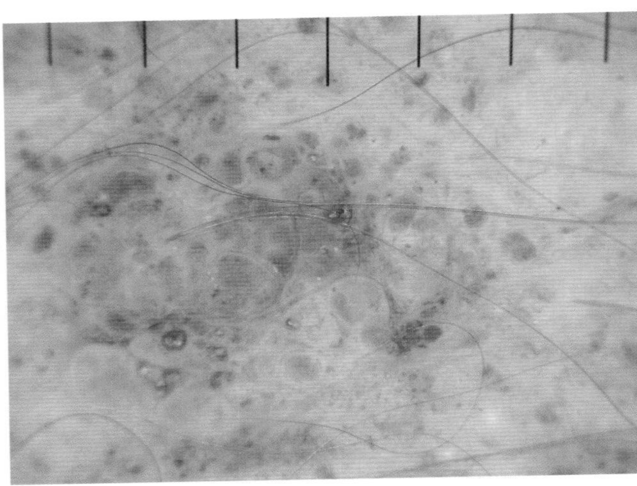

A 10 × 4 cm congenital naevus with multiple monomorphic hypo- and hyperpigmented papules on the abdomen of a 20-year-old woman: dermoscopy shows a globular and cobblestone morphology with comma vessels and hypertrichosis.

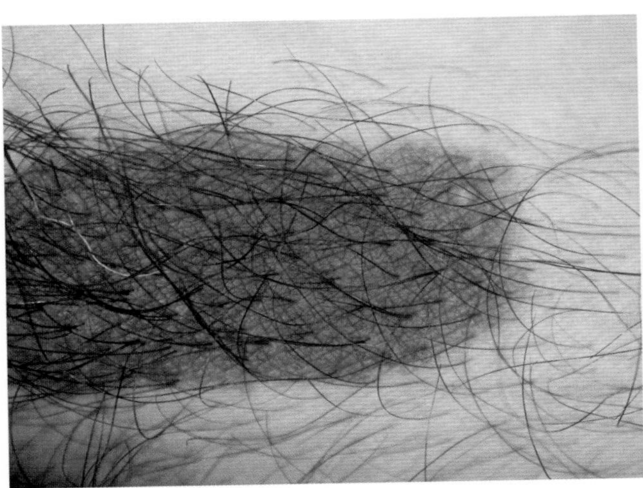

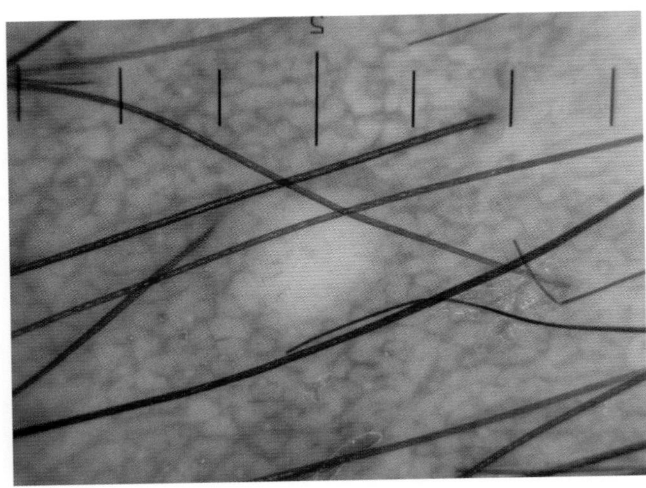

A naevus with hypertrichosis and a small eccentric hypopigmented papule on the back of a 30-year-old man: dermoscopy shows multiple terminal hairs, reticular pigmentation and focal hypopigmentation in this congenital naevus.

Cengiz, F.P. et al. Dermoscopic features of small, medium, and large-sized congenital melanocytic nevi. *Ann Dermatol*. 2017; 29(1): 26–32.

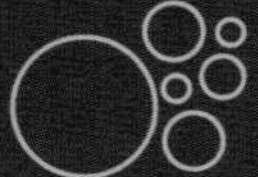

Agminated naevus and naevus spilus

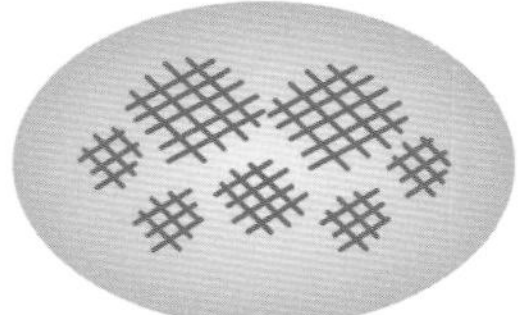

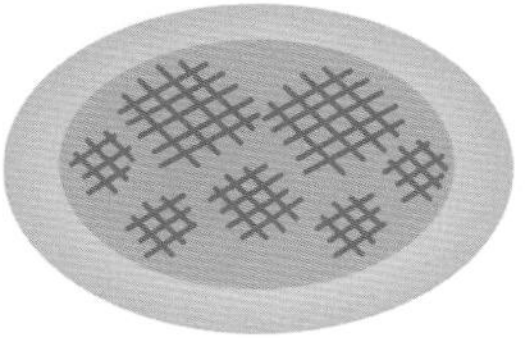

Agminated naevi are localised clusters of naevi without background pigment. Naevus spilus (or speckled lentiginous naevus), on the other hand, consists of a tan lentiginous background upon which multiple discrete macules and papules of naevi are distributed. The most common subtype of naevus is junctional with uniform reticular pigmentation on dermoscopy. Most cases tend to occur from birth or early childhood and are thus generally considered as a subtype of congenital naevus.

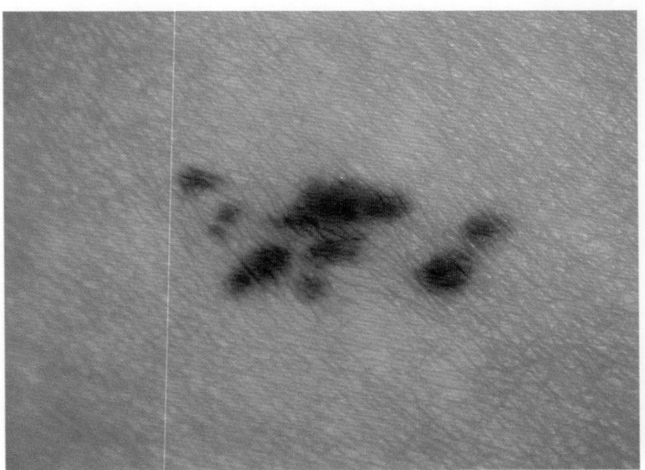

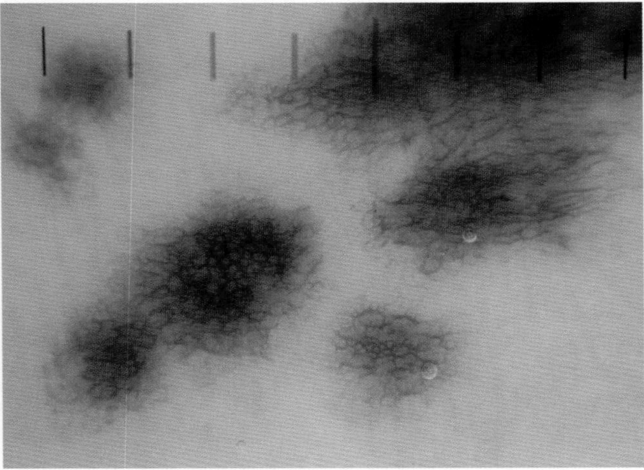

A long-standing stable pigmented group of macules on the lower back of a 40-year-old woman: dermoscopy shows multiple foci of reticular brown pigmentation upon a background of normal skin in this agminated naevus.

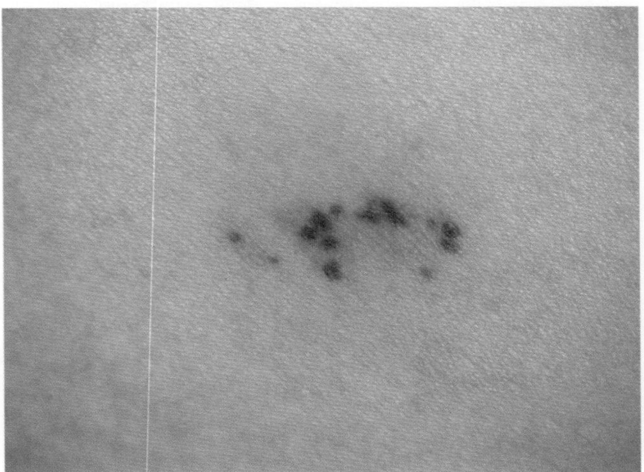

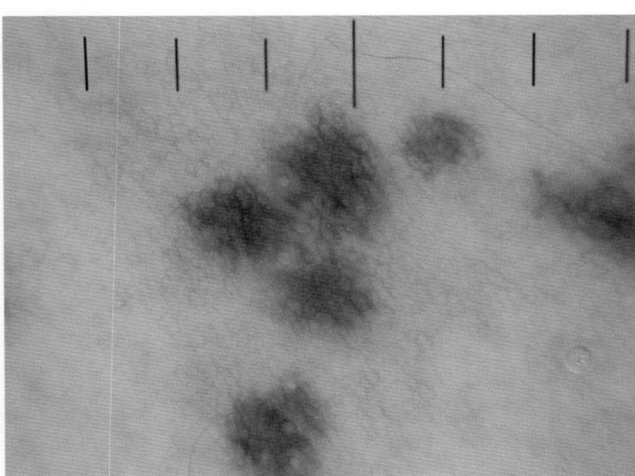

A long-standing stable pigmented macule with foci of hyperpigmentation on the back of a 30-year-old woman: dermoscopy shows multiple foci of reticular brown network upon a pale brown reticular background in this naevus spilus.

Larger segmental naevus spilus should be monitored for melanoma which may present as a focal area of change. Ly, L. et al. Melanoma(s) arising in large segmental speckled lentiginous nevi: a case series. *J Am Acad Dermatol*. 2011;64(6):1190–3.

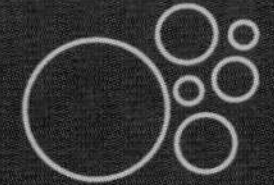

Reed naevus I

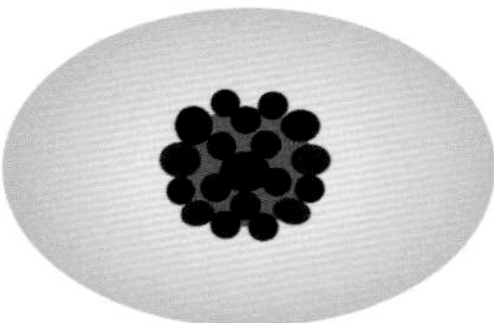

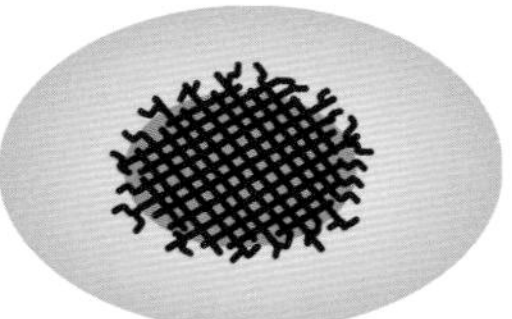

Reed naevus is a heavily pigmented variant of Spitz naevus. Clinically they present as hyperpigmented macules and may mimic melanoma. Reed naevi are dermoscopically dynamic. The pigmented variants often have a globular morphology initially, which may progress to become reticular and then homogeneous.

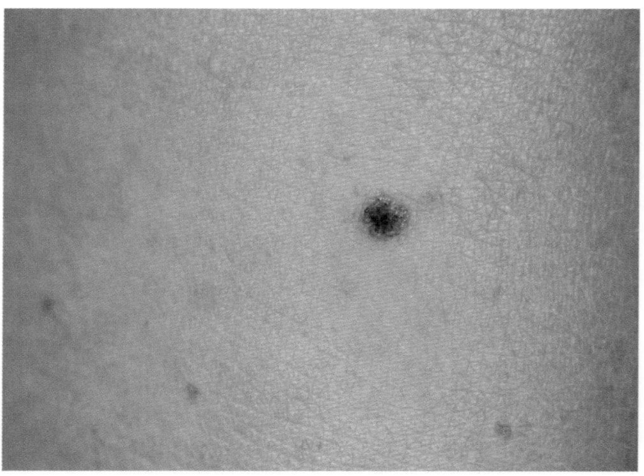

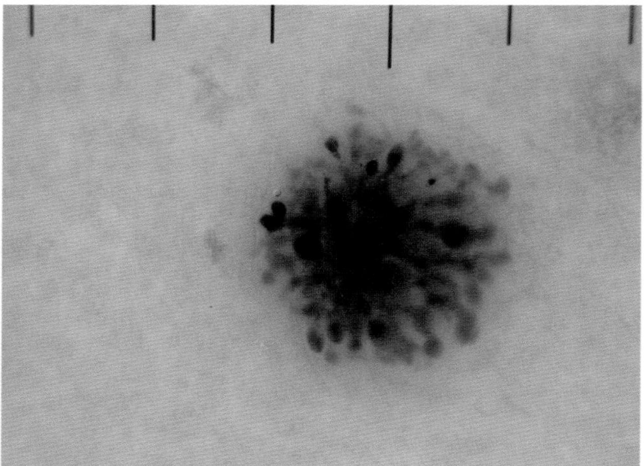

A new hyperpigmented macule on the deltoid of a 20-year-old woman: dermoscopy shows multiple, radiating pigmented globules of variable colours from brown to black in this histopathologically confirmed Reed naevus.

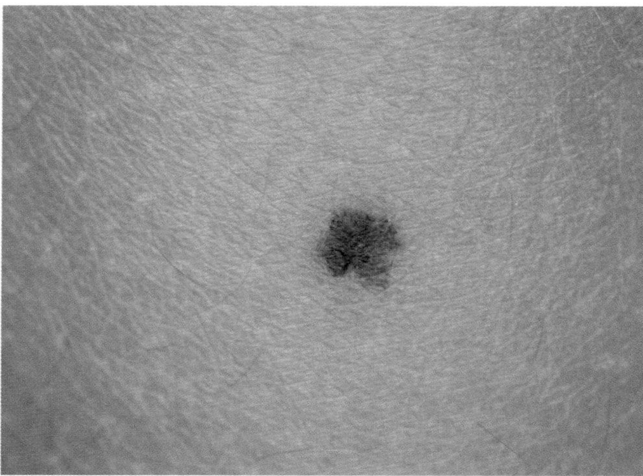

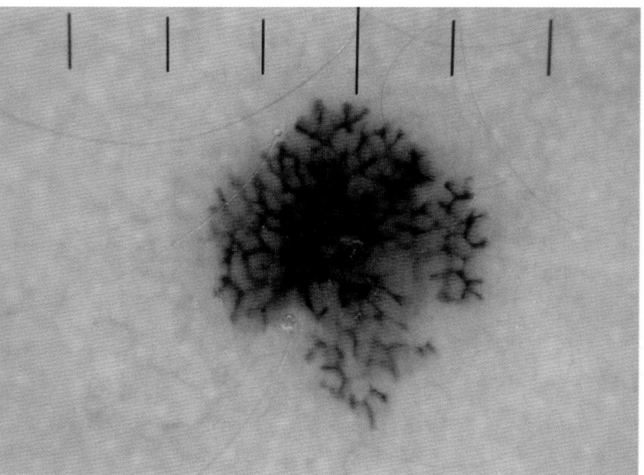

A new pigmented macule on the leg of a 30-year-old woman: dermoscopy shows broad reticular morphology with brown to black radial streaks in this histopathologically confirmed Reed naevus.

Lallas, A. et al. Update on dermoscopy of Spitz/Reed naevi and management guidelines by the International Dermoscopy Society. *Br J Dermatol*. 2017;177(3):645–655.

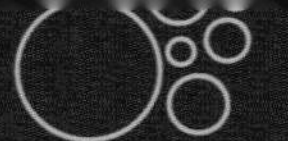

Reed naevus II

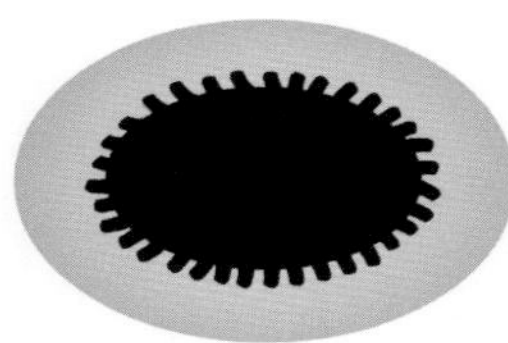

As Reed naevi develop, the central area becomes more homogeneous. The peripheral streaks may become more uniform, creating what has been described as a 'starburst' pattern. Clinically, this type of well-demarcated hyperpigmented plaque mimics melanoma. Whilst the starburst pattern is reassuring in a child, recognising this pattern in an adult is more concerning and pathology should always be obtained after excision.

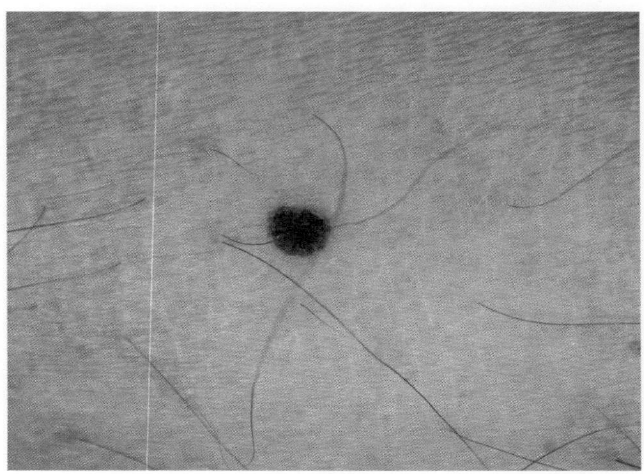

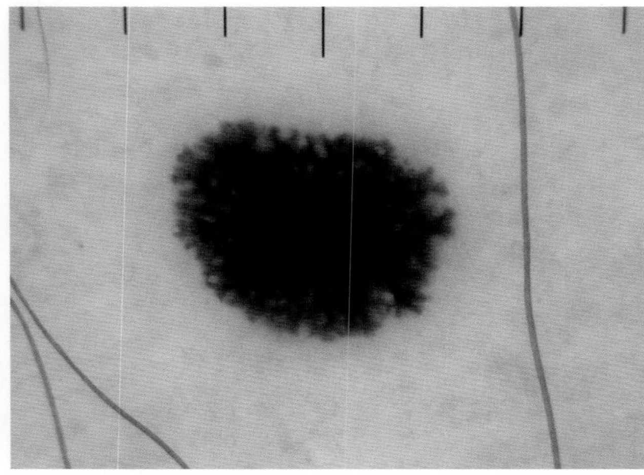

A hyperpigmented macule on the thigh of a 40-year-old man: dermoscopy shows a central black blotch, a broad hyperpigmented network and circumferential pigment streaks in this histopathologically confirmed Reed naevus.

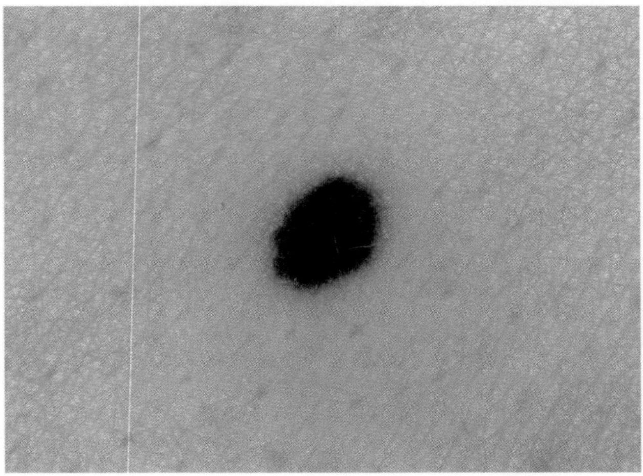

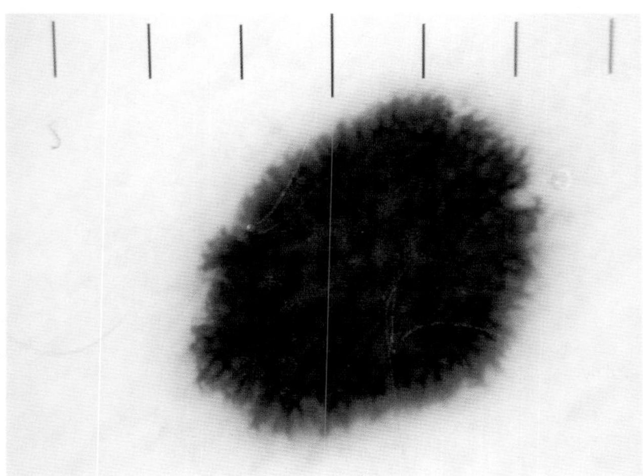

A new hyperpigmented macule on the back of a 30-year-old man: dermoscopy shows central homogeneous hyperpigmentation with circumferential pigment streaks in this histopathologically confirmed Reed naevus.

Reed naevi are dynamic and typically show evolving features on repeat imaging, up to the point that they stabilise, and cause ongoing clinical concern. It may therefore be practical to consider early excision rather than follow-up.

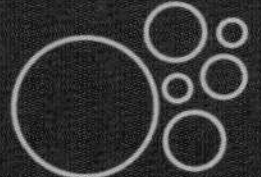

Pigmented Spitz naevus

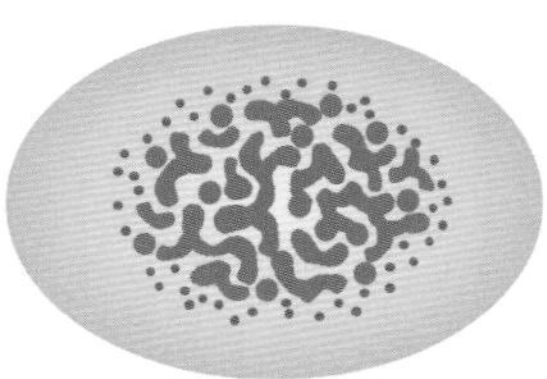

Additional to Reed naevus (the purely pigmented variant of Spitz naevus) is a pattern that comprises a blend of pigmented and non-pigmented structures. Pigment globules surrounded by a negative (inverse) pigment network and dotted vessels is a well-recognised pattern of Spitz naevi. The overlap of clinical and dermoscopic features with melanoma makes excision mandatory.

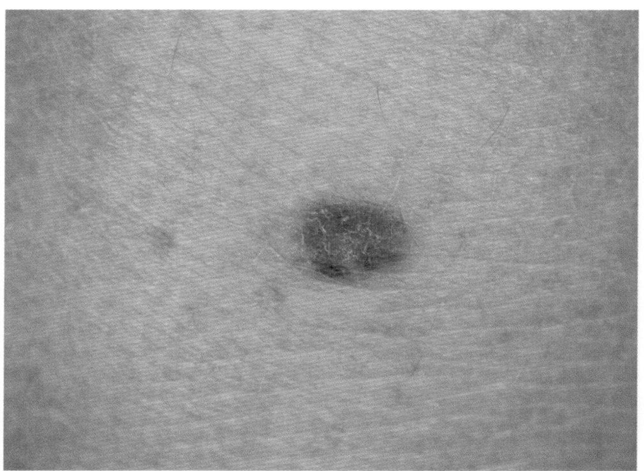

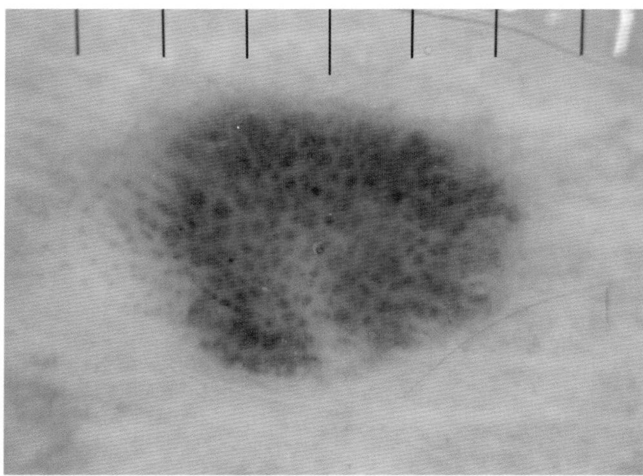

A suspicious pigmented plaque on the distal forearm of a 50-year-old woman: dermoscopy shows pigment globules, a negative network and eccentric dotted vessels in this histopathologically confirmed pigmented Spitz naevus.

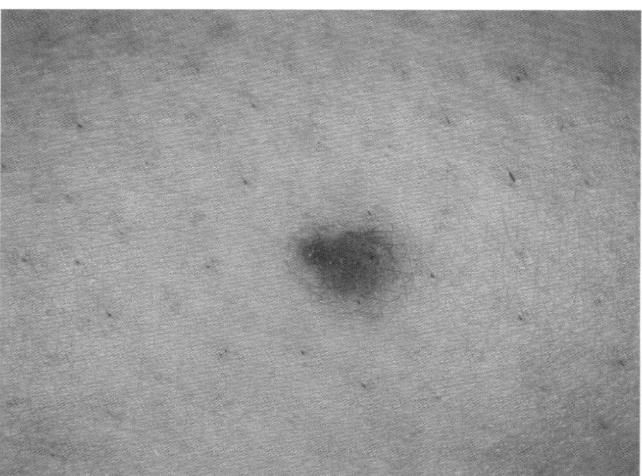

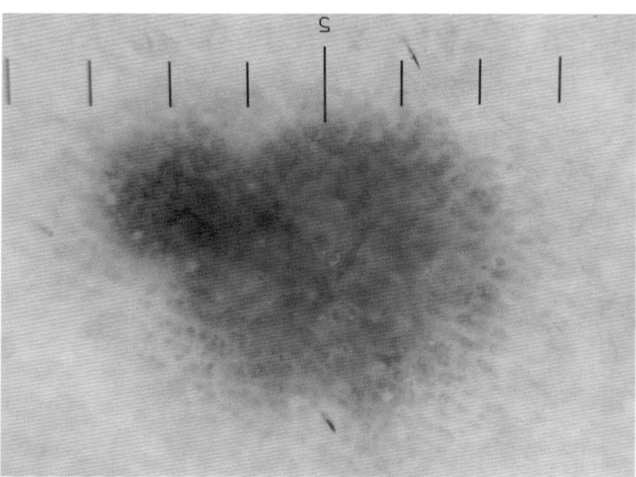

A new multicoloured plaque on the leg of a 50-year-old woman: dermoscopy shows blue-grey colour, brown globules, peripheral dotted vessels and negative network in this histopathologically confirmed pigmented Spitz naevus.

Consider excision for any Spitzoid skin lesion. Bowling, J. et al. Dermoscopy key points: recommendations from the International Dermoscopy Society. *Dermatology*. 2007;214(1):3–5.

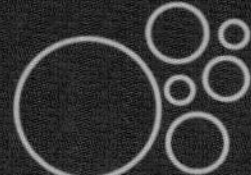

Hypomelanotic Spitz naevus I

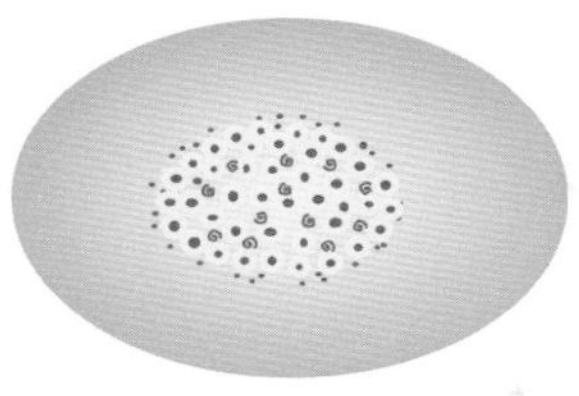

Hypomelanotic/hypopigmented Spitz naevi typically present as a solitary pink papule or nodule with dermoscopic features of erythema alone or with dotted and coiled or glomerular vessels and negative pigment network. There is significant overlap clinically with a number of diagnoses, particularly amelanotic nodular melanoma, so excision is mandatory.

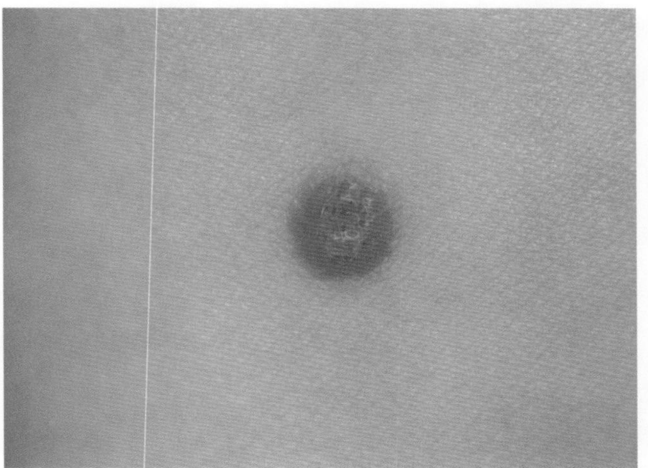

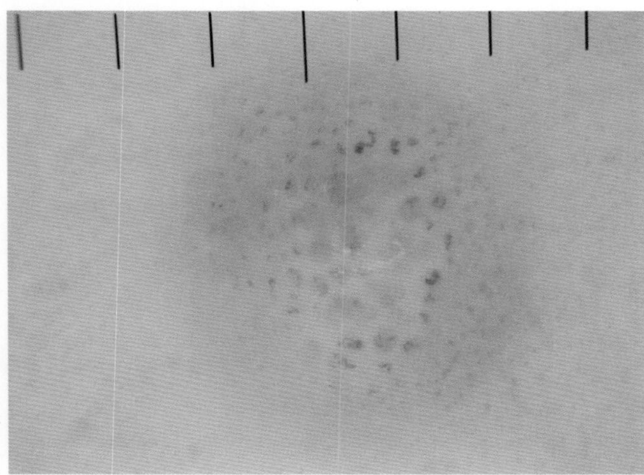

A pink papule on the arm of a 15-year-old girl: dermoscopy shows dotted and coiled or glomerular vessels with negative network in this histopathologically confirmed Spitz naevus.

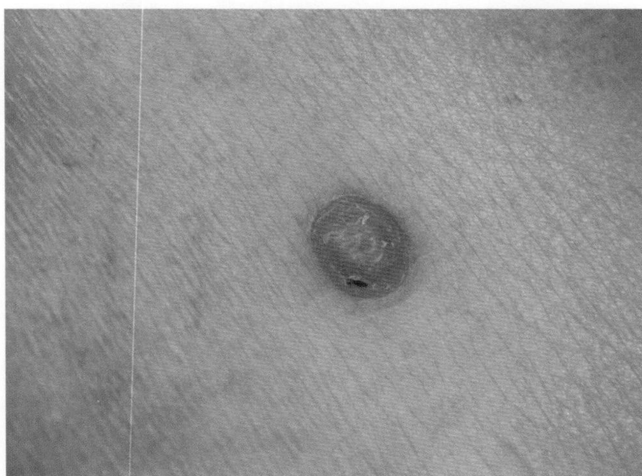

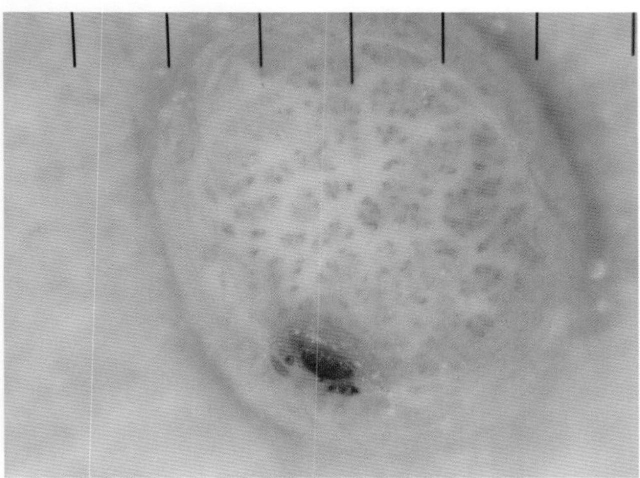

A pink nodule on the thigh of a 40-year-old woman: dermoscopy shows dotted and coiled or glomerular vessels, interspersed negative network and a focus of traumatic ulceration in this histopathologically confirmed Spitz naevus.

Consider excision for any growing solitary pink papule, plaque or nodule and ensure that the specimen is reported by an experienced dermatopathologist. Clinicopathologic correlation or multiple opinions are sometimes required for difficult cases.

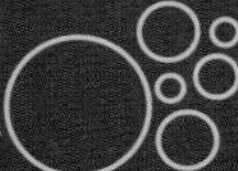

Hypomelanotic Spitz naevus II

Desmoplasia which represents dense fibrosis typically diminishes the features seen dermoscopically. Desmoplastic Spitz naevus presents as a pink papule or nodule and on dermoscopy shows bland, milky, pinkish erythema and an otherwise featureless background. There is significant clinical overlap with amelanotic and desmoplastic melanoma and therefore excision is mandatory.

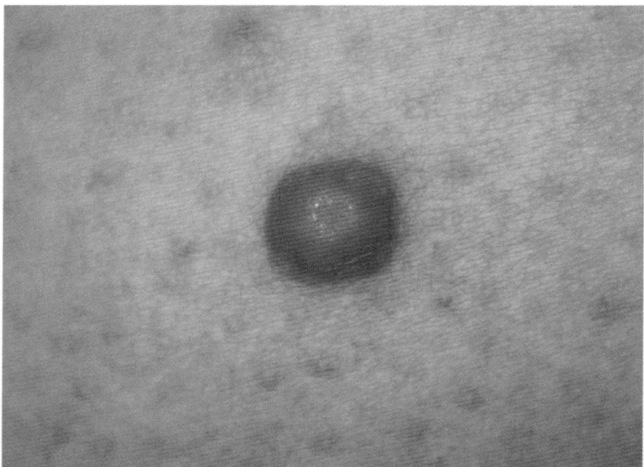

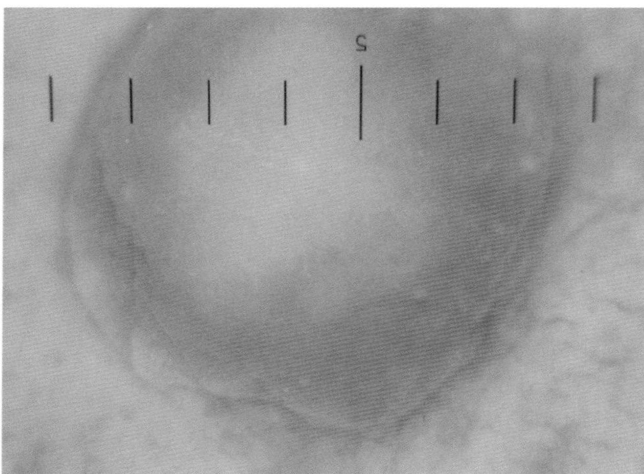

A pink nodule on the lower back of a 55-year-old woman: dermoscopy shows milky, pinkish erythema only and a featureless background in this histopathologically confirmed desmoplastic Spitz naevus.

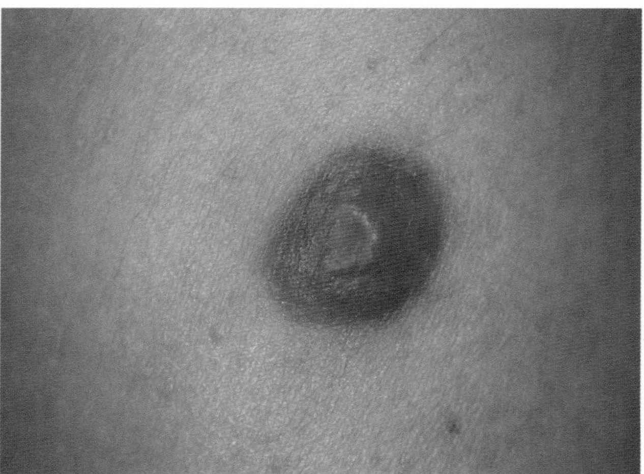

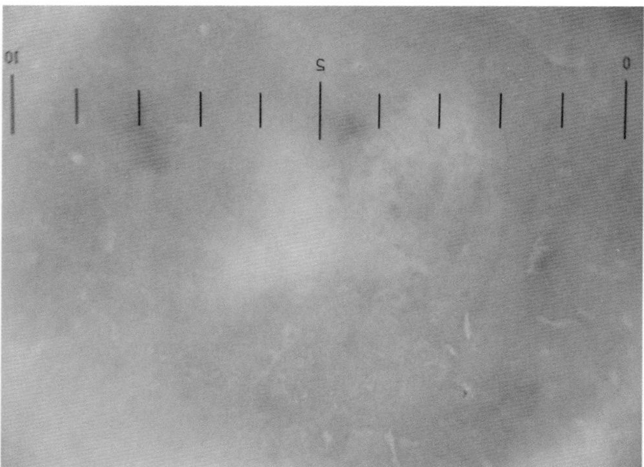

A pink nodule on the arm of a 40-year-old woman: dermoscopy shows milky, pinkish erythema only and a featureless background in this histopathologically confirmed desmoplastic Spitz naevus.

Spitz naevus poses a challenge for both the clinician and pathologist. Good clinicopathologic correlation, liaision with an experienced dermatopathologist and a low threshold for biopsy help to avoid missing Spitzoid melanoma.

3.1 Melanoma – clinical variants

Small diameter 40
Small diameter cases 41
Geometric border 42
Geometric border cases 43
Geographic border 44
Geographic border cases 45
Disordered polarity 46
Disordered polarity cases 47
Naevus-associated 48
Naevus-associated cases 49
Congenital melanocytic naevus-associated 50

Diagnostic Dermoscopy: The Illustrated Guide, Second Edition. Jonathan Bowling.

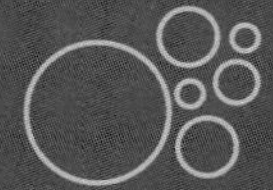

Small diameter

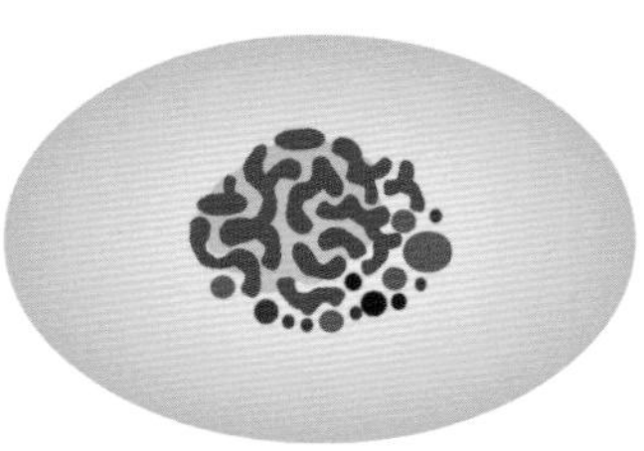

As melanomas evolve they develop more dermoscopic features. These same dermoscopic features may be seen in small diameter melanocytic lesions suggesting a diagnosis of melanoma. This principle also helps to identify melanomas on sequential dermoscopic imaging.

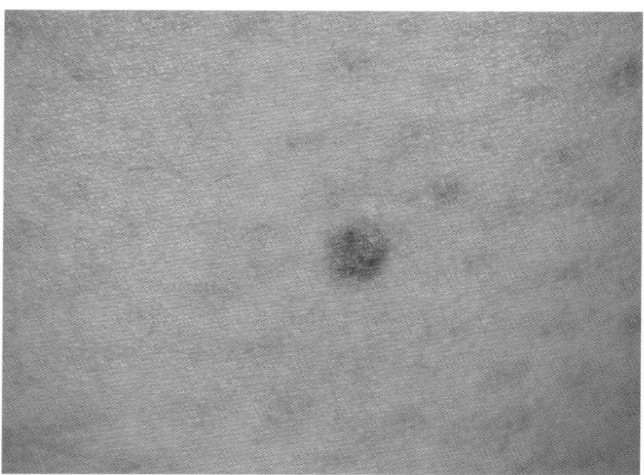

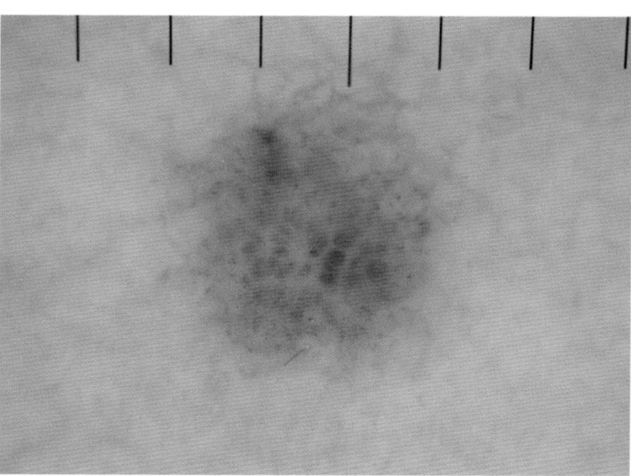

A 3 mm pink macule on the shoulder of a 19-year-old woman: dermoscopy shows irregular brown globules and dotted vessels in this 0.3 mm thick superficial spreading melanoma (SSM).

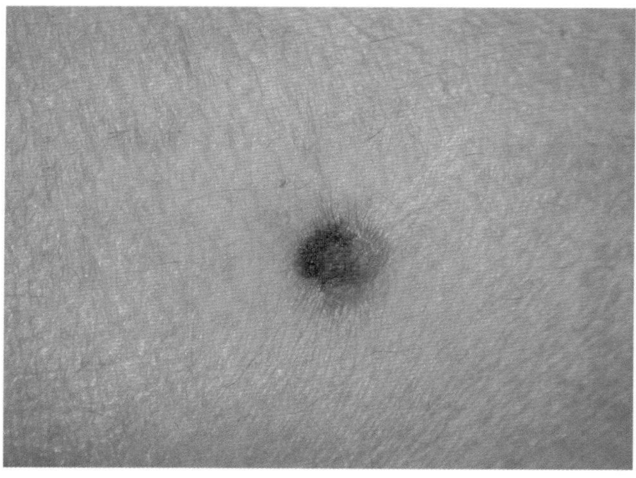

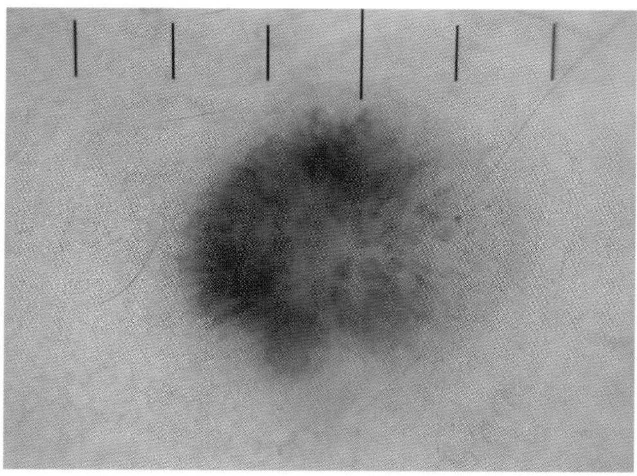

A 3 mm hyperpigmented macule on the back of a 30-year-old man: dermoscopy shows a disordered lesion with irregular brown globules, polymorphous vessels and peripheral streaks in this 0.6 mm thick SSM.

Seidenari, S. et al. Dermoscopy of small melanomas: just miniaturized dermoscopy? *Br J Dermatol*. 2014;171(5):1006–1013.

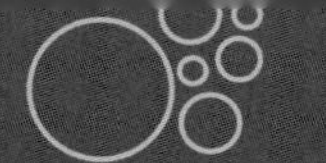

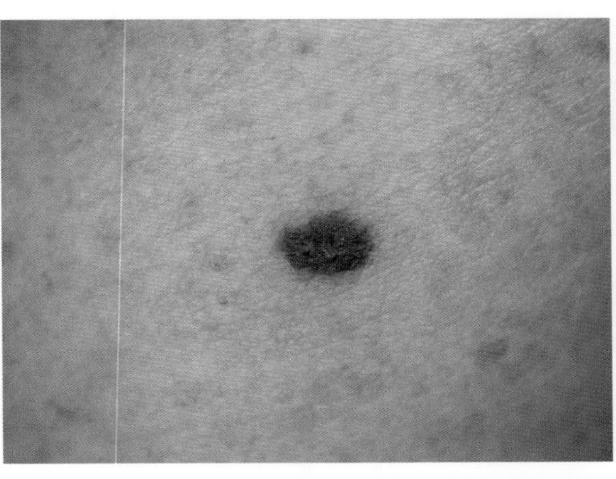

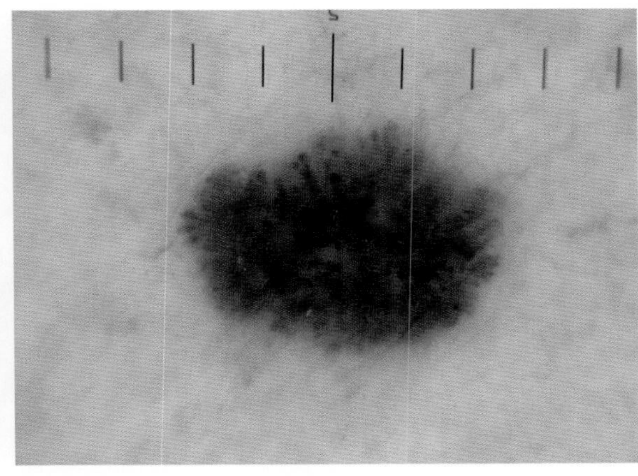

A 4 mm pigmented macule on the shoulder: dermoscopy shows irregular globules, peripheral streaks and a blue-whitish veil in this 0.3 mm thick SSM.

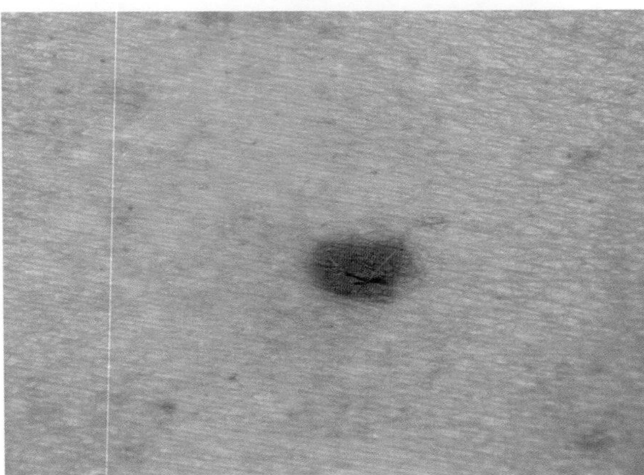

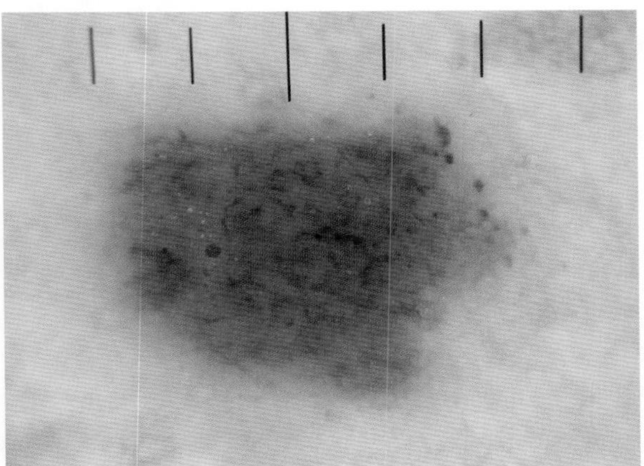

A 4 mm pigmented macule on the lower leg: dermoscopy shows eccentric irregular brown globules, dotted vessels and a blue-whitish veil in this 0.6 mm thick SSM.

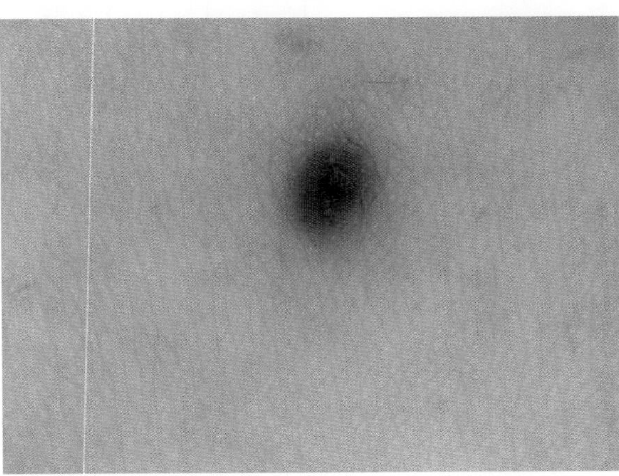

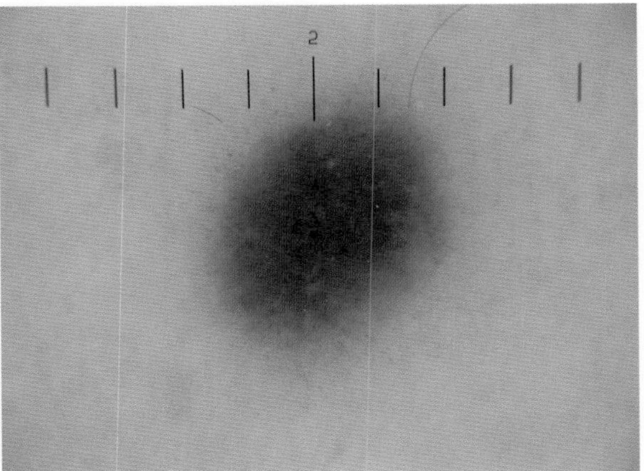

A 4 mm blue-brown macule on the back of a 20-year-old man: dermoscopy shows multiple colours including central ill-defined blue-whitish veil, shiny white streaks and diffuse dotted and linear vessels in this 0.4 mm thick SSM.

Dermoscopists need to use all of their acumen to identify small diameter melanomas, which can be invasive. Subtle small melanomas diagnosed on dermoscopy may not be very distinct clinically (so-called 'Little Red Riding Hood' sign).

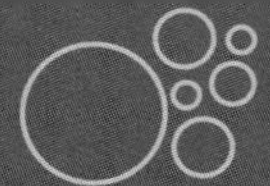

Geometric border

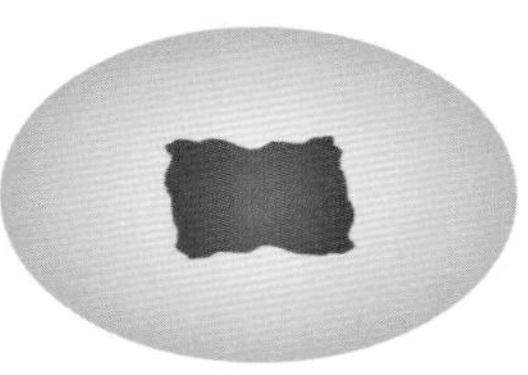

Benign melanocytic lesions are typically round or oval with multiple axes of symmetry. A solitary angulated or geometrically shaped melanocytic lesion should be closely examined for dermoscopic features of melanoma. The angulated margin may resemble an arrowhead.

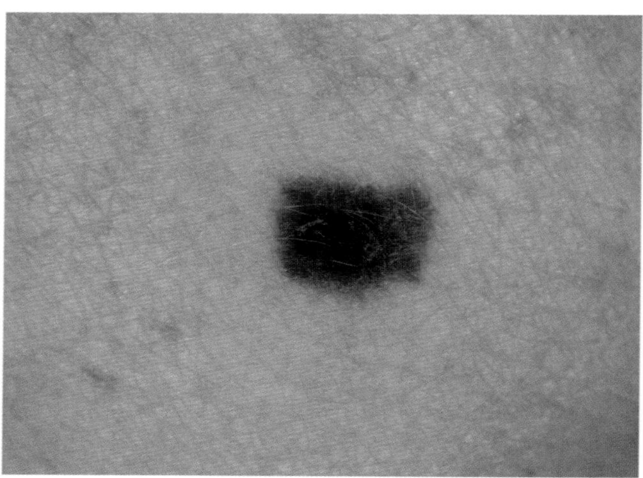

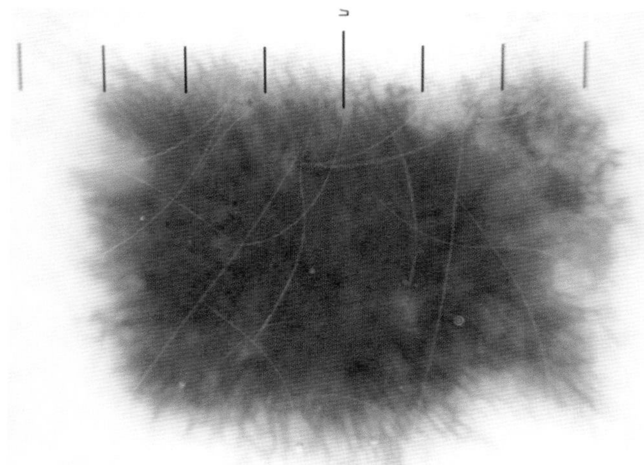

Hyperpigmented angulated/geometric macule on the shoulder of this 50-year-old woman: dermoscopy shows central hyperpigmentation, atypical pigment network and peripheral streaks in this melanoma in situ (MIS).

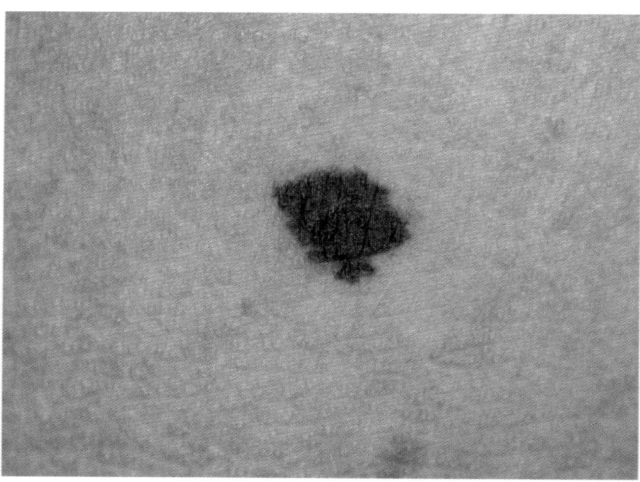

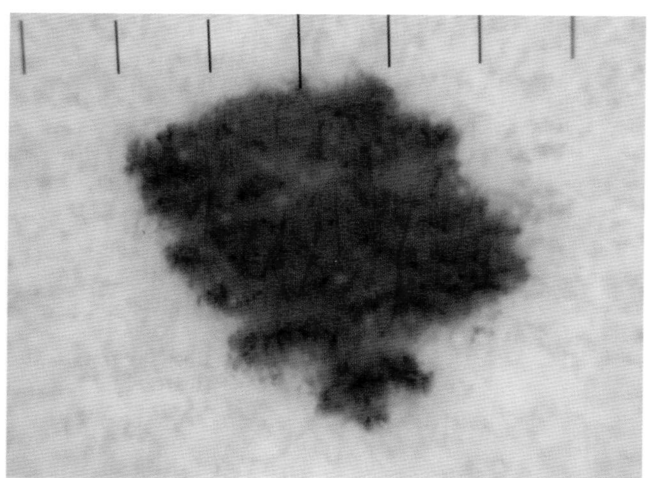

A hyperpigmented and geometric macule on the abdomen of a 40-year-old woman: dermoscopy shows multiple colours, black dots and streaks both centrally and focally at the margin in this 0.3 mm thick SSM.

Morris, AD. et al. Geometric Cutaneous Melanoma: A Helpful Clinical Sign of Malignancy? *Dermatol Surgery*. 2003;29:827–9.

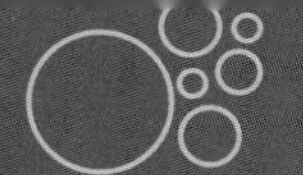

Geometric border cases

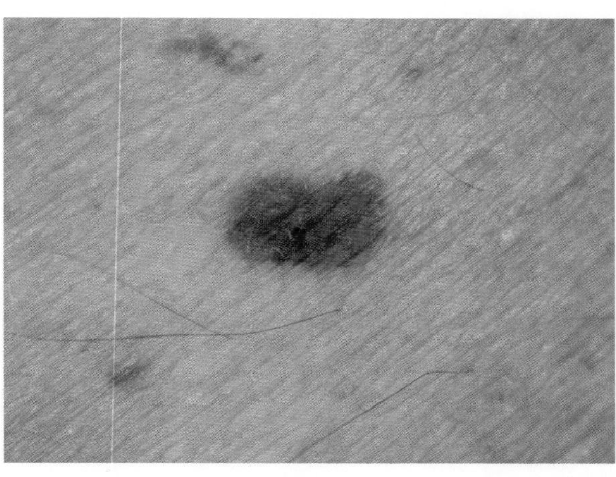

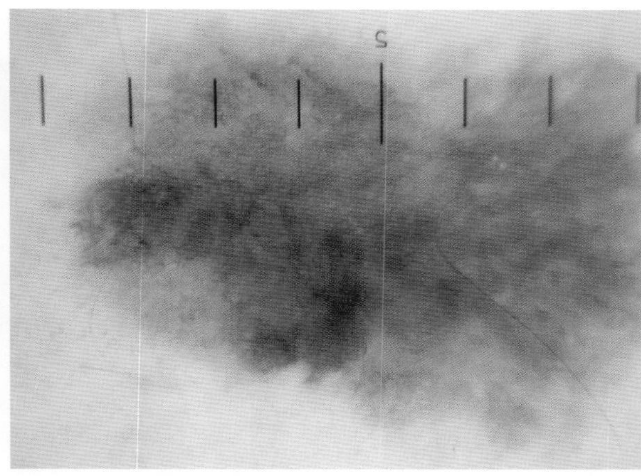

A rectangular tan-coloured 'ugly duckling' lesion: dermoscopy shows an eccentric focus of broadened atypical network involving one quadrant in this MIS.

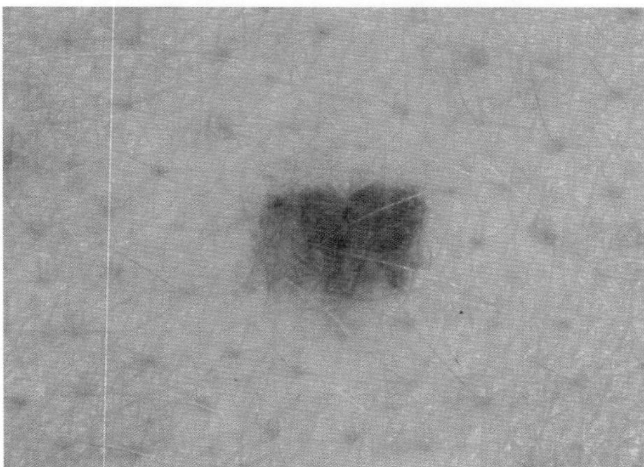

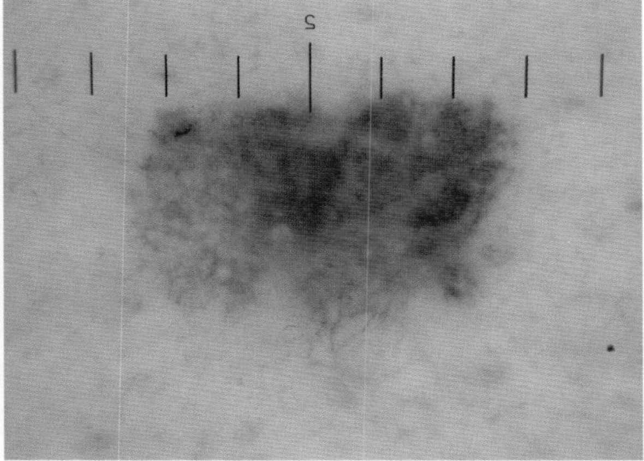

A rectangular tan macule on the lower back: dermoscopy shows irregular pigmentation and granular grey dots in this MIS.

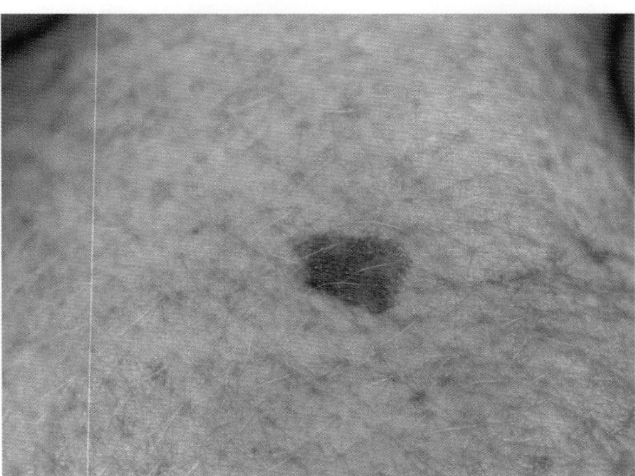

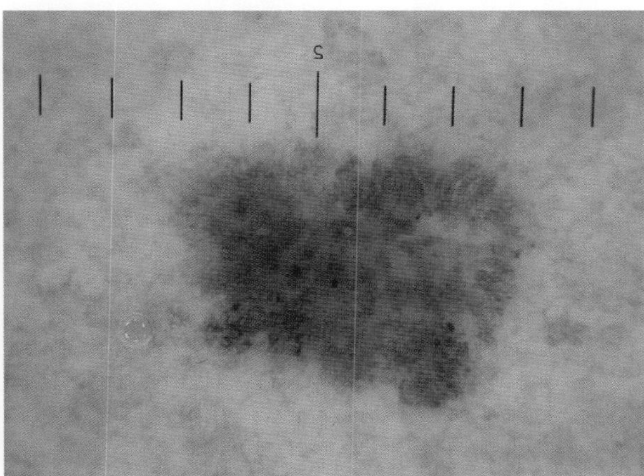

An angulated rectangular macule on the abdomen of a 60-year-old woman: dermoscopy shows atypical pigment network and irregular grey-brown globules in this 0.5 mm thick SSM.

Gachon, J. et al. First prospective study on the recognition process of melanoma in dermatological practice. *Arch Dermatol*. 2005;141(4):434–438.

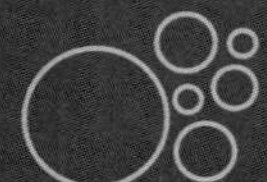

Geographic border

Similar to melanocytic lesions having geometric borders, one should also examine melanocytic lesions with geographic borders carefully to exclude dermoscopic features of melanoma.

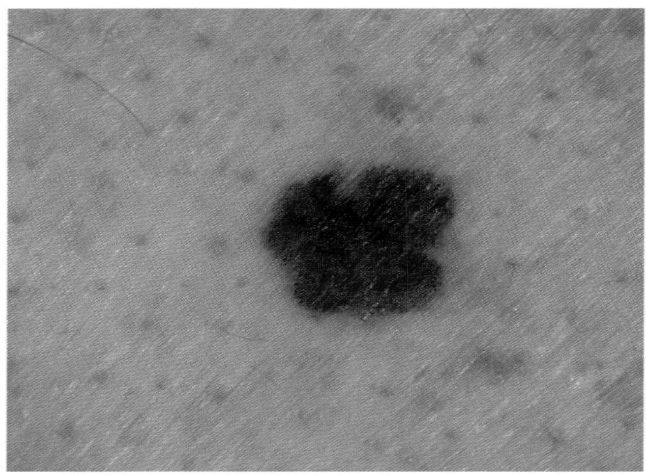

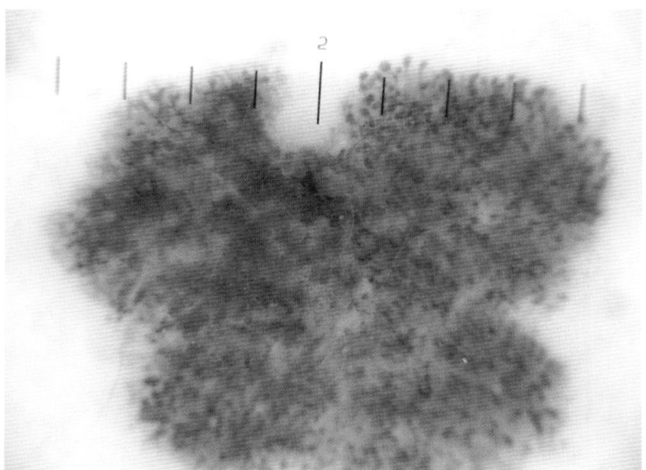

A hyperpigmented multilobed 0.5 mm thick SSM on the upper back: dermoscopy shows an irregular globular morphology with an eccentric focal blue-whitish veil.

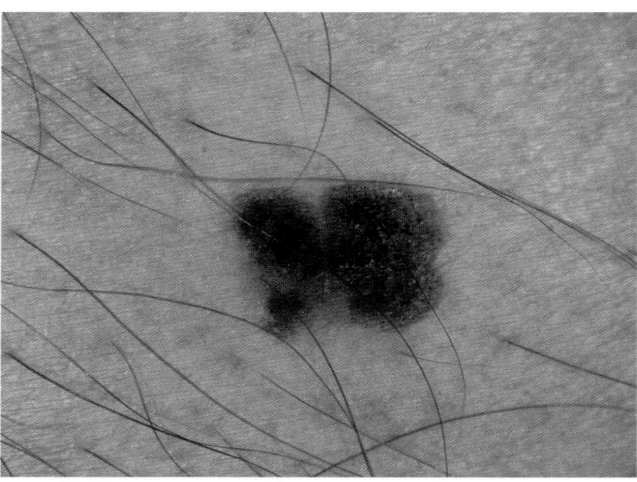

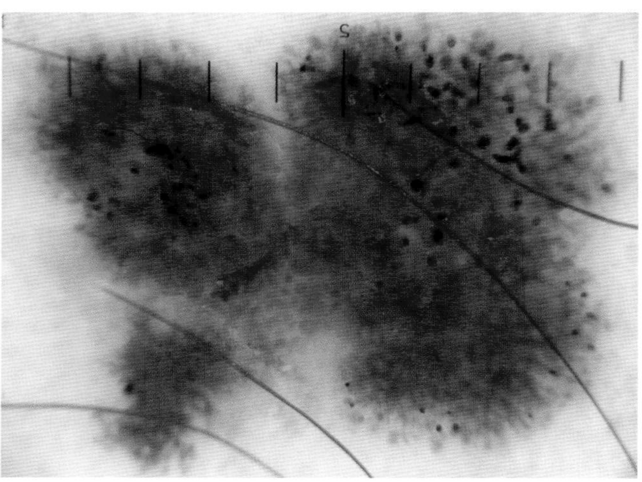

A hyperpigmented multilobed 0.7 mm thick SSM on the lower leg: dermoscopy shows an asymmetrical multicomponent pattern with irregular black dots and globules, atypical pigment network, a blue-whitish veil and a negative network.

Melanoma commonly presents as an irregularly shaped pigmented lesion. Whilst the ABCD rule applies well for radial growth phase melanomas, it does not always help for nodular melanoma.

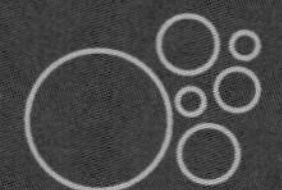

Geographic border cases

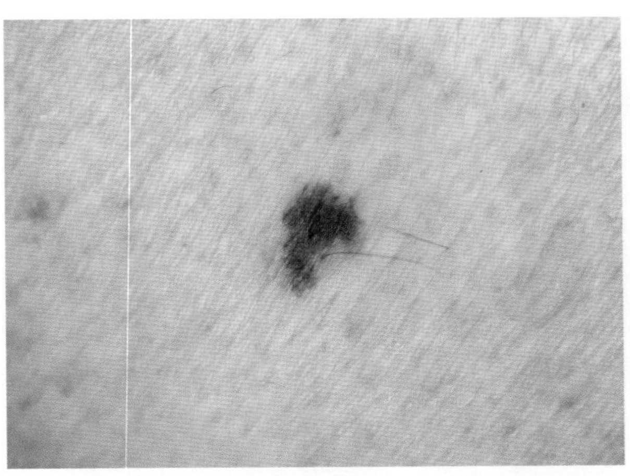

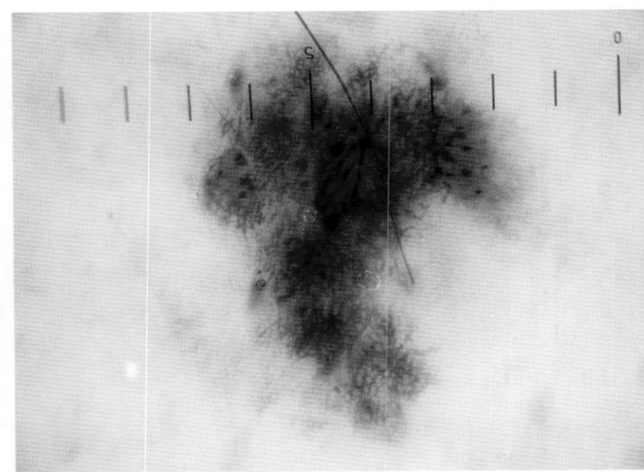

An 'ugly duckling' irregular and geographically shaped pigmented macule on the back of a 50-year-old man: dermoscopy shows irregularly distributed black dots and globules in this MIS.

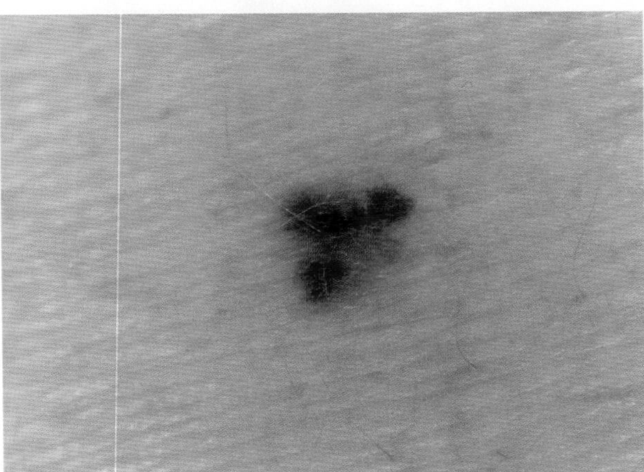

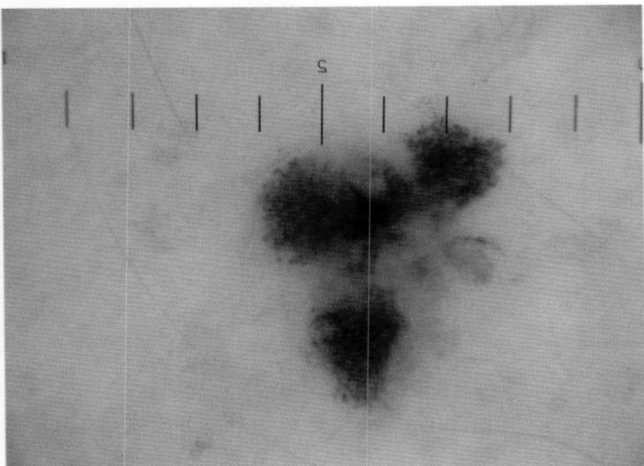

An 'ugly duckling' irregularly shaped macule on the thigh of a 65-year-old woman: dermoscopy shows a disordered lesion with black dots, granular pigmentation and focal focal peripheral streaks in this 0.2 mm thick SSM.

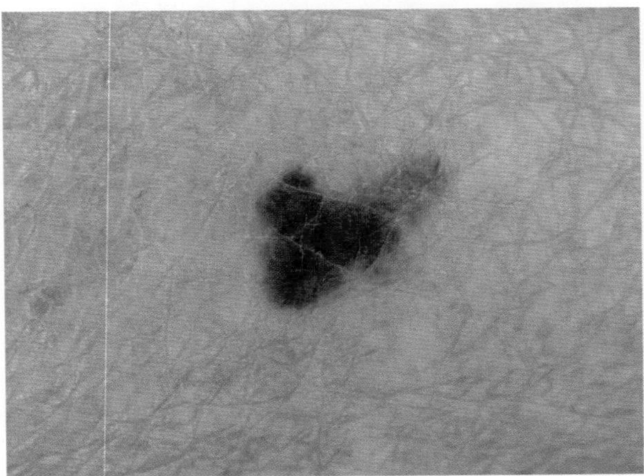

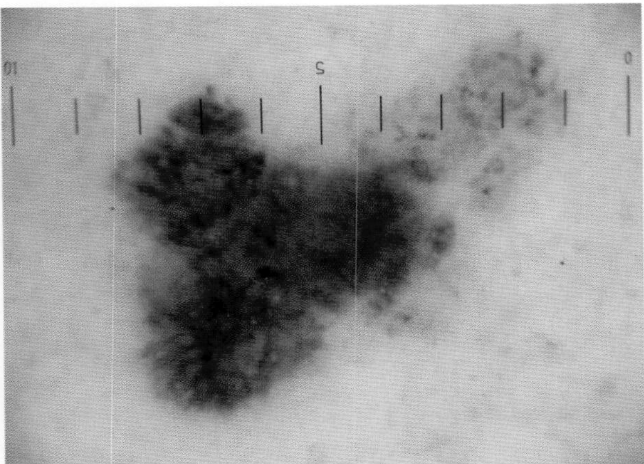

An 'ugly duckling' irregularly shaped macule on the thigh of a 70-year-old woman: dermoscopy shows a disordered lesion with atypical broadened pigment network and black dots in this 0.3 mm thick SSM.

Blum, A. et al. Rorschach dermoscopy. *Arch Dermatol.* 2012;148(11):1342.

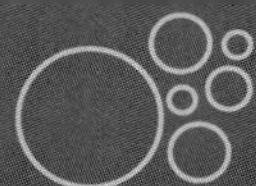

Disordered polarity

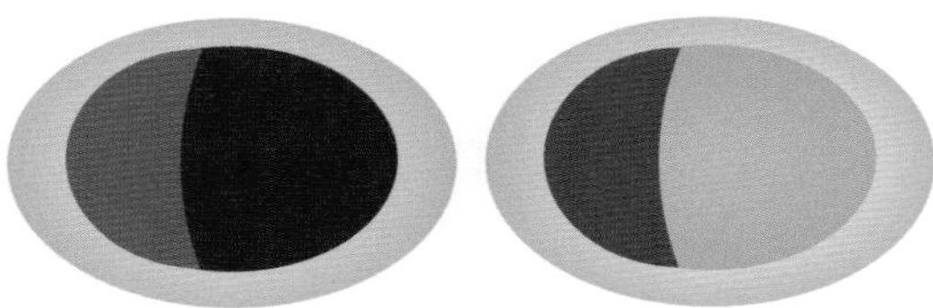

It is not unusual for some patients to present with multiple naevi with a combination of two tones of pigmentation. This may represent their signature naevus, an important concept. However, a solitary melanocytic lesion with polarity of pigmentation or dermoscopic features should be treated with suspicion.

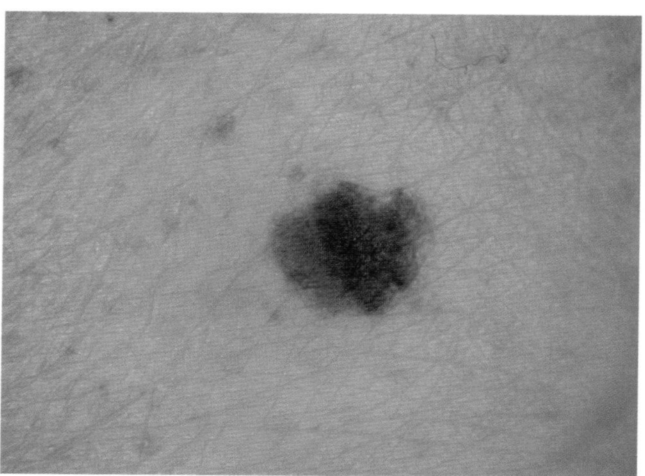

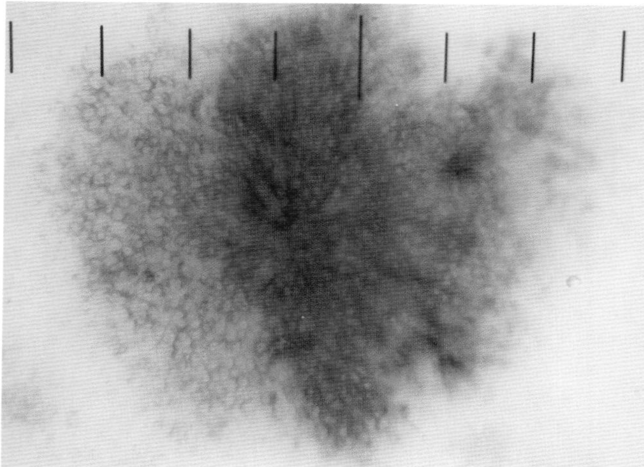

A two-toned pigmented macule on the upper back of a 50-year-old man: dermoscopy shows reticular tan pigmentation to one side and a darker broader network on the other side of this MIS.

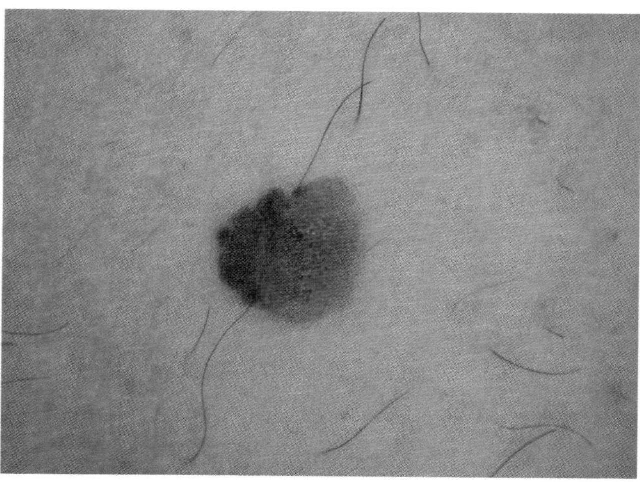

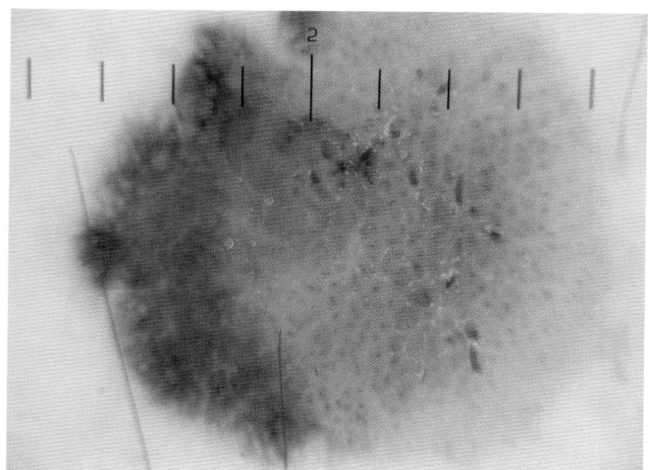

A two-toned pink-brown plaque on the popliteal fossa of a 60-year-old man: dermoscopy shows an atypical pigment network to one side and dotted vessels, erosions and negative network on the other side of this 0.9 mm thick SSM.

Be suspicious of the solitary two-toned melanocytic lesion. Sometimes this pattern may reflect dysplastic naevus only. The presence of negative or inverse network is a clue to naevus-associated melanoma.

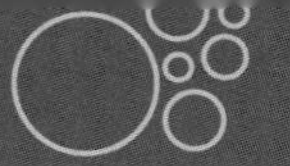

Disordered polarity cases

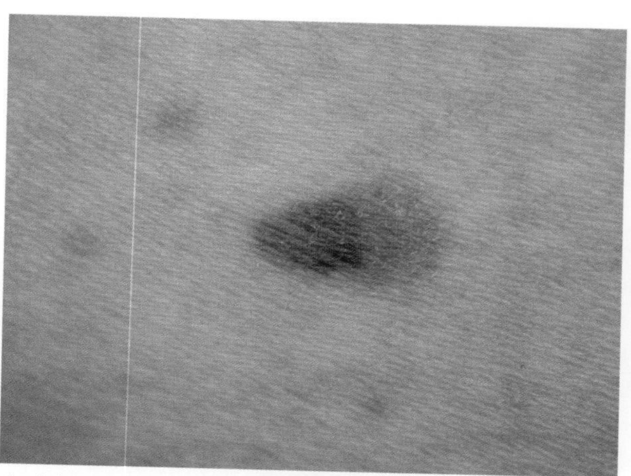

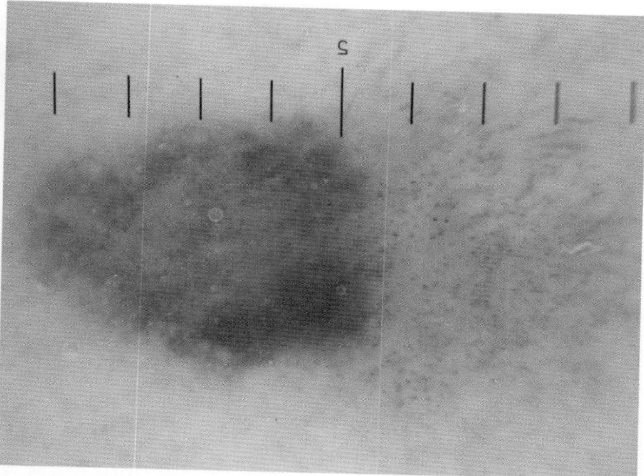

A pink-tan two-toned macule on the arm of a 40-year-old woman: dermoscopy shows polar variability in pigmentation with a tan homogeneous pole with a central structureless area and a pink pole with dotted vessels in this MIS.

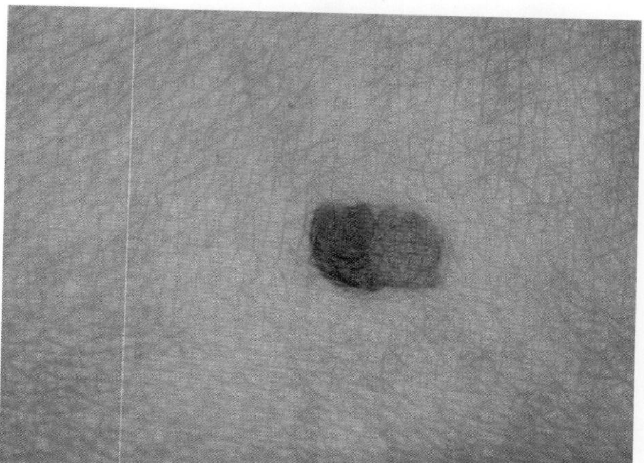

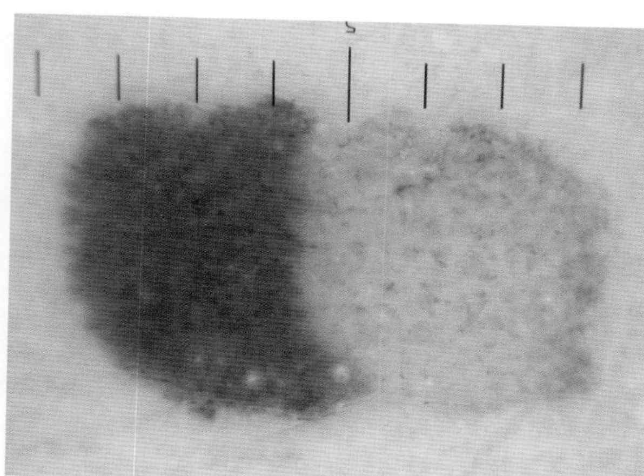

Pink-brown rectangular plaque on the arm of a 40-year-old woman: dermoscopy shows varying pigment patterns with streaks at one margin in this atypical Spitzoid tumour of uncertain malignant potential (STUMP).

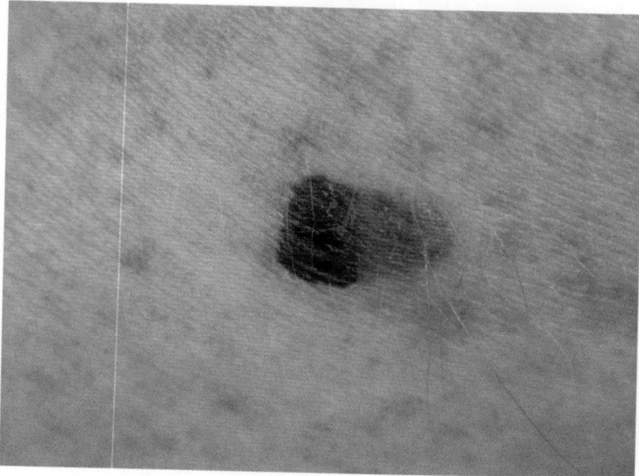

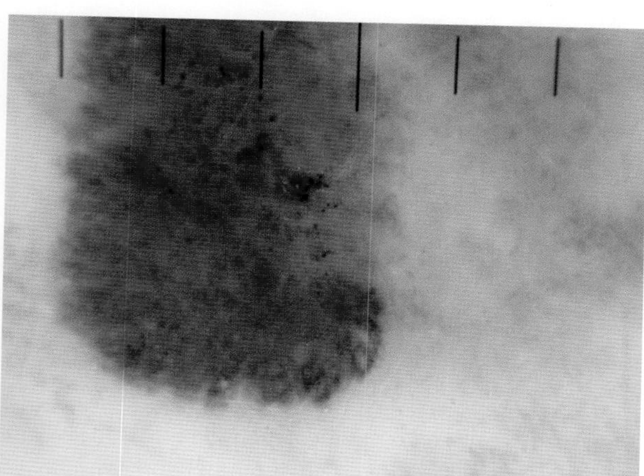

A variably pigmented plaque on the lower leg: dermoscopy shows multiple colours, atypical network, negative network and irregular dots and globules in this 0.9 mm thick SSM.

Polar pigmentation in a single melanocytic lesion can sometimes be simulated by a collision between two differently coloured nevi.

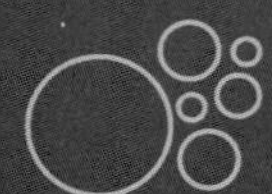

Naevus-associated

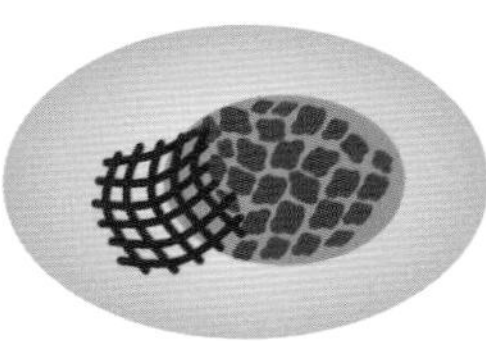

Although most melanomas arise *de novo*, approximately 30% develop within an existing naevus. In the early stages of naevus-associated melanoma, features of both the pre-existing naevus and the evolving melanoma may coexist. In later stages the features of melanoma dominate and the naevus features may only be seen on histopathology.

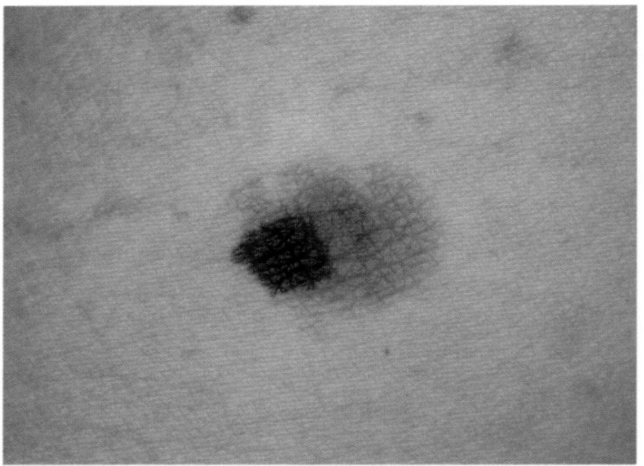

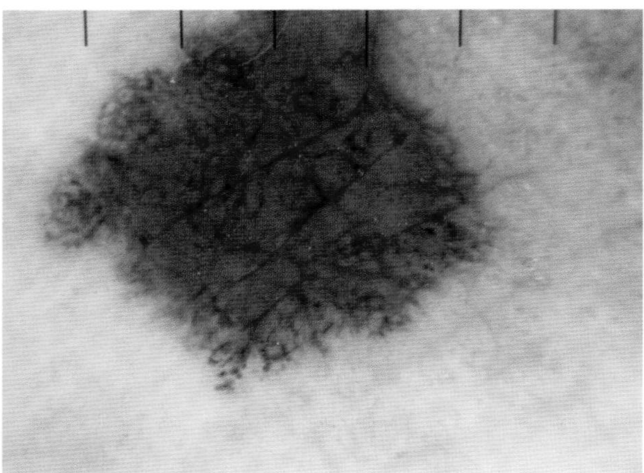

A pigmented macule with a hyperpigmented eccentric focus on the thigh of a 60-year-old woman: dermoscopy shows an eccentric focus of atypical pigment network, radial streaks and black dots in this MIS arising in a dysplastic naevus.

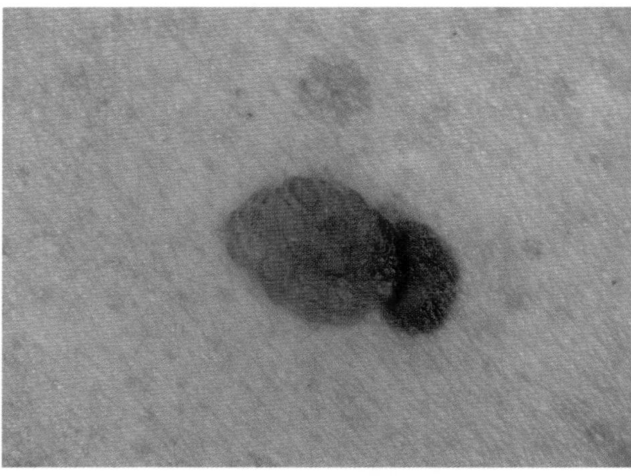

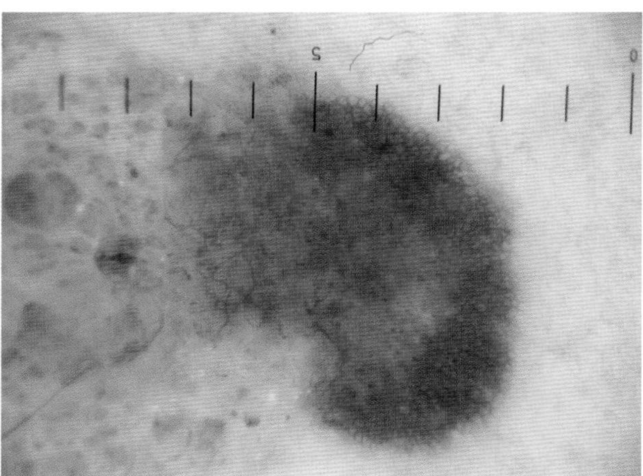

A tan plaque with an eccentric hyperpigmented macule in a 50-year-old man: dermoscopy shows cobblestone remnants and an eccentric focus of reticular tan network with focal grey dots in this MIS arising in a dermal naevus.

Zalaudek, I. et al. Clinical and dermoscopic characteristics of congenital and noncongenital naevus-associated melanomas. *J Am Acad Dermatol*. 2020;83(4):1080–1087.

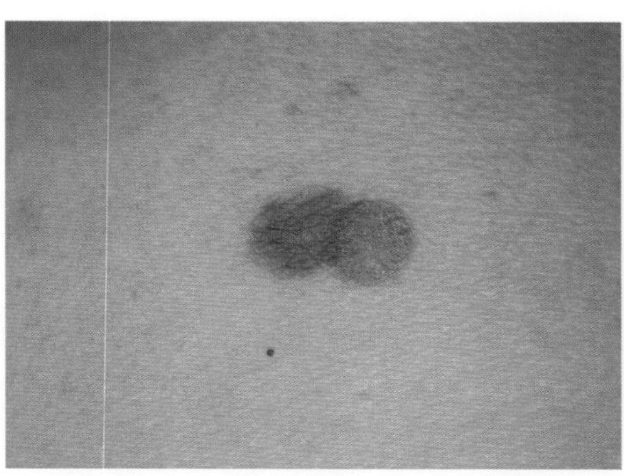

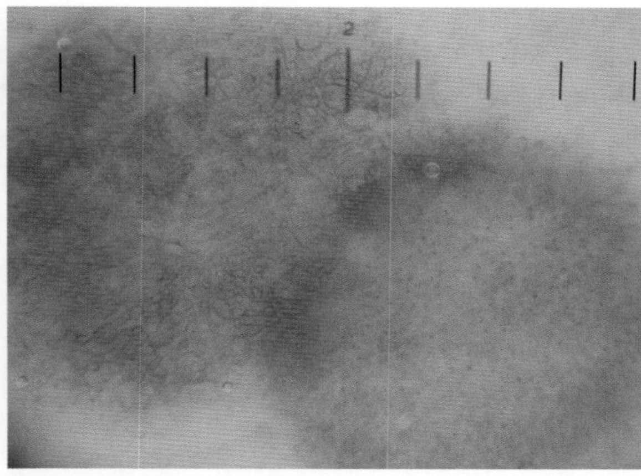

A bilobed pink and brown macule in a 70-year-old woman: dermoscopy shows a reticular lesion combined with an eccentric zone of dotted vessels and subtle negative network in this naevus-associated MIS.

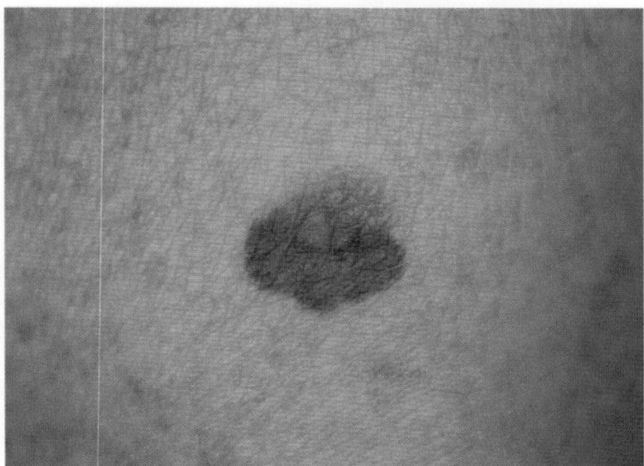

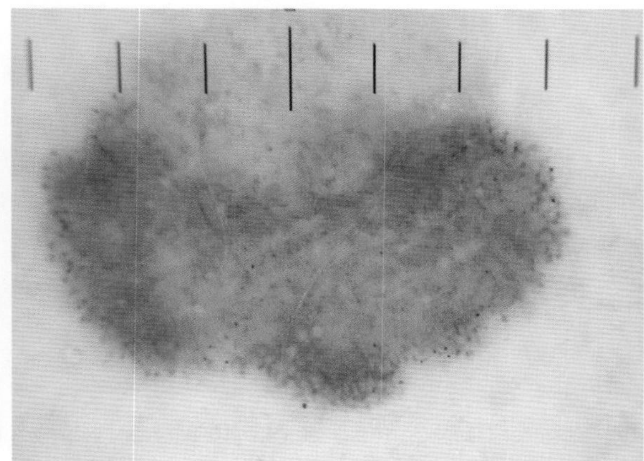

Variably pigmented macule on the arm of a 50 year old woman: dermoscopy shows a multicomponent pattern with peripheral brown globules and curvilinear vessels (superiorly) in this 0.3 mm thick naevus-associated SSM.

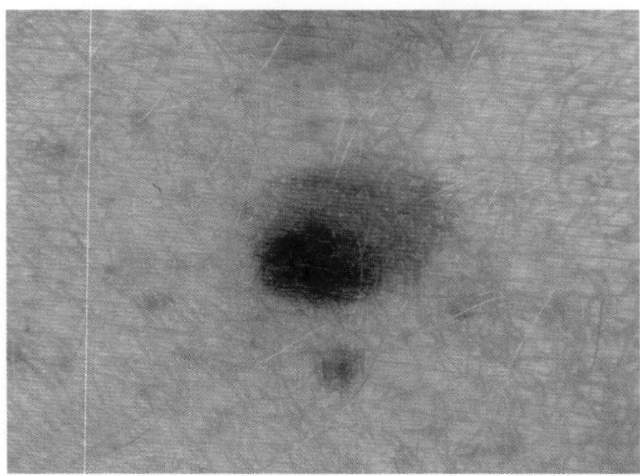

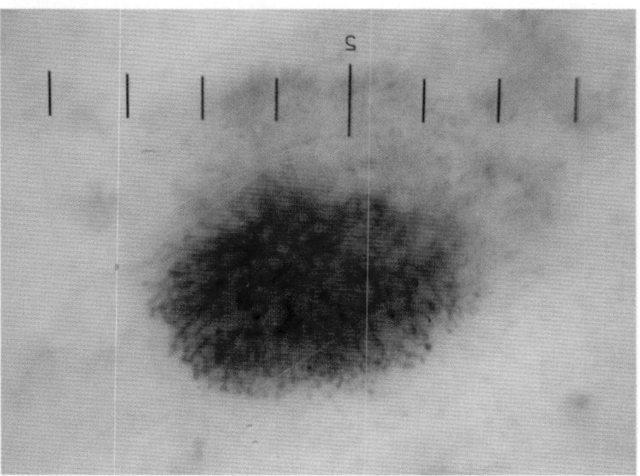

A variably pigmented plaque on the thigh of a 25-year-old man: dermoscopy shows a multicomponent pattern with atypical network, peripheral globules and structureless areas in this naevus-associated MIS.

Pampena, R. et al. A meta-analysis of nevus-associated melanoma: Prevalence and practical implications. *J Am Acad Dermatol.* 2017;77(5):938–945.e4.

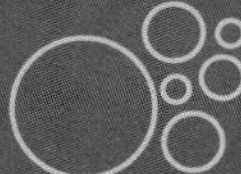

Congenital melanocytic naevus-associated

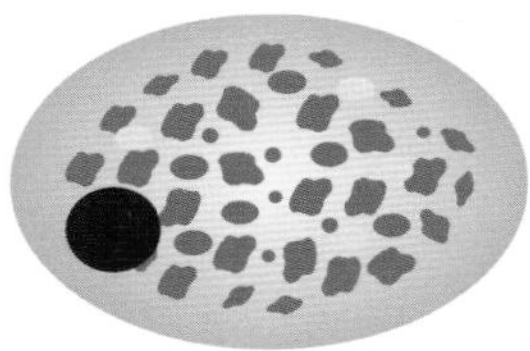

The risk of melanoma development within a congenital melanocytic naevus (CMN) is small but rises as the CMN increases in size. CMN can be categorised as small (<1.5 cm) medium (1.5 cm-20 cm) and large/giant (>20 cm). Dermoscopic features of melanoma, arising within a CMN, include focal eccentric pigment blotches, blue-whitish veil, ulceration and atypical vessels. Any change developing within a CMN should be considered high-risk.

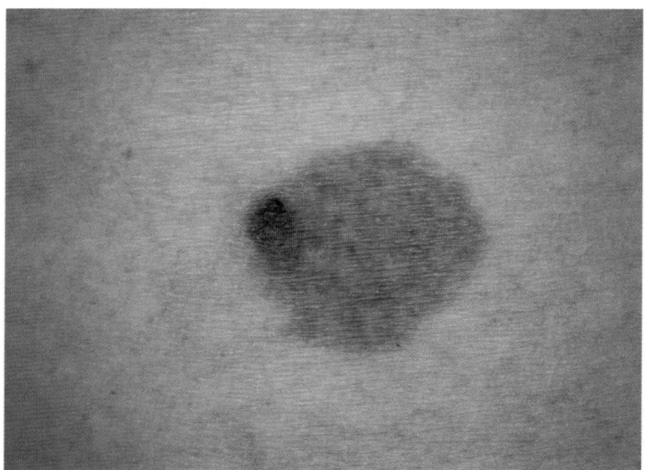

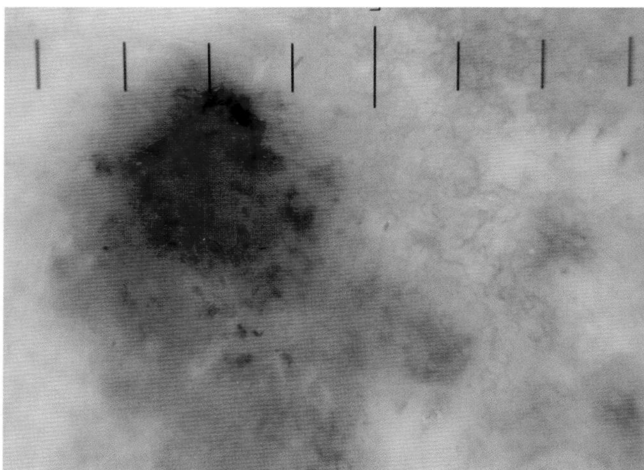

A 21-mm diameter CMN on the back of a 40-year-old woman: dermoscopy shows reticular background pigmentation with focal ulceration, haemorrhage, coiled vessels, a pigmented blotch and negative network in this 0.4 mm thick CMN-associated melanoma.

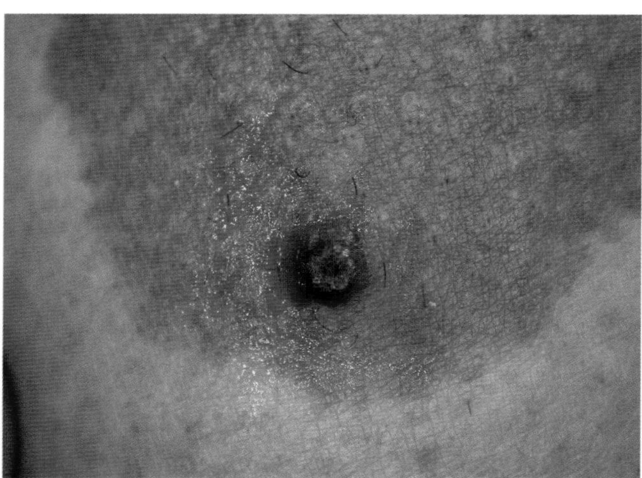

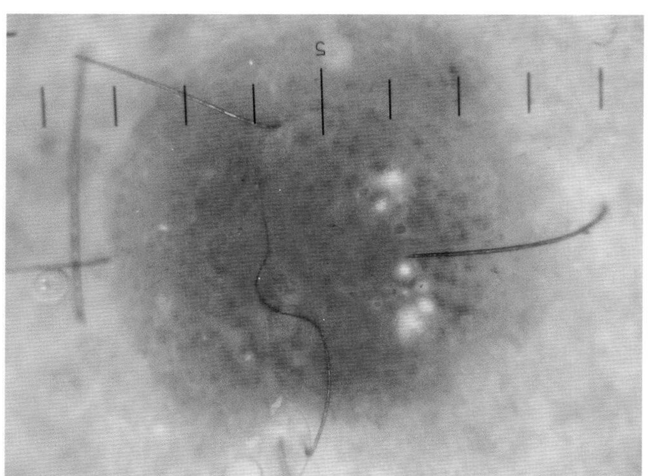

A CMN with a dark papule on the leg of a 60-year-old woman: dermoscopy shows irregular dark globules, dotted vessels and terminal hairs within the papule in this 1.4 mm thick CMN-associated melanoma.

Caccavale, S. et al. Cutaneous Melanoma Arising in Congenital Melanocytic Nevus: A Retrospective Observational Study. *Dermatology* 2021;237:473–478.

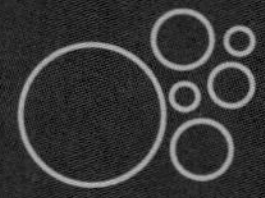

3.2 Melanoma – pigment variants

Multicoloured 52
Multicoloured cases 53
Multicomponent 54
Multicomponent cases 55
Hypermelanotic/hyperpigmented 56
Hypermelanotic/hyperpigmented cases 57
Amelanotic macules 58
Amelanotic macules – cases 59
Amelanotic papules 60
Amelanotic papules – cases 61
Hypomelanotic macules 62
Hypomelanotic macules – cases 63
Hypomelanotic tan plaques 64
Hypomelanotic tan plaques cases 65

Multicoloured

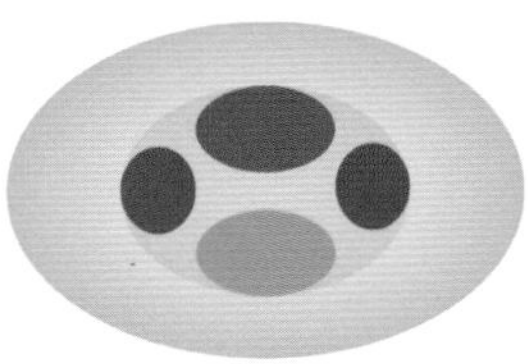

Multicoloured melanomas are usually invasive tumours. The variability in colour reflects the different depths infiltrated by malignant melanocytes. Pink areas may be a feature of neovascularisation and atypical vessels are best seen in these areas. Brown areas reflect epidermal melanocytes and blue pigmentation implies dermal involvement. Fewer colours are seen in very thick tumours as the boundaries between epidermal, dermal and vascular components become less distinct.

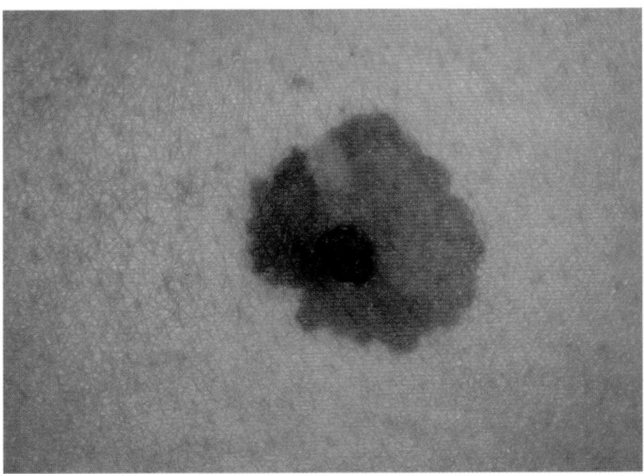

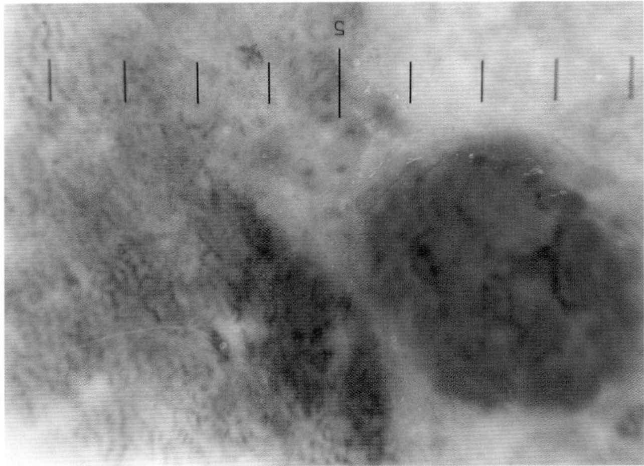

A multicoloured plaque on the back of a 60-year-old woman: dermoscopy shows a slate blue pigmented blotch, brown irregular pigmentation and focal brown globules in this 0.9 mm thick superficial spreading melanoma (SSM).

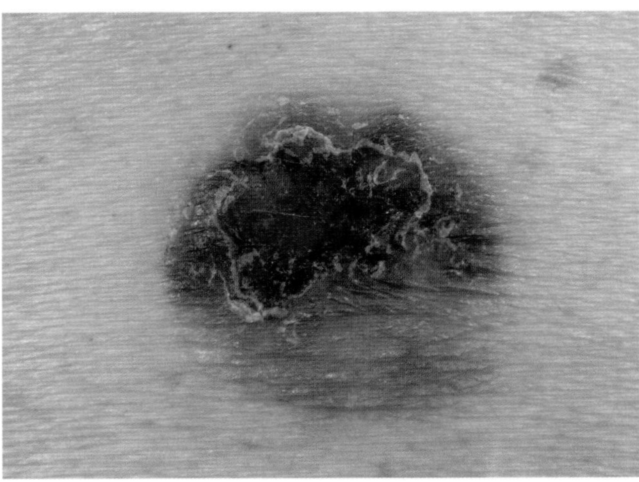

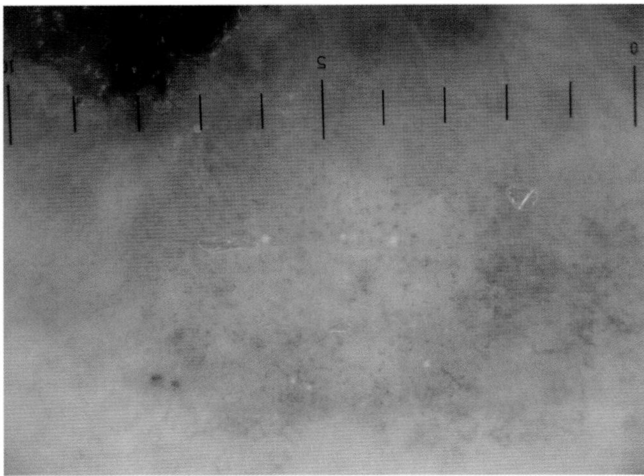

A multicoloured and eroded plaque on the lower back of a 40-year-old man: dermoscopy shows blue-whitish veil and prominent dotted vessels in this 1.0 mm thick SSM.

The colours seen on dermoscopy can help predict the histopathological depth of the melanoma. Pink-red colour is due to angiogenesis typically associated with invasion.

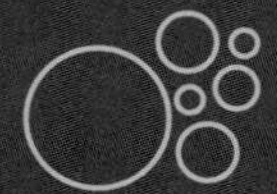

Multicoloured cases

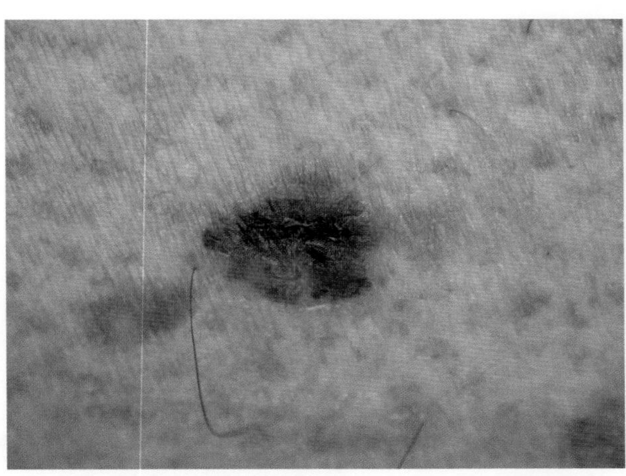

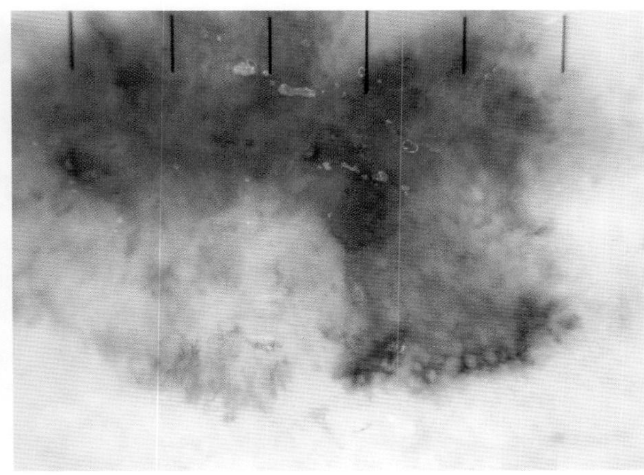

A multicoloured plaque on the back of a 60-year-old man: dermoscopy shows blue-whitish veil, hypopigmented structureless areas and focal atypical pigment network in this 1.0 mm thick SSM.

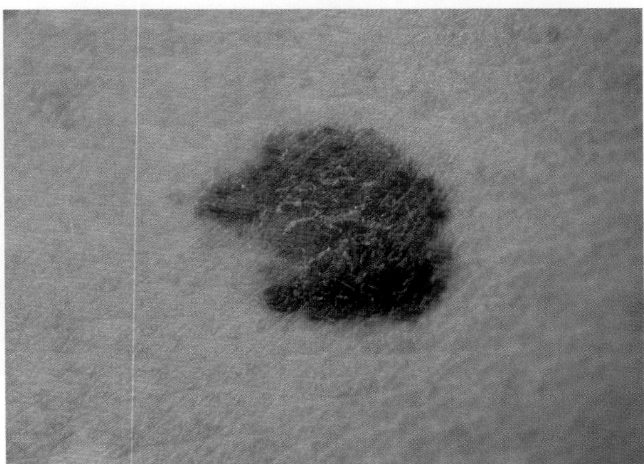

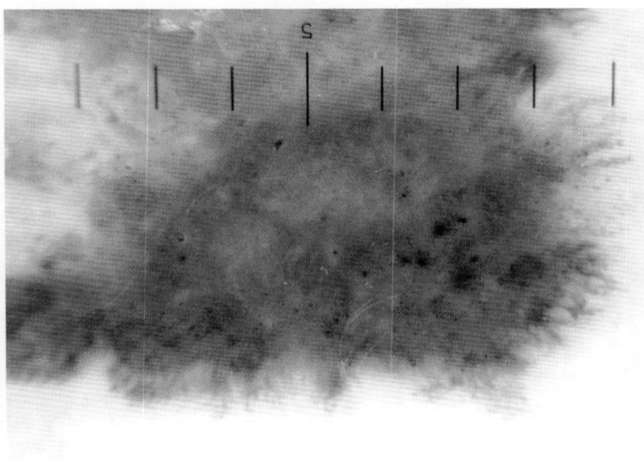

A multicoloured plaque on the lower back of a 40-year-old woman: dermoscopy shows variable zones of blue, pink and brown pigmentation, and atypical network in this 1.0 mm thick SSM.

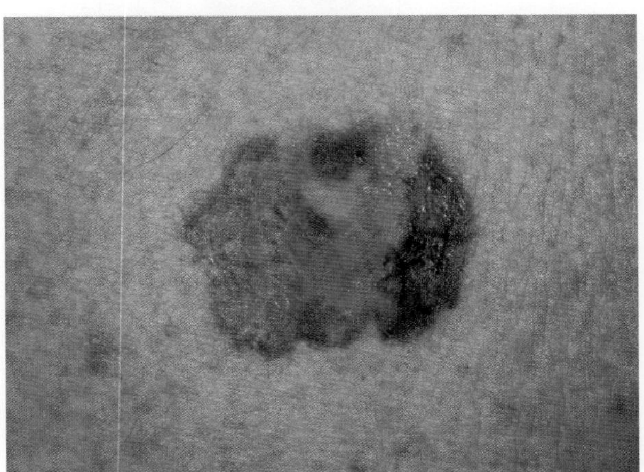

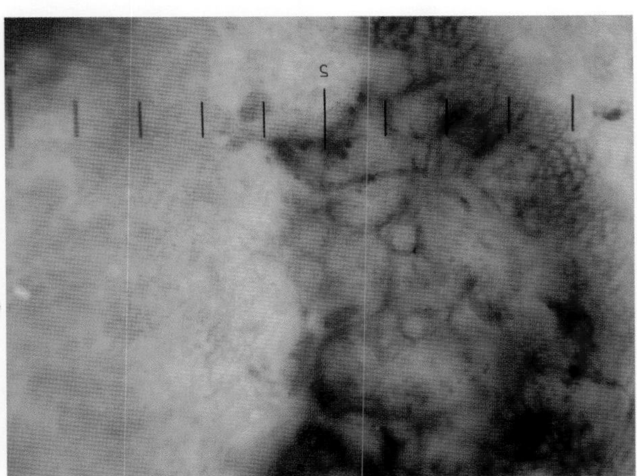

A large multicoloured patch on the upper back a 50-year-old man: dermoscopy shows a mixture of pink, browns and blue colours with polymorphous vessels, atypical network and focal blue-whitish veil in this 0.4 mm thick SSM.

The more colours present in a melanocytic lesion the more likely it is melanoma. The presence of 5 colours is very suggestive of melanoma in fact.

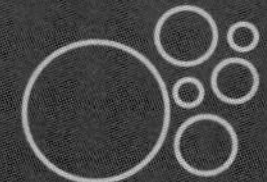

Multicomponent

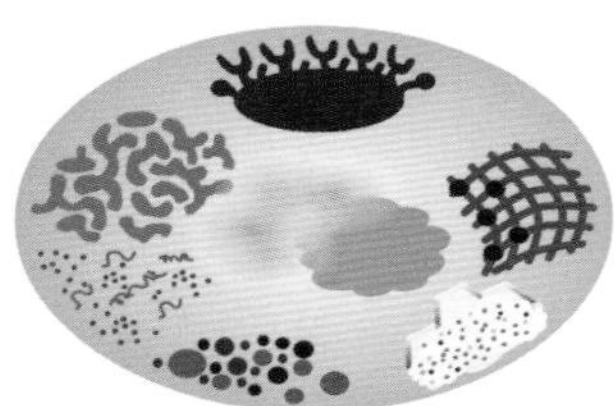

Melanomas that have had years to develop may show multiple structural components, diagnostic for melanoma, at the time of presentation. Typically they have an irregular shape and border, and multiple colours. On dermoscopy, multiple different diagnostic features can be seen across the melanoma.

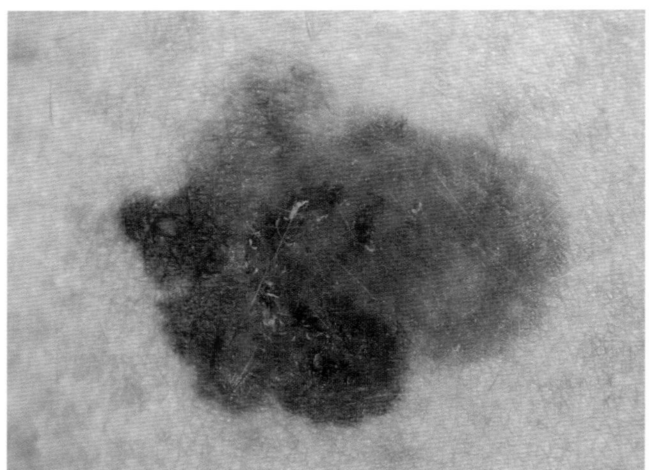

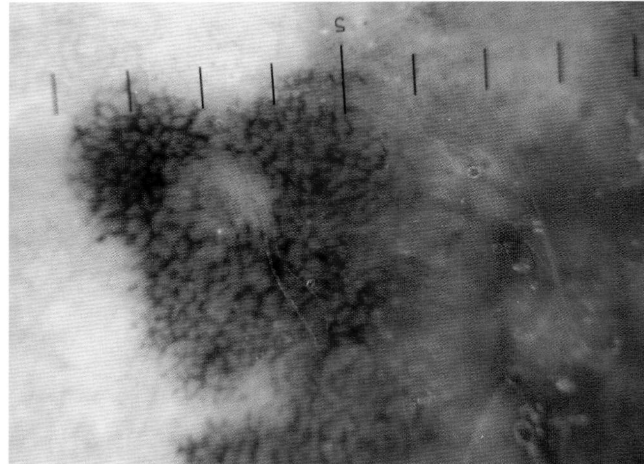

A large complex multicoloured plaque on the back: dermoscopy shows a close-up of the atypical pigment network regression and blue-whitish dermal pigmentation in this 0.8 mm thick SSM.

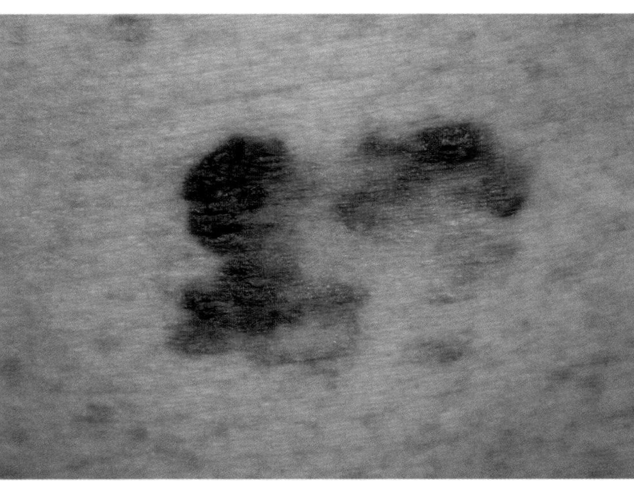

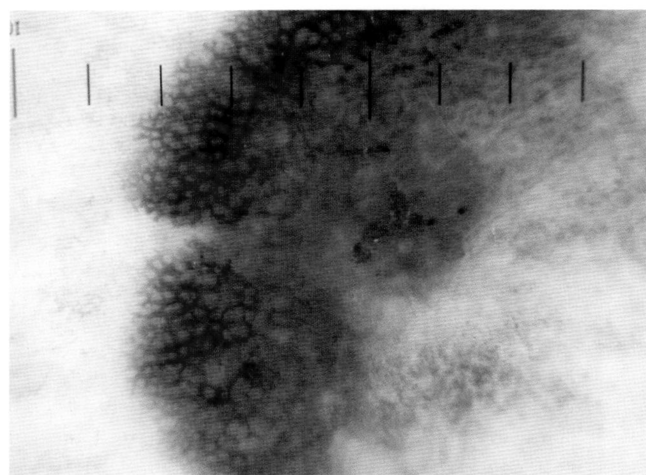

A large complex pigmented plaque with extensive regression on the back of a 60-year-old man: dermoscopy shows atypical pigment network and extensive regression with grey dots/peppering in this 0.8 mm thick SSM.

Melanoma commonly presents as an irregularly shaped, multicomponent melanocytic lesion.

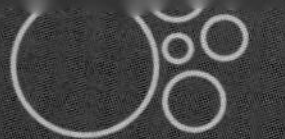

Multicomponent cases

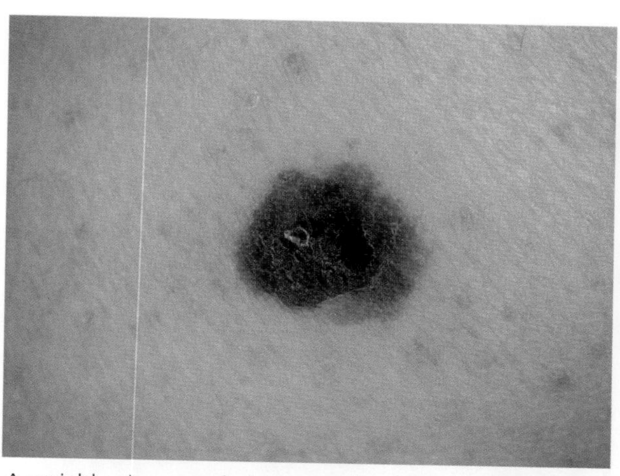

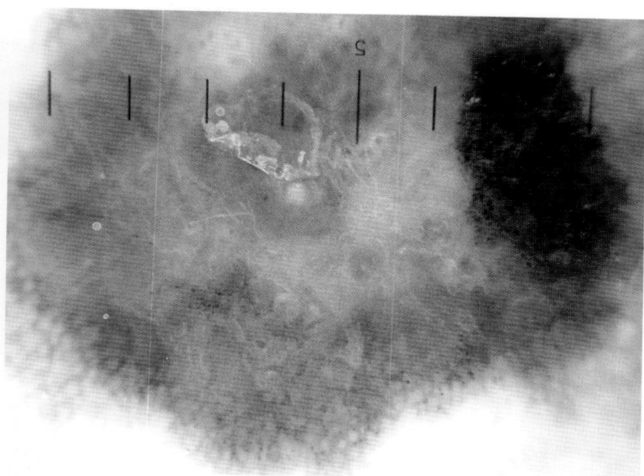

A variably pigmented plaque on the thigh of a 50-year-old woman: dermoscopy shows a central blue-whitish veil, dense black dots and peripheral brown reticular pigmentation in this 1.0 mm thick SSM.

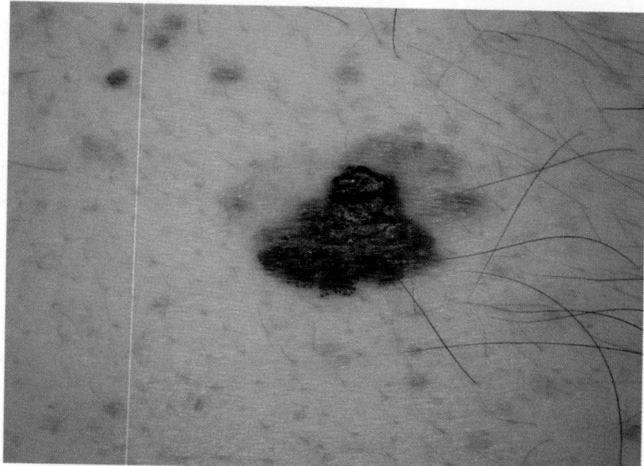

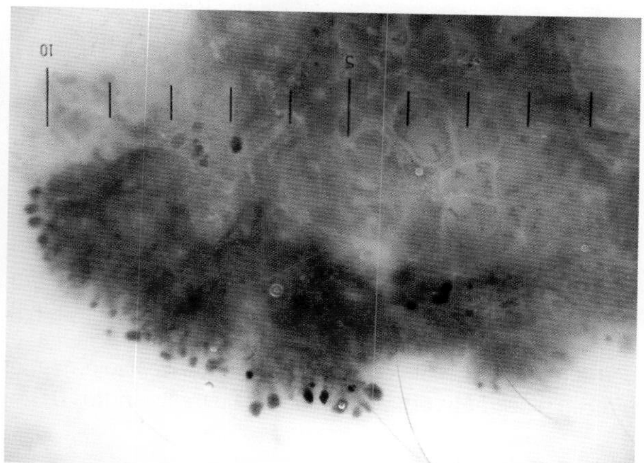

An irregular hyperpigmented plaque on the abdomen of a 50-year-old man: dermoscopy shows a chaotic pattern with focal globules, brown homogeneous areas, blue-whitish veil and polymorphous vessels in this 1.3 mm thick SSM.

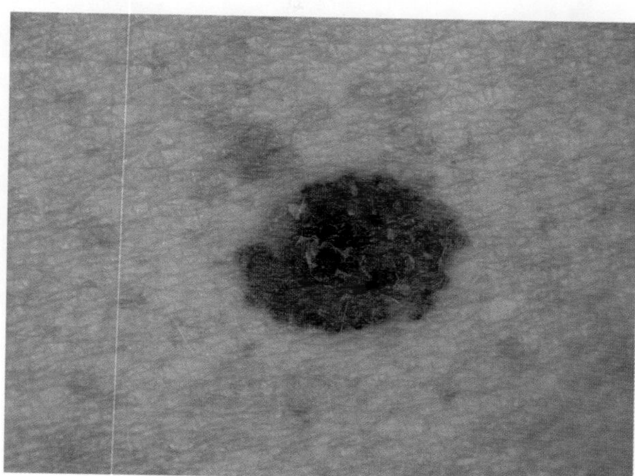

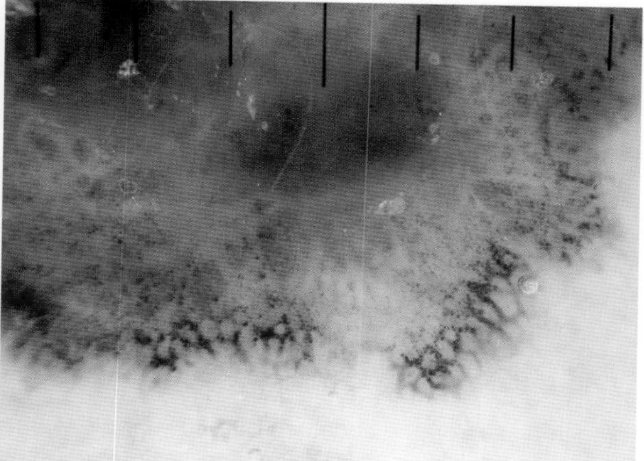

A variably pigmented plaque on the lower leg: dermoscopy shows an atypical peripheral granular pigmented network, blue homogeneous and milky pink/red areas with irregular vessels in this 1.2 mm thick SSM.

Melanocytic lesions are considered to have a multicomponent pattern when displaying 3 or more dermoscopic patterns.

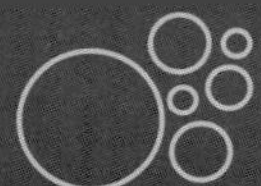

Hypermelanotic/hyperpigmented

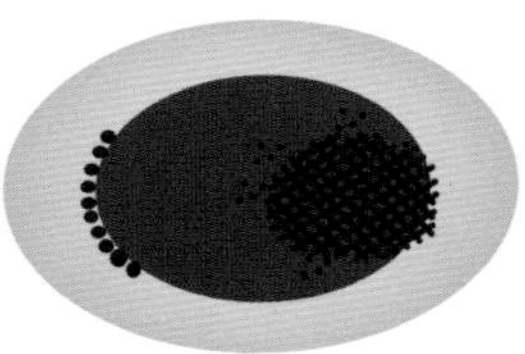

In hyperpigmented melanoma, the diagnostic features are often only seen at the peripheral margin of the tumour at the junction with normal skin.

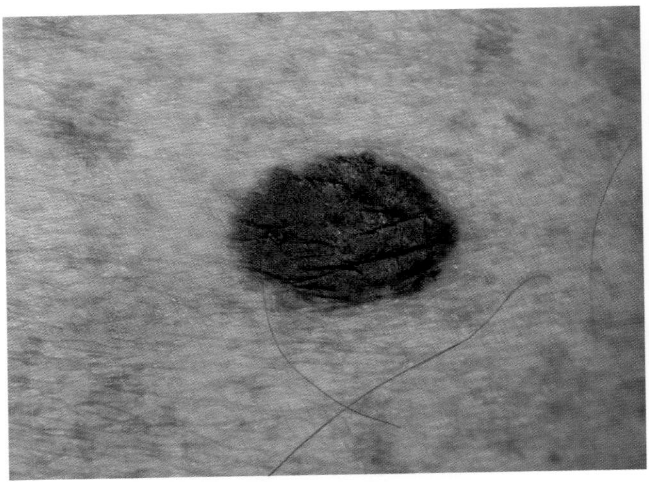

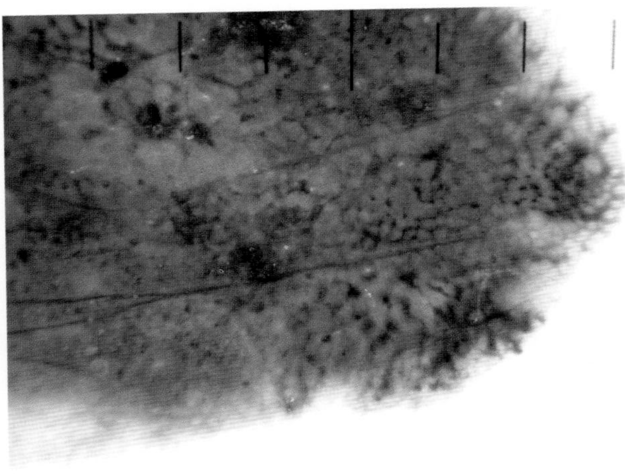

A hyperpigmented macule on the back of a 50-year-old man: dermoscopy shows blue-whitish veil, black dots and globules, and a superficial black network with peripheral streaks in this 0.3 mm thick SSM.

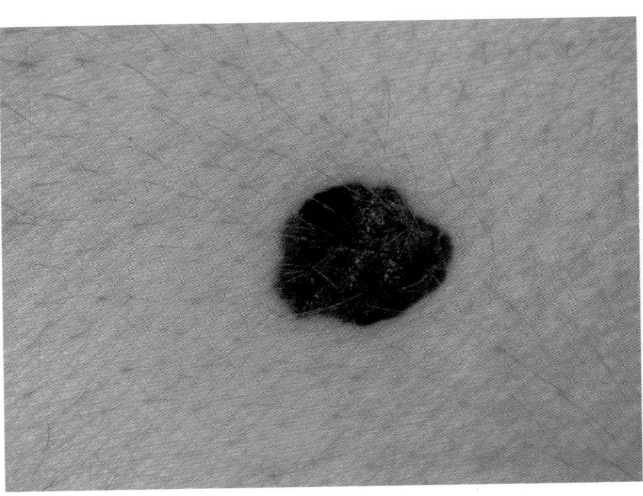

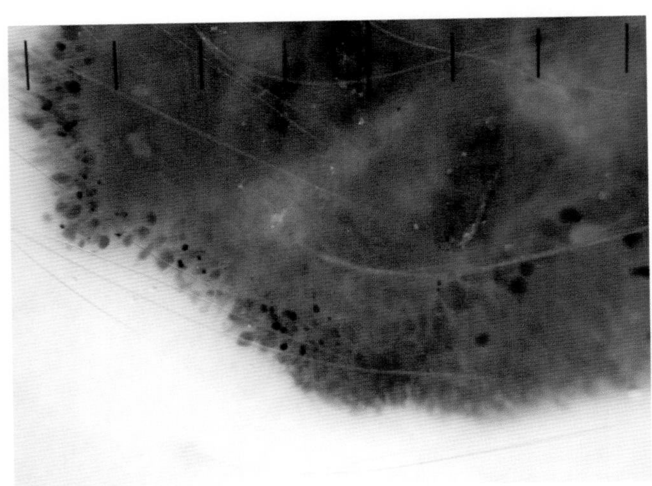

A blackened plaque on the abdomen of a 30-year-old woman: dermoscopy shows a central blue-whitish veil as well as hyperpigmented dots and globules in this 1.0 mm thick SSM.

Hyperpigmented melanomas typically do not cause diagnostic uncertainty, although the hyperpigmentation may make the clinical judgement of Breslow thickness difficult to predict.

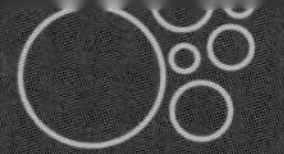

Hypermelanotic/hyperpigmented cases

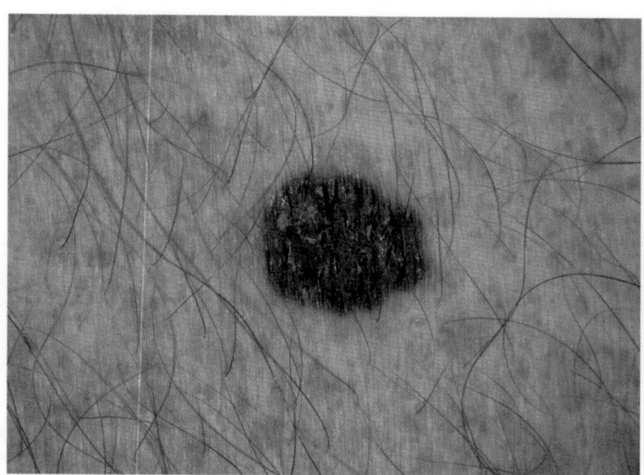

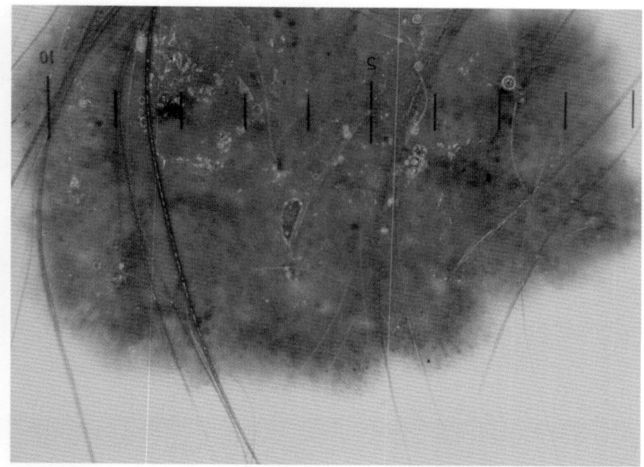

A hyperpigmented plaque on the upper back: dermoscopy shows blue-whitish veil centrally, multiple black and brown dots, and peripheral brown globules in this 1.0 mm thick SSM.

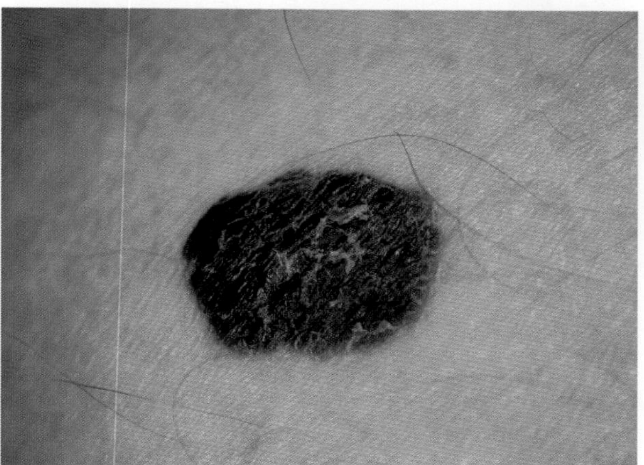

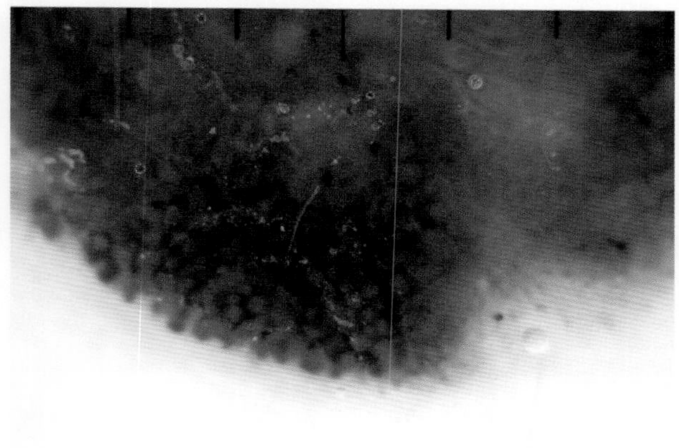

Hyperpigmented plaque on the thigh: dermoscopy shows blue-whitish veil, blackened network, peripheral bluish globules and hyperpigmented granular pigmentation in this 1.1 mm thick SSM.

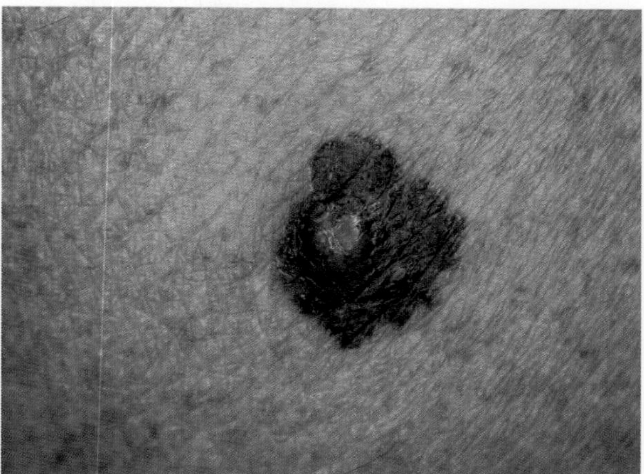

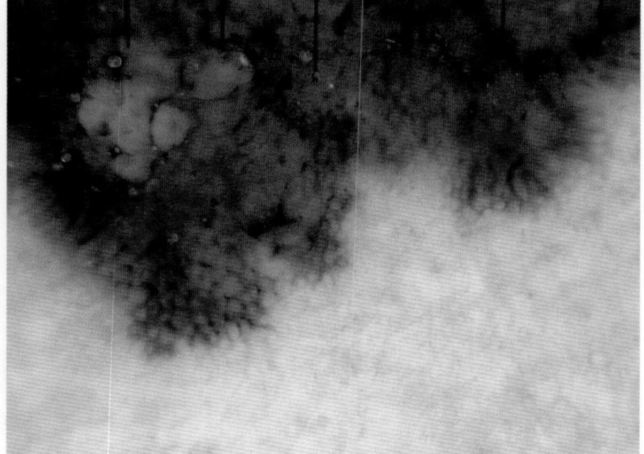

A hyperpigmented plaque on the upper back: dermoscopy of the edge shows an atypical hyperpigmented network, black dots and globules and structureless blue-grey areas in this 1.9 mm thick SSM.

Examine the margin in hyperpigmented melanocytic lesions.

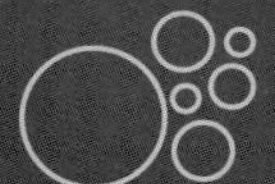

Amelanotic macules

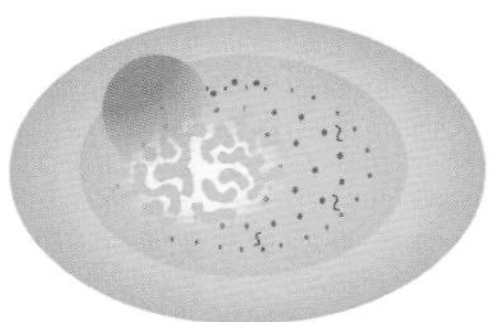

In patients with light skin, a solitary pink macule should always be regarded as potential melanoma. The dermoscopic features may be subtle and typical pigmented features of melanoma are often absent. Truly amelanotic melanoma is rare. In hypomelanotic melanomas, discrete brown pigment remnants are often seen at the periphery.

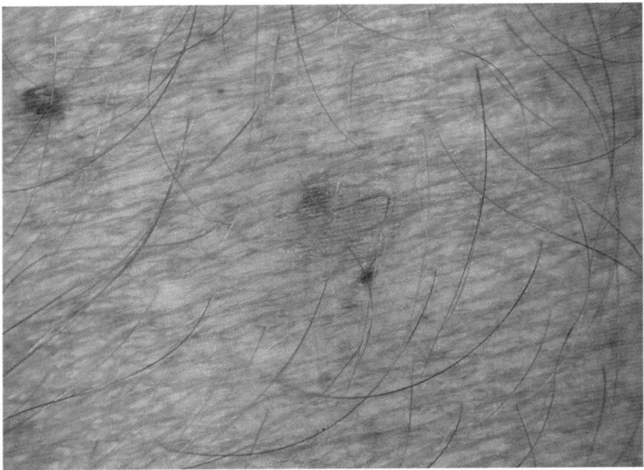

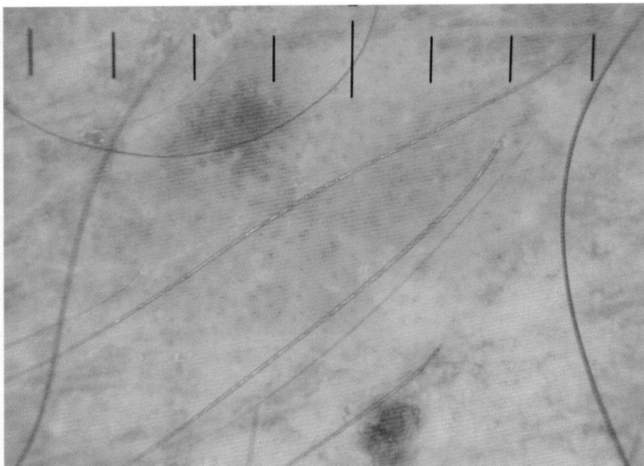

A pink plaque on the knee of a 50-year-old man: dermoscopy shows dotted vessels, negative network and eccentric tan network in this melanoma in situ (MIS).

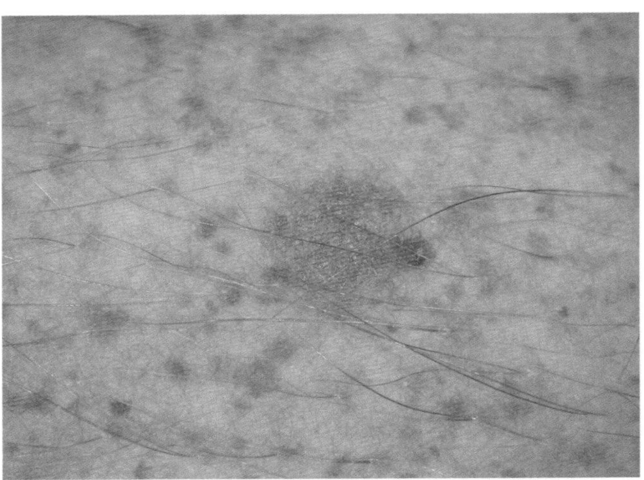

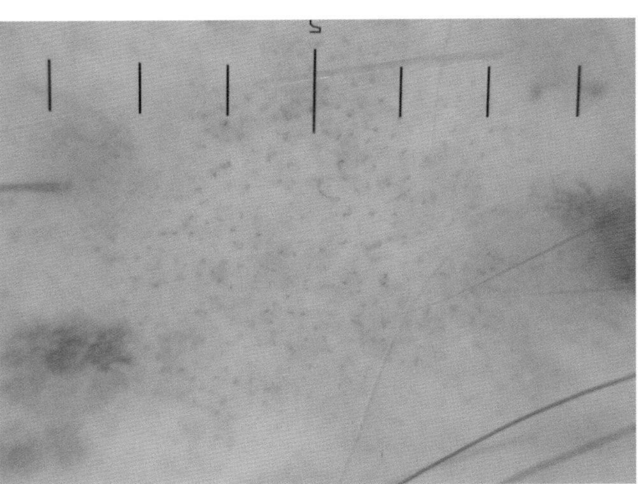

A solitary pink macule on the abdomen of a 40-year-old man: dermoscopy shows predominantly dotted vessels and a few linear irregular vessels plus a small remnant of eccentric pigment network in this MIS.

If the 'ugly duckling' is pink, melanoma is the tumour to think!

Amelanotic macules – cases

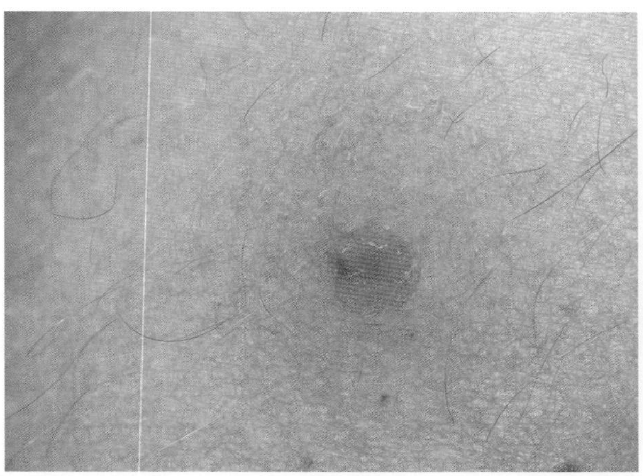
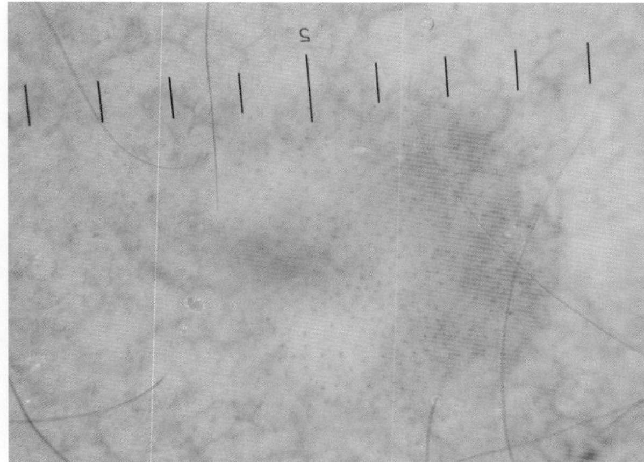

A solitary pink macule ('ugly duckling') on the back of a 25-year-old man: dermoscopy shows uniform dotted vessels and a small focus of eccentric tan pigmentation in this 0.7 mm thick SSM.

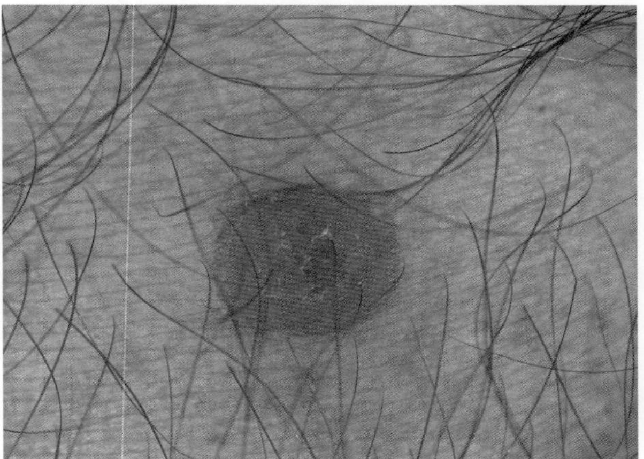
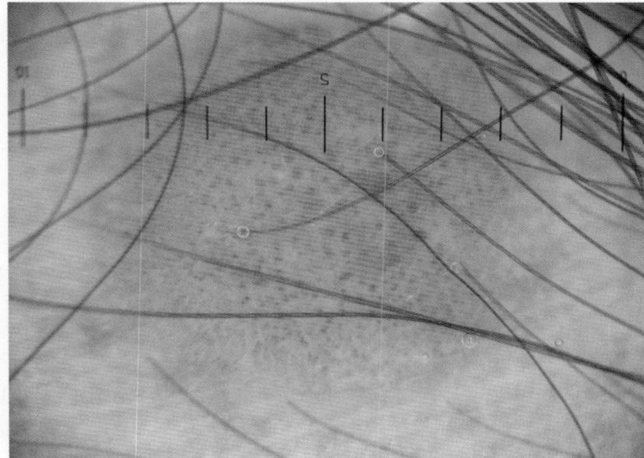

A solitary pink plaque ('ugly duckling') on the knee of a 45-year-old man: dermoscopy shows regular dotted vessels larger red globules and some focal peripheral negative network in this 0.8 mm thick Spitzoid SSM.

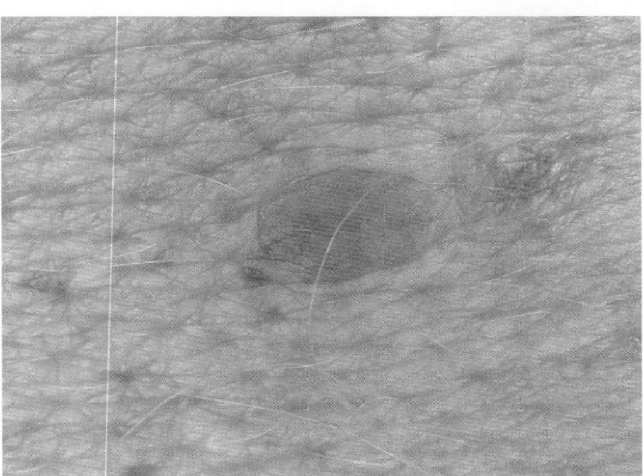
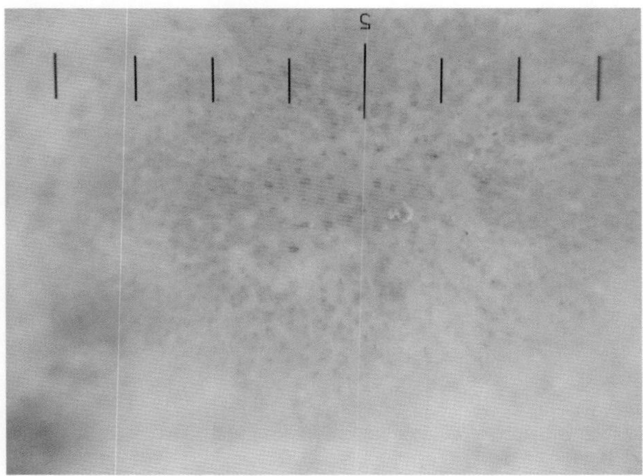

A solitary pink plaque on the lower back of a 60-year-old man with light skin: dermoscopy shows regular dotted vessels and a peripheral negative network in this 0.9 mm thick Spitzoid SSM.

Spitzoid lesions may show a primarily vascular pattern or negative network. Histopathology is required to distinguish Spitz naevi from melanoma.

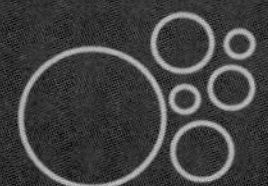

Amelanotic papules

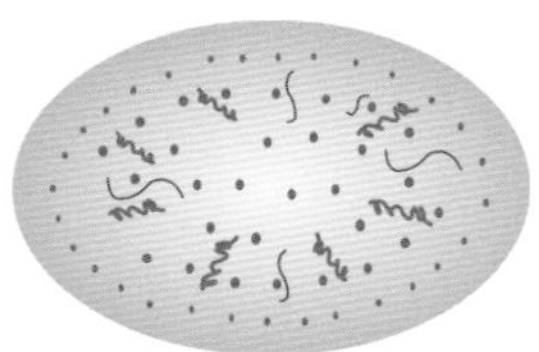

A solitary pink papule should be considered as a highly suspicious skin lesion. On dermoscopy the presence of linear irregular vessels is an indicator of angiogenesis in a skin tumour and surgical excision is required to classify this skin tumour.

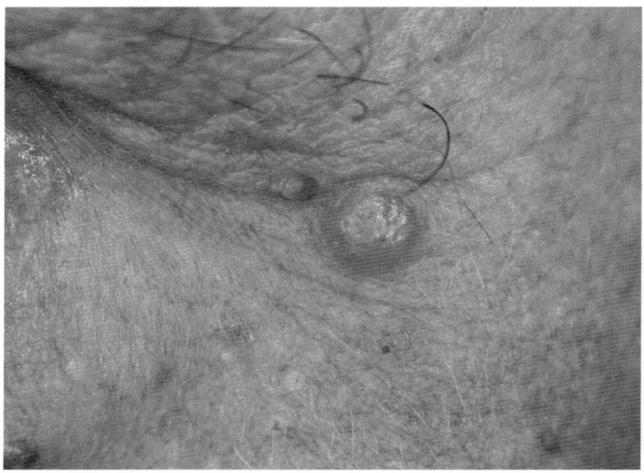

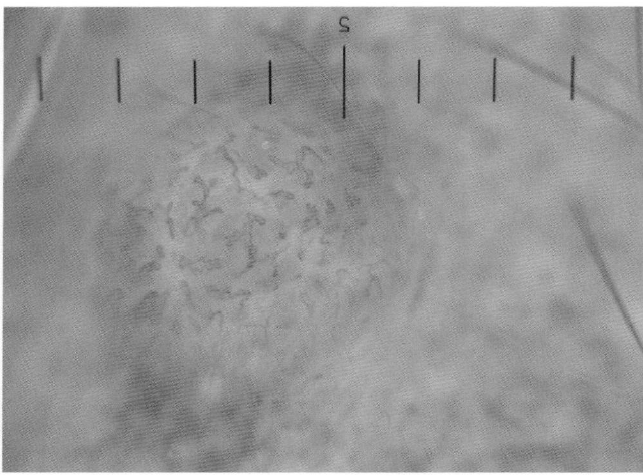

A solitary enlarging pink papule on the lateral canthus of an 80-year-old man: dermoscopy shows multiple linear irregular vessels (polymorphous vascular pattern) in this 1.0 mm thick melanoma.

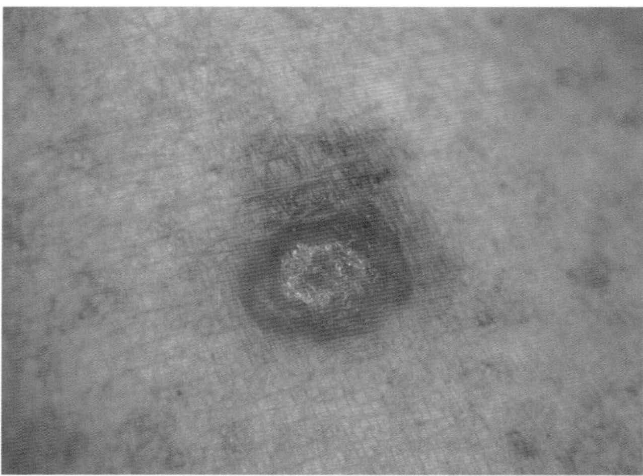

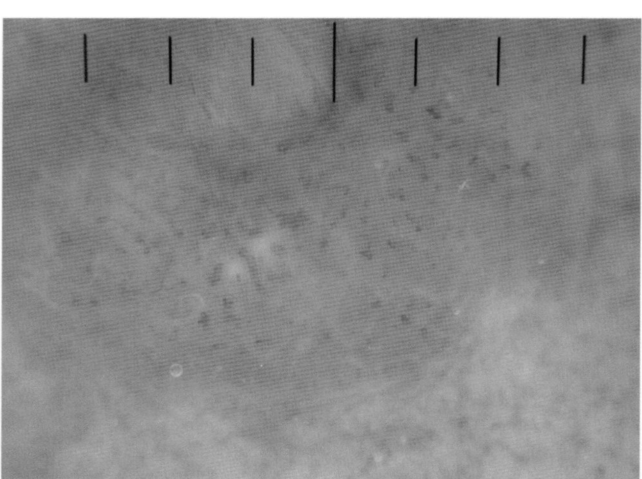

A solitary pink papule on the upper arm of a 70-year-old man: dermoscopy shows multiple atypical/polymorphous vessels (including linear irregular, dotted, coiled and corkscrew vessels), in this 1.7 mm thick SSM.

Beware of a solitary pink papule. Whilst there are many benign simulants, early diagnosis of hypomelanotic melanoma saves lives.

Amelanotic papules – cases

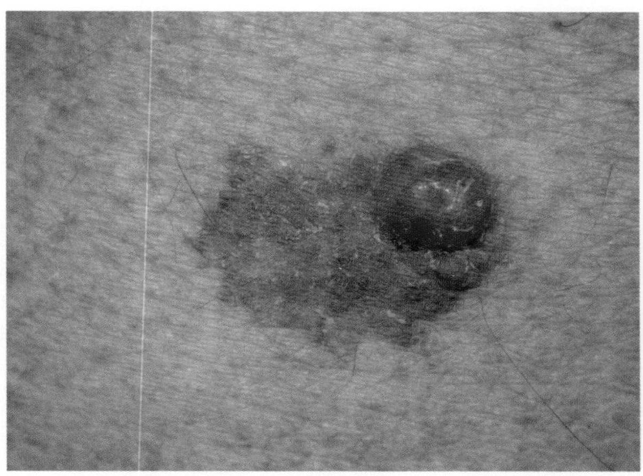

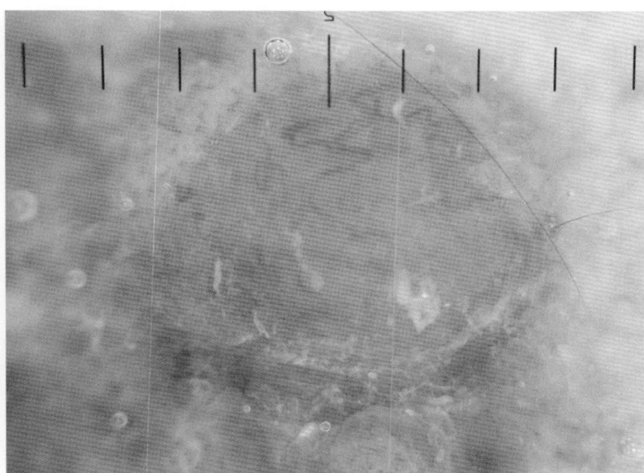

Variably pigmented plaque with an eccentric pink papule on the upper back of a 70-year-old man: dermoscopy shows polymorphous vessels and variegated blue, grey and brown pigmentation in this 1.7 mm thick SSM.

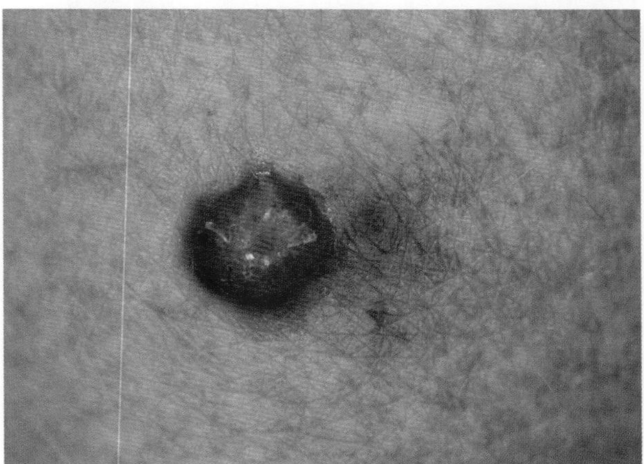

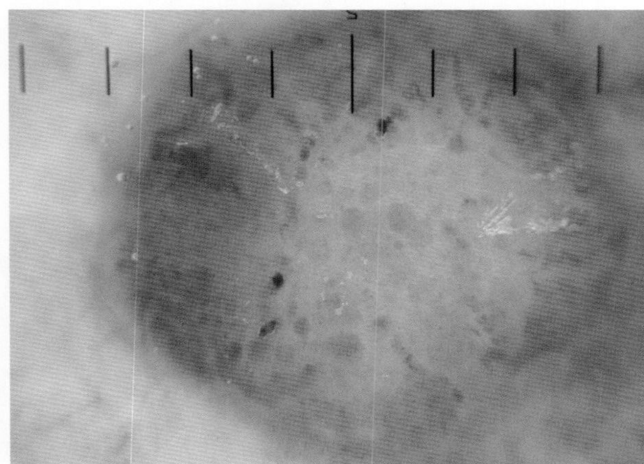

Pink papule with an eccentric pigmented macule on the leg of a 60-year-old woman: dermoscopy shows micro-erosions, atypical vessels, tan and pink globules, and an eccentric purple blotch in this 2.4 mm thick SSM.

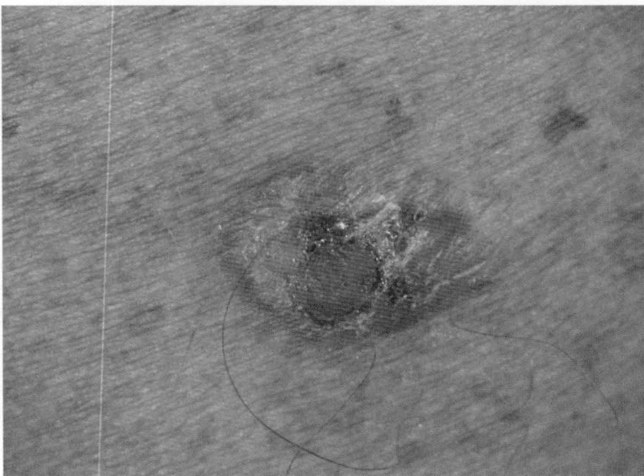

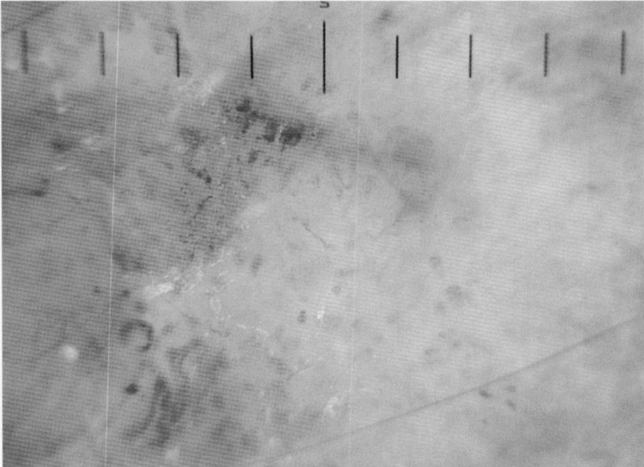

Ulcerated pink plaque on the upper chest in a 60-year-old man: dermoscopy shows ulceration and polymorphous vessels (both fine and large calibre) in this 3.4 mm thick amelanotic SSM.

Carefully assess amelanotic papules. Small foci of pigment also point to melanoma. Amelanotic papules arising within these areas indicate increased growth rate and invasion.

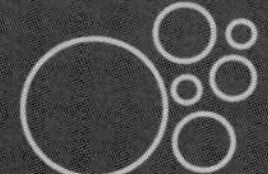

Hypomelanotic macules

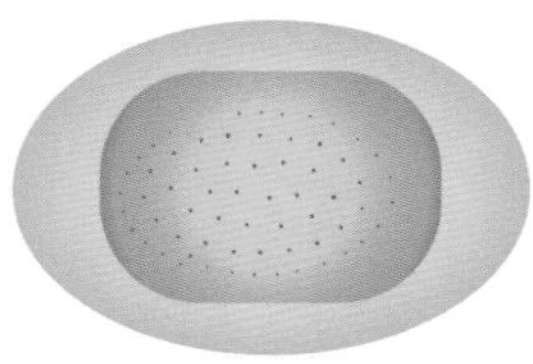

In slightly darker skin, eumelalin is the dominant pigment and we are therefore primed to perceive melanoma as a solitary irregular pigmented macule. However, in patients with light skin, phaeomelanin predominates, and their naevi will typically be less pigmented. In these patients detection of a solitary larger pink-tan macule should be considered suspicious. Dermoscopic features may be subtle and typical pigmented structures of melanoma are often absent.

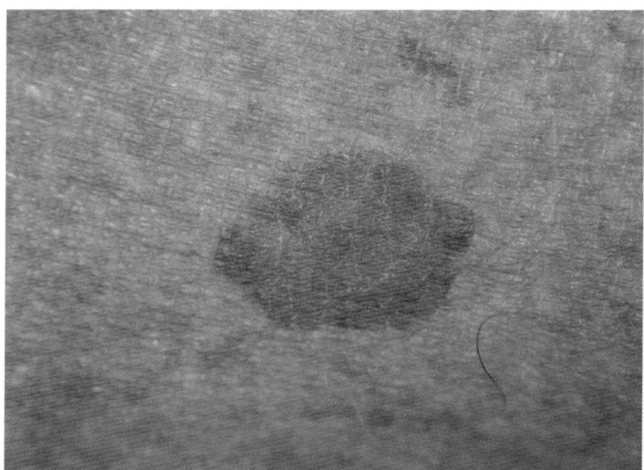

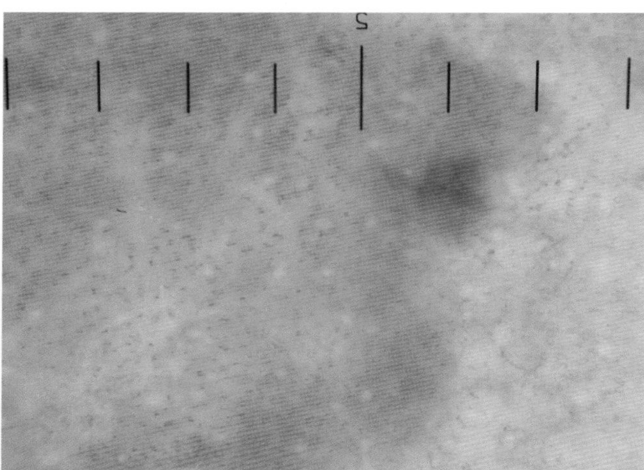

A large tan macule on the upper arm of a 40-year-old man: dermoscopy shows only dotted vessels and eccentric tan pigmentation in this MIS.

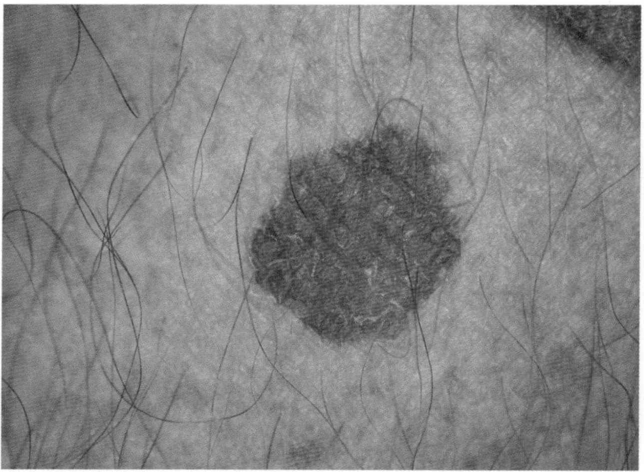

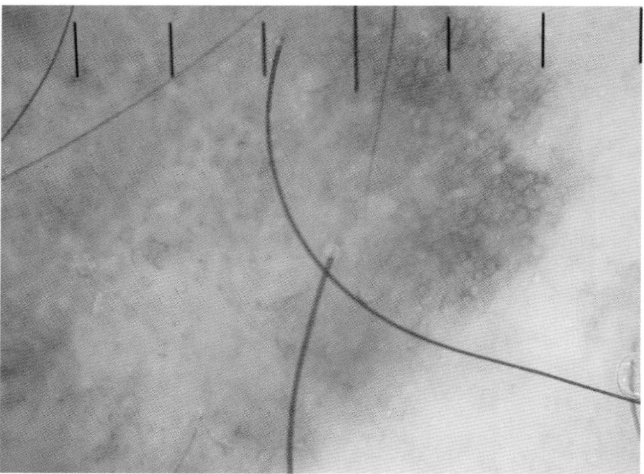

A large tan macule on the upper arm of a 50-year-old man: dermoscopy shows few dotted and short linear irregular vessels, early negative network centrally and an eccentric pigmented network in this MIS.

"Pink and brown should make you frown!".

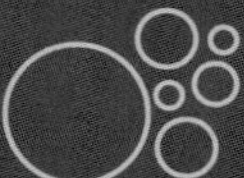

Hypomelanotic macules – cases

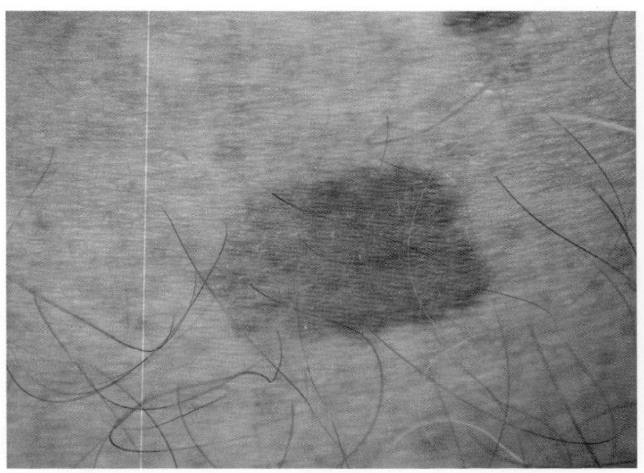

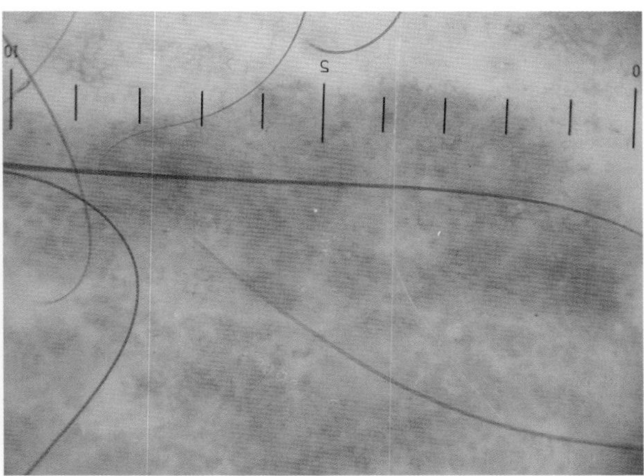

A pink and tan macule on the lower back of a 50-year-old man: dermoscopy shows a tan pigment network superiorly, dotted vessels and a faint negative pigment network (best appreciated at the lateral limits) in this 0.3 mm thick SSM.

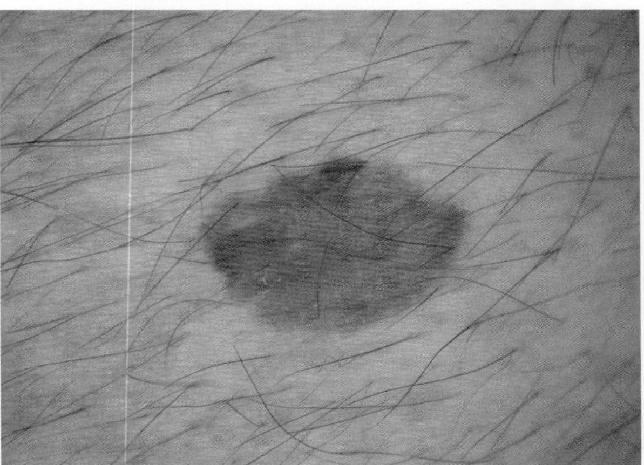

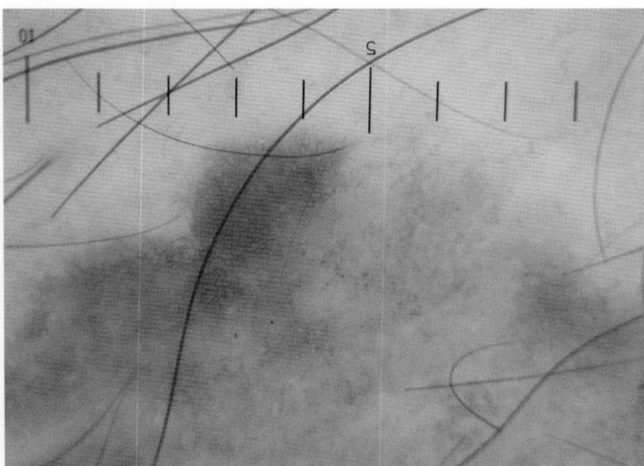

A pink and tan macule on the abdomen of a 30-year-old man: dermoscopy shows a tan pigment network, dotted and linear irregular vessels and a faint negative pigment network in this 0.3 mm thick SSM.

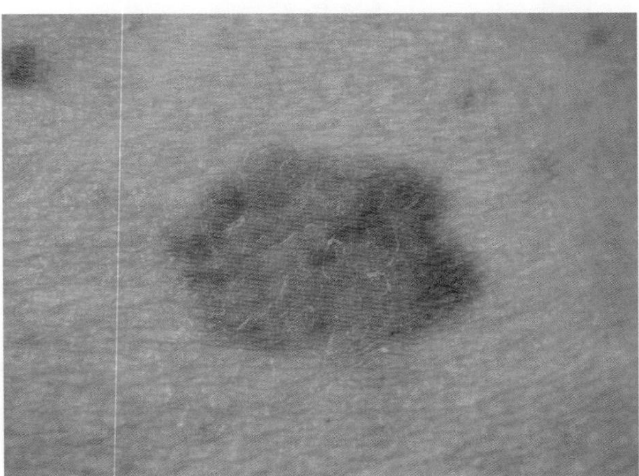

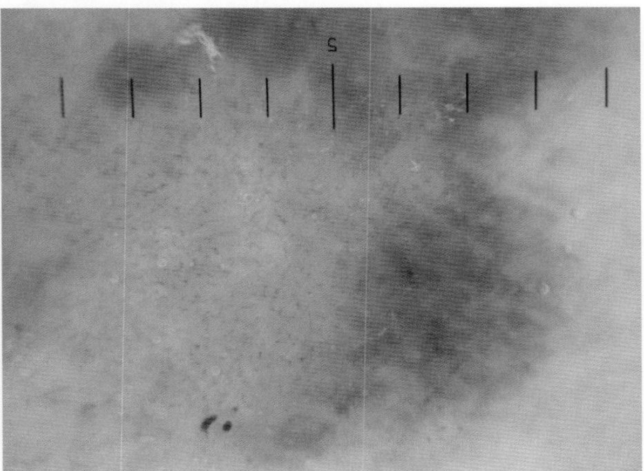

A pink and tan macule on the arm of a 60-year-old woman: dermoscopy shows tan homogeneous eccentric pigmentation with extensive polymorphous vessels (dotted, linear irregular and looped) in this 0.4 mm thick SSM.

In patients with light skin, a solitary stand-out pink-tan macule, may only show subtle dermoscopic clues to melanoma (i.e. vascular or shiny white structures) and should be viewed with a high index of suspicion.

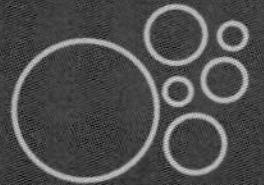

Hypomelanotic tan plaques

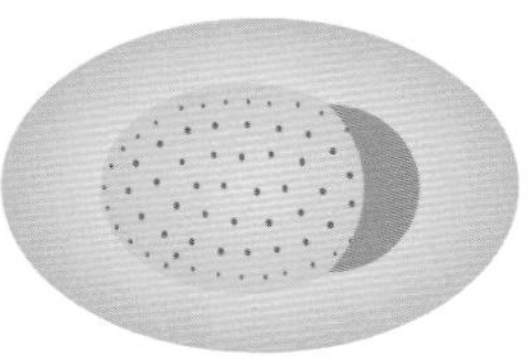

In patients with light skin, the clinical scenario of a solitary pink-tan plaque should be assessed carefully as possible for melanoma. The dermoscopic features may be subtle and typical pigmented structures of melanoma are often absent. In hypopigmented melanoma it can be difficult to predict the Breslow thickness on clinical and dermoscopic examinations alone.

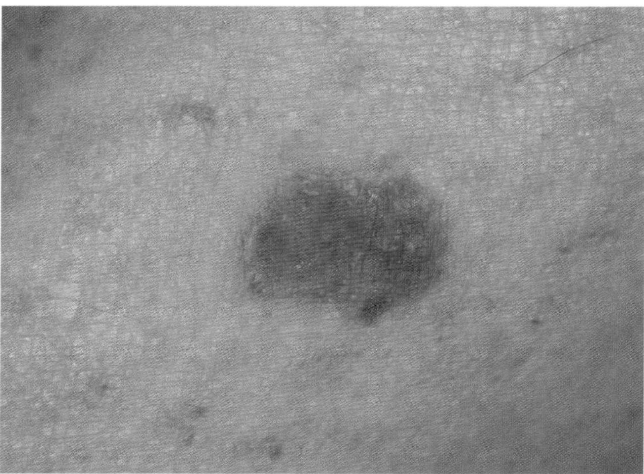

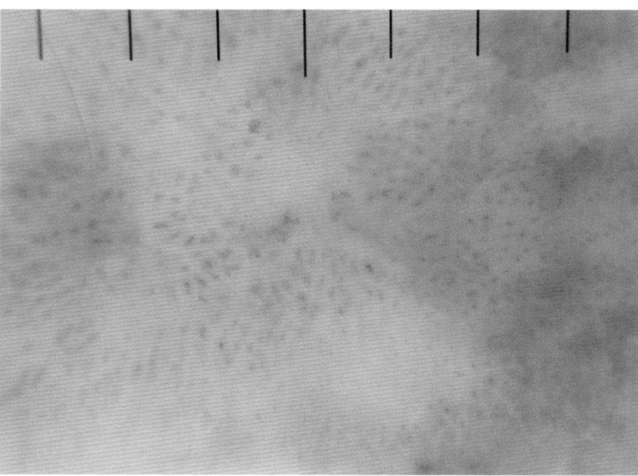

A pink-tan plaque on the knee of a 60-year-old woman: dermoscopy shows dotted and linear irregular vessels creating a negative network appearance along with eccentric tan pigment in this 0.6 mm thick SSM.

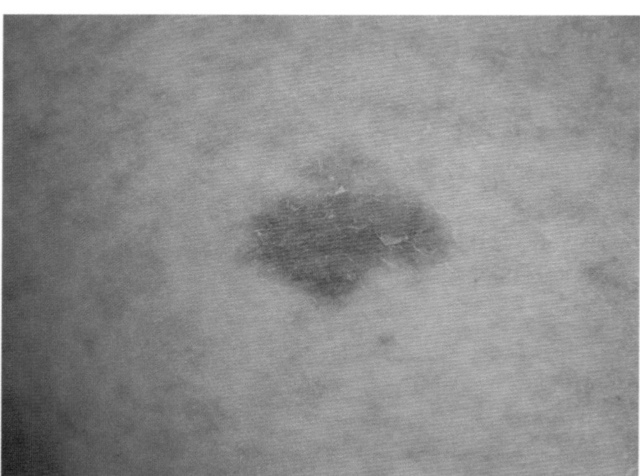

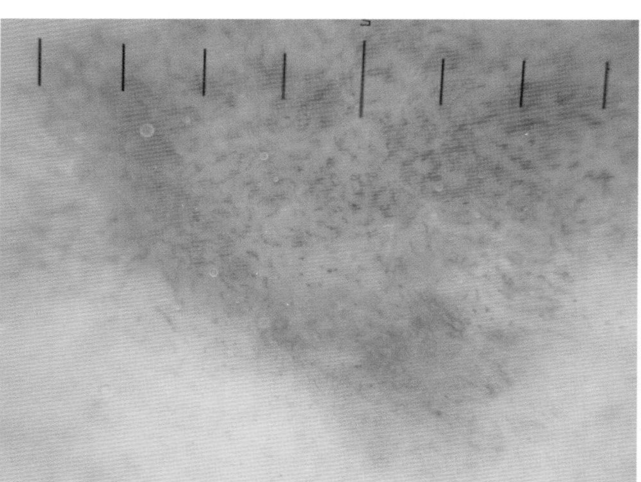

A tan macule with an evolving pink component on the elbow of a 40-year-old woman: dermoscopy shows extensive dotted and linear irregular vessels and eccentric tan pigmentation in this 0.6 mm thick hypomelanotic SSM.

Use pressure to see the pigment and avoid pressure (or use non-contact polarising mode) to see the vessels. Hypomelanotic melanomas are always subtle.

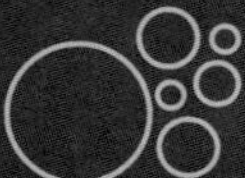

Hypomelanotic tan plaques cases

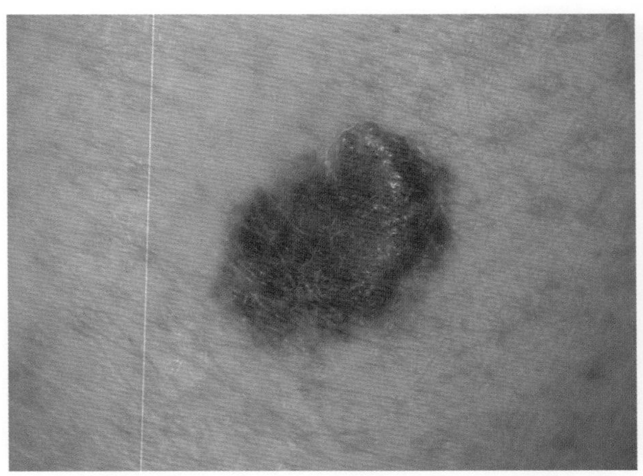

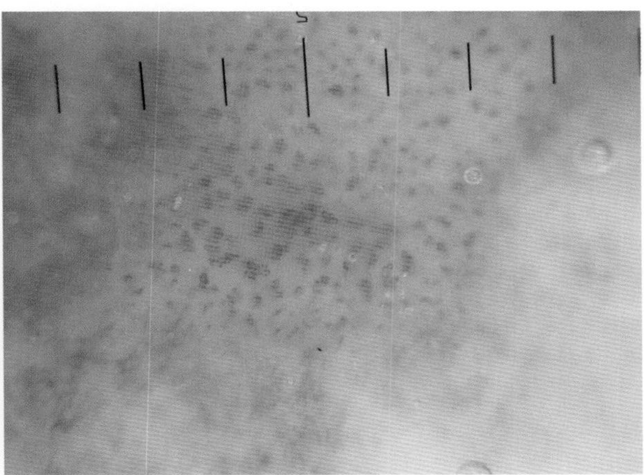

A tan macule with superimposed pink plaque on the leg of a 40-year-old woman: dermoscopy shows tan homogeneous pigmentation and a focal zone of polymorphous vessels (dotted, looped and highly tortuous) in this 0.8 mm thick SSM.

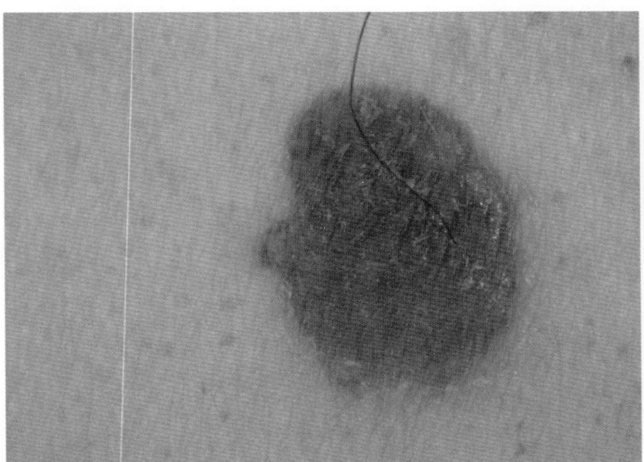

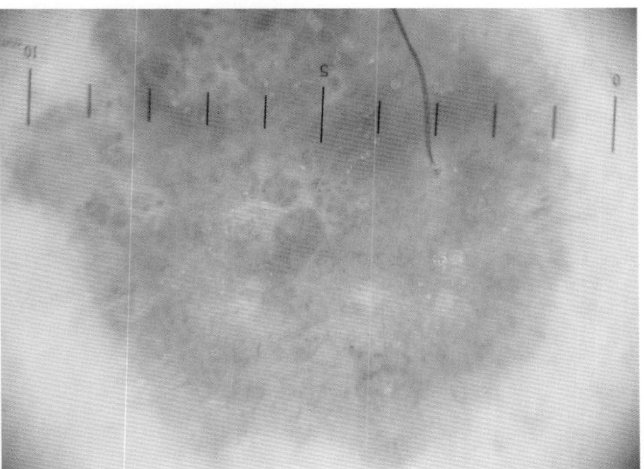

A pink-tan plaque on the upper back of a 60-year-old man: dermoscopy shows tan homogeneous eccentric pigment, milky erythema and negative network in this 1.0 mm thick SSM.

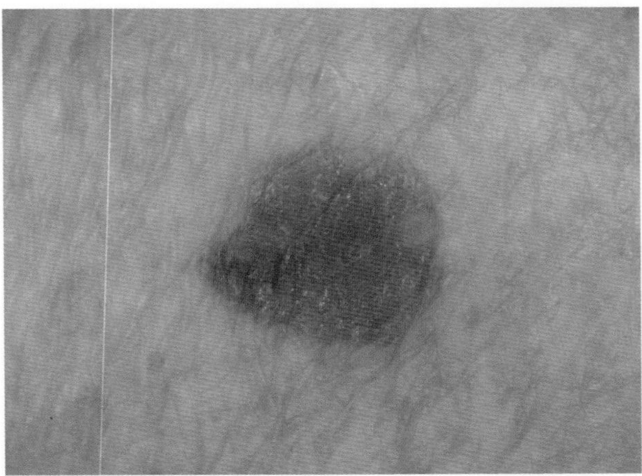

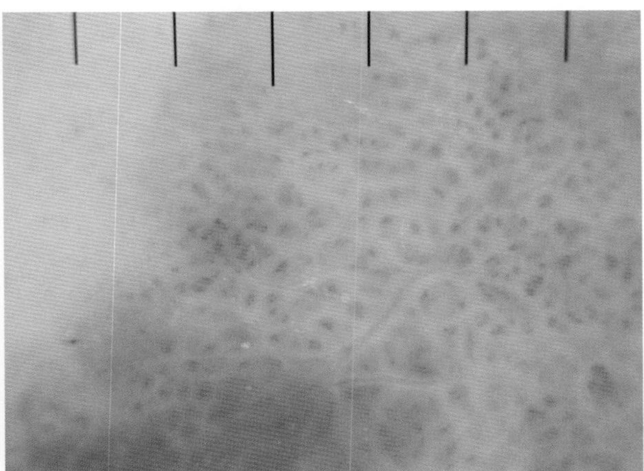

A pink-tan plaque on the lower calf of a 65-year-old woman: dermoscopy shows tan homogeneous eccentric pigmentation with dotted vessels creating a negative network in this 1.8 mm thick SSM.

Pizzichetta, M. et al. Dermoscopic of amelanotic/hypomelanotic melanoma. *Br J Dermatol*. 2017:177(2):538–540.

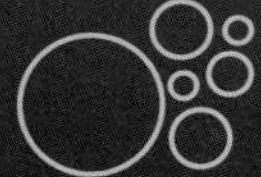

3.3 Melanoma – dermoscopic features

Melanoma-specific features	67
Atypical network – focal	68
Atypical network – focal cases	69
Atypical network – multifocal	70
Atypical network – multifocal cases	71
Atypical beaded network	72
Atypical beaded network cases	73
Black dots and globules	74
Black dots and globules cases	75
Eccentric brown blotch	76
Eccentric brown blotch – cases	77
Eccentric black blotch	78
Eccentric black blotch – cases	79
Eccentric grey blotch	80
Eccentric grey blotch – cases	81
Angulated lines	82
Angulated lines cases	83
Negative network	84
Negative network cases	85
Extensive regression	86
Extensive regression cases	87
Focal regression	88
Focal regression cases	89
Blue-whitish veil	90
Blue-whitish veil cases	91
Dermal pigmentation	92
Dermal pigmentation cases	93
Polymorphous vessels	94
Polymorphous vessels cases	95
Skin surface markings	96
Skin surface markings cases	97

Diagnostic Dermoscopy: The Illustrated Guide, Second Edition. Jonathan Bowling.

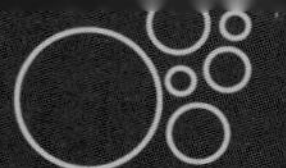

Melanoma-specific features

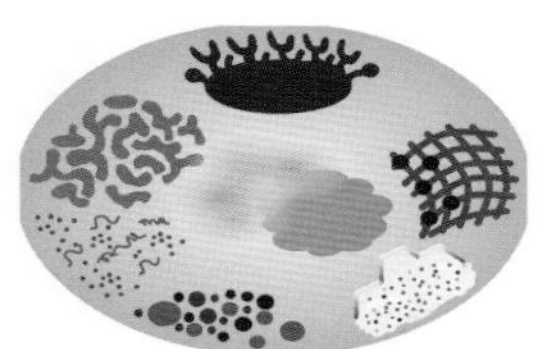

Clinical examination allows identification of melanoma with overt variations in shape, size, and colour combinations. Dermoscopic examination enhances available information by the additional identification of recognised structures in the skin which have a high specificity for melanoma. Melanoma in situ (MIS) may present with relatively few dermoscopic structures. Invasive superficial spreading melanoma (SSM) will typically have a more variable combination of structures seen compared with MIS.

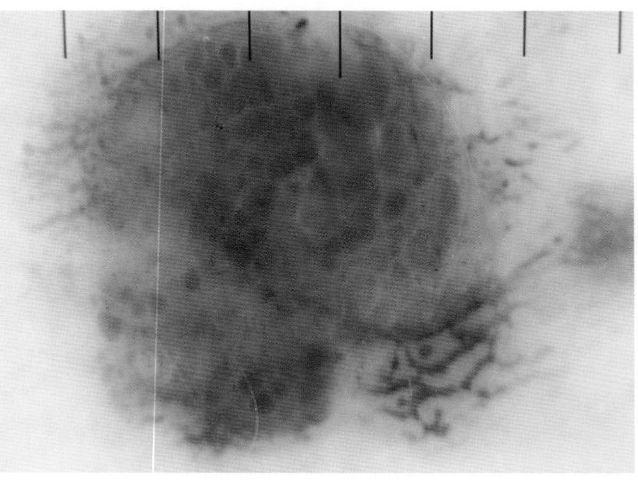

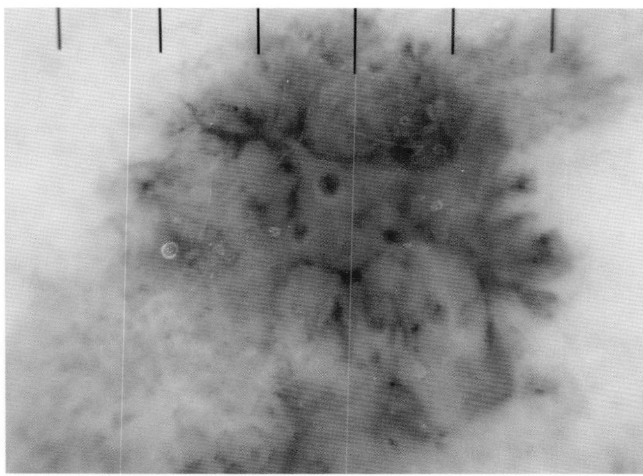

Atypical pigment network, blue-whitish veil, pigment streaks, shiny white structures, irregular dots and globules and a negative network can be seen in these two <1.0 mm thick SSM.

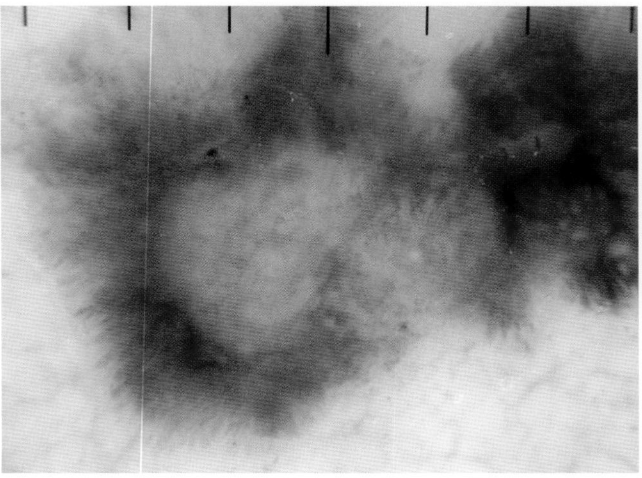

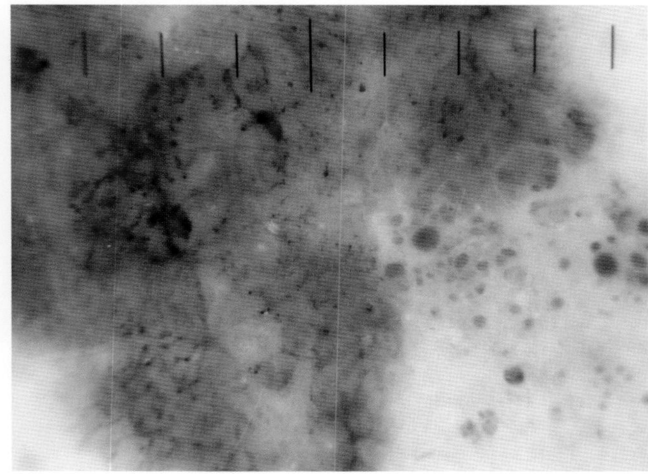

An atypical pigment network, pigment streaks, black dots and globules, regression structures, irregular linear vessels and irregular pigmented globules can be seen in these two < 0.5 mm thick SSM.

Early identification of SSM is key in reducing morbidity and mortality.

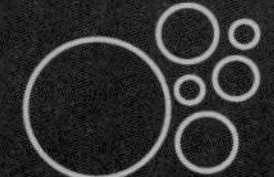

Atypical network – focal

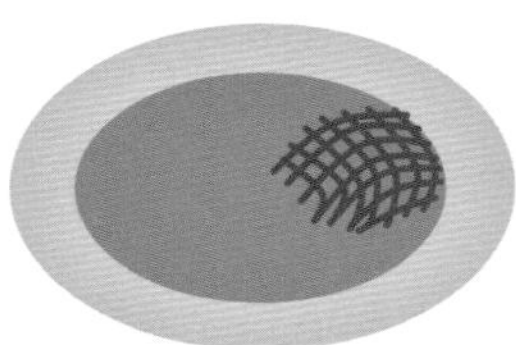

Eccentric epidermal pigmentation is an important clinical sign of melanoma. The presence of a focal eccentric atypical pigment network on dermoscopy in a solitary melanocytic lesion should warrant further investigation. The histopathological correlate of an atypical pigment network includes fusion of the rete ridges creating a broad pigment network.

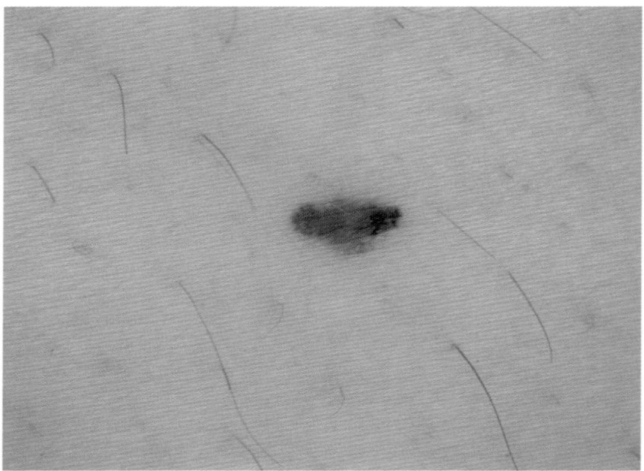

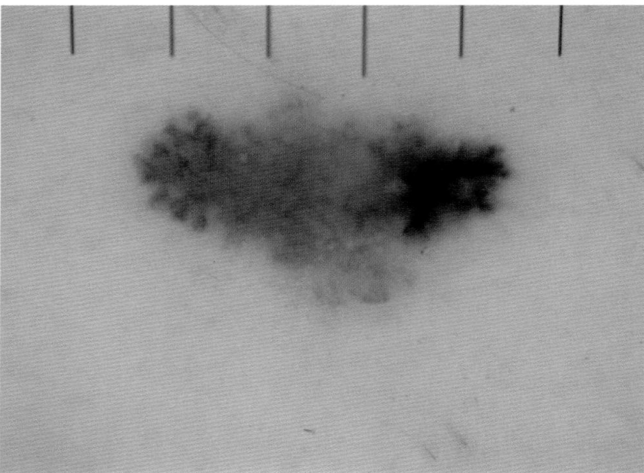

A tan and blackened 4 × 2 mm macule on the lower leg of a 30-year-old woman: dermoscopy shows eccentric hyperpigmented streaks at the polar end in this 0.2 mm thick SSM.

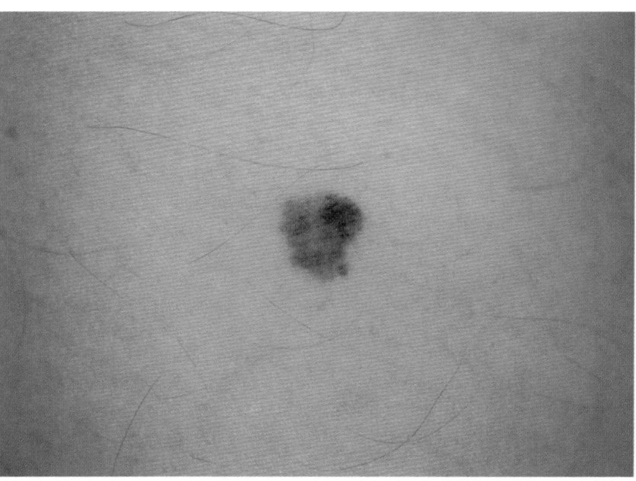

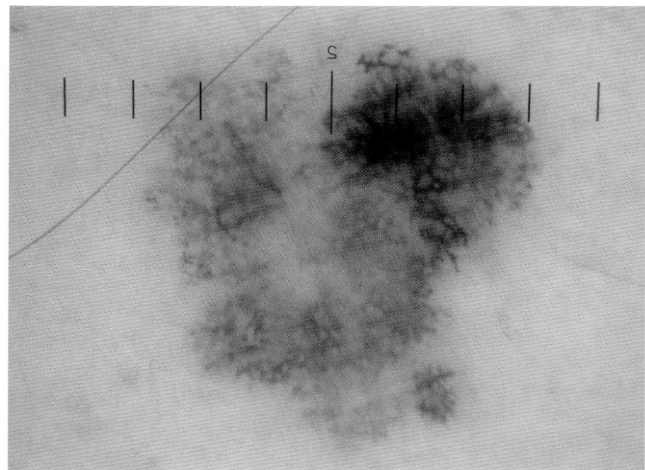

Variably pigmented 6 mm macule on the upper leg of a 60-year-old man: dermoscopy shows reticular pigmentation with an eccentric focus of atypical pigment network in this 0.3 mm thick SSM.

Consider excision for the solitary melanocytic lesion with eccentric epidermal pigmentation.

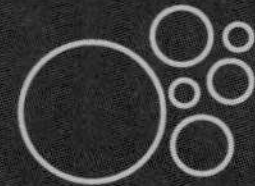

Atypical network – focal cases

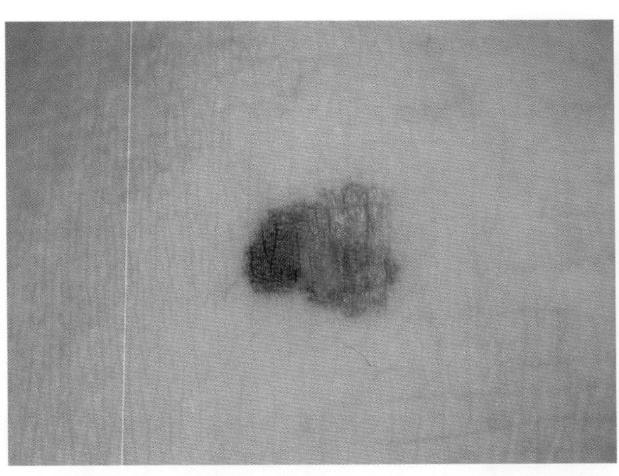

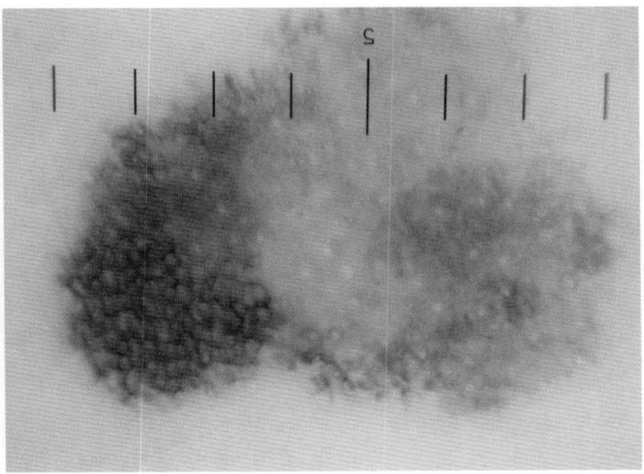

Variably pigmented macule on the dorsum of the foot in a 50-year-old woman: dermoscopy shows an eccentric focus of atypical pigmented network in this MIS.

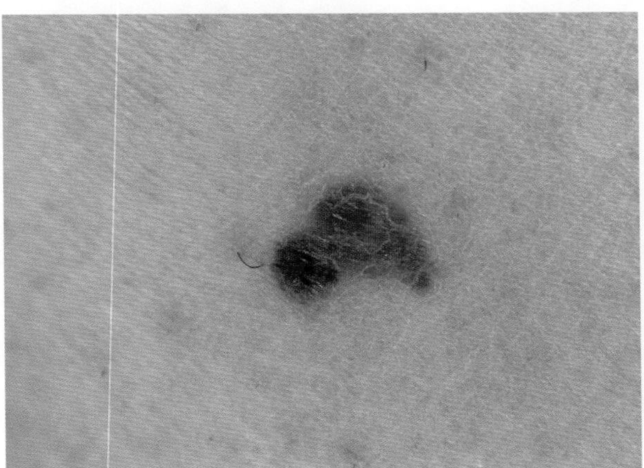

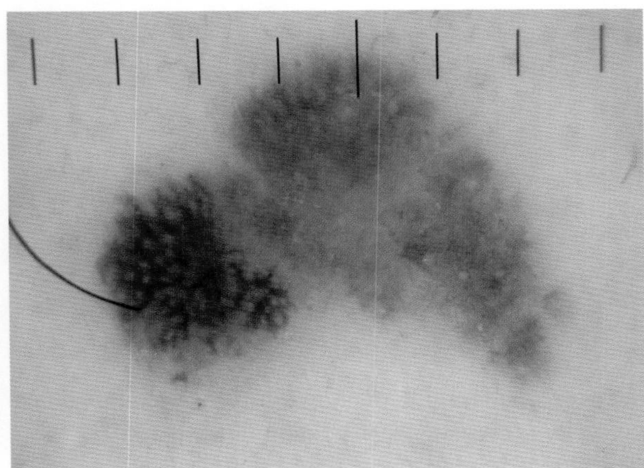

A pigmented macule on the lower leg of a 60-year-old woman: dermoscopy shows an eccentric focus of atypical pigmented network in this MIS.

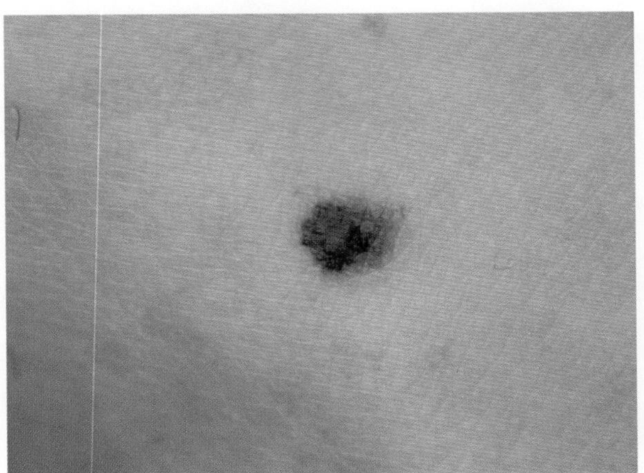

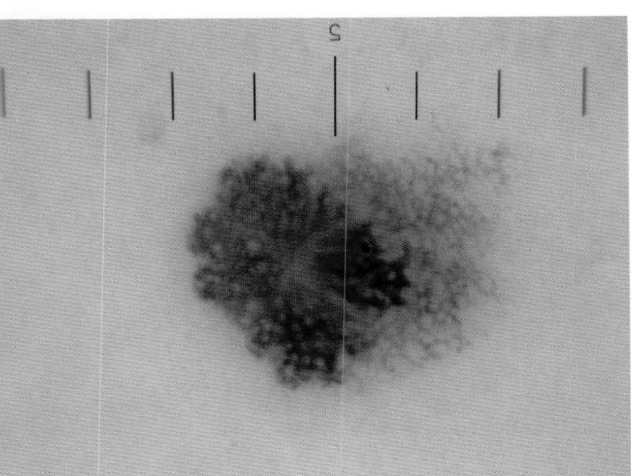

A pigmented macule on the lower leg of a 40-year-old woman: dermoscopy shows an eccentric focus of atypical pigmented network in this 0.2 mm thick SSM.

When a focus of atypical network is the only melanoma-specific feature found in a melanoma, the lesion will most probably be in situ or thin invasive.

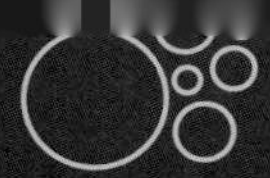

Atypical network – multifocal

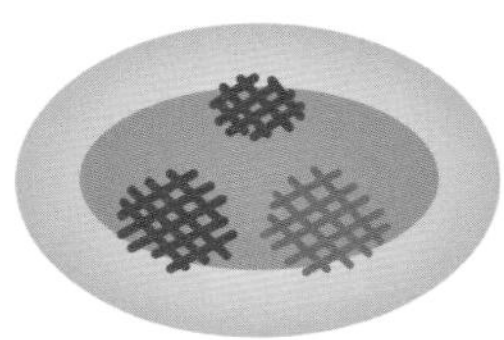

An irregularly shaped solitary melanocytic lesion with multifocal pigmented areas is an indicator of unpredictable histopathology. The foci of pigmentation may be similar or show different dermoscopic patterns. Consider excision for the solitary melanocytic lesion with multifocal asymmetrical pigmentation.

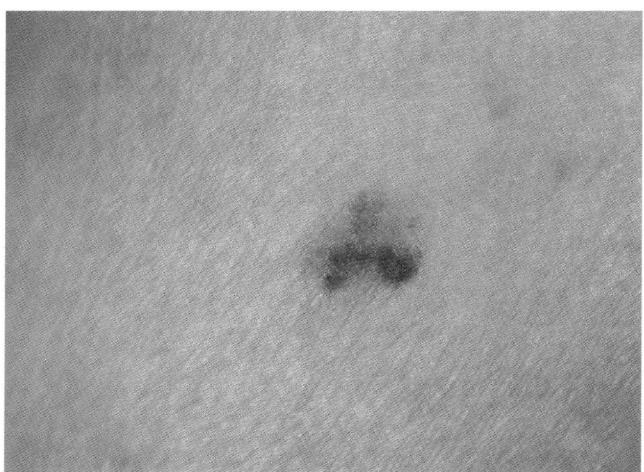

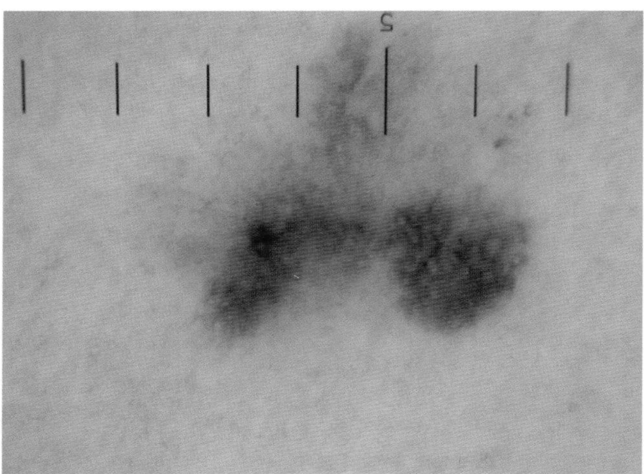

A 4 mm pigmented macule on the calf of a 50-year-old woman: dermoscopy shows a multicomponent trilobed melanocytic lesion with two foci of atypical pigment network in this MIS.

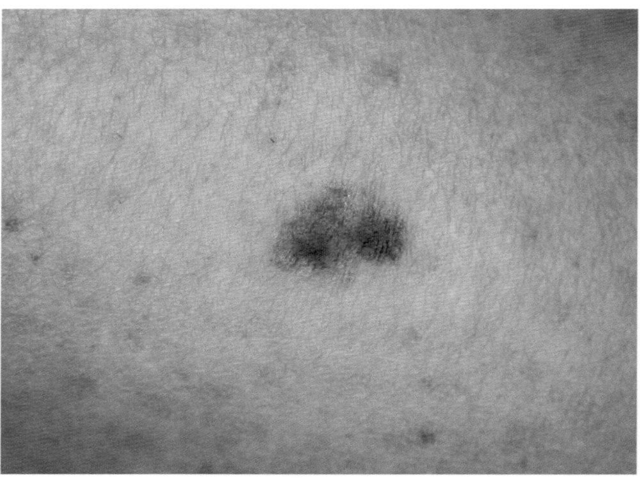

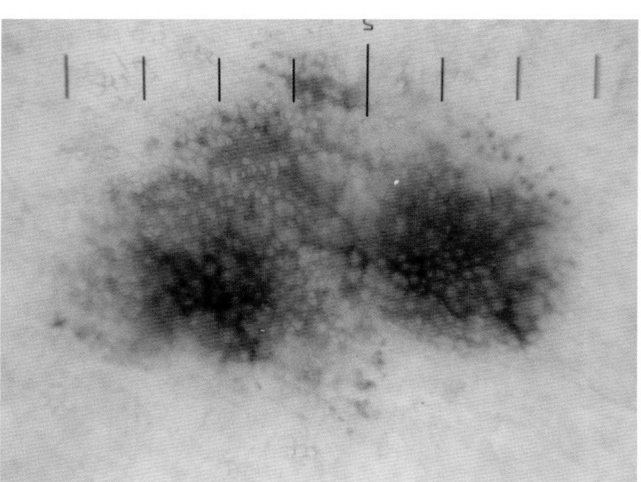

An irregular 7 mm macule on the lower leg of a 50-year-old woman: dermoscopy shows a dual focus of an atypical broad pigmented network with peripheral asymmetrical brown globules in this MIS.

Shi, K. et al. A retrospective cohort study of the diagnostic value of different subtypes of atypical pigment network on dermoscopy. *J Am Acad Dermatol*. 2020;83(4):1028–1034.

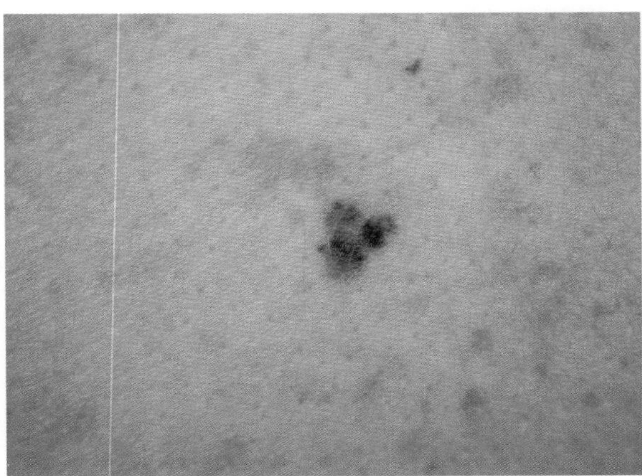
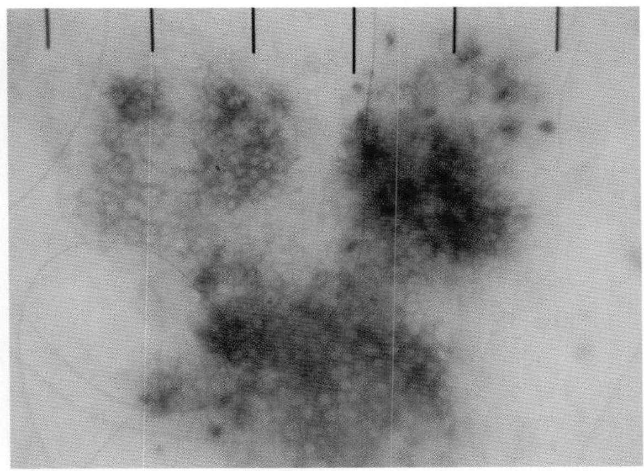

An irregularly pigmented macule on the upper back of a 50-year-old woman: dermoscopy shows multifocal zones of a pigment network with eccentric brown globules in this 0.2 mm thick SSM.

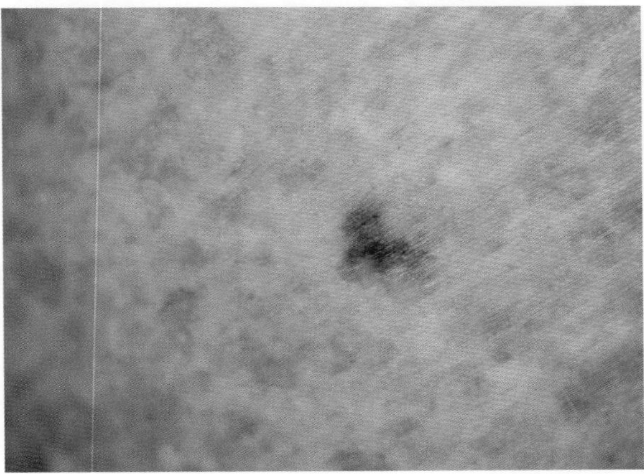
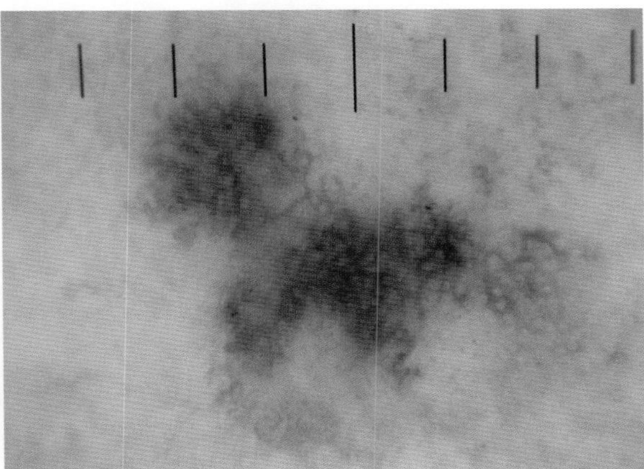

An irregularly pigmented macule on the upper arm of a 50-year-old woman: dermoscopy shows multifocal zones of atypical pigment network, brown globules centrally and eccentric dotted vessels in this 0.3 mm thick SSM.

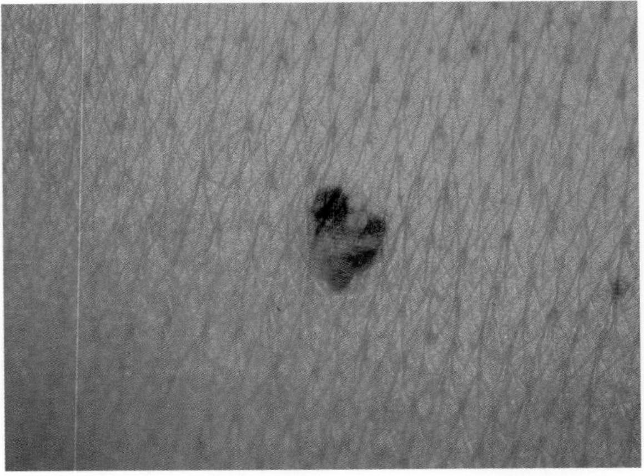
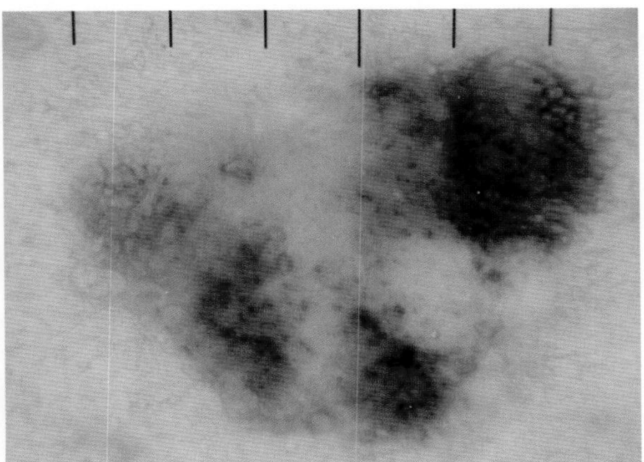

An irregularly pigmented plaque on the back of a 40-year-old woman: dermoscopy shows multiple foci of atypical pigmented network, atypical globules and structureless areas with dotted vessels in this 0.6 mm thick SSM.

Be suspicious of any solitary melanocytic lesion with multiple eccentric foci of reticular pigmentation.

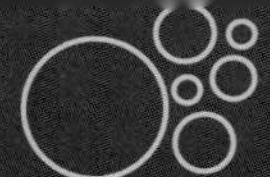

Atypical beaded network

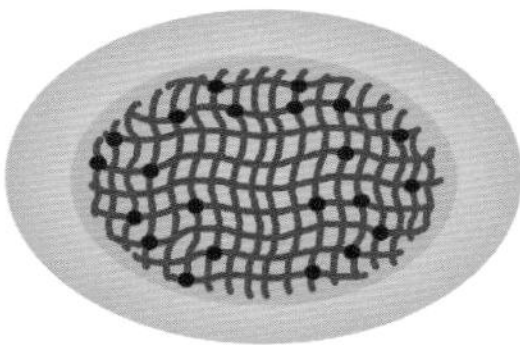

Hyperpigmented melanomas may show pigmented dots overlying the junction of the pigment network, giving a 'beaded' appearance. The hyperpigmented dots are due to nests of melanocytes high in the epidermis.

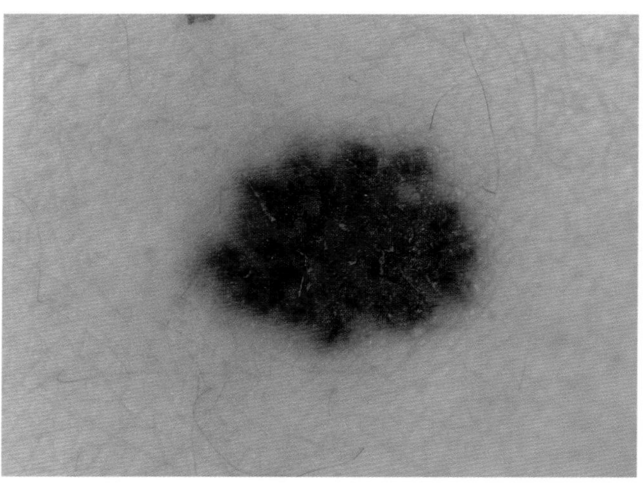

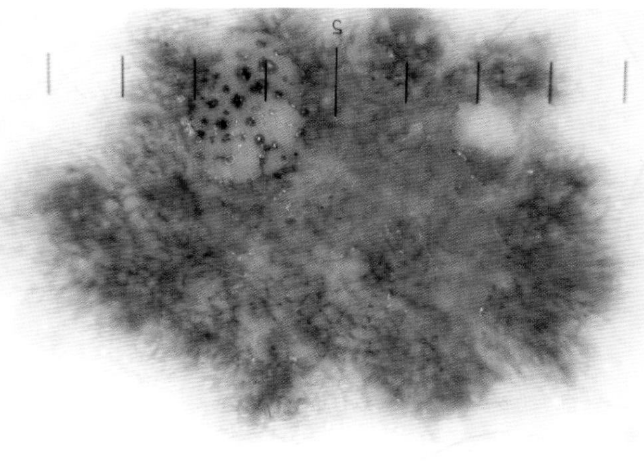

A hyperpigmented macule on the abdomen of a 50-year-old man: dermoscopy shows reticular pigmentation with foci of hyperpigmented dots overlying the junctions of the network and a structureless zone with black dots in this MIS.

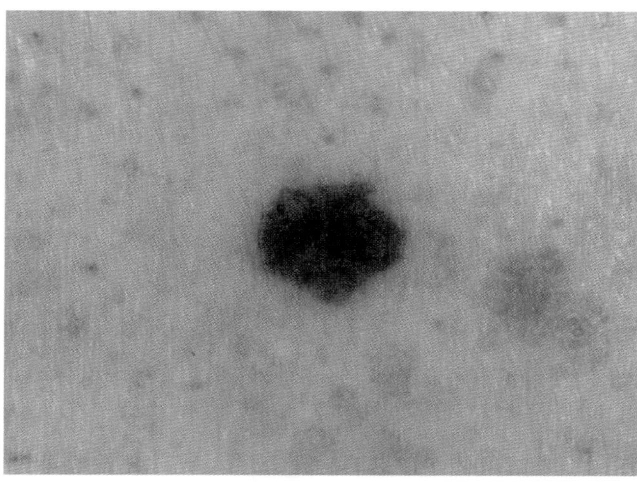

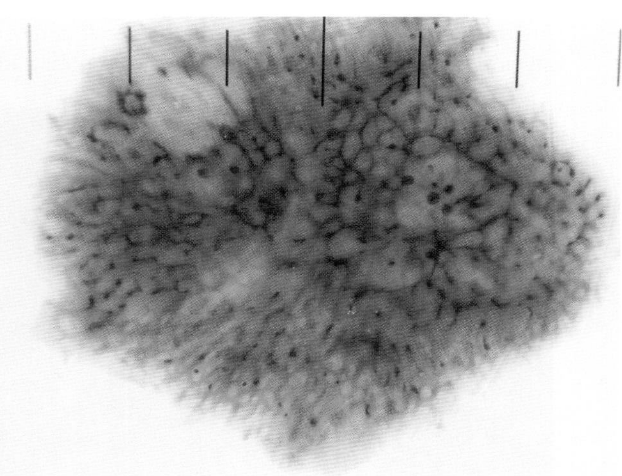

A hyperpigmented macule on the back of a 50-year-old woman: dermoscopy shows streaks and an atypical pigment network with multiple hyperpigmented dots and globules overlying the junctions of the network in this MIS.

Be suspicious of a beaded network with haphazard 'beading' across the lesion and highly suspicious if the 'beading' is eccentric.

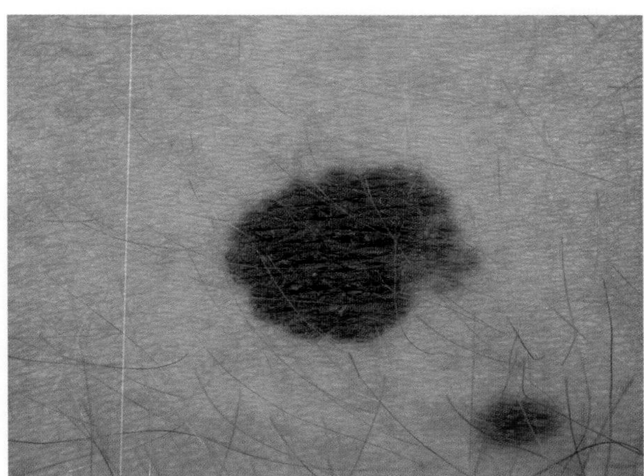

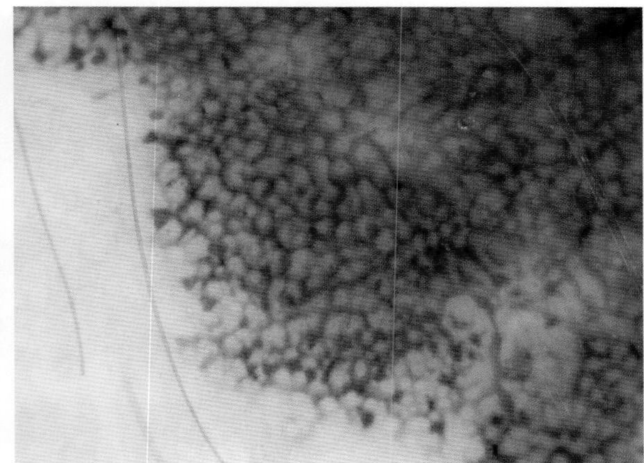

Large asymptomatic pigmented macule on the lower back: dermoscopy shows irregular pigment network with focal dots and globules in keeping with a beaded network in this MIS.

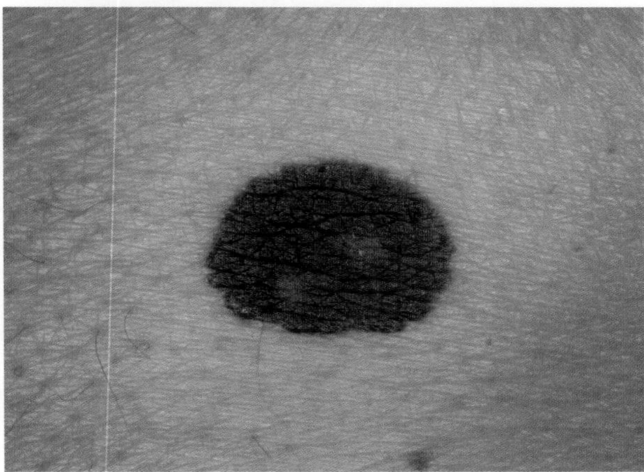

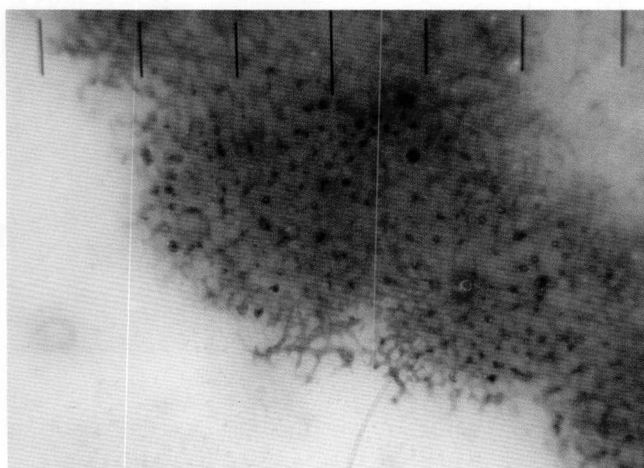

Large asymptomatic pigmented macule on the lower back: dermoscopy shows pigmented dots overlying the atypical pigment network, creating a beaded network in this MIS.

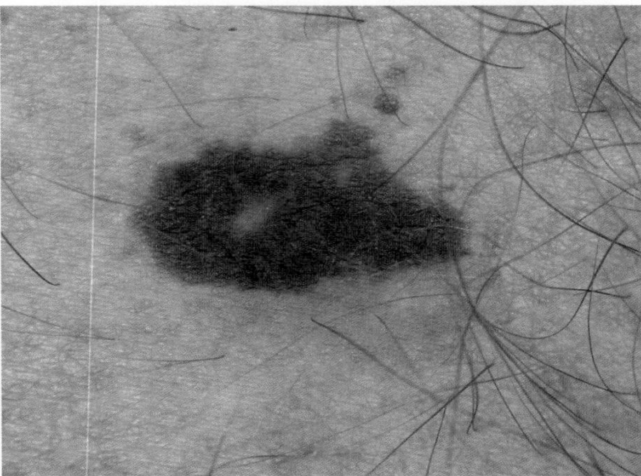

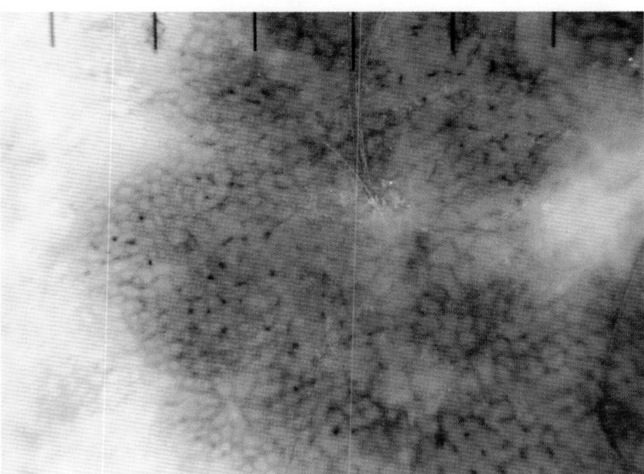

Large asymptomatic pink, brown and black patch on the abdomen: dermoscopy shows pigmented dots overlying the atypical pigment network creating a beaded network along with polygonal structures in this MIS.

An atypical 'beaded' network may also be described as an atypical network combined with irregular dots, which in itself is a sign indicative of melanoma.

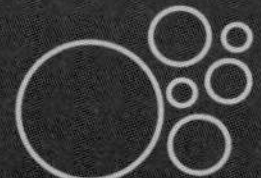

Black dots and globules

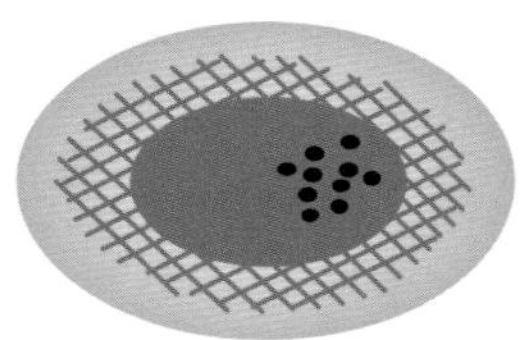

Hyperpigmented melanomas may show verrucous features with keratin structures mimicking the comedo-like openings of seborrhoeic keratosis.

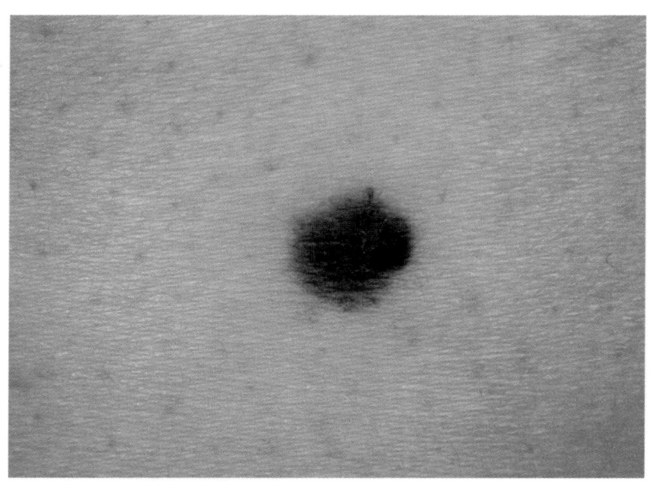

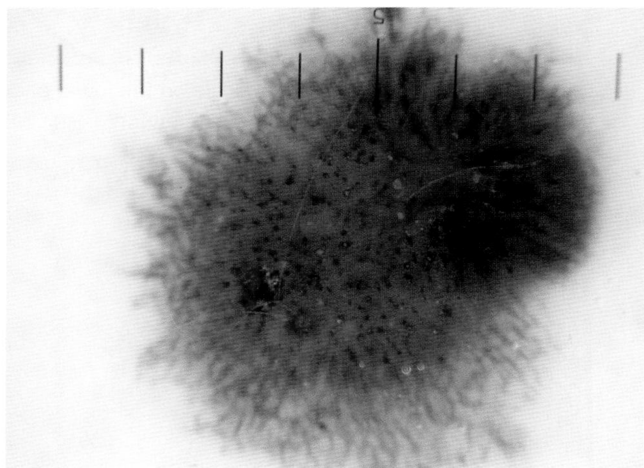

A hyperpigmented macule on the back of a 30-year-old woman: dermoscopy shows reticular pigmentation with central grey and black hyperpigmentation with multiple pigmented dots, globules and comedo-like openings in this MIS.

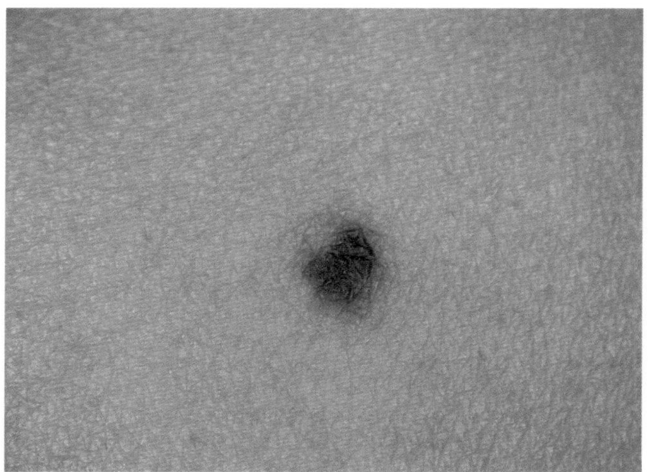

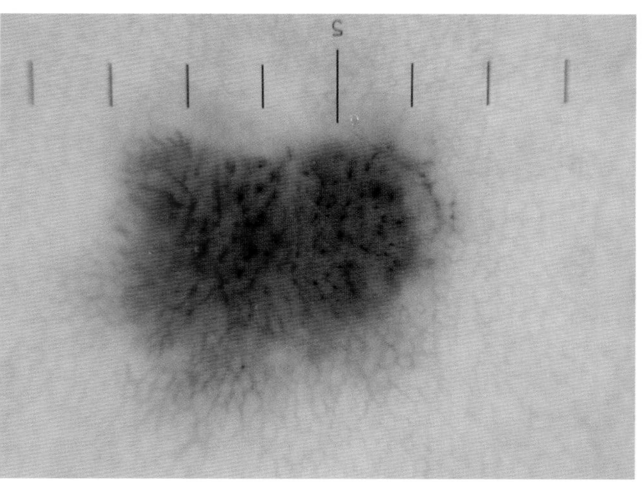

A hyperpigmented macule on the shoulder of a 40-year-old woman: dermoscopy shows atypical pigment network with multiple black dots and globules overlying blue-grey pigmentation in this 0.2 mm thick SSM.

Carrera, C. et al. Dermoscopic clues for diagnosing melanomas that resemble seborrhoeic keratosis. *JAMA Dermatol.* 2017;153(6):544–551.

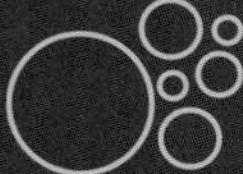

Black dots and globules cases

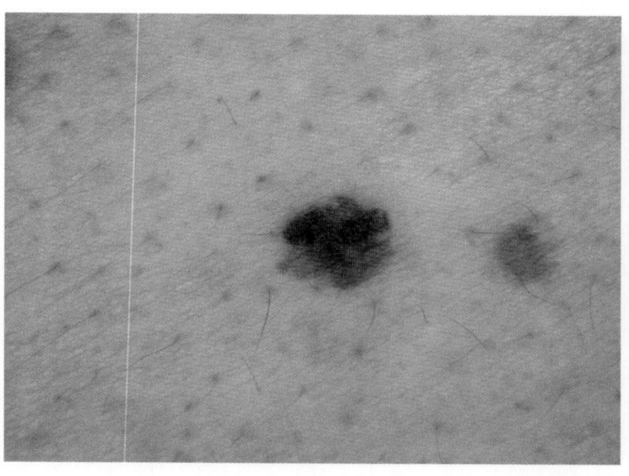

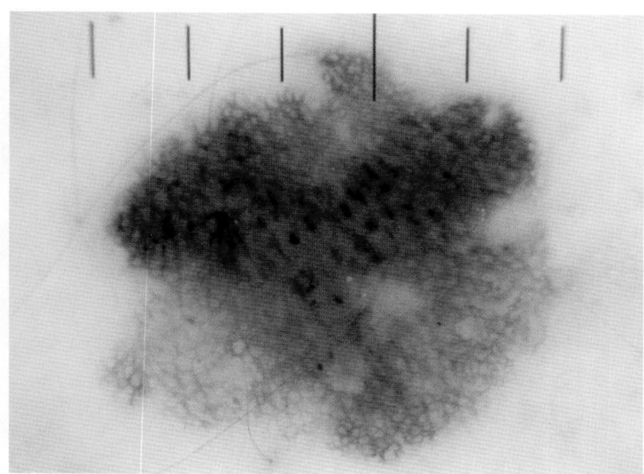

Pigmented macule on the thigh of a 60-year-old woman: dermoscopy shows irregular pigmented network and multiple black globules in the central grey structureless area within this MIS.

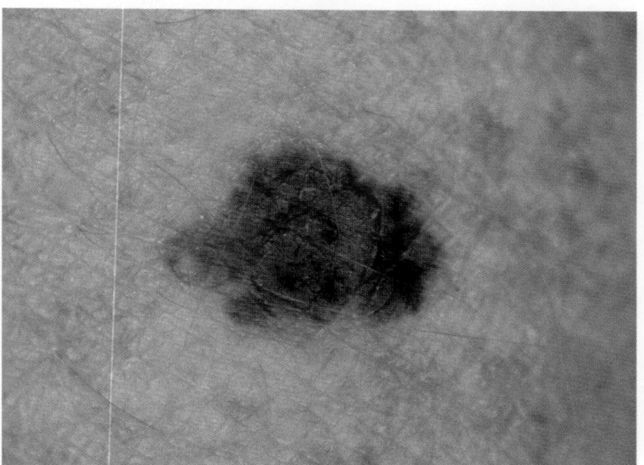

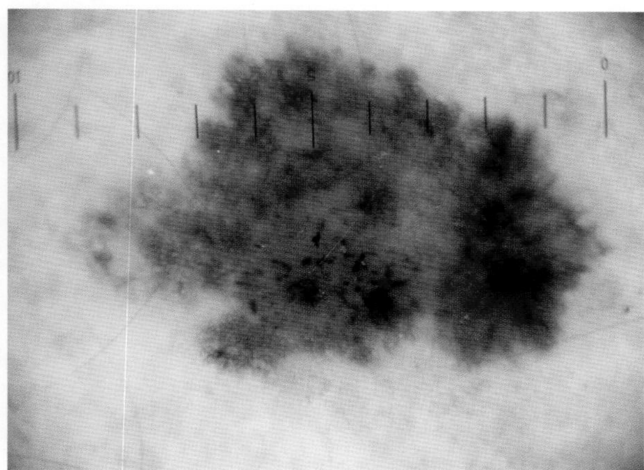

Large pigmented macule on the lower back of a 65-year-old man: dermoscopy shows irregular pigmentation including a grey structureless area with black dots and globules in this 0.3 mm thick SSM.

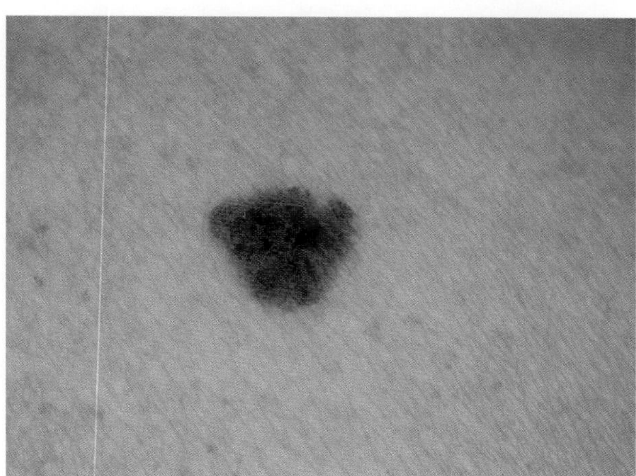

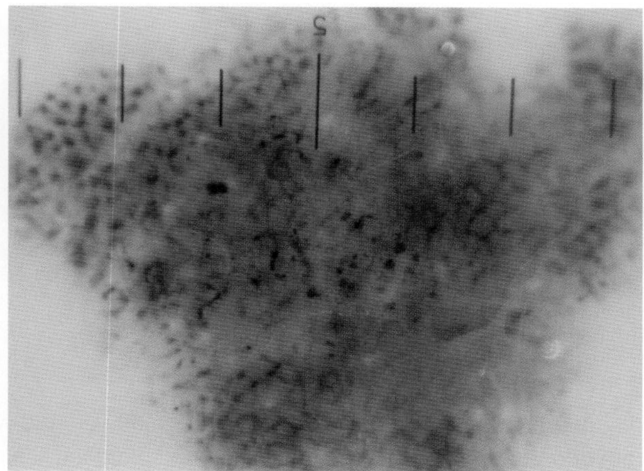

Pigmented macule on the shoulder in a 50-year-old woman: dermoscopy shows an atypical network and atypical black dots and globules overlying a grey structureless area in this 0.6 mm thick SSM.

Xu, J. et al. Analysis of globule types in malignant melanoma. Arch Dermatol. 2009;145(11):1245–51.

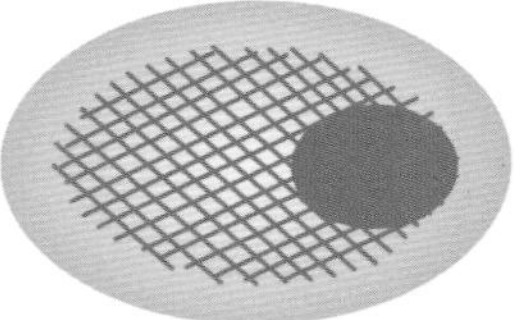

Eccentric epidermal pigmentation is an important clinical sign of melanoma. The presence of an eccentric blotch of pigmentation on dermoscopy in a solitary melanocytic lesion should warrant further investigation.

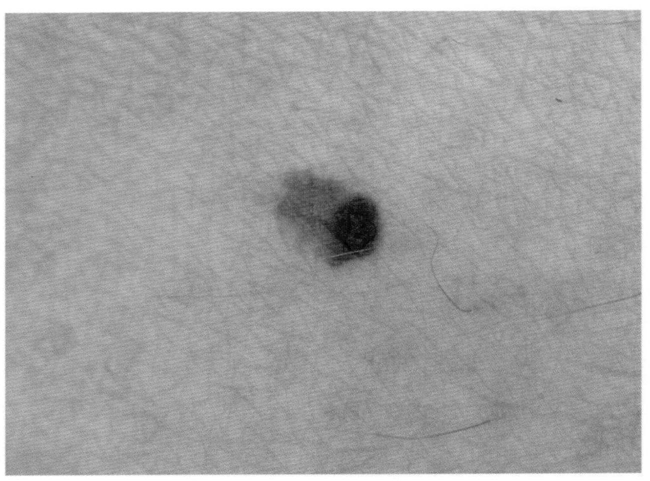

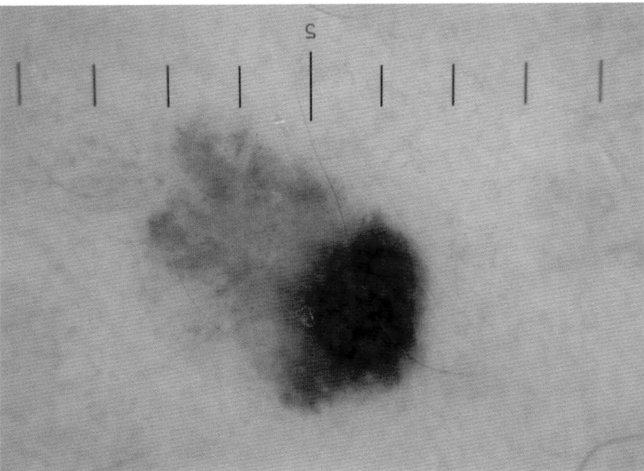

A variegated brown 4 mm macule on the posterior thigh of a 40-year-old woman: dermoscopy shows an eccentric pigmented blotch at the polar end of this 0.3 mm thick SSM.

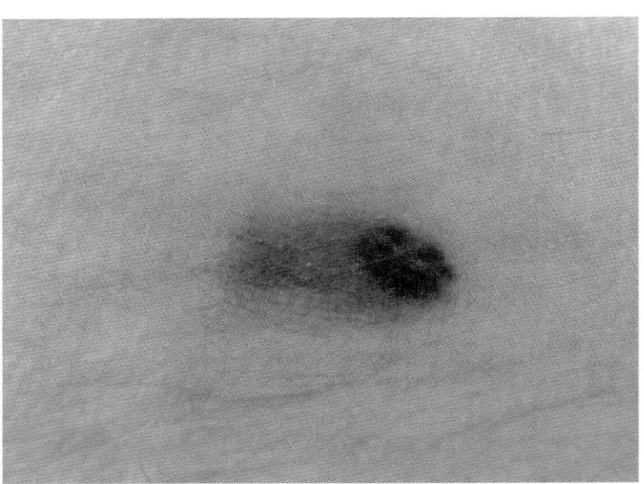

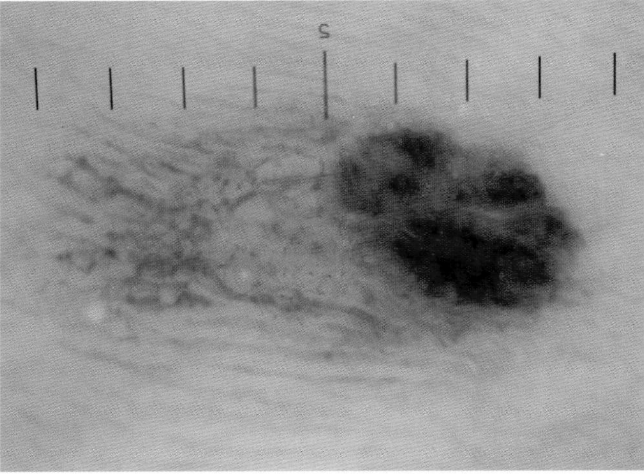

A variegated brown macule on the abdomen of a 60-year-old woman: dermoscopy shows eccentric elongated lentiginous network at one polar end and a hyperpigmented blotch at the other polar end in this 0.5 mm thick SSM.

Borsari, S. et al. Dermoscopic island: a new descriptor for thin melanoma. *Arch Dermatol.* 2010;146(11):1257–62.

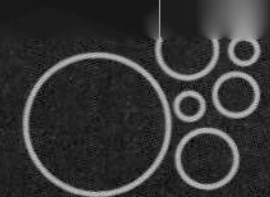

Eccentric brown blotch – cases

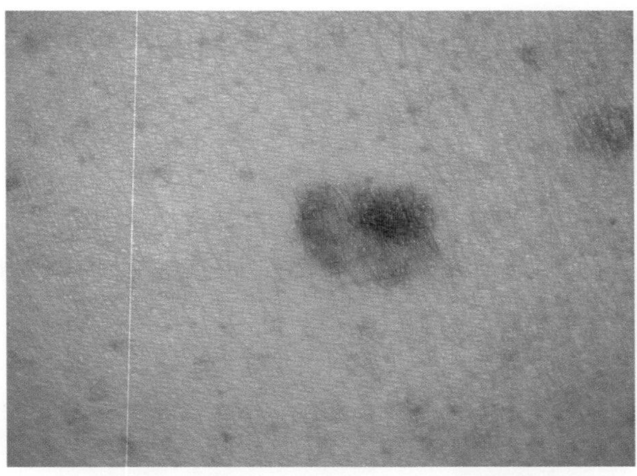

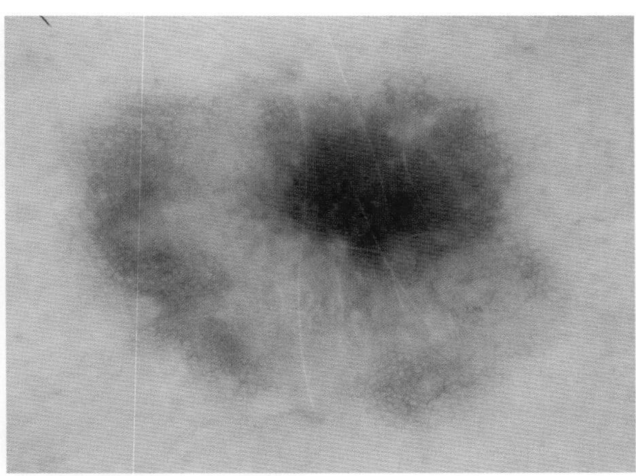

Variably pigmented macule on the back of a 40-year-old man: dermoscopy shows an eccentric brown blotch along with polymorphous vessels within a hypopigmented structureless area in this MIS.

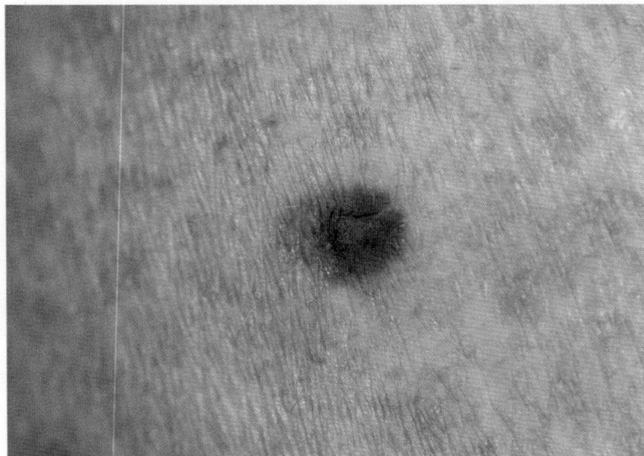

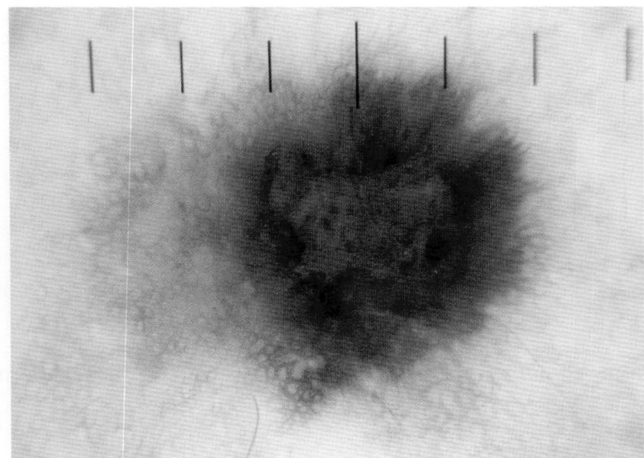

A pigmented macule on the back of a 60-year-old man: dermoscopy shows polarity of pigmentation and a large eccentric brown blotch in this MIS.

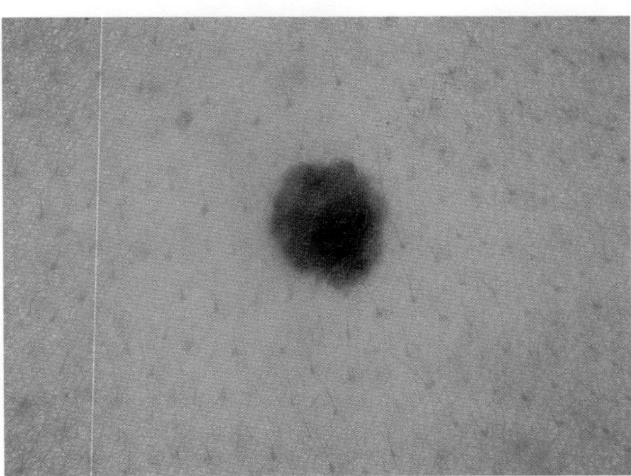

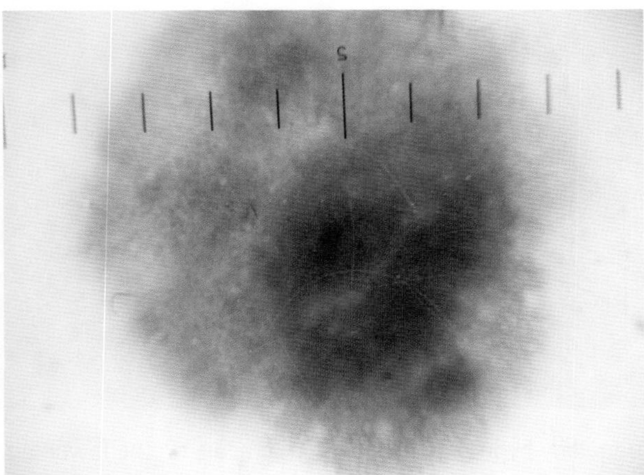

Pigmented macule on the back of a 30-year-old woman: dermoscopy shows a large eccentric brown blotch in this 0.2 mm thick SSM.

A brown eccentric blotch in a melanoma indicates that the lesion is either in situ or thin invasive in this area.

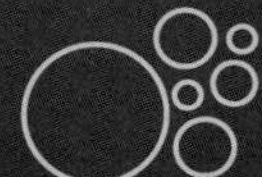

Eccentric black blotch

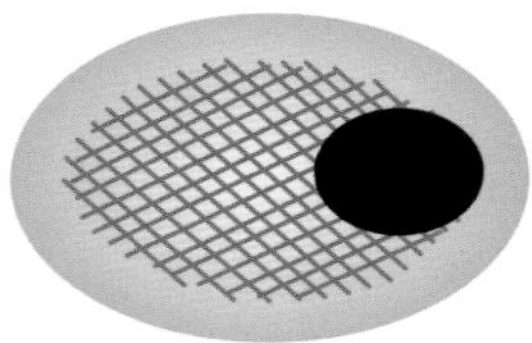

Eccentric black hyperpigmentation is an indicator of an unpredictable melanocytic lesion. The focus of hyperpigmentation typically represents a focus of globules, network, streaks or pigment blotch.

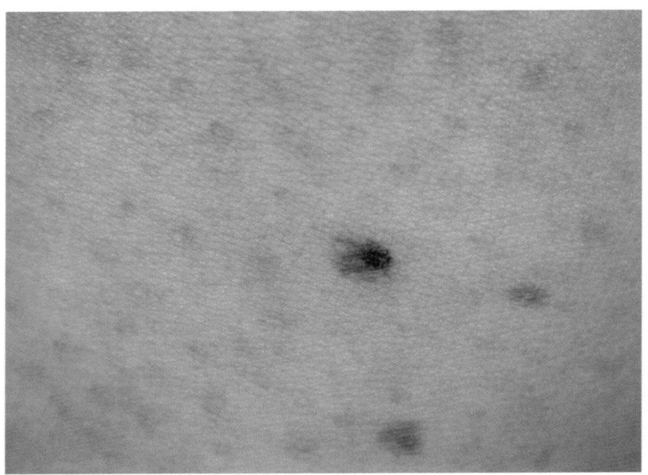

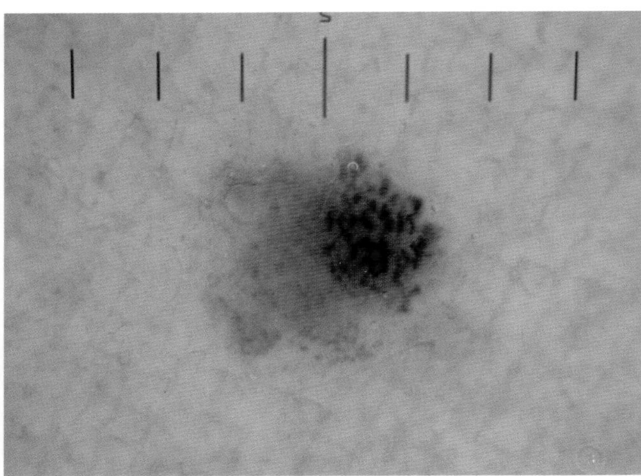

A 3 mm pigmented macule on the triceps of a 60-year-old woman: dermoscopy shows a 1 mm focus of eccentric hyperpigmented globular pigmentation in this MIS.

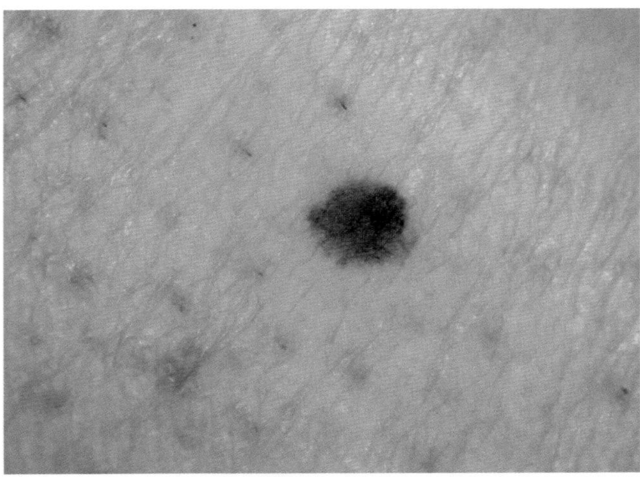

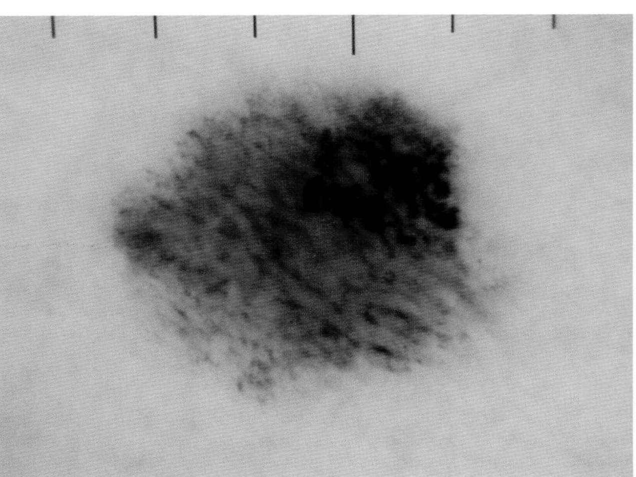

An irregularly hyperpigmented 4 mm macule on the lower leg of a 40-year-old woman: dermoscopy shows irregular globular and homogeneous pigmentation with an eccentric focus of hyperpigmented globules in this MIS.

Consider excision for the solitary melanocytic lesion with eccentric black hyperpigmentation.

Eccentric black blotch – cases

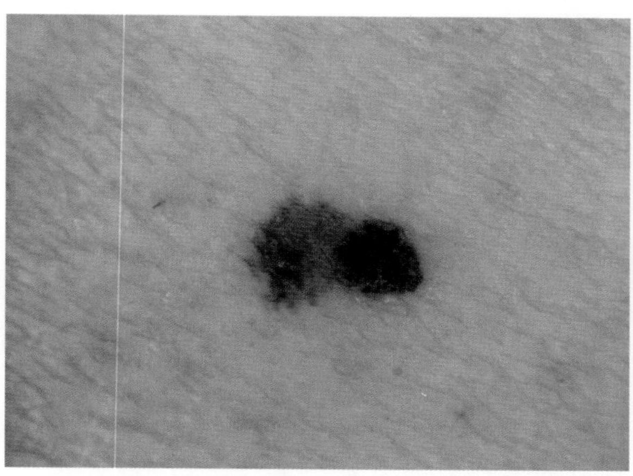

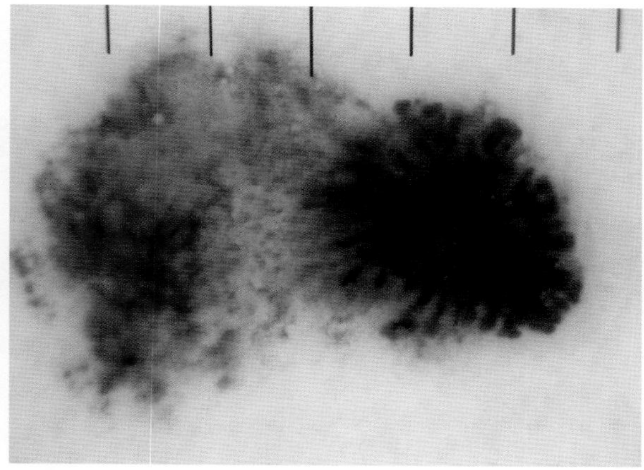

An irregularly pigmented macule on the shin in a 40-year-old woman: dermoscopy shows multicomponent morphology, irregular globules with an eccentric blotch with atypical streaks forming a starburst pattern in this 0.2 mm thick SSM.

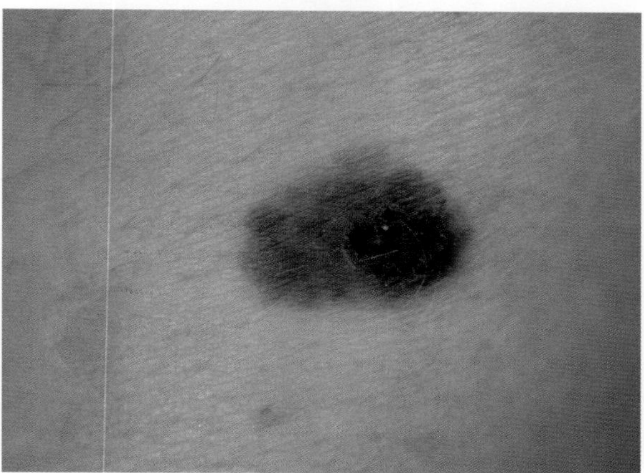

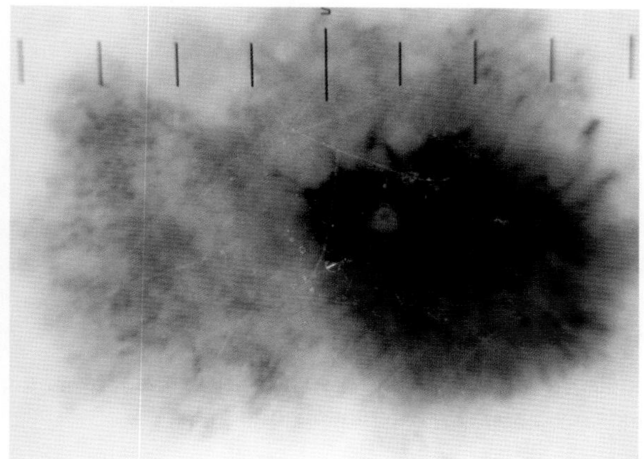

An irregularly pigmented plaque on the forearm of a 60-year-old woman: dermoscopy shows a multicomponent morphology with an eccentric hyperpigmented blotch, atypical streaks and black globules in this 0.5 mm thick SSM.

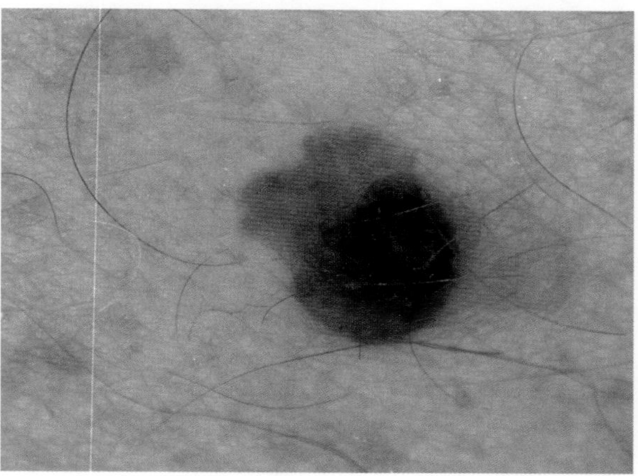

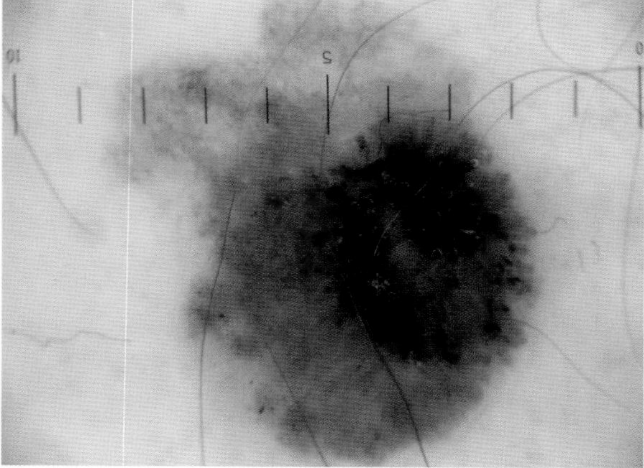

An irregularly pigmented plaque on the upper thigh of a 70-year-old man: dermoscopy shows a multicoloured lesion with an eccentric hyperpigmented blotch with black dots and globules in this 1.5 mm thick SSM.

An eccentric focus of any colour in a melanocytic lesion makes it suspicious for melanoma.

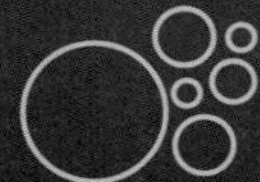

Eccentric grey blotch

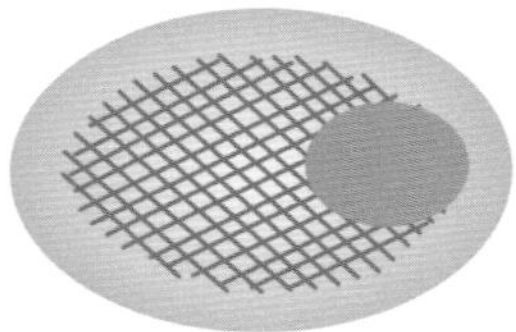

Eccentric grey (papillary dermal pigmentation) is an indicator of an unpredictable melanocytic lesion. The grey pigmentation may represent dermal involvement and/or regression.

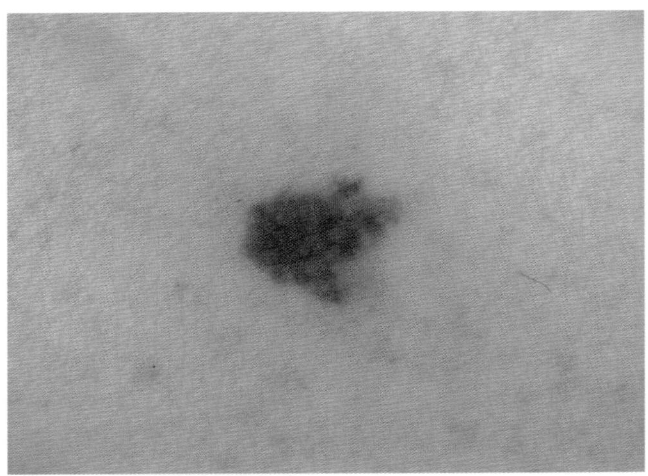

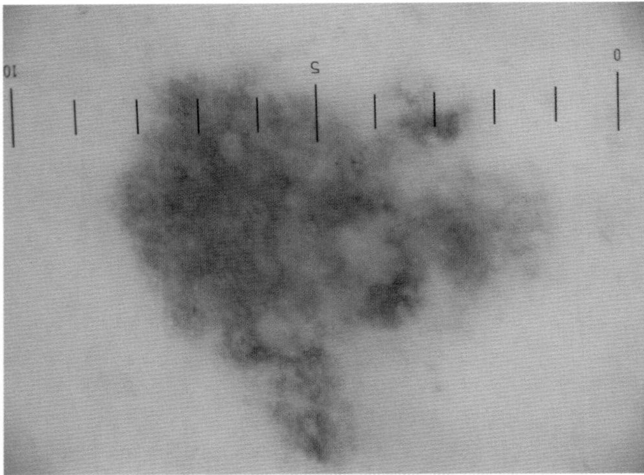

An irregularly shaped tan-grey macule on the leg of a 60-year-old woman: dermoscopy shows reticular pigmentation with eccentric grey granular pigmentation in this MIS.

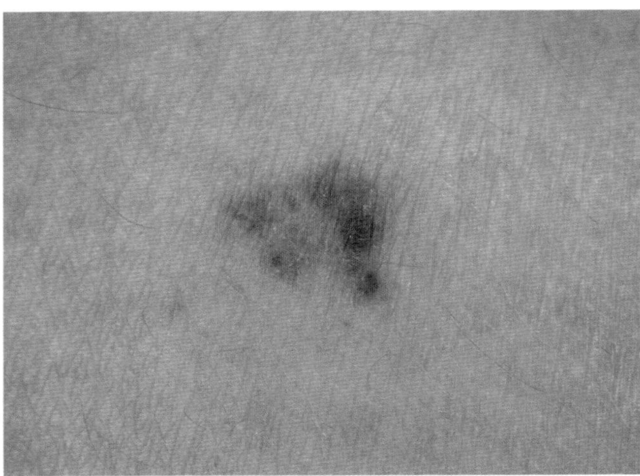

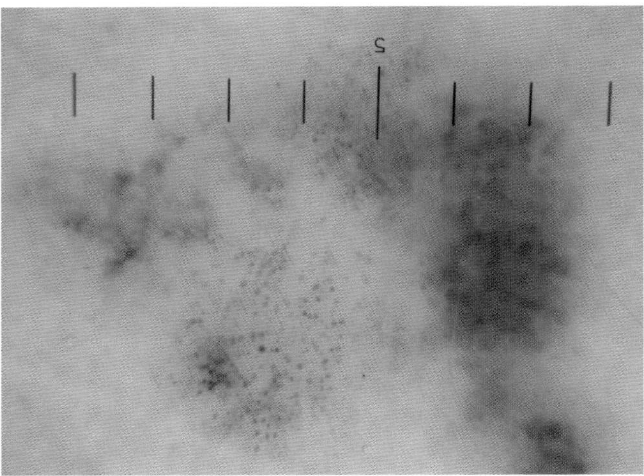

An irregular tan-grey pigmented macule on the thigh of a 30-year-old woman: dermoscopy shows irregular globules and a grey-brown eccentric granular and globular pigmentation in this 0.6 mm thick SSM.

Consider excision for the solitary melanocytic lesion with eccentric grey pigmentation.

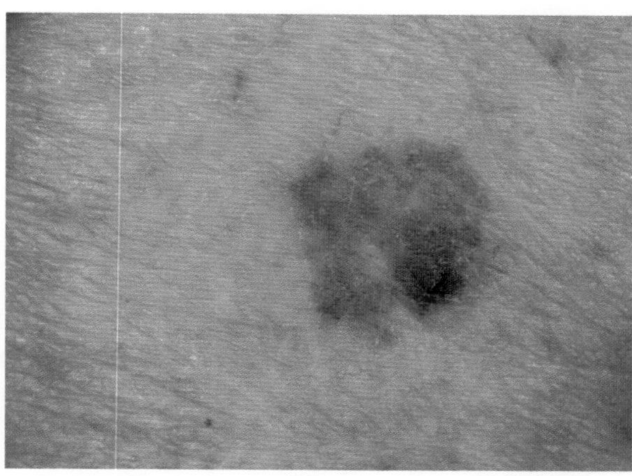

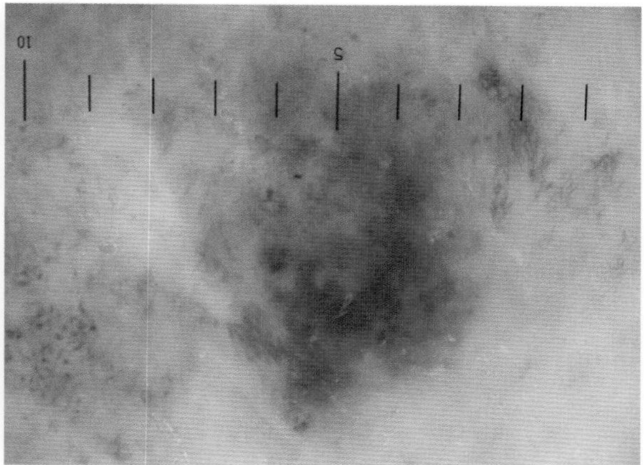

An irregularly pigmented macule on the back of a 70-year-old man: dermoscopy shows an eccentric focus of grey granular globular pigmentation and irregular globules in this 0.4 mm thick SSM.

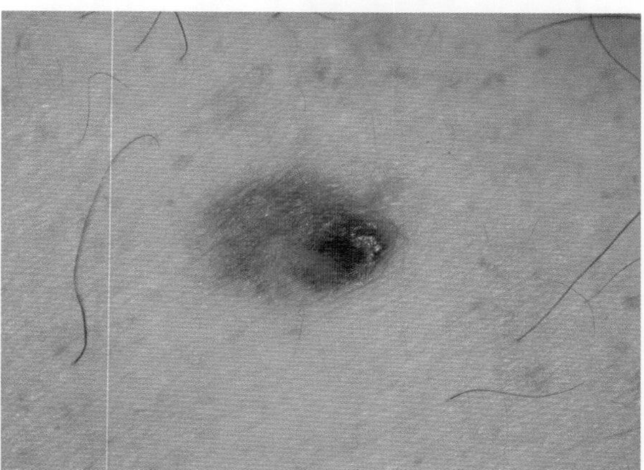

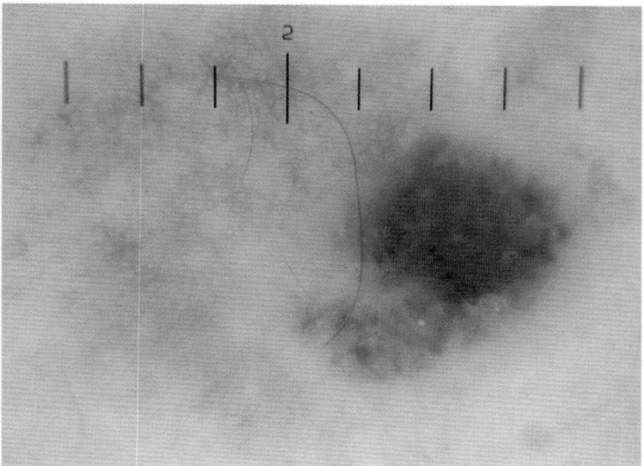

An irregularly pigmented plaque on the back of a 60-year-old man: dermoscopy shows an eccentric blotch of grey granular and structureless pigment in this 0.5 mm thick SSM.

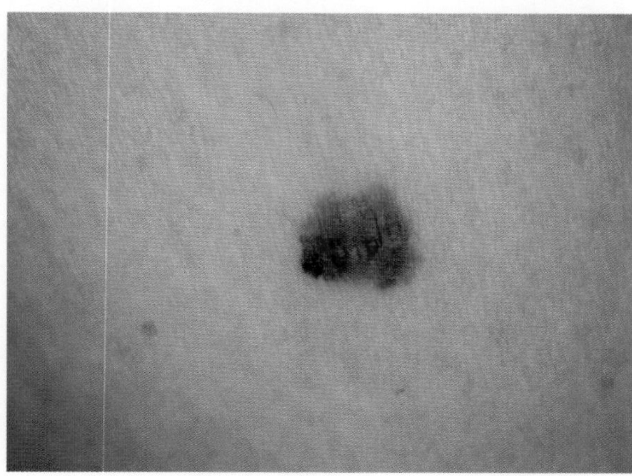

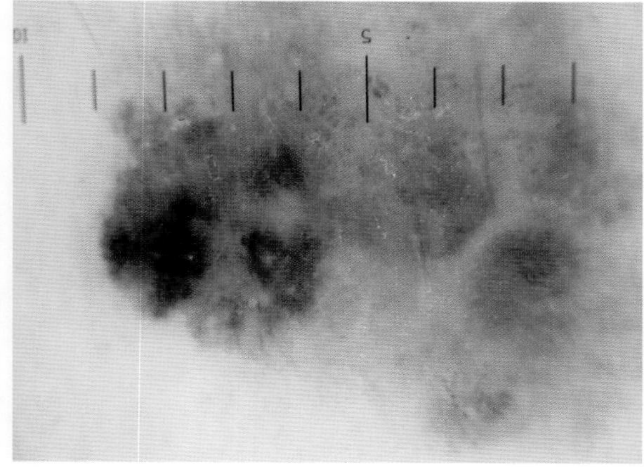

An irregularly pigmented plaque on the arm of a 30-year-old woman: dermoscopy shows multiple foci of irregular brown and black pigmentation and a large focus of grey structureless and globular pigmentation in this 0.9 mm thick SSM.

Grey granular pigmentation (otherwise known as 'peppering') is often indicative of regression correlating with melanophages in the upper papillary dermis.

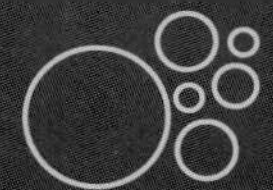

Angulated lines

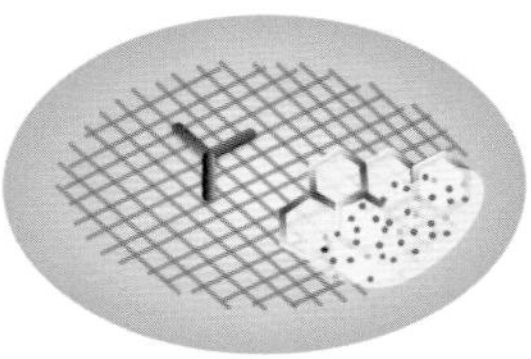

When lentigo maligna (LM) occurs on non-facial skin, it tends to lack the typical features of facial LM. This is due to the reduction in the density of follicular units and the increase in contours at the dermoepidermal junction on non-facial skin. This subtype of melanoma is more common in the elderly with a high degree of photodamage. Angulated lines are a feature that may be seen in LM, lentiginous melanoma and SSM.

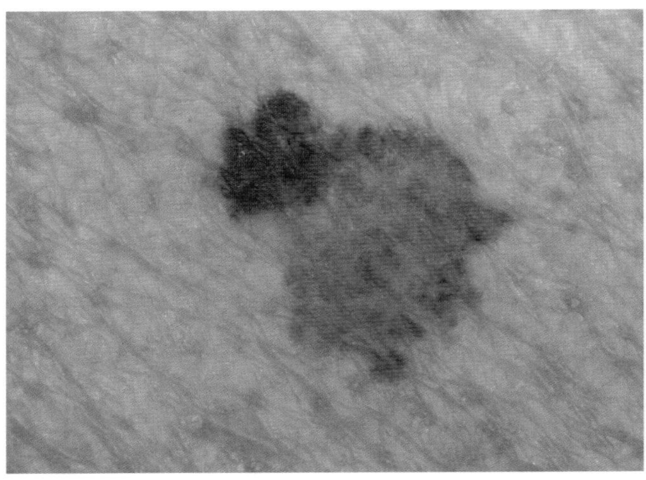

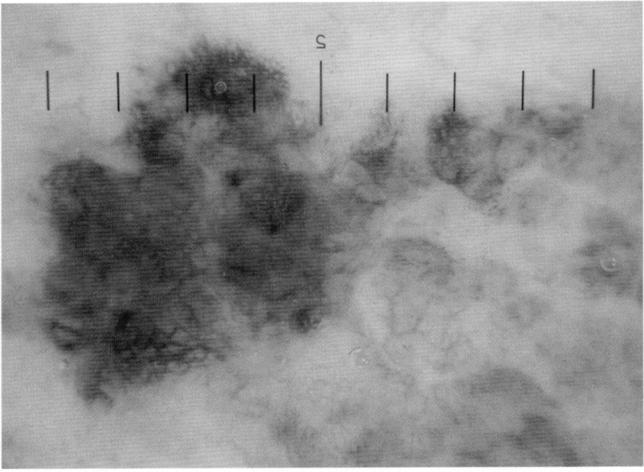

Irregularly pigmented macule with eccentric hyper pigmentation on the upper back of an 85-year-old man: dermoscopy shows irregular reticular pigmentation and structureless areas with angulated lines in this extrafacial lentigo maligna.

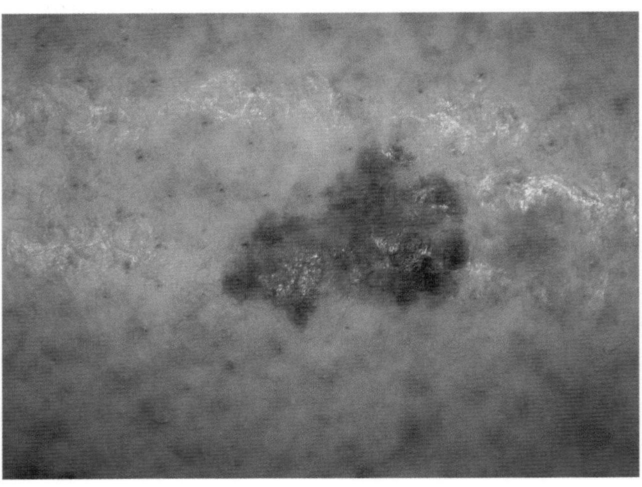

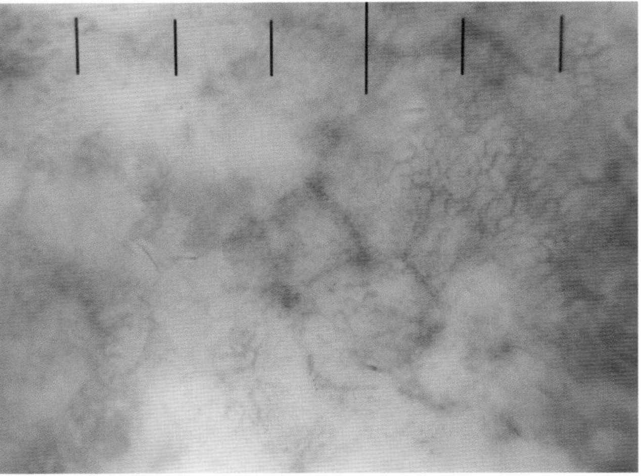

A variably pigmented patch on the upper shin of a 70-year-old woman: dermoscopy shows granular grey pigmented angulated lines (forming polygonal structures) and background reticular pigmentation in a lentiginous MIS.

Angulated lines can also be referred to as polygonal structures, zig-zag lines or rhomboidal structures.

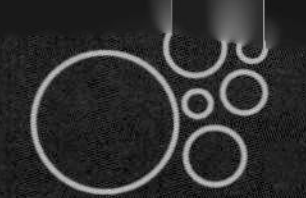

Angulated lines cases

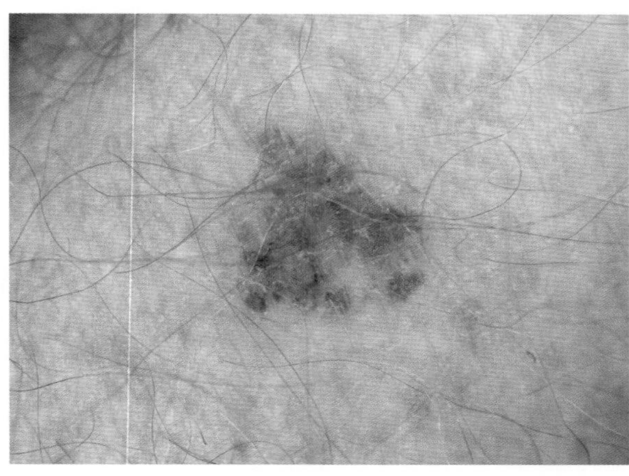

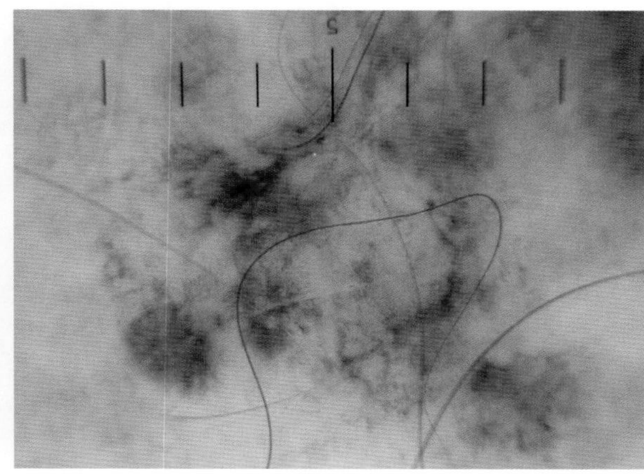

A variably pigmented macule on the lower leg: dermoscopy shows angulated lines with irregular skin surface markings in this lentiginous MIS.

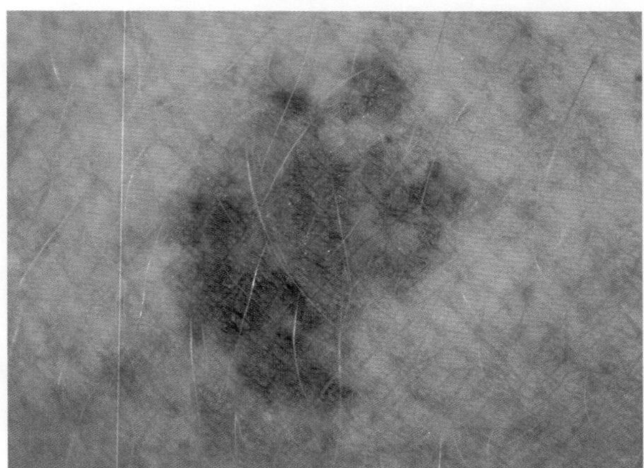

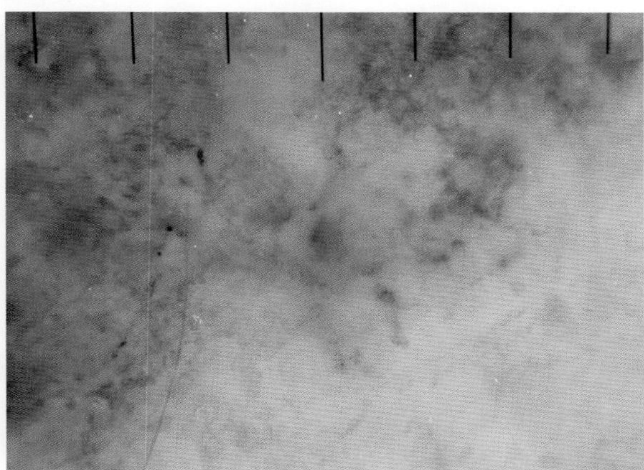

A variably pigmented patch on the thigh: dermoscopy shows angulated lines of granular grey pigmentation in this lentiginous MIS.

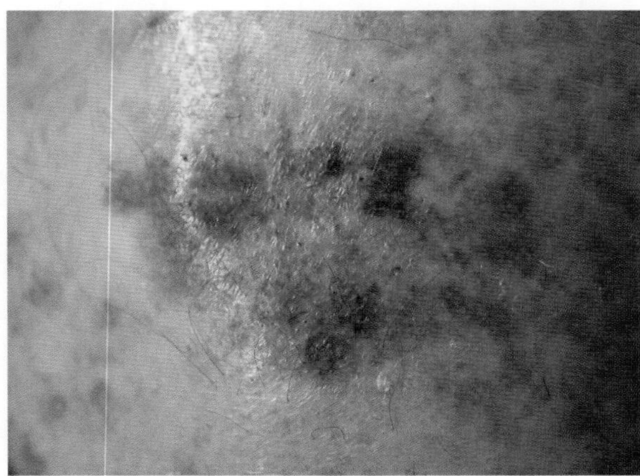

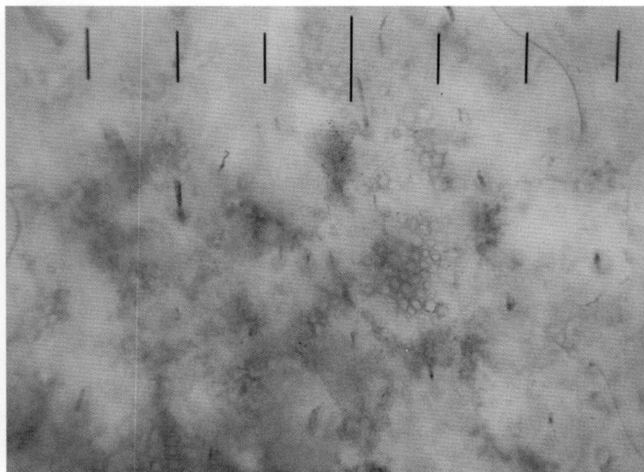

A variably pigmented patch on the vertex of the scalp: dermoscopy shows multiple angulated grey granular lines creating polygonal structureless areas in this lentiginous MIS.

Multiple angulated lines create polygonal structures indicative of melanoma of a lentiginous subtype arising on chronically sun-damaged skin.

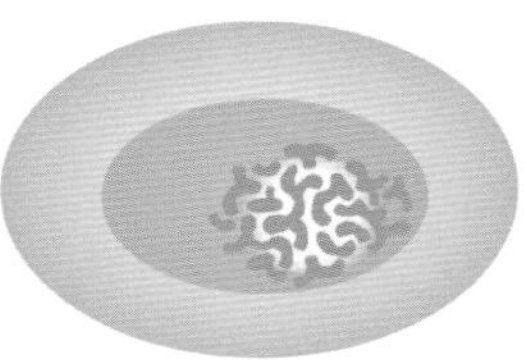

A negative or 'inverse' network may be seen in melanomas and Spitz naevi. It comprises depigmented lines or cords that intersect separating islands of globular and ovoid pigment. Rarely it may be the sole dermoscopic feature indicating melanoma. A histopathological correlate is difficult to establish but may represent thick and elongated rete ridges with hyperkeratosis/hypergranulosis and dermal fibrosis.

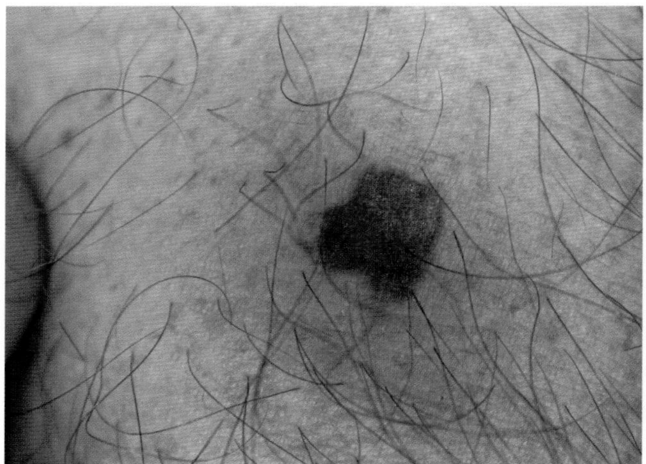

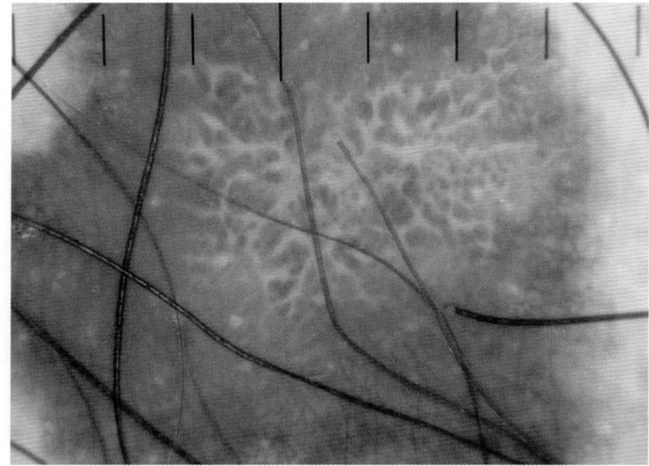

An angulated hyperpigmented macule in a 60-year-old man: dermoscopy shows a clear focus of a negative network in this MIS.

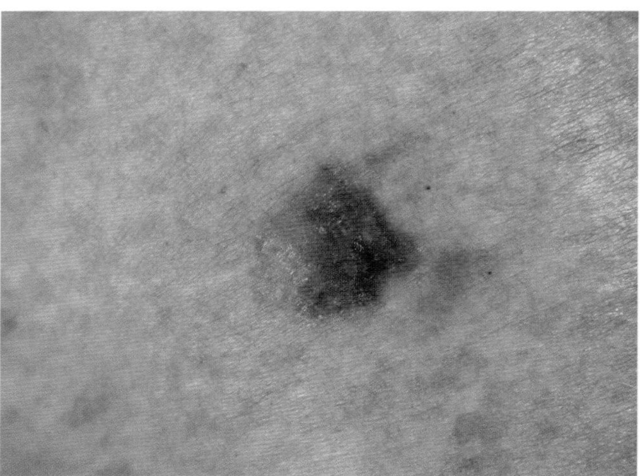

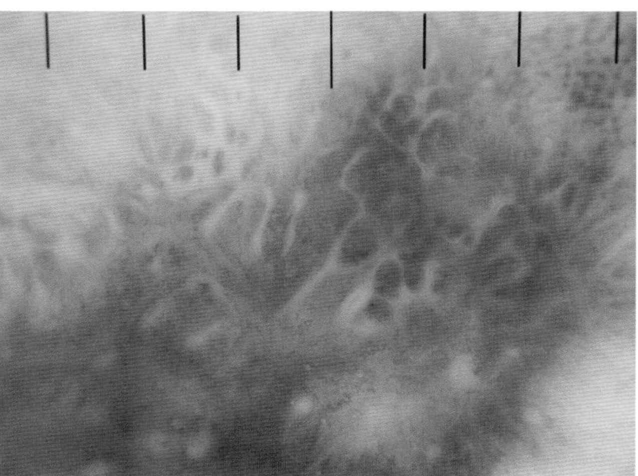

An angulated pigmented plaque on the upper back of a 60-year-old man: dermoscopy shows a clear negative network outlining the pigmented globules and ovoid structures, irregular pigmentation and atypical vessels in this 0.8 mm thick SSM.

Russo, T. et al. Dermoscopy pathology correlation in melanoma. *J Dermatol*. 2017;44(5):507–514.

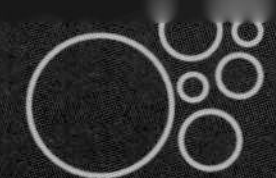

Negative network cases

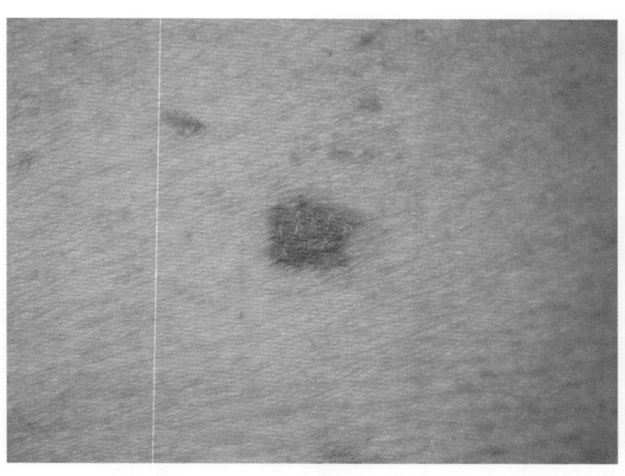

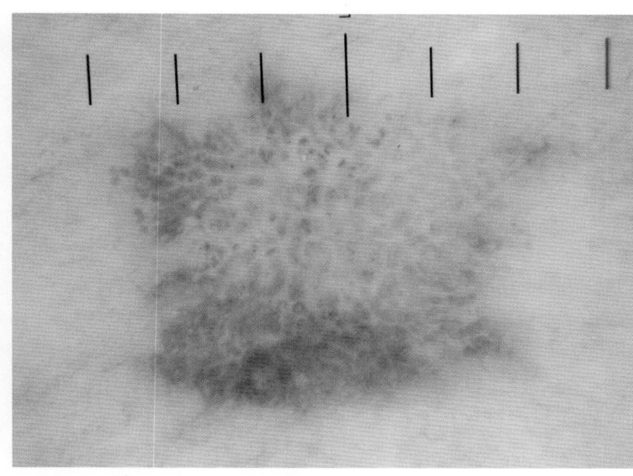

A tan macule on the lower back of a 70-year-old woman: dermoscopy shows a negative network across most of this MIS.

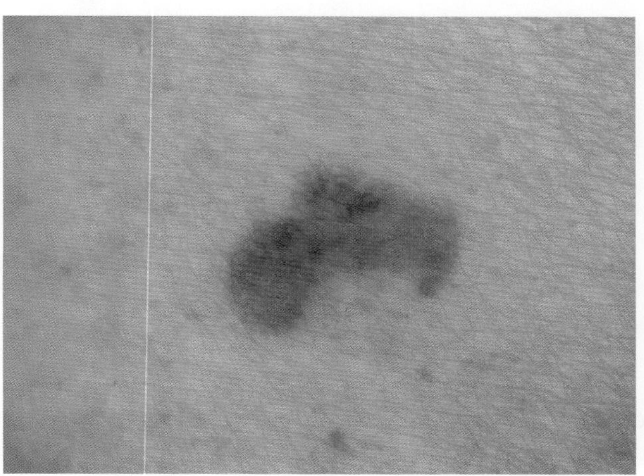

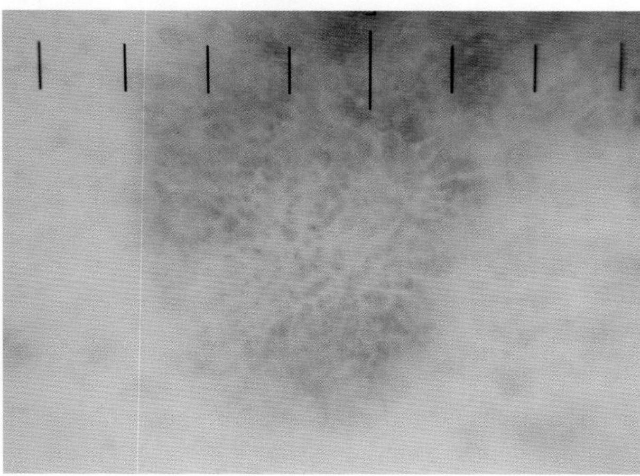

An irregularly shaped pigmented pink-brown macule on the thigh of a 60-year-old woman: dermoscopy shows widespread negative network in this MIS.

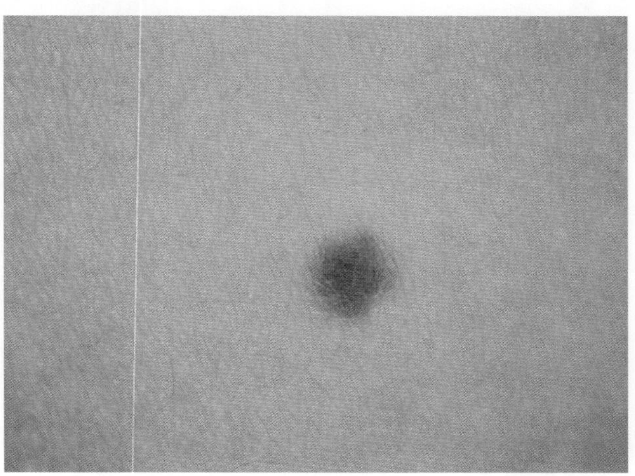

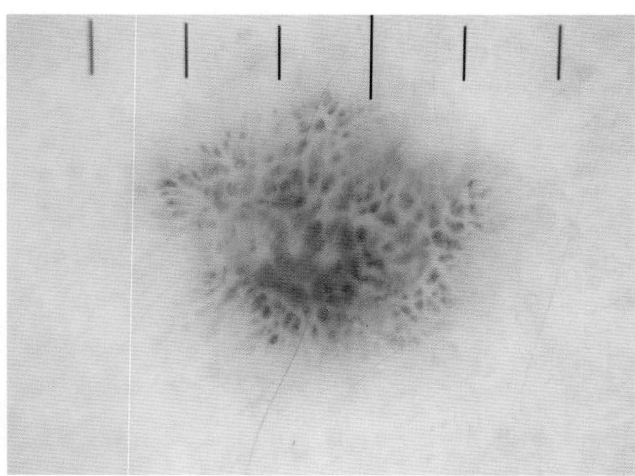

A tan pigmented macule on the shoulder of a 40-year-old woman: dermoscopy shows a negative network in this 0.5 mm thick SSM.

Inspect small pink-tan macules cautiously for subtle clues of melanoma such as a negative network.

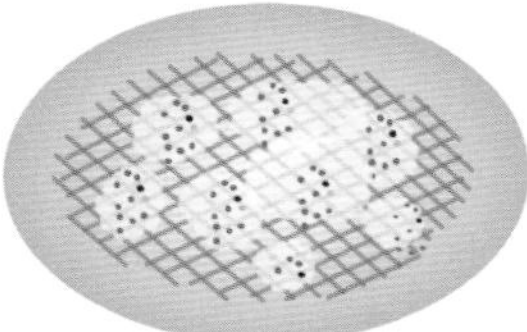

Regression in melanoma may be focal or extensive. On dermoscopy, characteristic white areas with a pink hue and blue-grey granular pigmentation ('peppering') are typically seen. Regression is an active immunological response that is sometimes complete only leaving tumoral melanosis. Early regression may show a disruption of typical dermoscopic structures and late regression may show complete destruction of any residual dermoscopic features with scar formation.

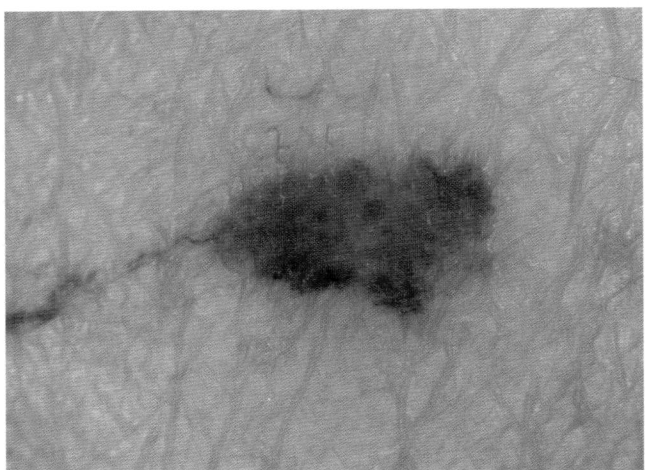

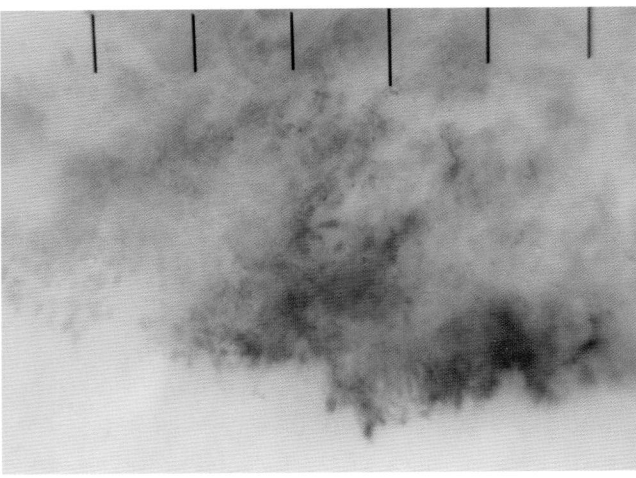

An irregularly pigmented macule on the upper back of an 80-year-old man: dermoscopy shows extensive blue-grey granules in a pink-white structureless areas surrounded by residual pigment structures in this MIS.

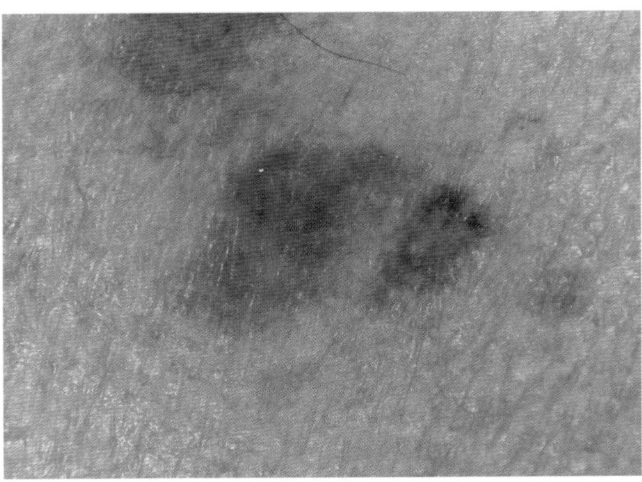

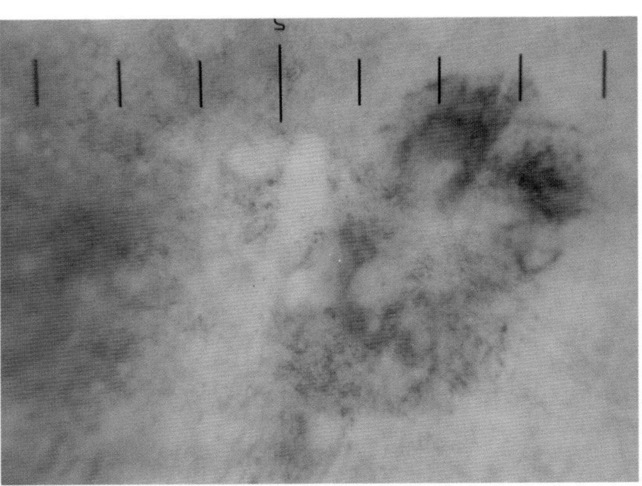

An irregularly pigmented macule on the upper arm of a 70-year-old man: dermoscopy shows a diffuse grey granular pigmentation and residual atypical network in this MIS.

Aung, PP. et al. Regression in primary cutaneous melanoma: aetiopathogenesis and clinical significance. *Lab Invest*. 2017; 97:657–668.

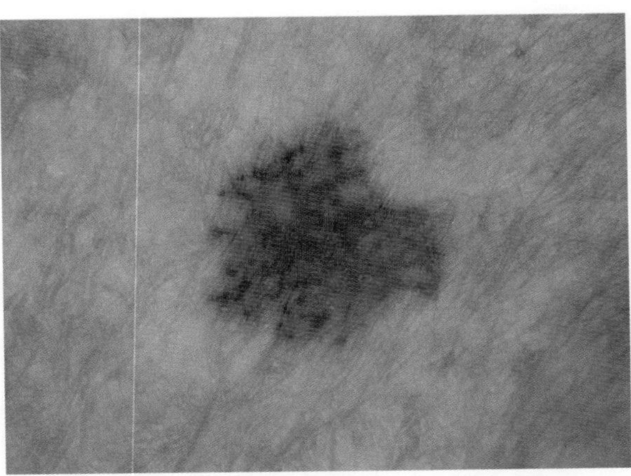

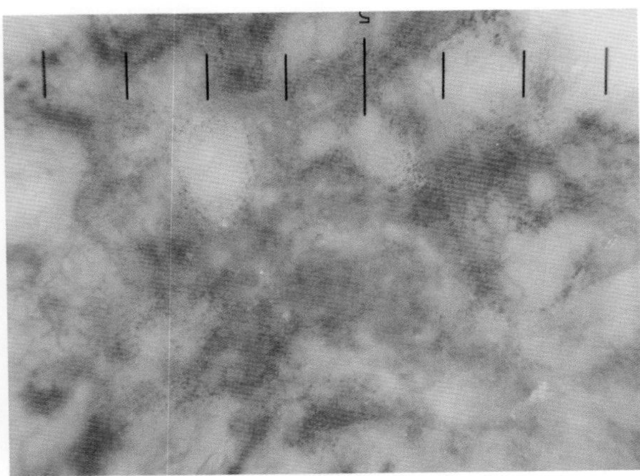

A multicoloured macule on the chest of an 80-year-old woman: dermoscopy shows a widespread grey granular and tan pigmentation with extensive regression on histopathology in this MIS.

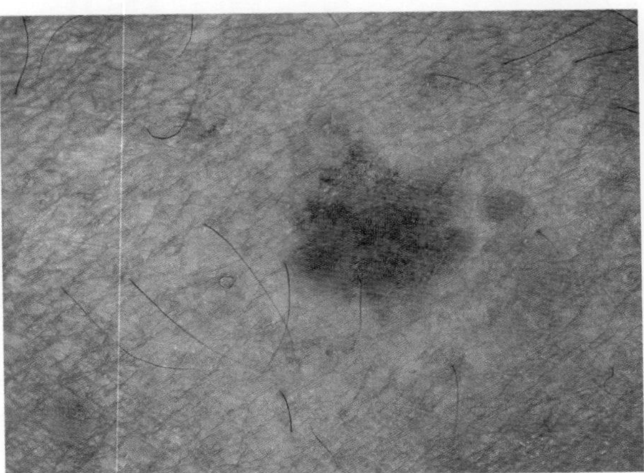

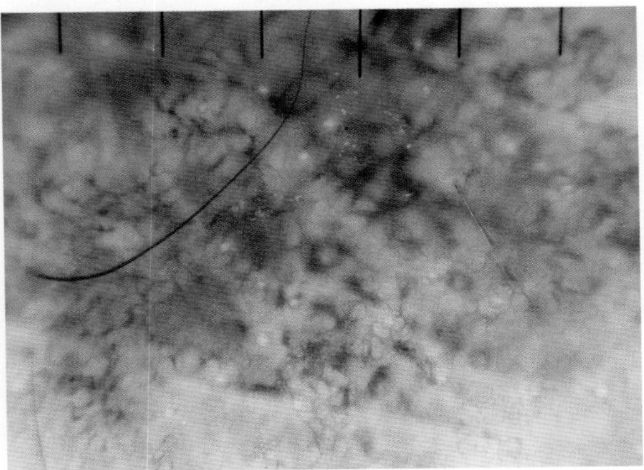

An irregularly pigmented macule on the leg of a 70-year-old man: dermoscopy shows multifocal grey granules and polygonal structures with extensive regression on histopathology in this 0.2 mm thick LM.

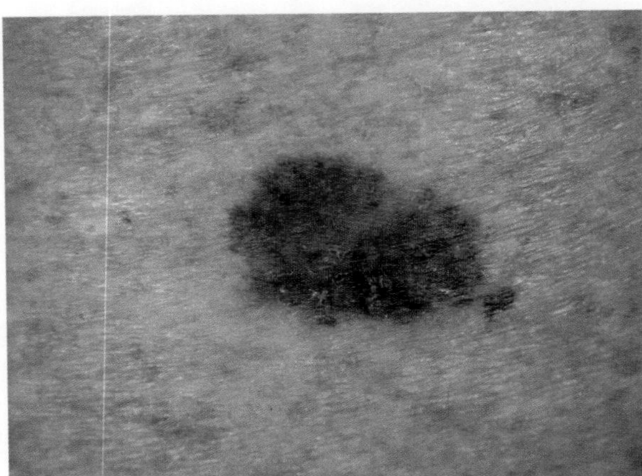

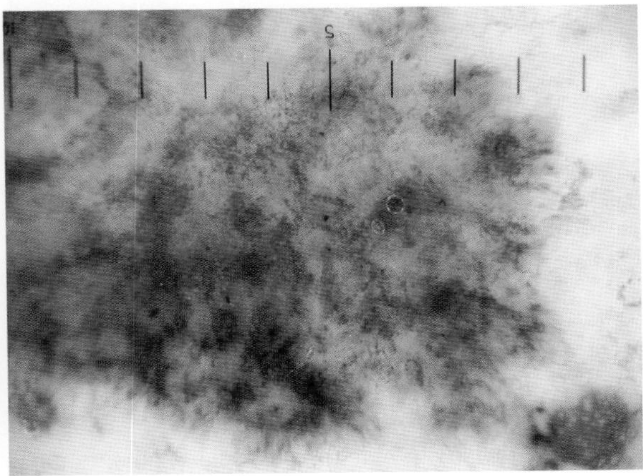

A hyperpigmented macule on the shoulder of an 80-year-old man: dermoscopy shows widespread hyperpigmented grey granular pigmentation with extensive regression on histopathology in this 0.4 mm thick SSM.

Widespread regression can create hyperpigmented grey granular pigmentation along with pale structureless scar-like zones.

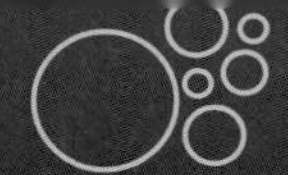

Focal regression

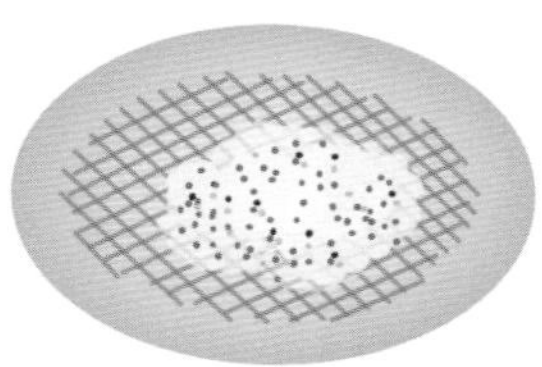

Regression in melanoma may be focal and more obvious in a specific area of the lesion. Dermoscopy reveals hypopigmentation or scar-like areas with variable erythema and/or peppering.

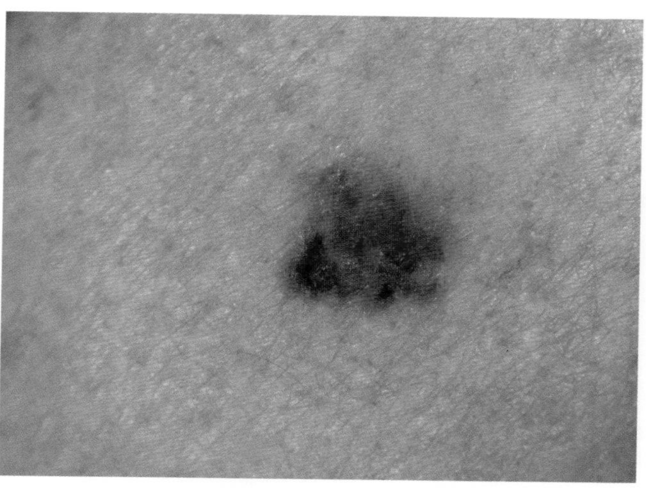

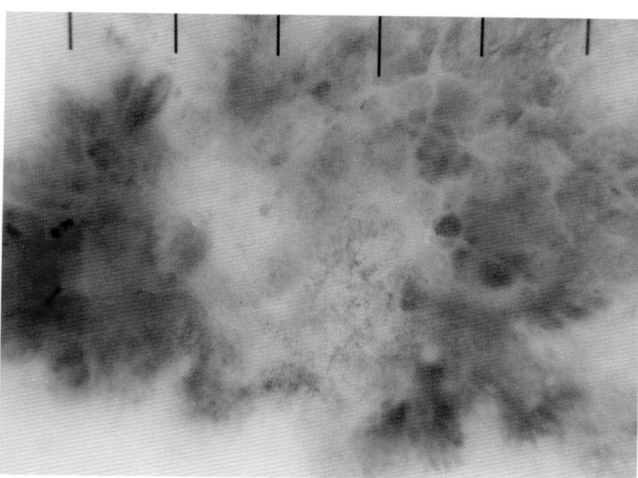

An irregularly pigmented macule on the upper arm of a 70-year-old woman: dermoscopy shows negative network, irregular globules, streaks and blotches plus central focal regression with grey-blue granular pigmentation in this 0.4 mm thick SSM.

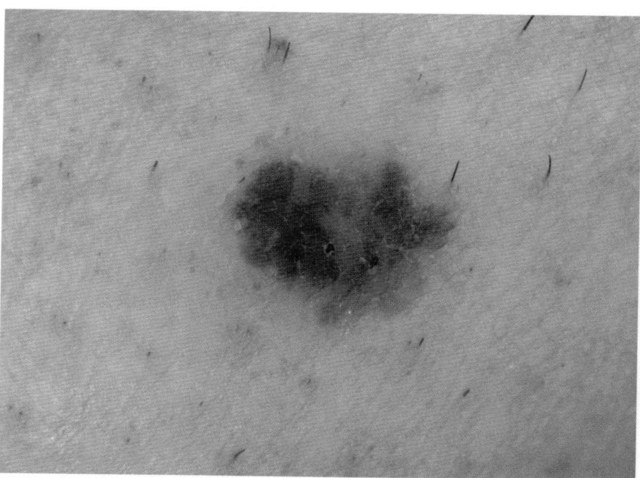

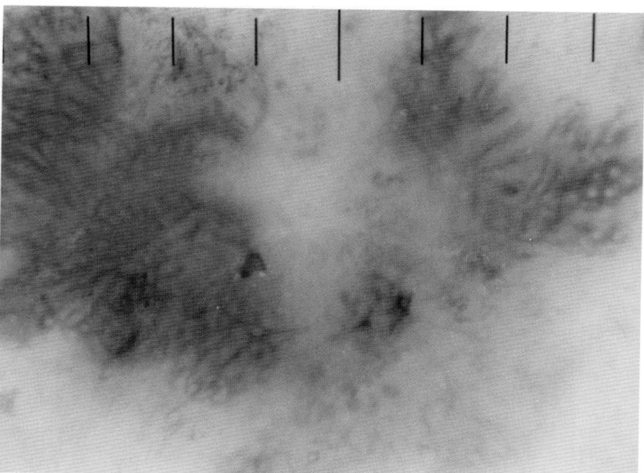

An irregularly pigmented macule on the lower leg of a 50-year-old woman: dermoscopy shows atypical pigment network and central focal regression with blue-grey granular pigmentation in this 0.4 mm thick SSM.

Moscarella, E. et al. Pigmented skin lesions displaying regression features: Dermoscopy and reflectance confocal microscopy criteria for diagnosis. *Exp Dermatol*. 2019;28(2):129–135.

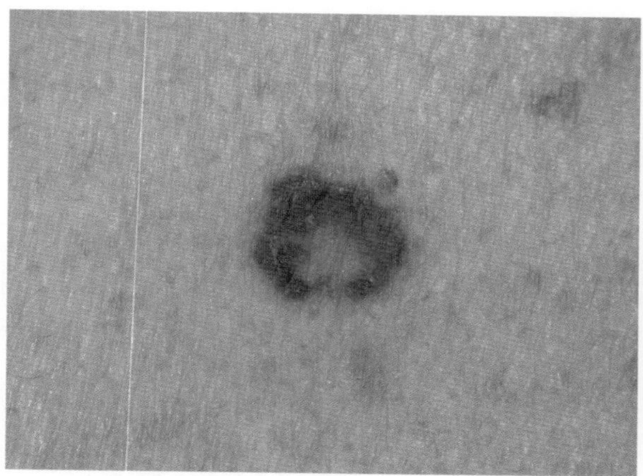

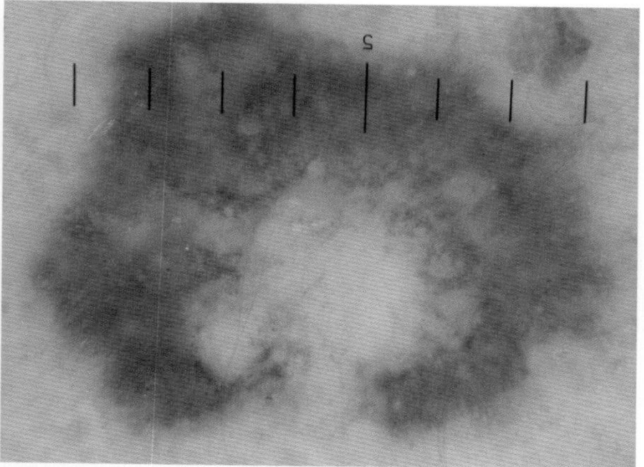

Annular pigmented macule on the back of a 70-year-old man: dermoscopy shows a focal hypopigmented structureless area with grey granular pigmentation in this MIS.

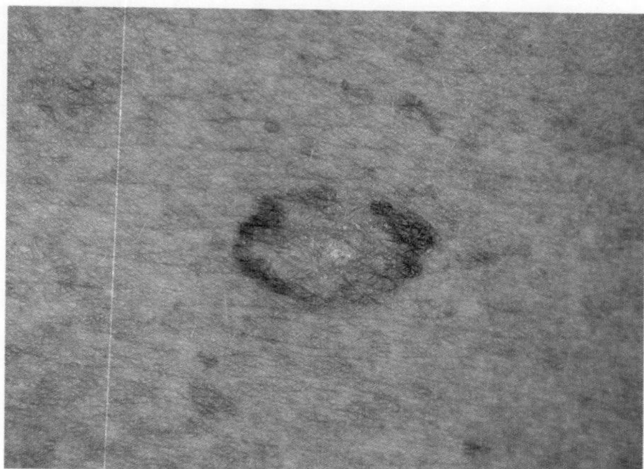

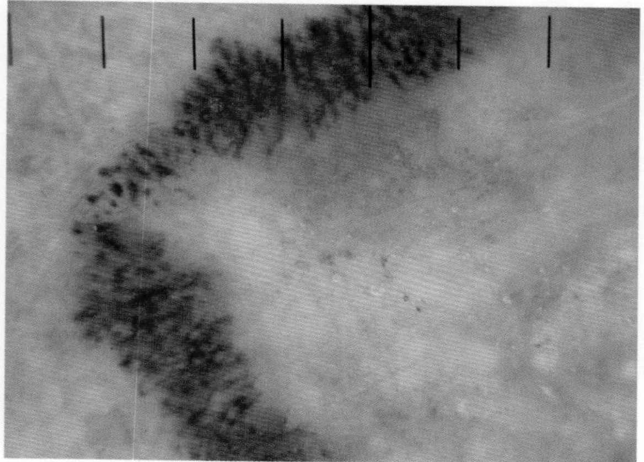

Annular hyperpigmented macule on the chest of a 60-year-old woman: dermoscopy shows peripheral irregular globular-reticular pigmentation with central structureless pink and subtle grey peppering in this 0.3 mm thick SSM.

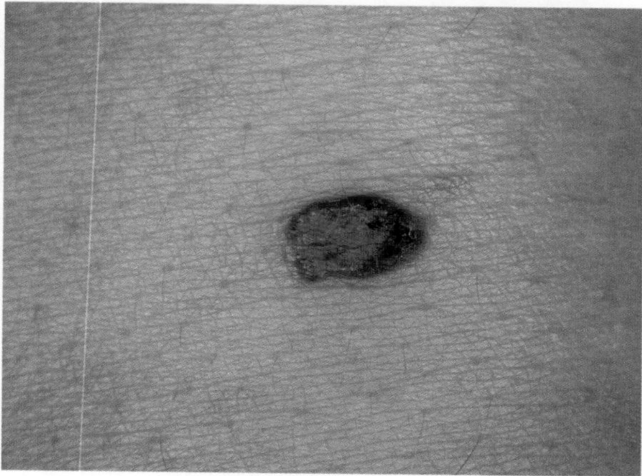

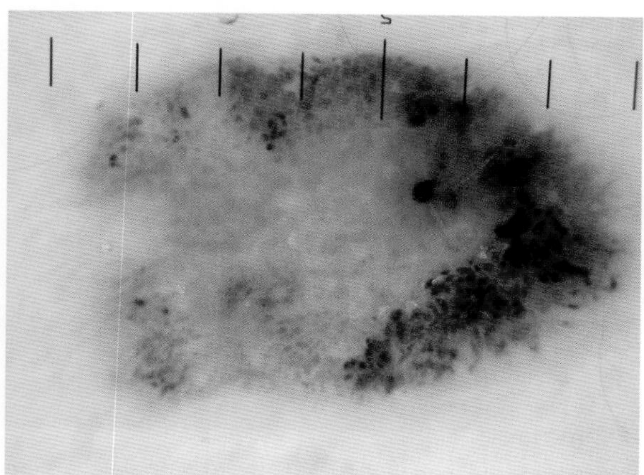

A hyperpigmented macule on the shoulder of a 50-year-old woman: dermoscopy shows peripheral pigmented globules and streaks and central structureless pink and grey granular pigmentation in this 0.6 mm thick SSM.

Using polarised dermoscopy, regressed lesions can show shiny white lines which is a marker of remodelled dermal collagen.

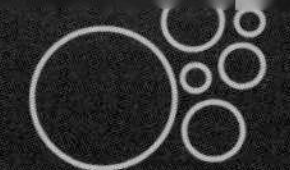

Blue-whitish veil

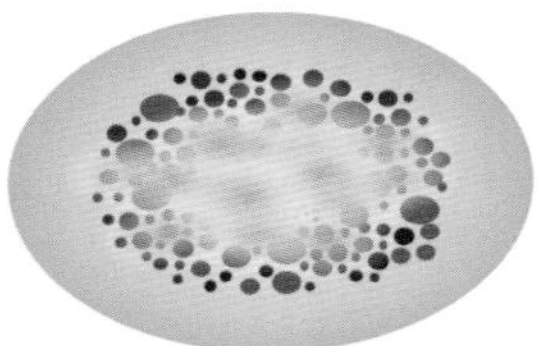

The presence of a blue-whitish veil in a melanocytic lesion is highly indicative of a diagnosis of invasive melanoma. The histopathologic correlate of a blue-whitish veil is an acanthotic epidermis with compact orthokeratosis overlying heavy dermal pigment.

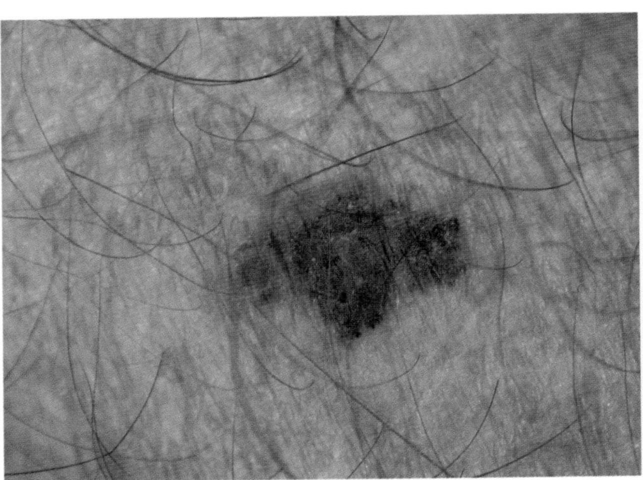

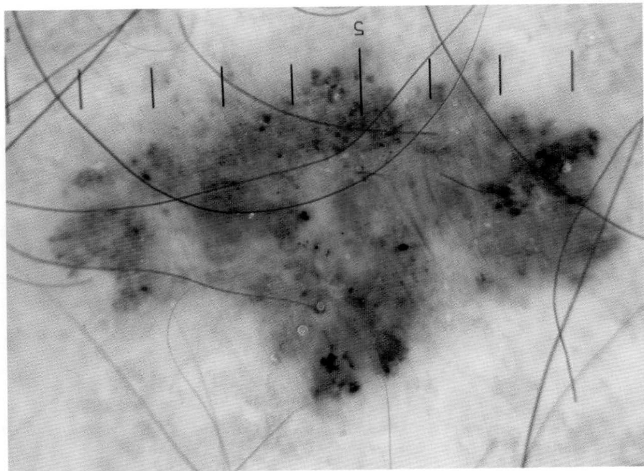

A hyperpigmented macule on the forearm of a 50-year-old man: dermoscopy shows a disordered multicoloured lesion with multiple hyperpigmented globules and a central blue-whitish veil in this 0.4 mm Breslow SSM.

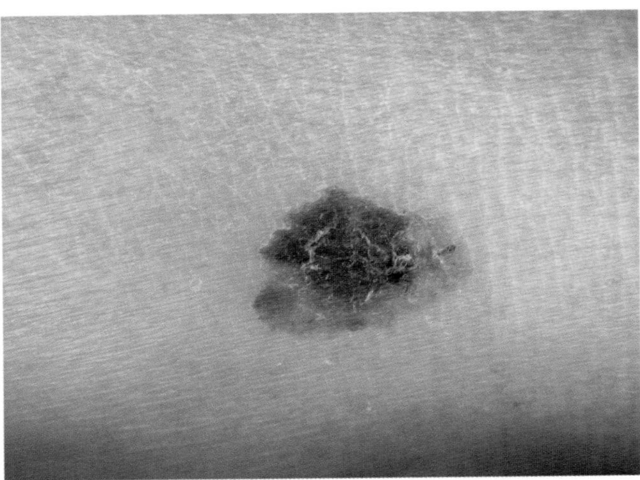

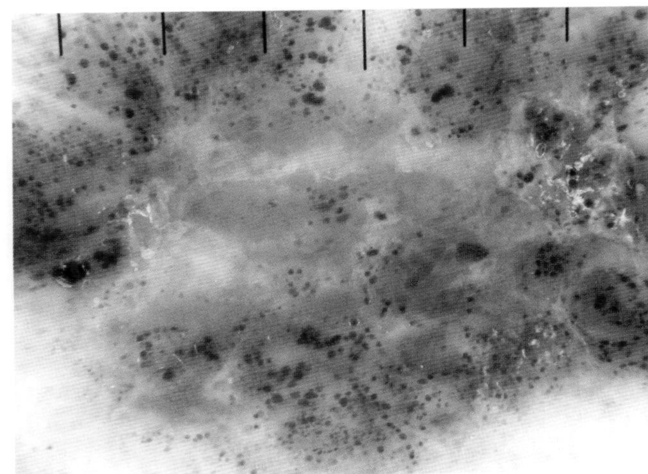

A variably pigmented macule on the ankle of a 60-year-old woman: dermoscopy shows multiple irregular globules, background erythema and a central blue-whitish veil in this 0.8 mm thick SSM.

Massi, D. et al. Diagnostic significance of the blue hue in dermoscopy of melanocytic lesions: a dermoscopic-pathologic study. *Am J Dermatopathol.* 2001;23(5):463–469.

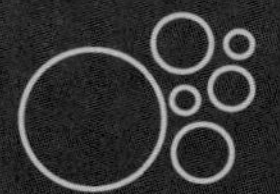

Blue-whitish veil cases

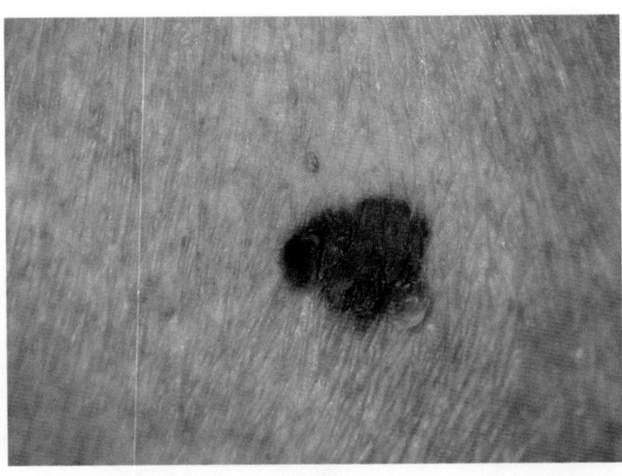

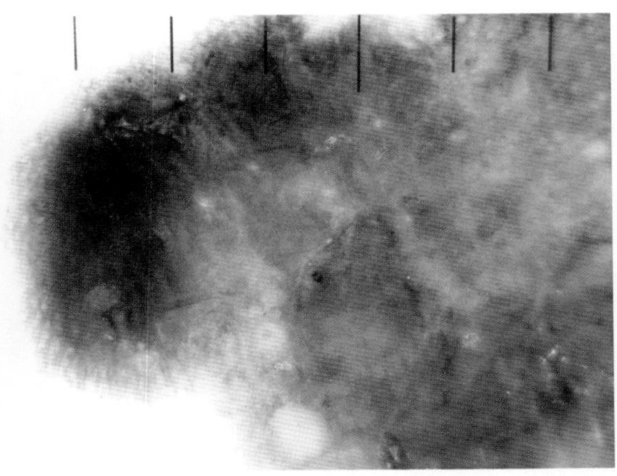

Hyperpigmented macule on the back of a 70-year-old man: dermoscopy shows irregular pigmentation and a blue-whitish veil in this 0.2 mm thick SSM.

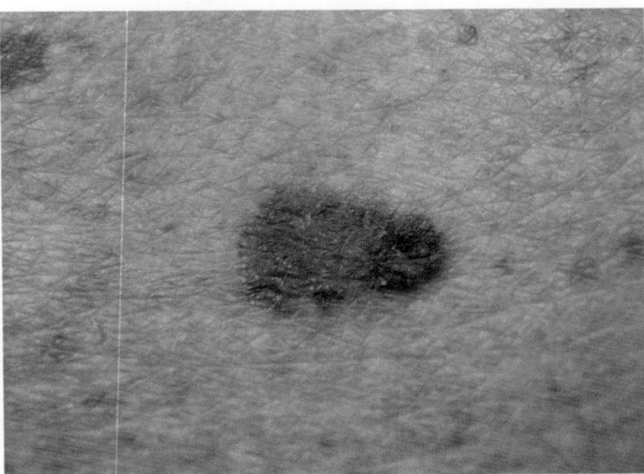

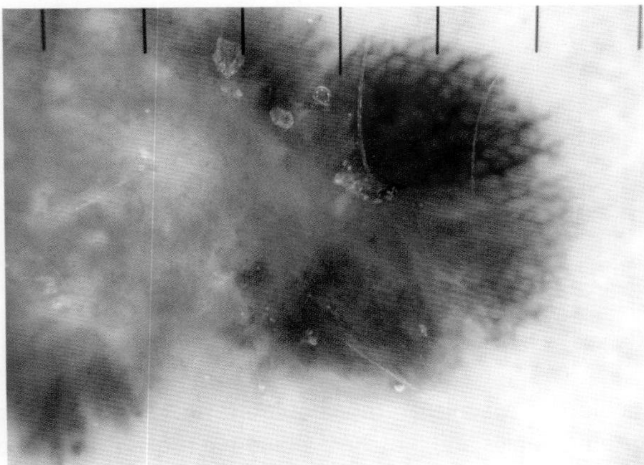

A hyperpigmented macule on the back of a 50-year-old man: dermoscopy shows irregular pigment network and a blue-whitish veil in this 0.7 mm thick SSM.

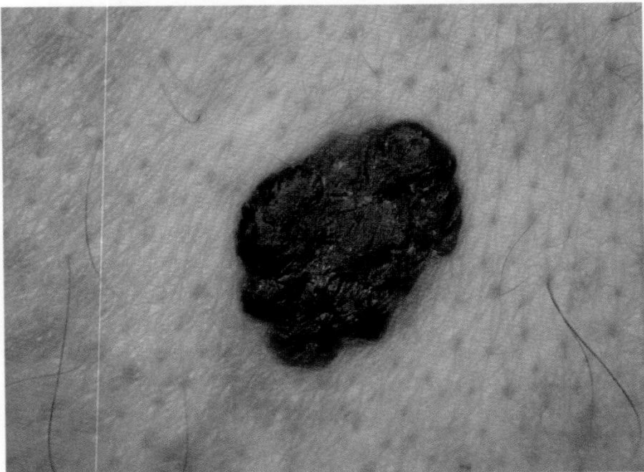

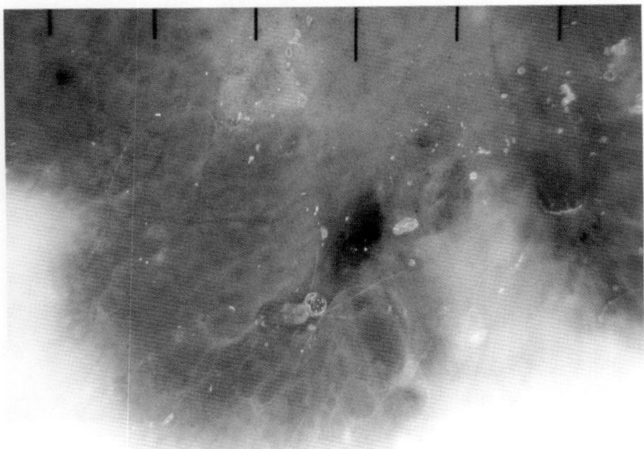

Blackened plaque on the back of a 70-year-old man: dermoscopy shows irregular pigment globules, negative network, black dots and a blue-whitish veil in this 1.2 mm thick nodular melanoma.

The blue-whitish veil in invasive melanomas usually corresponds to the area of greatest Breslow thickness. This sign is regarded as the most sensitive clue to melanoma.

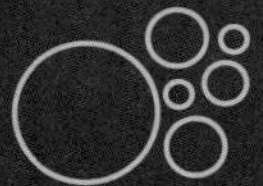

Dermal pigmentation

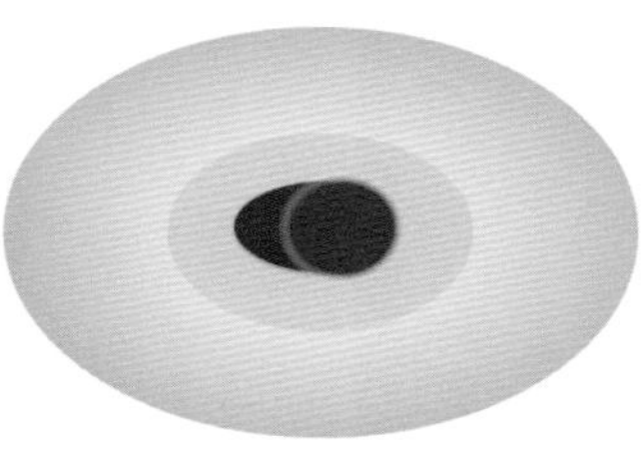

Melanomas may present with an obvious dermal component on dermoscopy. This feature of invasive melanoma should be reflected in the histopathology report.

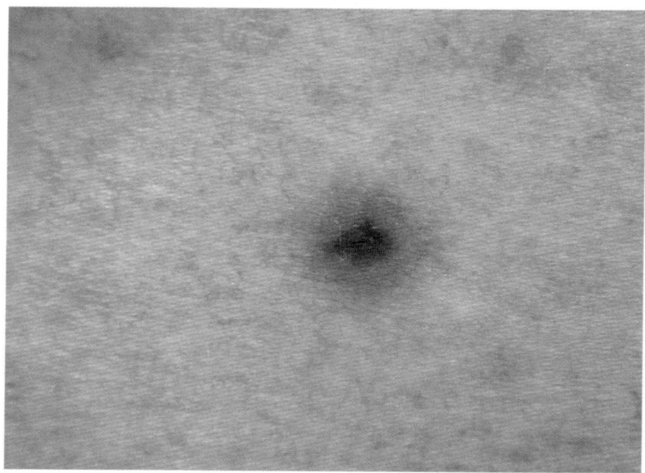

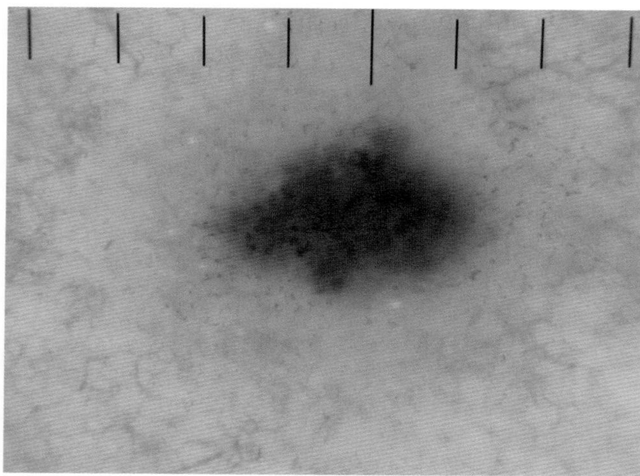

A multicoloured macule on the shoulder of a 50-year-old woman: dermoscopy shows central brown and slate blue pigmented globules and blotches, a blue-whitish veil and peripheral dotted vessels in this 0.3 mm thick SSM.

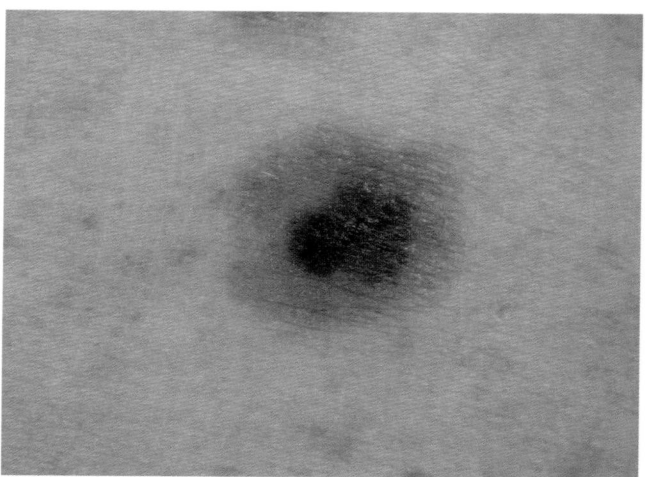

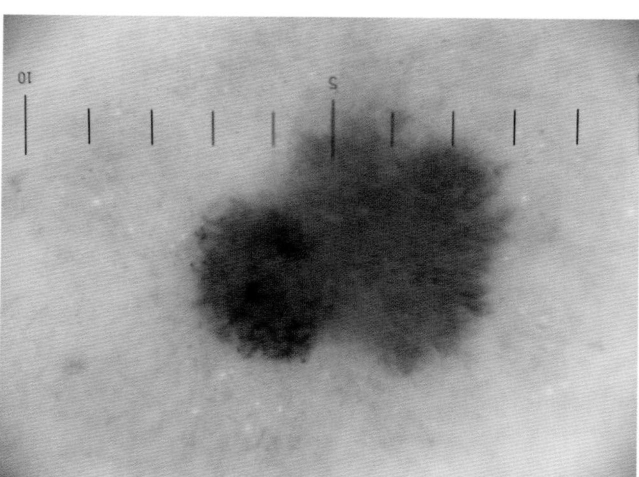

An irregularly pigmented macule on the abdomen of a 50-year-old woman: dermoscopy shows a central hyperpigmented blotch, dots and streaks, a blue-whitish veil and peripheral dotted vessels in this 0.4 mm thick SSM.

Dermal pigmentation in melanomas is blue in dermoscopy due to the Tyndall effect in which shorter-wavelength blue light is reflected back more than longer-wavelength red light.

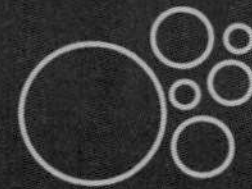

Dermal pigmentation cases

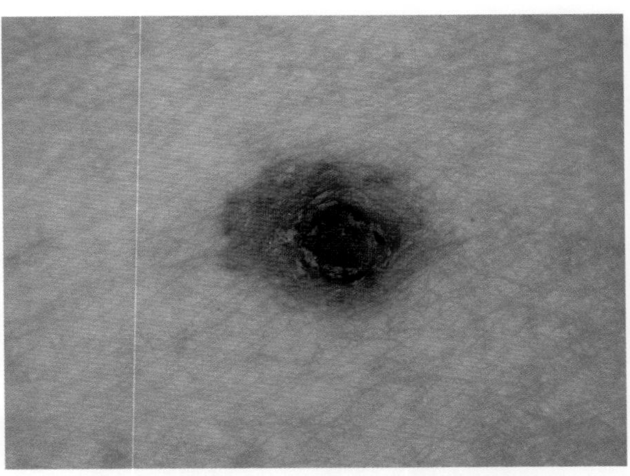

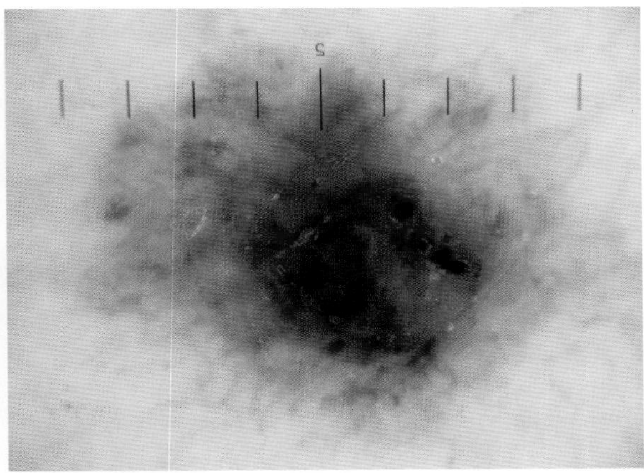

An 8 mm multicoloured macule on the back: dermoscopy shows central blue-purple irregular pigmentation corresponding to dermal pigmentation with surrounding erythema and pigment network in this 0.6 mm thick SSM.

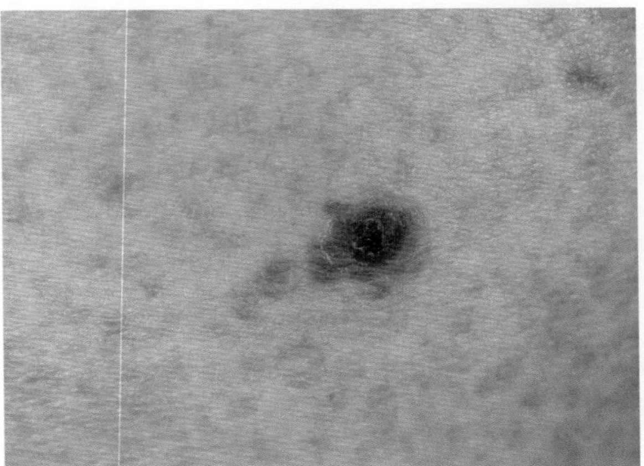

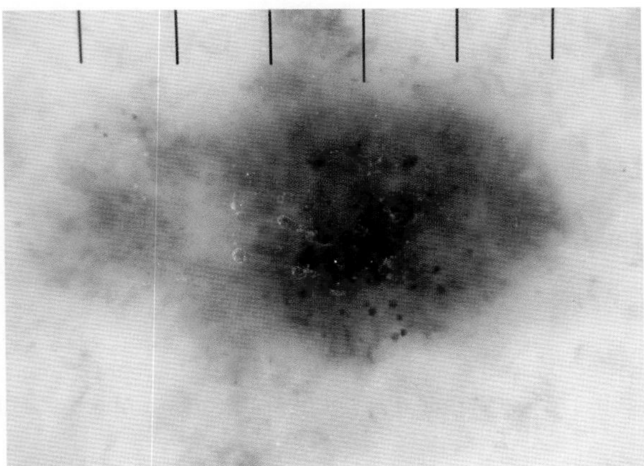

A 6 mm multicoloured centrally hyperpigmented macule on the upper arm: dermoscopy shows focal brown globules within a blue-whitish veil in this 0.8 mm Breslow SSM.

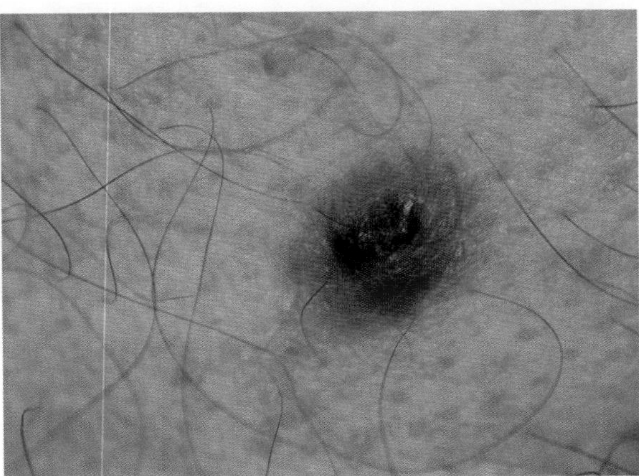

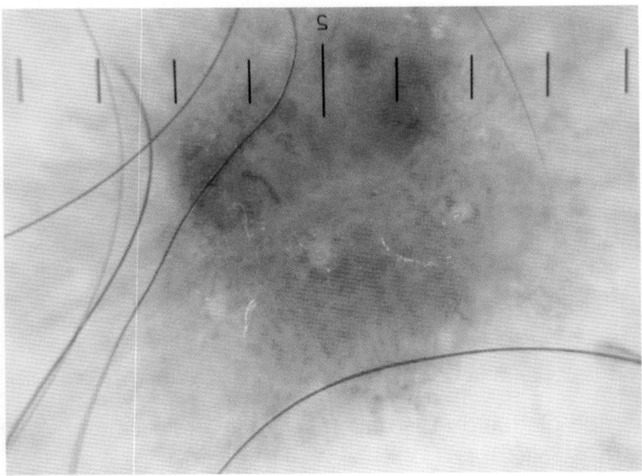

An 8 mm reddish-purple plaque on the leg: dermoscopy shows central slate blue hyperpigmentation with surrounding erythema and polymorphous vessels extending throughout this 1.8 mm thick SSM.

Central blue-purple hyperpigmentation can indicate invasive melanoma.

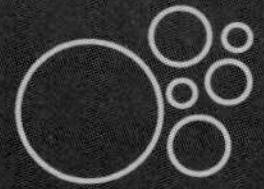

Polymorphous vessels

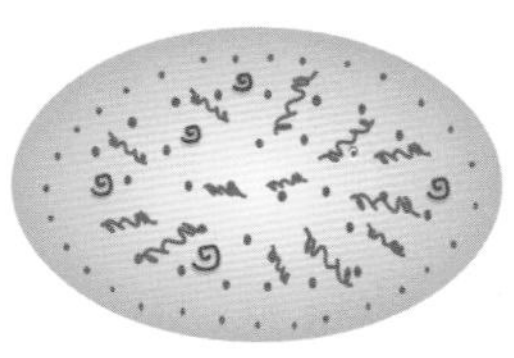

Melanomas may present with an obvious vascular component on dermoscopy. This feature of neoangiogenesis is highly indicative of invasive melanoma. Vessels in melanomas can be dotted, linear-irregular, corkscrew-like or polymorphous.

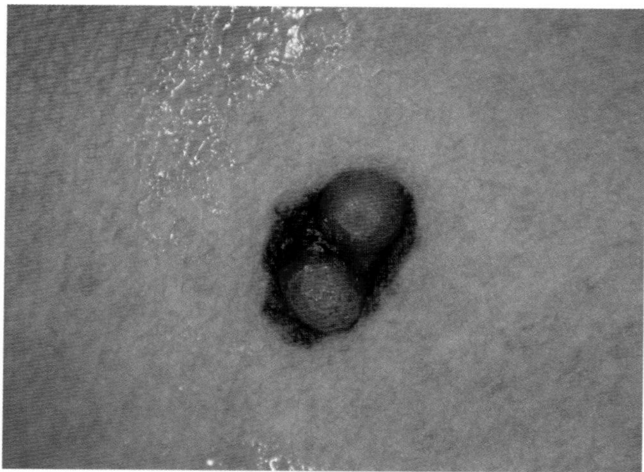

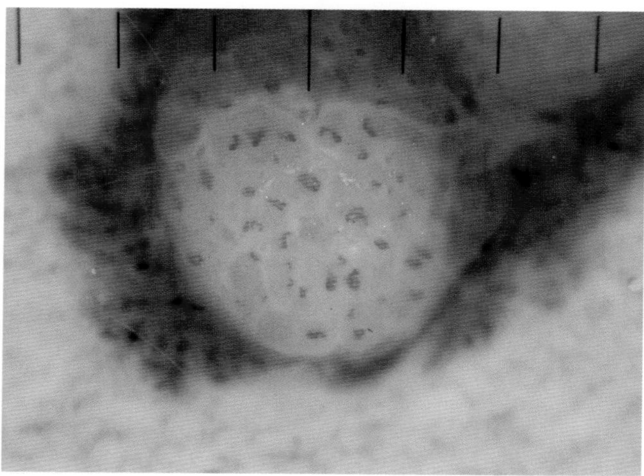

A pigmented papular plaque on the neck of a 20-year-old man: dermoscopy shows polymorphous vessels surrounded by white septae in the raised papule and peripheral pigment and black globules in this 1.8 mm SSM.

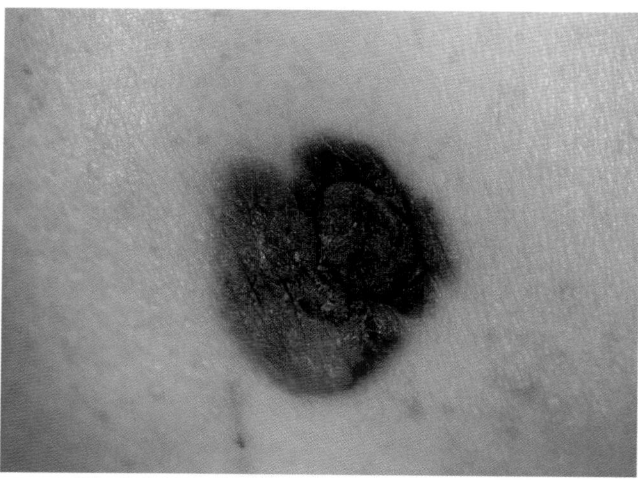

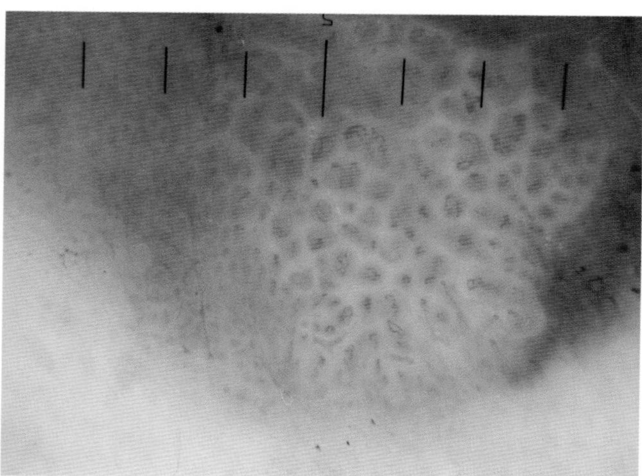

A pigmented plaque on the back of a 30-year-old woman: dermoscopy shows atypical vessels within a negative network in this 1.4 mm thick SSM.

Argenziano, G. et al. Vascular structures in skin tumours: a dermoscopy study. *Arch Dermatol* 2004;140(12):1485–1489.

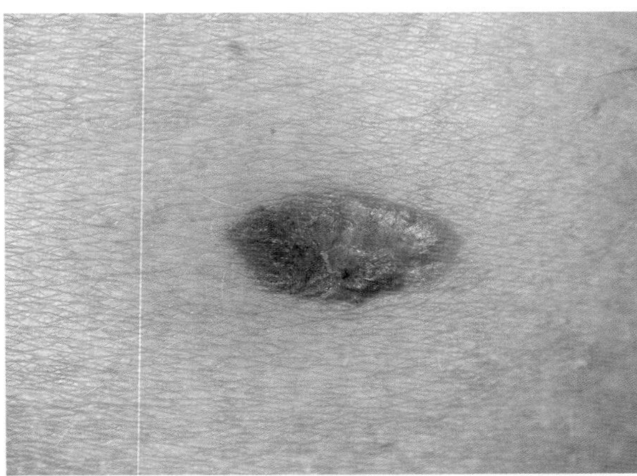
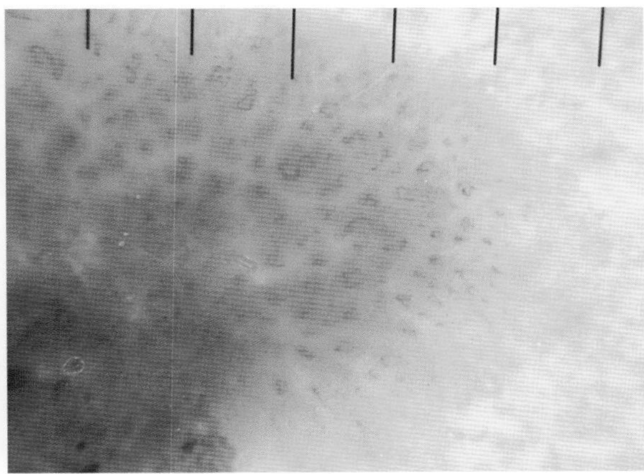

A multicoloured plaque on the upper arm: dermoscopy shows irregular pigmentation and multiple polymorphous vessels in this 1.4 mm thick SSM.

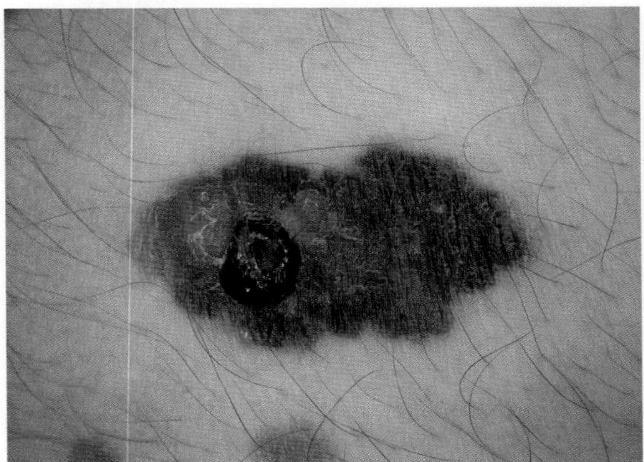
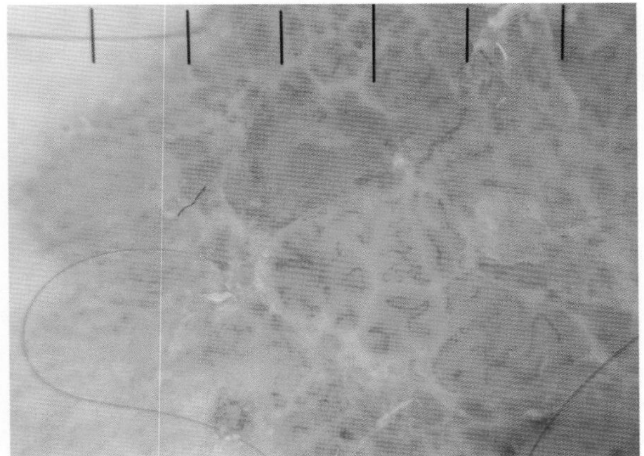

A thick multicolored melanoma on the abdomen with hyper- and hypopigmented papules: dermoscopy shows polymorphous vessels within the hypopigmented papular component in this 2.8 mm thick SSM.

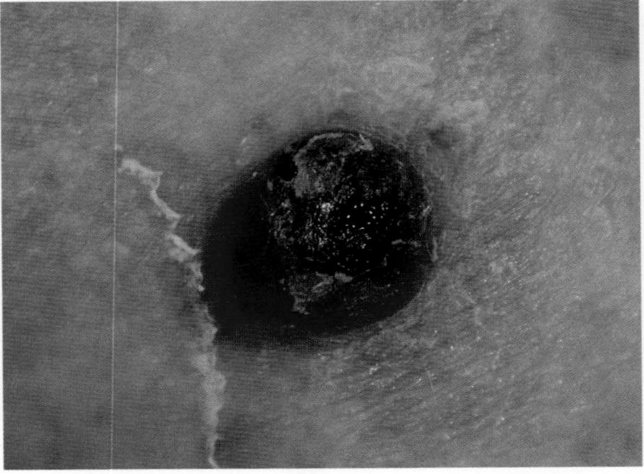
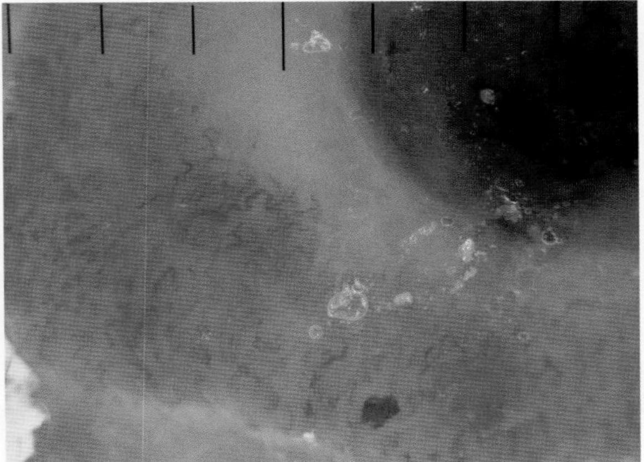

A thick ulcerated nodular melanoma on the right upper arm: dermoscopy shows multiple polymorphous vessels and central hypo- and hyperpigmentation in this 4.5 mm nodular melanoma.

Polymorphous vessels are more commonly seen in thick tumours on an erythematous or hypopigmented base.

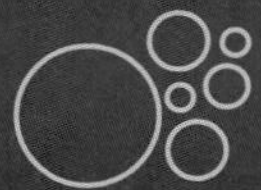

Skin surface markings

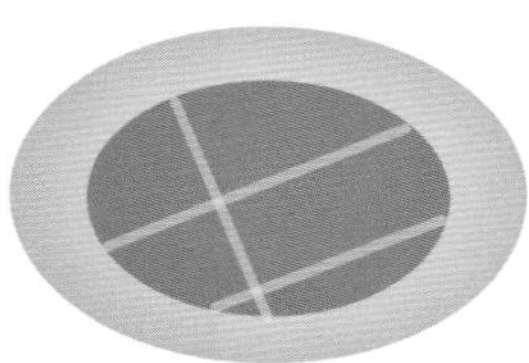

Skin surface markings (linear intersecting furrows) are frequently seen in naevi and solar lentigines. These are hypopigmented straight lines that criss-cross the skin and may run perpendicular to each other. In melanocytic lesions with either an atypical clinical appearance (ugly duckling) or with a history of change and/or symptoms, this feature should not provide false reassurance. Skin surface markings may be a feature of MIS and are lost as thicker tumours grow thicker and consume them.

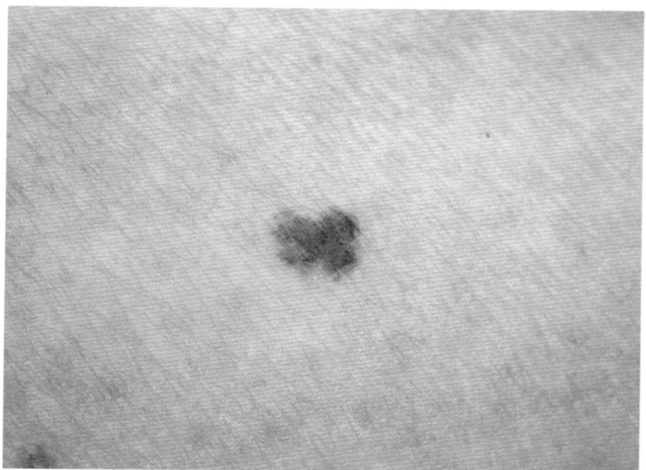

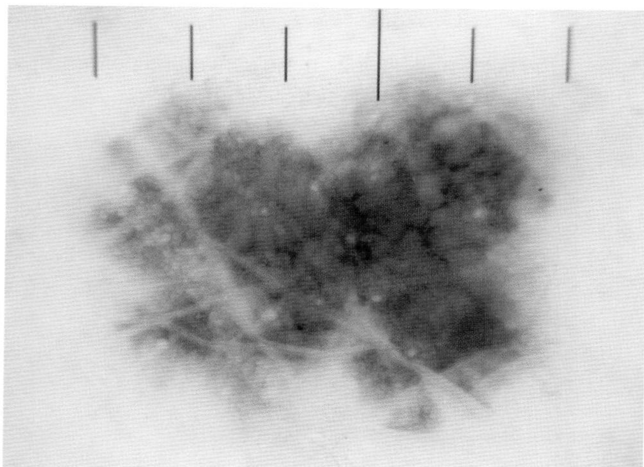

An irregularly pigmented macule on the knee of a 50-year-old woman: dermoscopy shows atypical pigment network and foci of hyperpigmentation with prominent skin surface markings in this MIS.

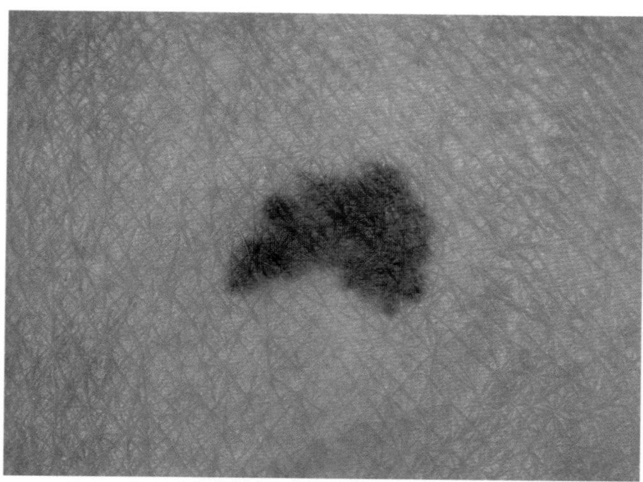

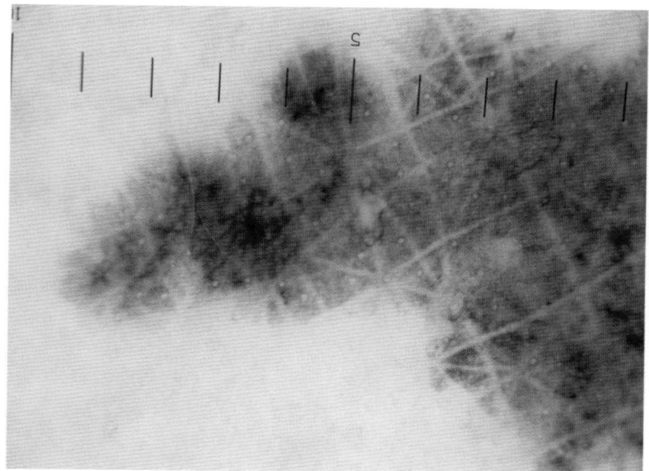

An irregularly pigmented macule on the upper arm of a 40-year-old man: dermoscopy shows an atypical pigment network and multiple skin surface markings in this MIS.

Lallas, A. et al. Accuracy of dermoscopic criteria for the diagnosis of melanoma in situ. *JAMA Dermatol.* 2018;154(4):414–419.

Skin surface markings cases

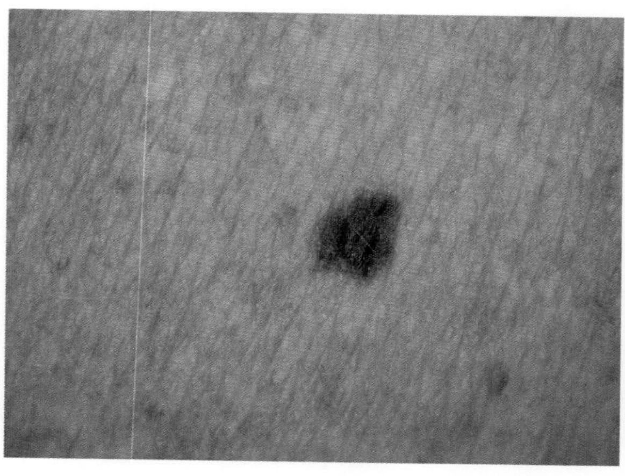

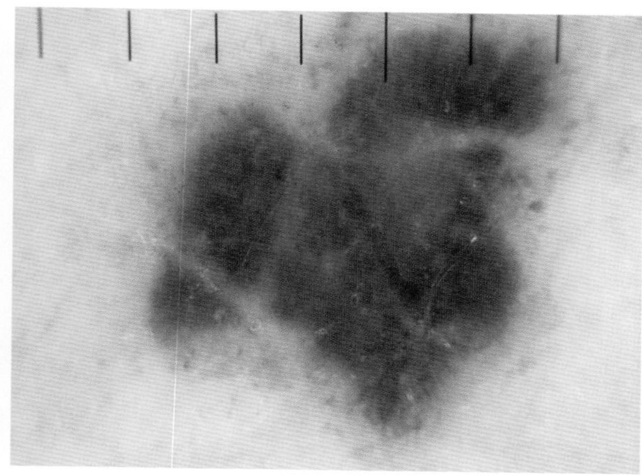

'Ugly duckling' tan macule on the back of a 70-year-old man: dermoscopy shows eccentric peripheral globules and hyperpigmented blotches separated by prominent skin surface markings in this MIS.

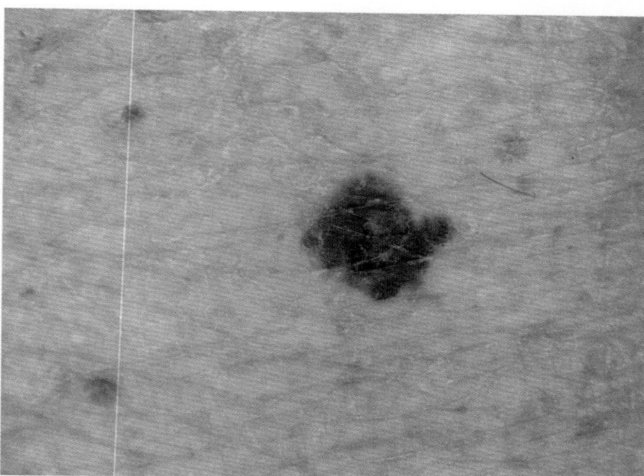

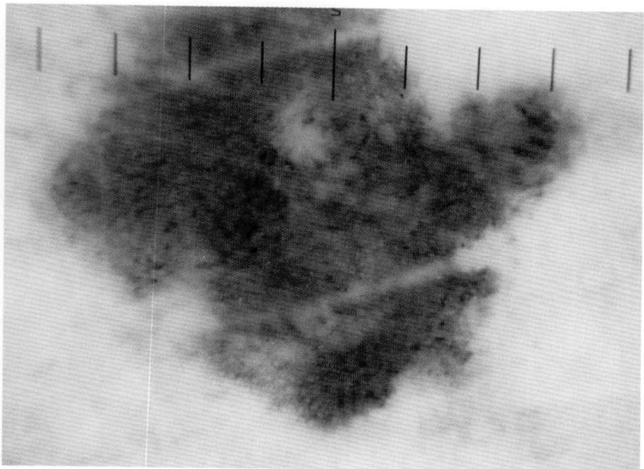

Angulated 'ugly duckling' hyperpigmented macule on the leg of a 70-year-old woman: dermoscopy shows an atypical beaded network with black dots and prominent skin surface markings in this MIS.

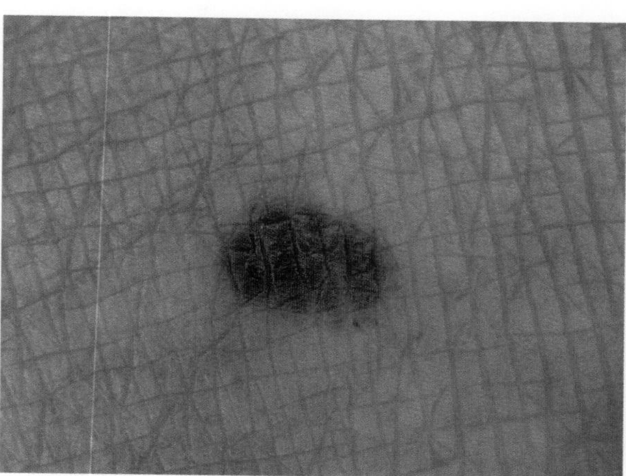

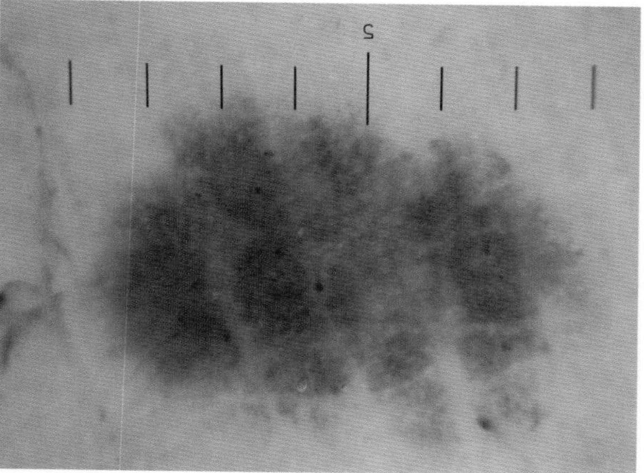

Tan macule on the leg of a 50-year-old woman: dermoscopy shows multicomponent morphology with an atypical network, brown dots and globules and prominent skin surface markings in this 0.2 mm thick SSM.

Skin surface markings may not be a reassuring feature in melanocytic lesions if clinical suspicion of melanoma exists.

5.4 Melanoma – high-risk scenarios

Late features of melanoma	99
Feature-poor melanoma	100
Feature-poor melanoma cases	101
Nodular melanoma	102
Nodular melanoma cases	103
Amelanotic nodular melanoma	104
Amelanotic nodular melanoma cases	105
Metastatic melanoma	106
Metastatic melanoma cases	107
Rare melanoma subtypes	108
Synchronous melanoma	109

Diagnostic Dermoscopy: The Illustrated Guide, Second Edition. Jonathan Bowling.

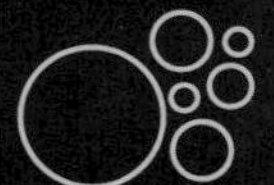

Late features of melanoma

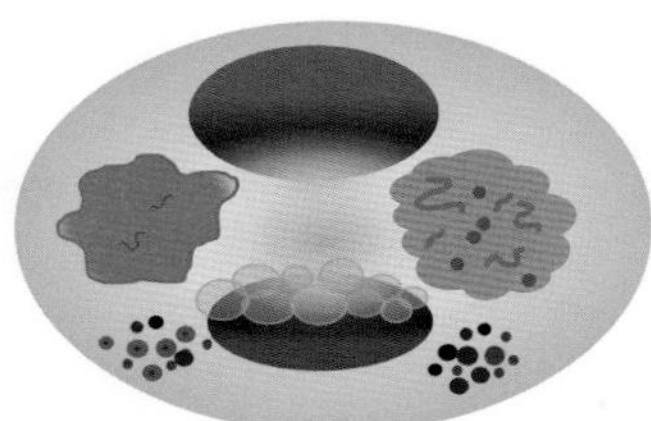

As melanomas increase in thickness the subtle dermoscopic features of an atypical network, streaks and angulated lines may be replaced with structureless hyperpigmented globules, ulceration and polymorphous vessels (neoangiogenesis). Ulceration and neoangiogenesis are features that are associated with a worse prognosis for melanoma. Rarely separate globular aggregates of pigment may be seen in keeping with in-transit metastatic deposits..

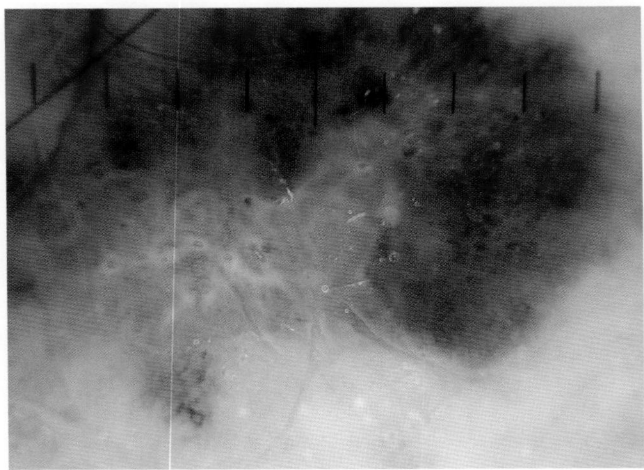

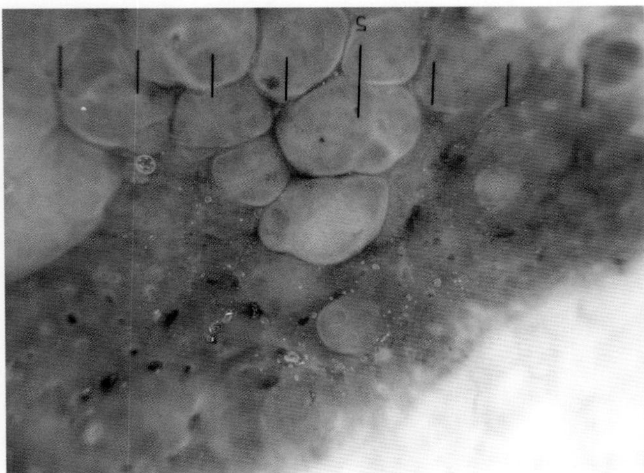

Polymorphous vessels, hyperpigmented blotches, blue-whitish veil and irregular globules are seen in these two >1 mm thick superficial spreading melanomas (SSM).

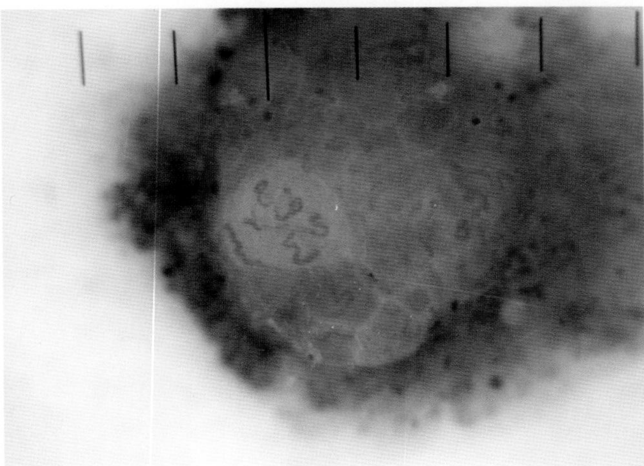

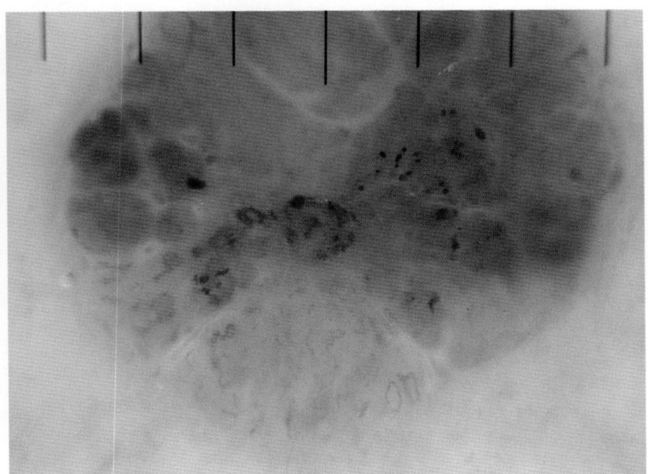

Irregular hyperpigmented globules, polymorphous vessels and ulceration are seen in these two > 1 mm thick SSM.

Take a close look at the surrounding skin, for signs of in-transit metastatic deposits, when melanoma presents with high risk features.

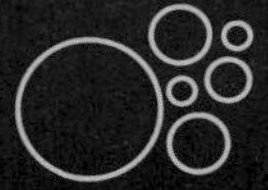

Feature-poor melanoma

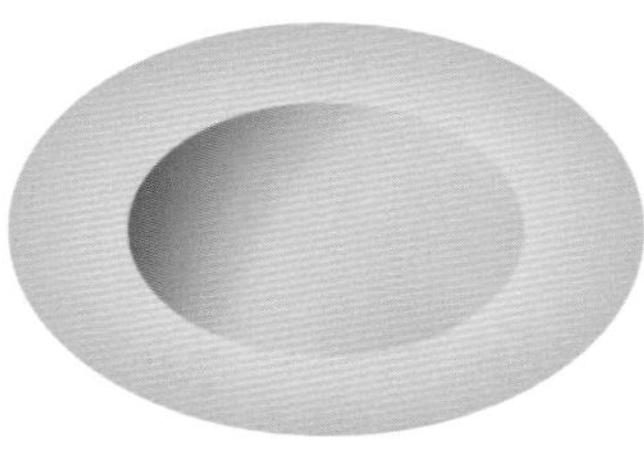

Melanomas that lack the overt clinical and dermoscopic features ("melanoma incognito") pose a diagnostic challenge. A truly featureless melanoma is uncommon. More commonly subtle features may be seen on close dermoscopic examination. Features to look for include areas of non-specific, ill-defined or variable pigmentation, a negative network or alternatively an atypical vascular pattern.

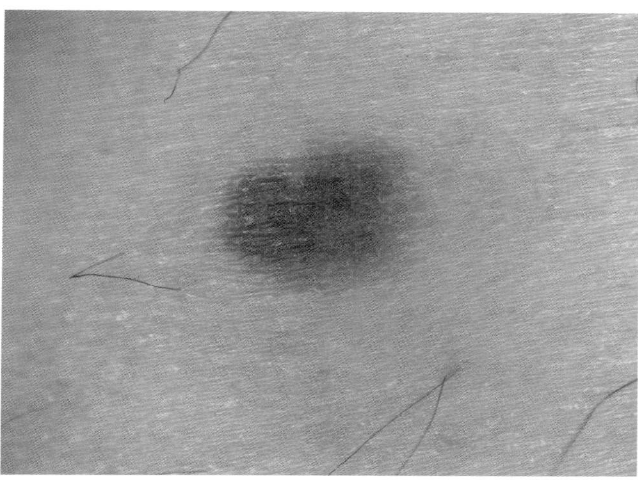

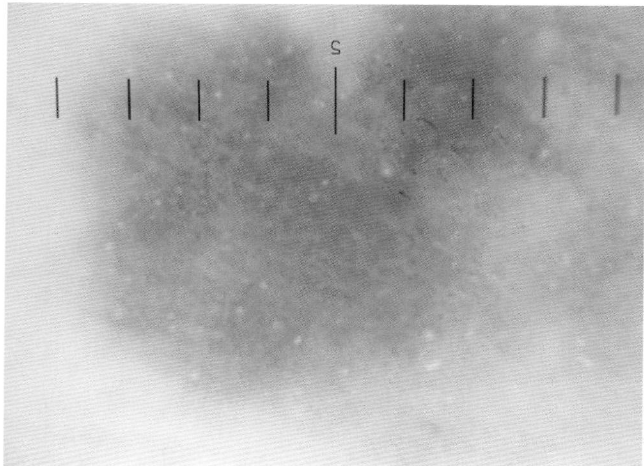

A uniformly pigmented macule on the buttock of a 60-year-old man: dermoscopy shows a faint negative network and structureless tan pigmentation in this melanoma in situ (MIS).

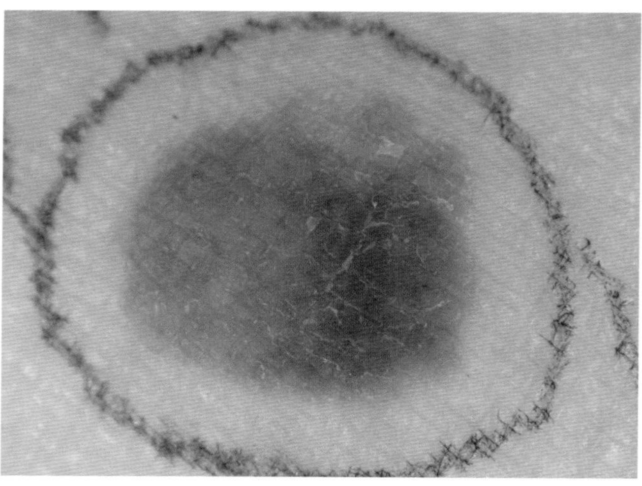

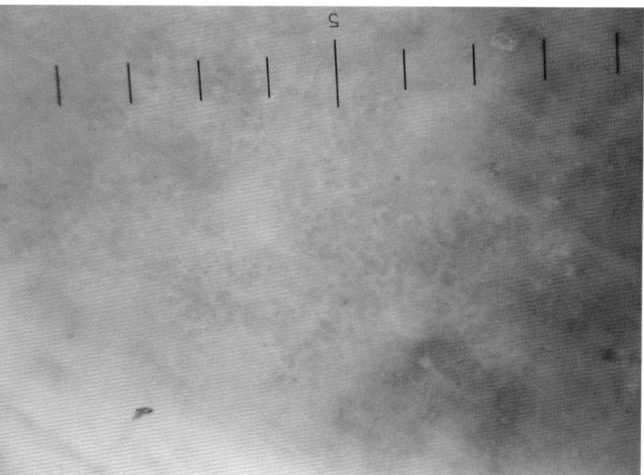

A large pigmented macule on the thigh of a 70-year-old man: dermoscopy shows a faint negative network and structureless tan pigmentation in this 0.6 mm thick SSM.

Argenziano, G. et al Dermocopy features of melanoma incognito: indications for biopsy. *J Am Acad Dermatol*. 2007;56(3): 508–13.

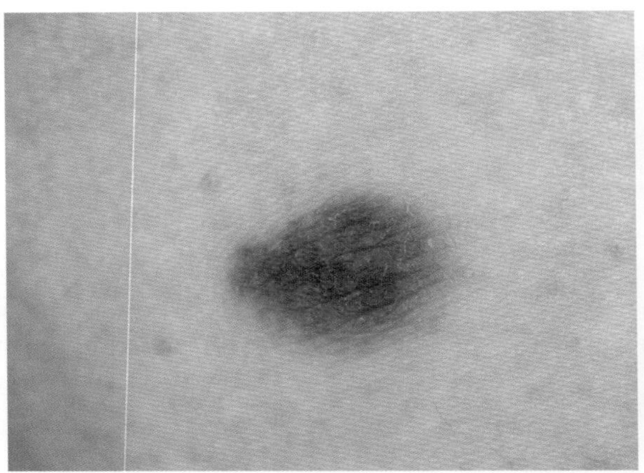

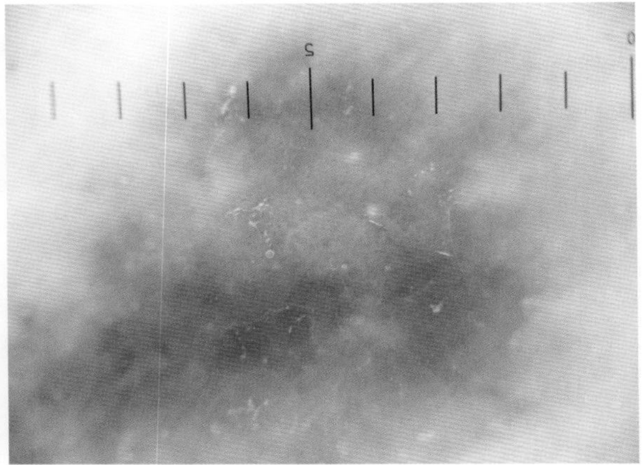

An irregularly pigmented macule on the buttock of a 60-year-old woman: dermoscopy shows ill-defined pink-brown structureless/featureless pigmentation in this 0.6 mm thick SSM.

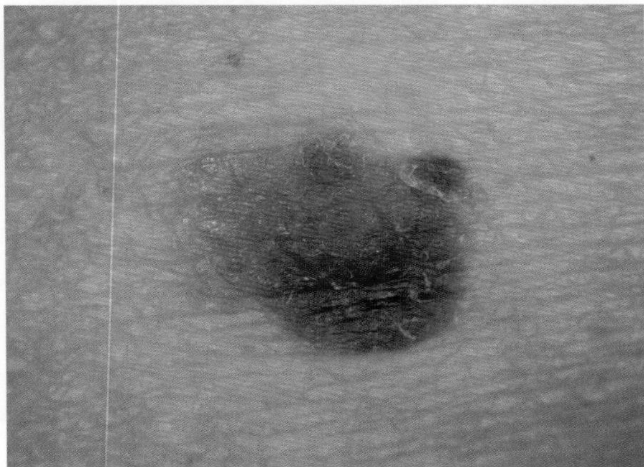

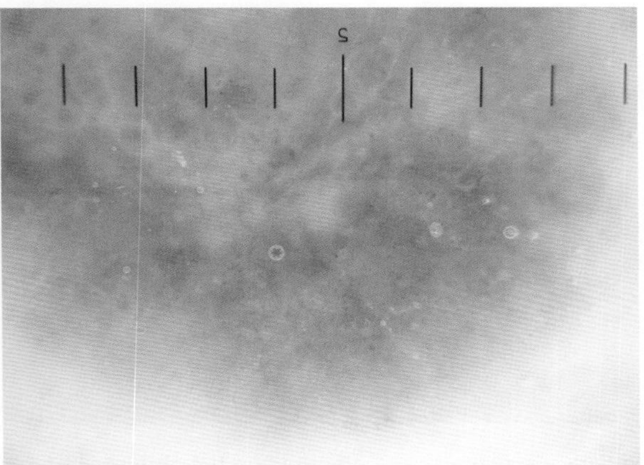

An irregularly pigmented pink and brown plaque on the lower back of a 50-year-old woman: dermoscopy shows pink, brown and purple pigmentation with focal vessels centrally and negative network in this 0.6 mm thick SSM.

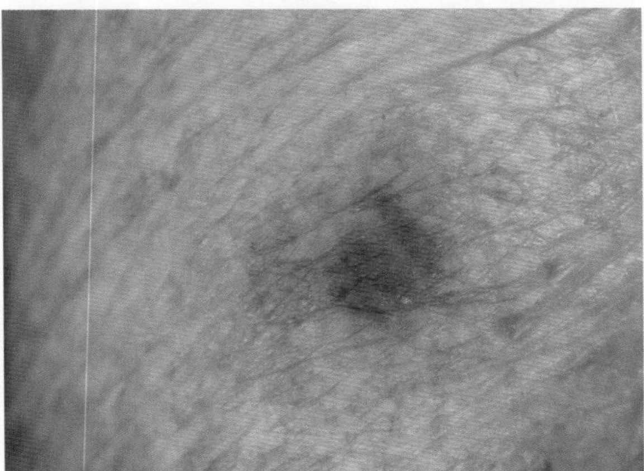

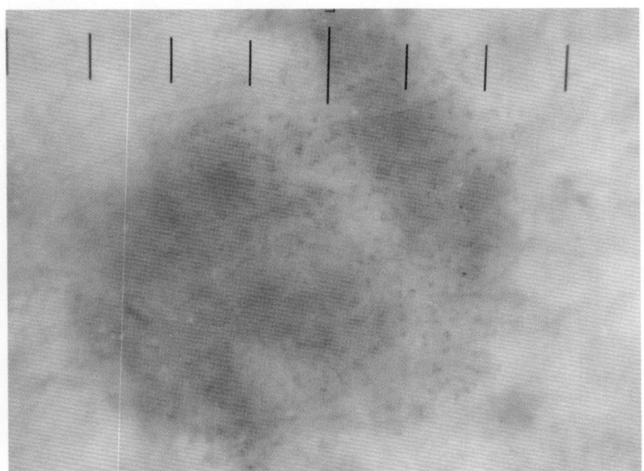

An irregularly pigmented macule on the upper arm of a 70-year-old woman: dermoscopy shows ill-defined brown pigmentation and milky erythema with irregular vessels in this 0.8 mm thick naevoid melanoma.

Diagnosis is a summation of risk factors, history, clinical appearance and dermoscopic features. Therefore, lack of dermoscopic features alone cannot reliably exclude melanoma in otherwise suspicious cases.

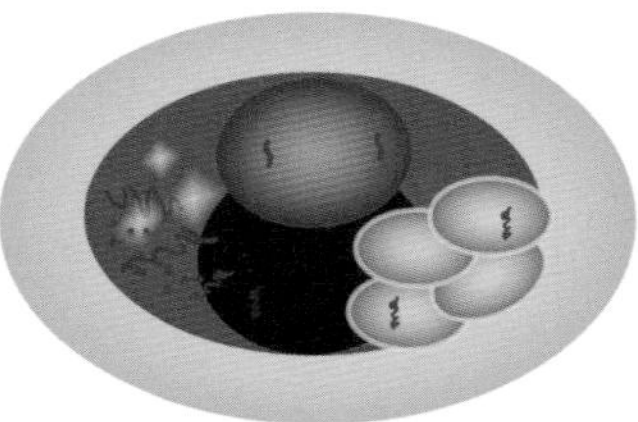

Nodular melanomas (NM) share many of the features associated with thicker SSM, such as pigmented structureless areas, irregular vessels, ulceration and a blue-whitish veil. However, they typically lack the peripheral epidermal features of SSM (streaks, atypical network and globules). A common feature of NM is negative network with whitish septae around variably coloured (polygonal) globules, where tumour aggregates are seen with granular pigmentation and irregular vessels.

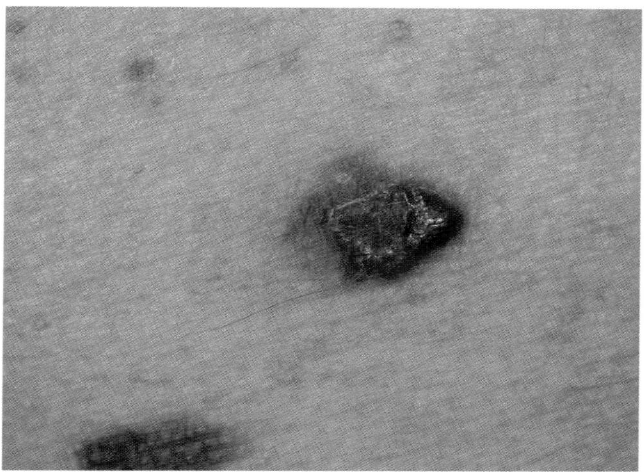

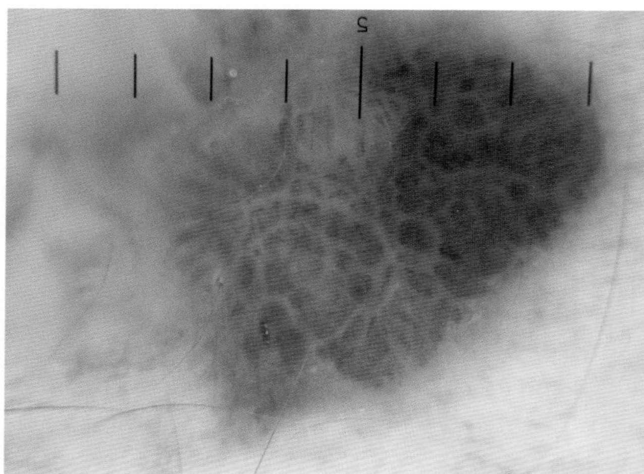

An irregularly pigmented plaque/nodule on the abdomen of a 50-year-old man: dermoscopy shows multiple polygonal globules with brown granules separated by white lines/septae and polymorphous vessels in this 1.5 mm thick NM.

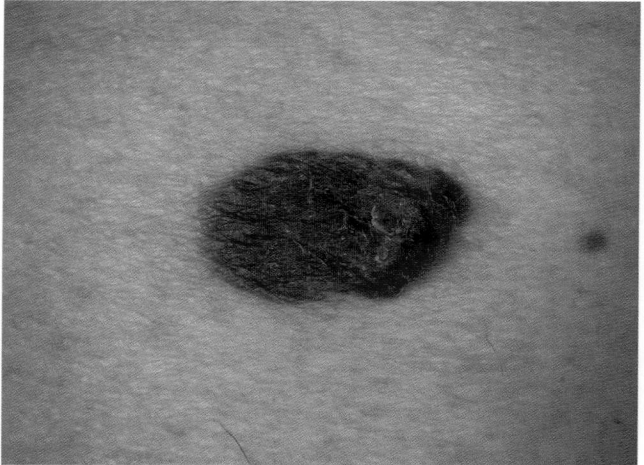

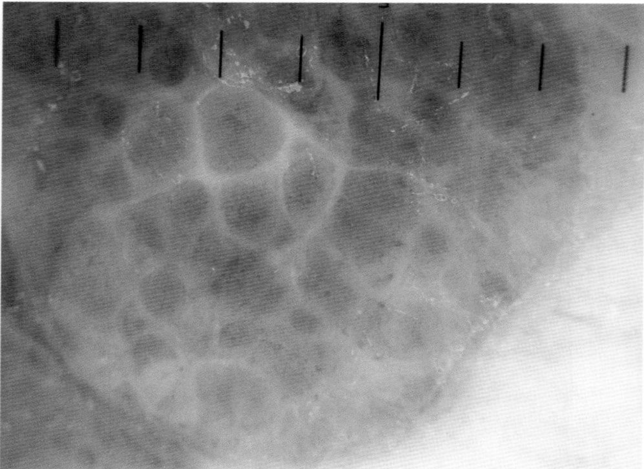

An irregularly pigmented plaque on the back of a 40-year-old man: dermoscopy shows large polygonal globules with granular pigmentation and irregular vessels separated by whitish septae in this 2.5 mm thick NM.

Menzies, S.W. et al. Dermoscopic evaluation of nodular melanoma. *JAMA Dermatol*. 2013;149(6):699–709.

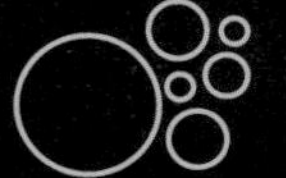

Nodular melanoma cases

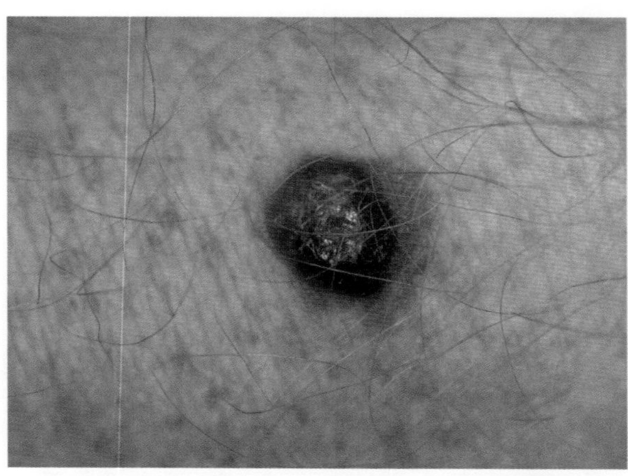

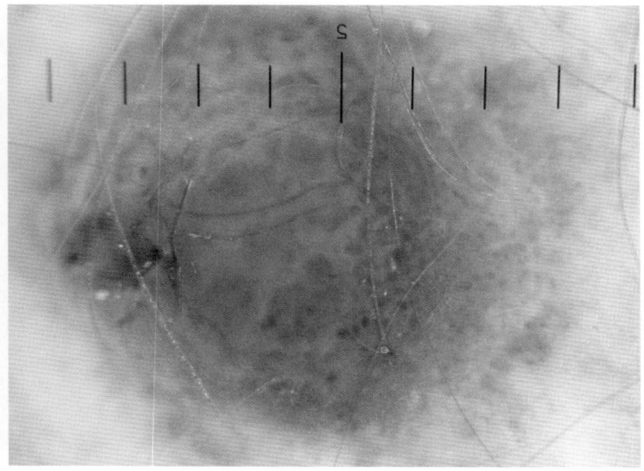

A dark purple nodule on the upper arm of a 70-year-old man: dermoscopy shows multiple colours, erosions, blue-whitish veil and atypical ill-defined vessels in this 1.9 mm thick NM.

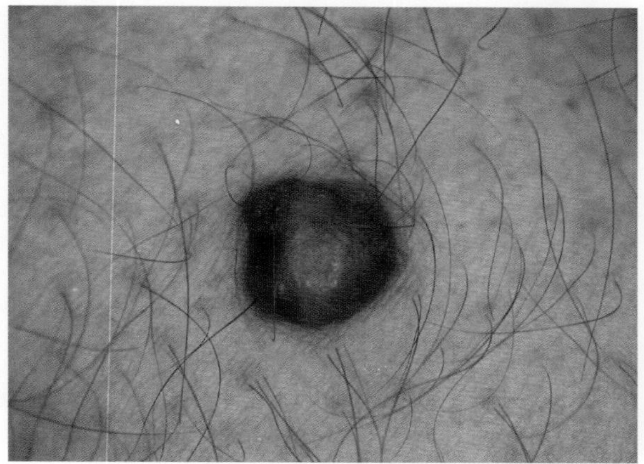

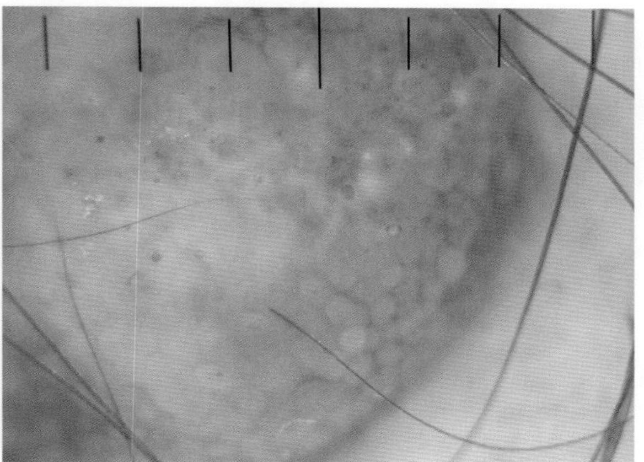

A dark crimson-coloured nodule on the lower leg of a 60-year-old man: dermoscopy shows homogeneous structureless globular morphology, scattered light brown globules and an atypical vascular pattern (red globules) in this 2.5 mm NM.

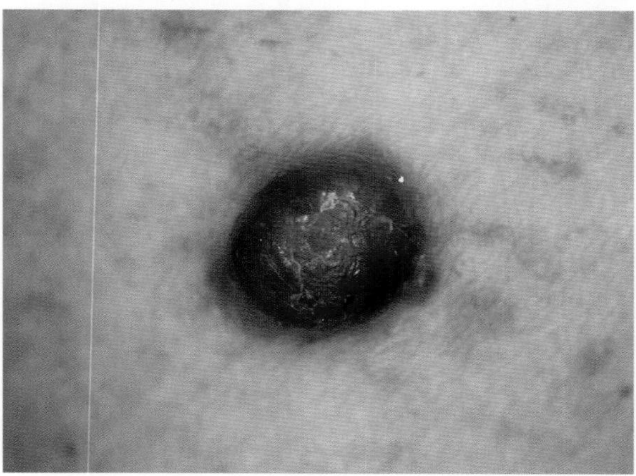

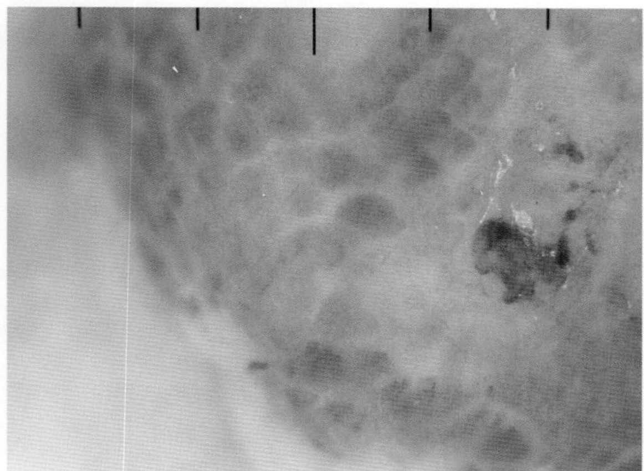

A dark crimson-coloured nodule on the upper arm of a 65-year-old woman: dermoscopy shows ill-defined structureless purple globules, whitish septae, peripheral irregular vessels and erosions in this 5.1 mm thick NM.

Sgouros, D. et al. Dermatoscopic features of thin (2 mm Breslow thickness) vs. thick (>2 mm Breslow thickness) nodular melanoma (abbrev.). *J Eur Acad Dermatol Venereol*. 2020;34(11):2541–2547.

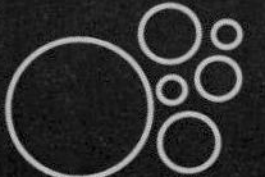

Amelanotic nodular melanoma

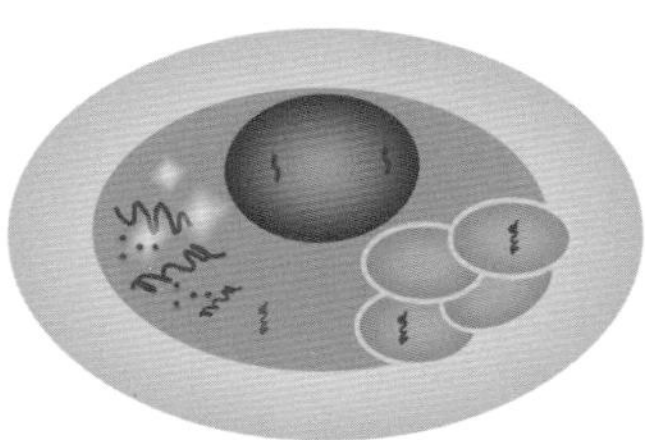

Hypomelanotic/amelanotic NM remains a clinical challenge as it often presents late. Typical features include pink structureless areas, atypical vessels, ulceration and milky red globules. They also typically lack the peripheral epidermal features of SSM (streaks, atypical network and globules). Additional dermoscopic features include polygonal globules separated by whitish septae or a negative network.

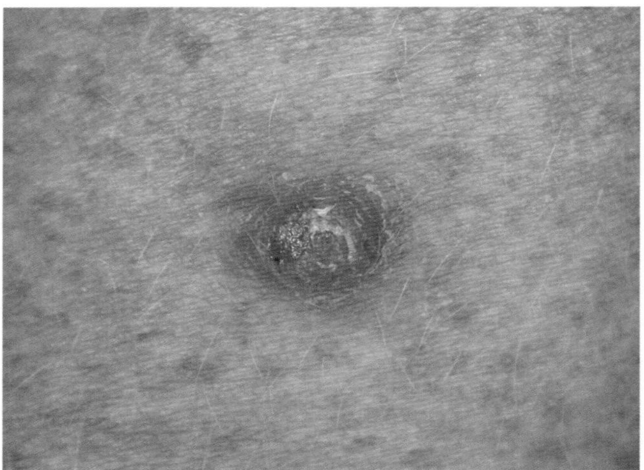

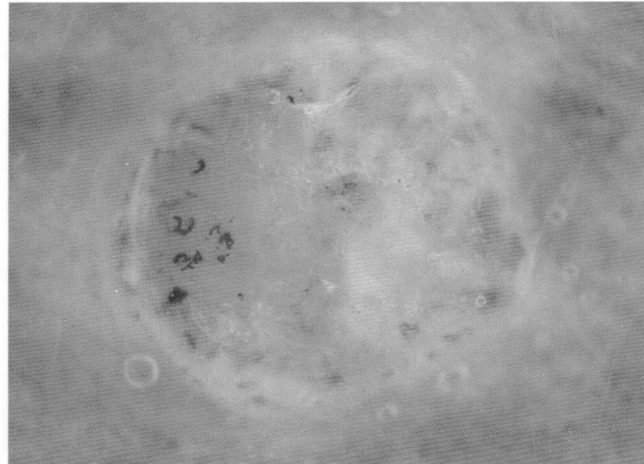

An ulcerated pink nodule on the upper arm of a 40-year-old woman: dermoscopy shows ulceration, structureless areas and irregular vessels in this 1.9 mm thick amelanotic NM.

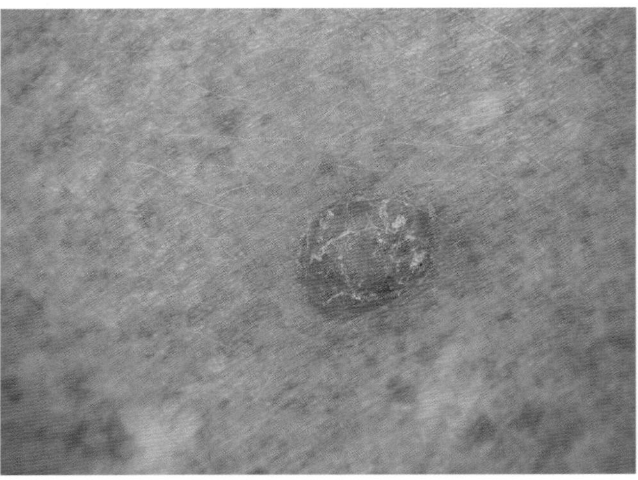

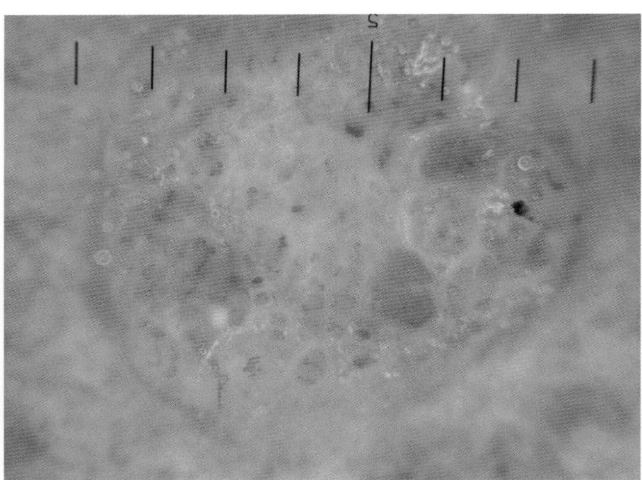

A solitary pink scaly nodule on the forearm of a 60-year-old woman: dermoscopy shows polygonal globules, with polymorphous vessels separated by whitish septae in this 2.6 mm thick amelanotic NM.

Cavicchini, S. et al. Dermoscopic vascular patterns in nodular 'pure' amelanotic melanoma. *Arch Dermatol.* 2007;143(4):556.

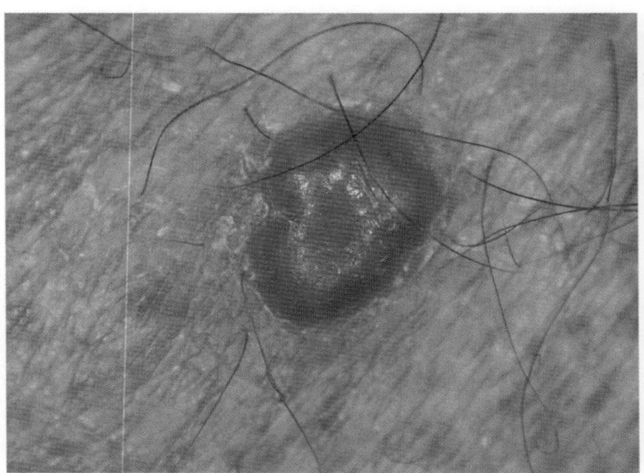

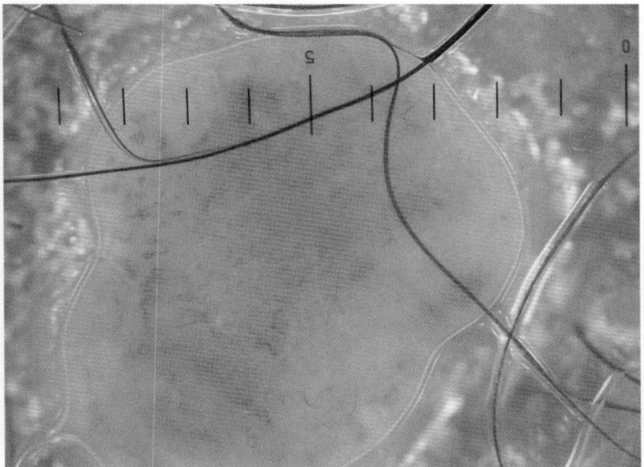

Pink amelanotic nodule on the forearm of a 60-year-old man: dermoscopy shows a homogeneous pink background with multiple small linear irregular vessels in this 1.9 mm thick amelanotic NM.

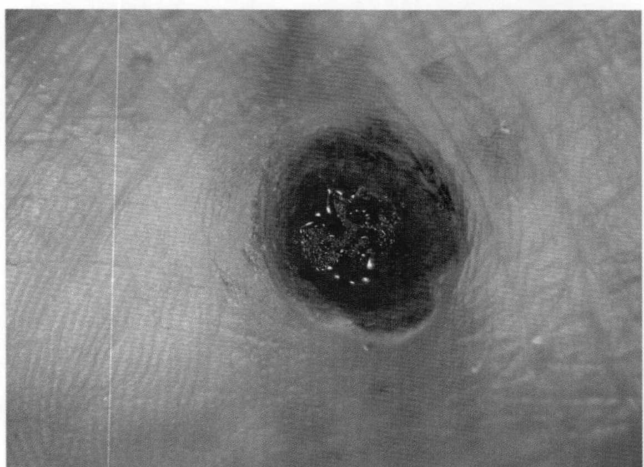

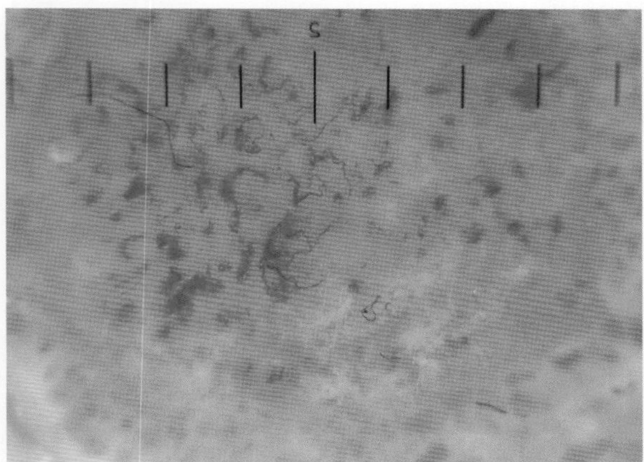

Ulcerated nodule on the sole of a 65-year-old woman: dermoscopy shows linear irregular vessels, erosions and ulceration with adherent fibres in this 2.8 mm thick amelanotic acral NM.

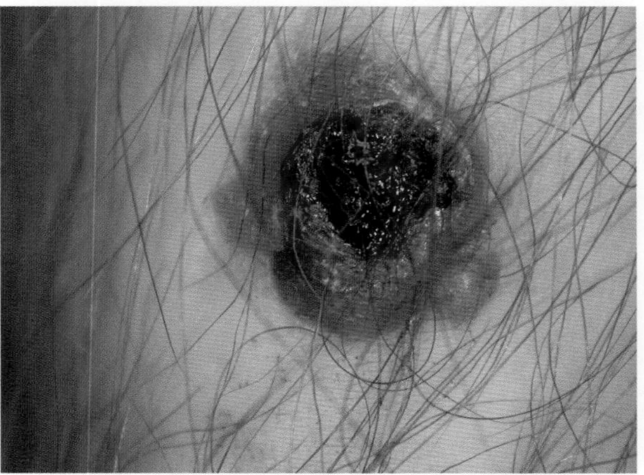

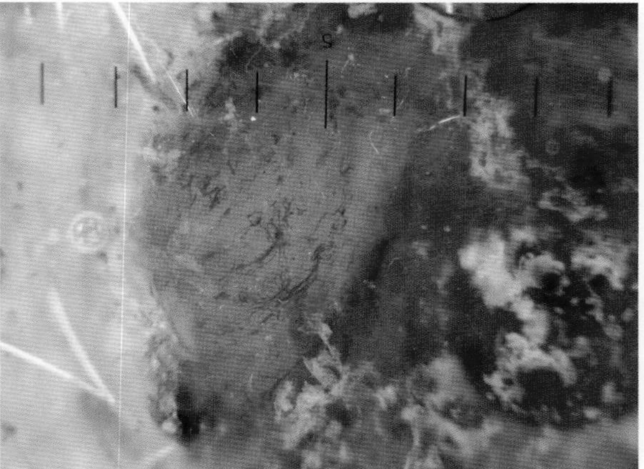

A large ulcerated tumour on the calf of a 25-year-old man: dermoscopy shows ulceration, irregular vessels and an absence of epidermal features in this 3.9 mm amelanotic NM.

Thick NMs lack the more varied dermoscopic features seen in thinner tumours and predominantly tend to show ulceration, structureless pink or milky red areas and irregular vessels.

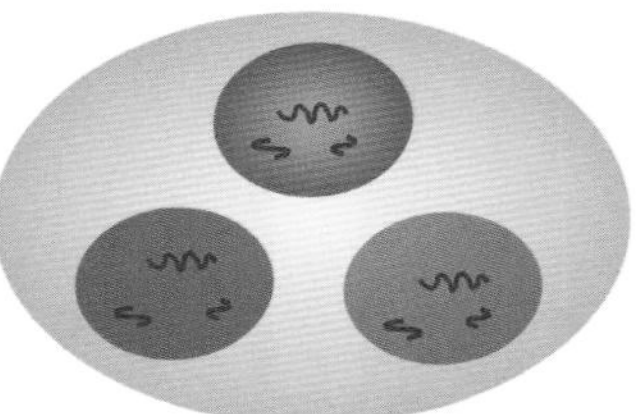

Metastatic deposits from cutaneous melanoma may be macroscopic or microscopic, localised, regional or widespread. Epidermal features of radial growth phase melanomas are usually absent. They typically present as pink, brown, blue, black or purple papules or nodules with features including structureless areas, atypical vessels, milky red globules, granular pigmentation or polygonal globules seperated by whitish septae.

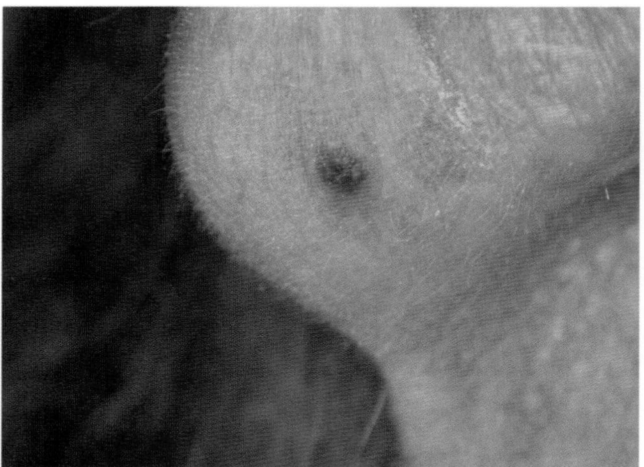

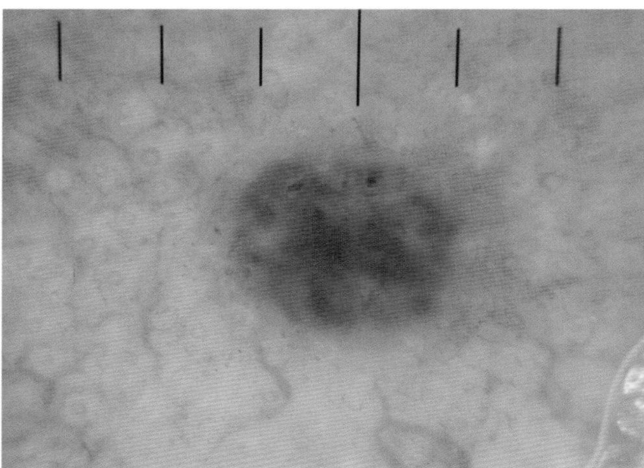

A papule on the posterior ear lobe of a 70-year-old man with a history of melanoma on the neck: dermoscopy shows aggregates of brown granular and bluish pigmentation and few linear vessels. Histopathology confirmed metastatic melanoma.

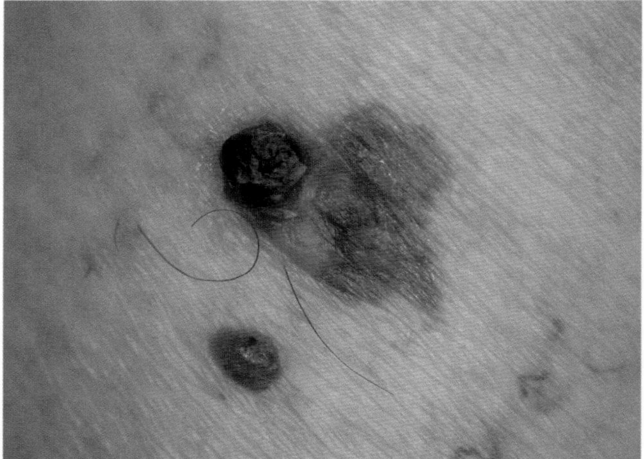

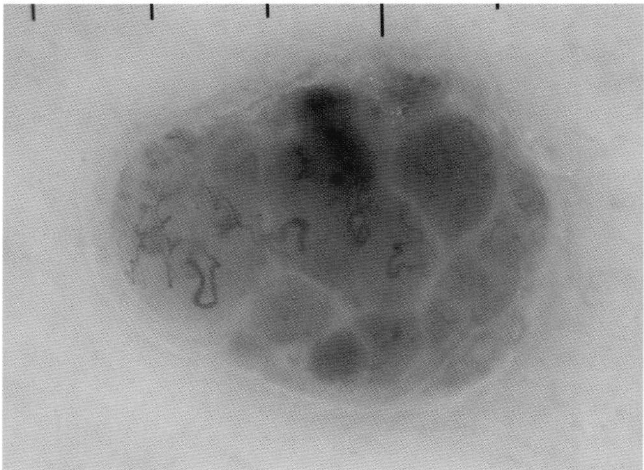

A pink papule inferior to a multicoloured plaque on the knee of a 60-year-old man: dermoscopy of the papule shows whitish septae, large polygonal globules with granular pigmentation and irregular vessels in this in-transit metastatic deposit.

Suspect melanoma metastasis when encountering one or more 'ugly duckling' papules or nodules in a patient with a personal history of melanoma.

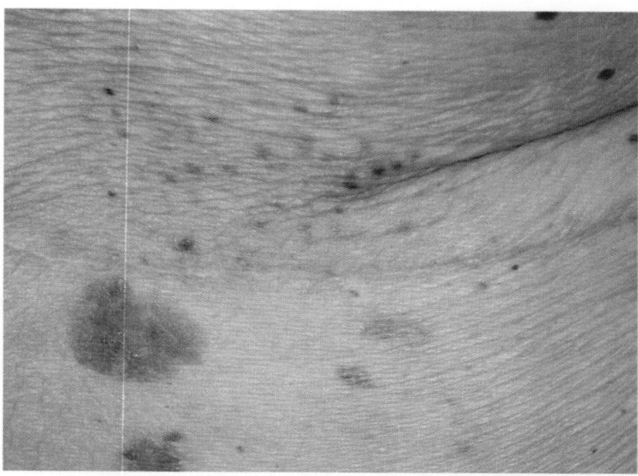
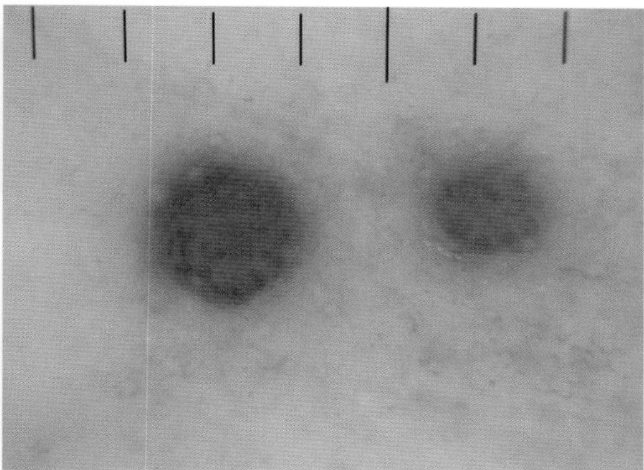

Cutaneous melanoma metastases presenting as multiple papules in the groin of a 70-year-old woman: dermoscopy shows tan granular pigmentation and minimal vascular features.

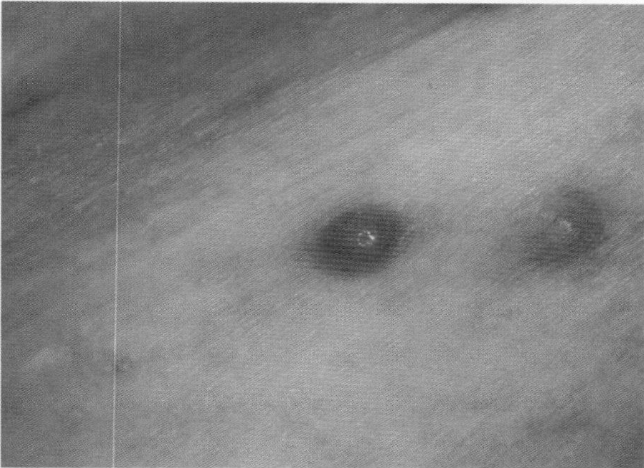
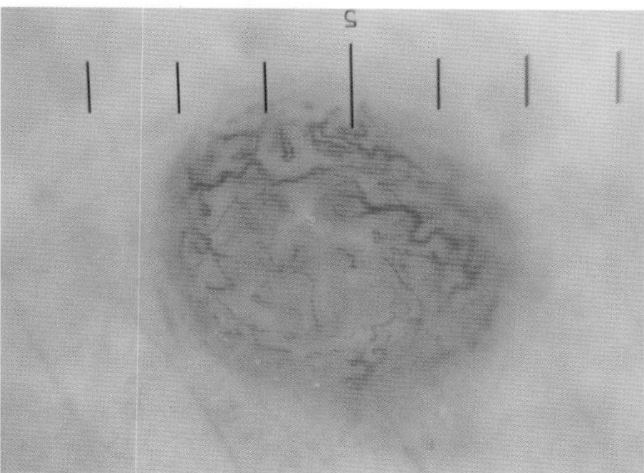

Cutaneous in-transit melanoma metastases presenting as vascular papules on the arm of a 60-year-old man: dermoscopy shows polymorphous linear irregular and looped or hairpin vessels.

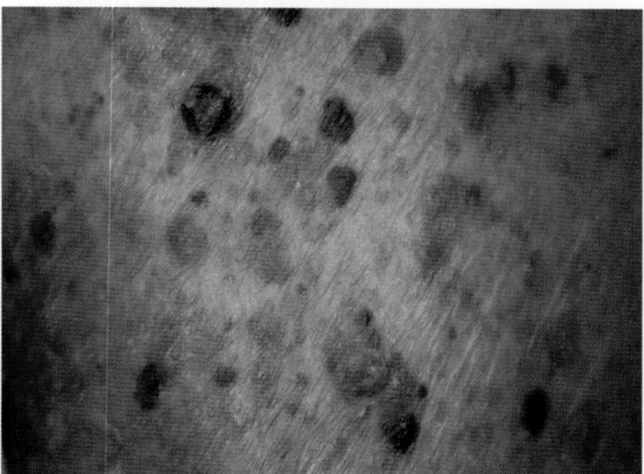
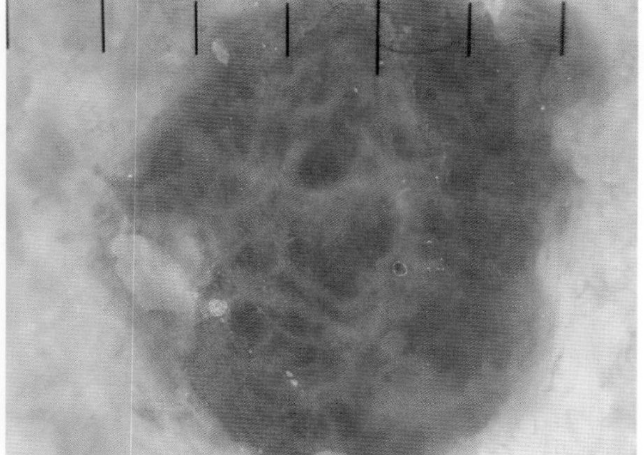

Extensive locoregional cutaneous melanoma metastases on the lower limb of a 75-year-old woman: dermoscopy shows purple-brown pigmentation and whitish lines within a blue-whitish veil.

Costa, J. et al. Dermoscopic patterns of melanoma metastases: inter-observer consistency and accuracy for metastases recognition. *Br J Dermatol*. 2013;169(1):91–99.

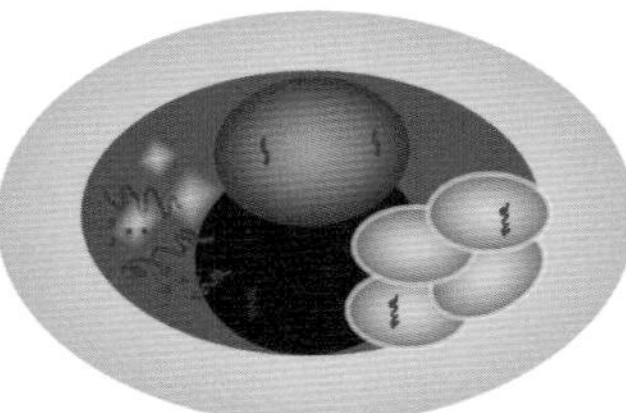

There are a number of NM histopathological subtypes that evade a confident clinical diagnosis. The specific subtype diagnosis is usually confirmed on histopathology as they share features with more typical melanomas.

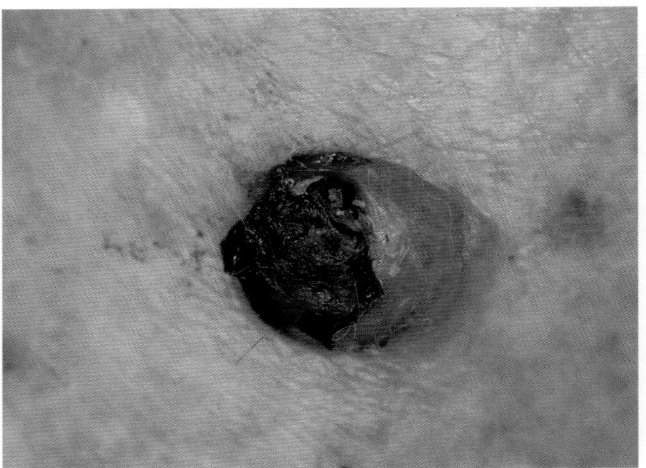

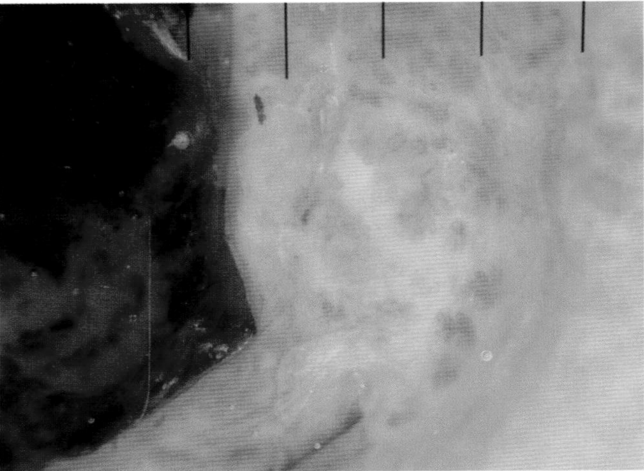

An ulcerated pink nodule on the leg of a 70-year-old woman: dermoscopy shows ulceration, milky red structureless areas with multiple foci of coiled or glomerular and linear vessels in this 2.6 mm thick balloon cell melanoma.

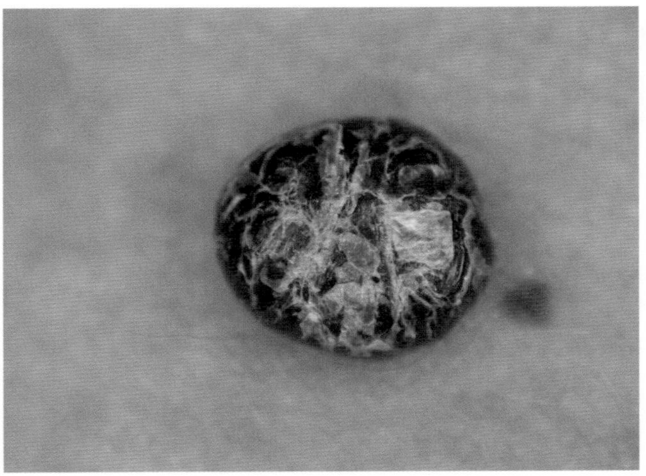

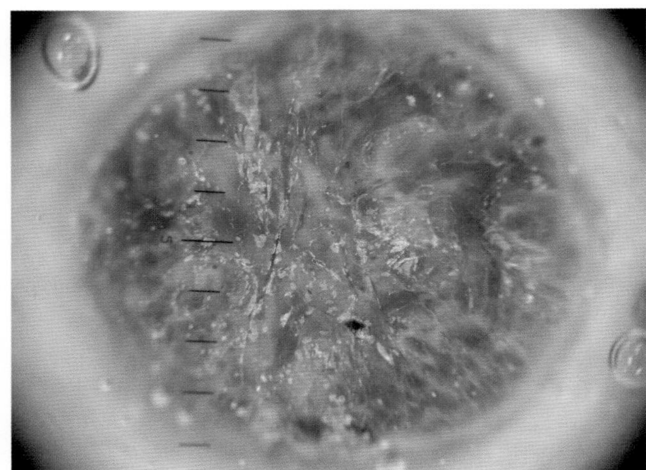

A hyperpigmented nodule on the upper back of a 50-year-old woman: dermoscopy shows blue, black and white uniform blue pigmentation with diffuse whitish lines in this 4.3 mm Breslow 'animal-type' NM.

Maher, J. et al. Balloon cell melanoma: a case report with polarized dermatoscopy and dermatopathology. *Dermatol Pract Concept*. 2014;4(1):6973.

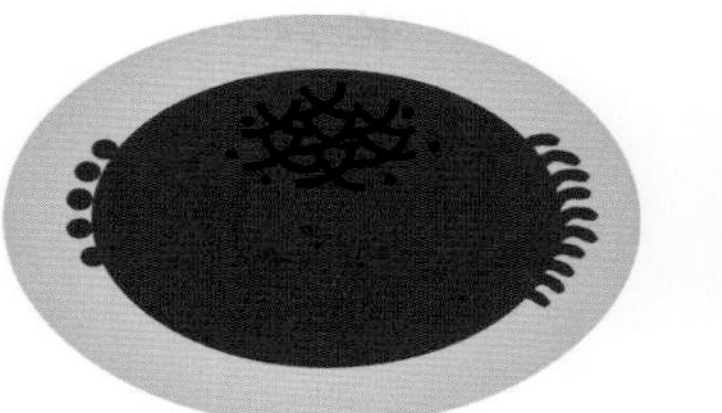
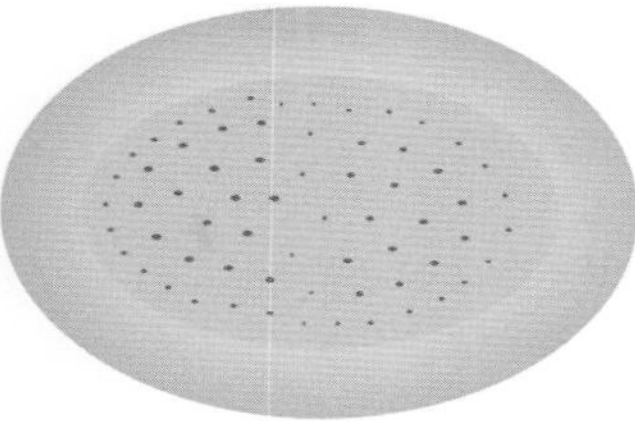

In addition to the index lesion, patients may have more than one melanoma on their skin at the time of presentation, known as a synchronous melanoma. The presence of a synchronous melanoma should be sought at the time of presentation.

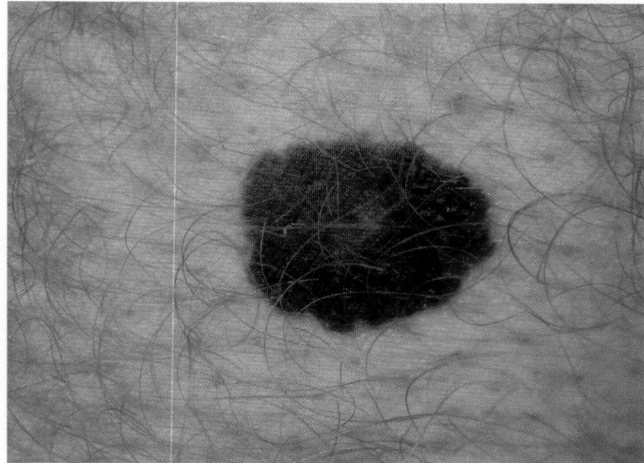
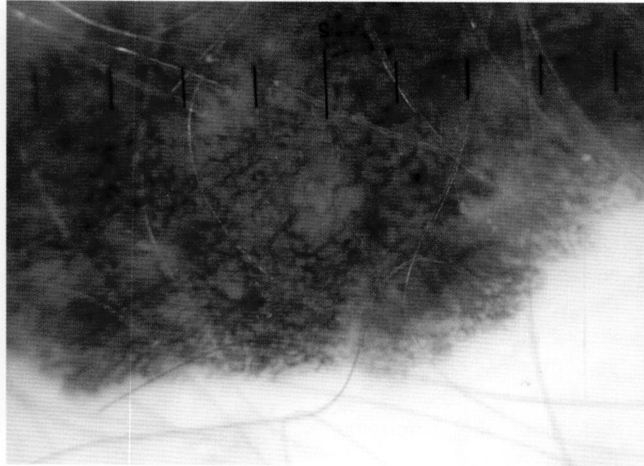

A 30-year-old man with light skin with a pigmented macule on the lateral thigh: dermoscopy shows an atypical beaded network in this 0.3 mm thick SSM.

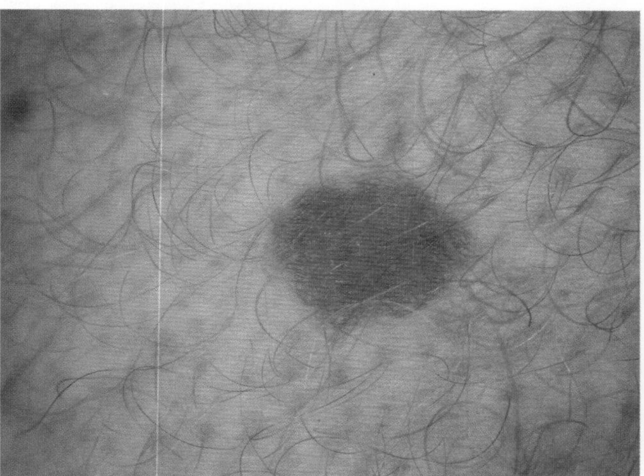
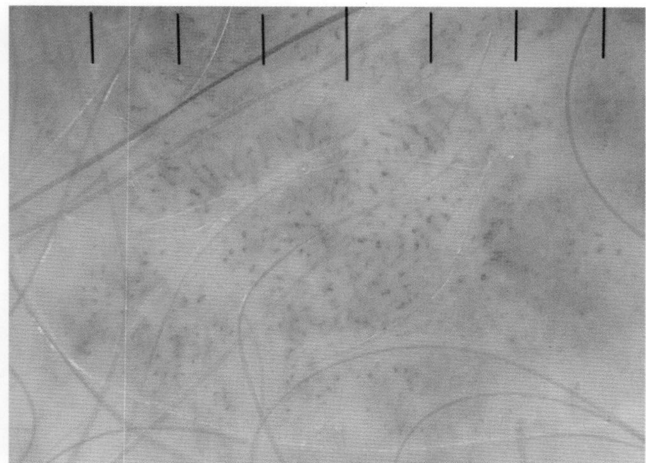

The same 30-year-old man at presentation had an additional pink macule on the anterior thigh: dermoscopy showed dotted and linear irregular vessels with peripheral tan pigmentation in this 0.5 mm SSM.

There is no guarantee that the additional synchronous melanoma follows the same morphology of the index lesion.

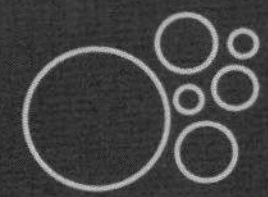

4 Non-melanocytic lesions

Macrocomedone 111
Solar lentigo – fingerprint pattern 112
Solar lentigo – homogeneous pattern 113
Solar lentigo – reticular pattern 114
Solar lentigo – hyperpigmented 'ink spot' 115
Solar lentigo – evolving seborrhoeic keratosis 116
Seborrhoeic keratosis – cerebriform pattern 117
Seborrhoeic keratosis – homogeneous pattern 118
Seborrhoeic keratosis – keratotic pattern 119
Seborrhoeic keratosis – hyperpigmented 120
Seborrhoeic keratosis – hypopigmented 121
Seborrhoeic keratosis – irritated 122
Seborrhoeic keratosis – traumatised 123
Seborrhoeic keratosis – clonal 124
Clear cell acanthoma 125
Benign lichenoid keratosis – inflammatory phase 126
Benign lichenoid keratosis – post-inflammatory phase 127
Dermatofibroma 128
Dermatofibroma – hypopigmented 129
Dermatofibroma – hyperpigmented 130
Dermatofibroma – atypicall 131
Dermatofibrosarcoma protuberans 132
Neurofibromas 133
Porokeratosis 134
Porokeratosis cases 135
Epidermal naevus 136
Epidermal naevus cases 137
Cutaneous T-cell lymphoma 138
Pseudolymphoma 139
Eccrine poroma 140

Diagnostic Dermoscopy: The Illustrated Guide, Second Edition. Jonathan Bowling.

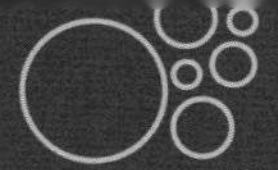

Macrocomedone

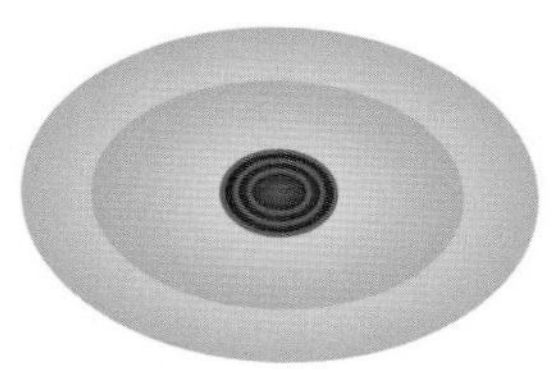

Macrocomedones rarely cause diagnostic concern although they may present to the clinician due to patient concern. Hyperkeratosis within an enlarged ostium of the sebaceous gland shows multiple concentric rings of laminated keratin on dermoscopy.

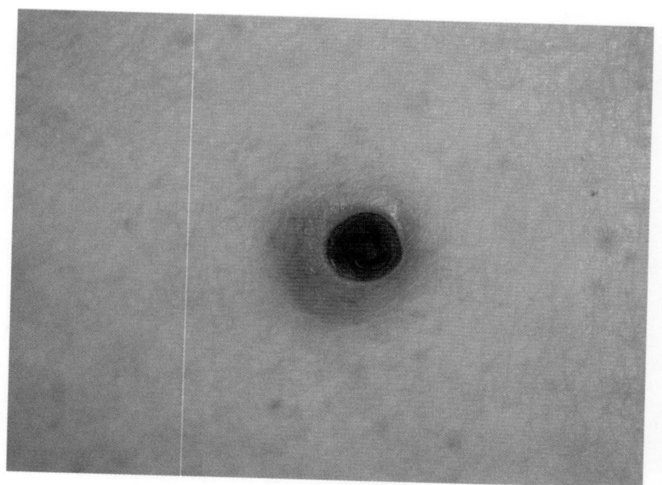

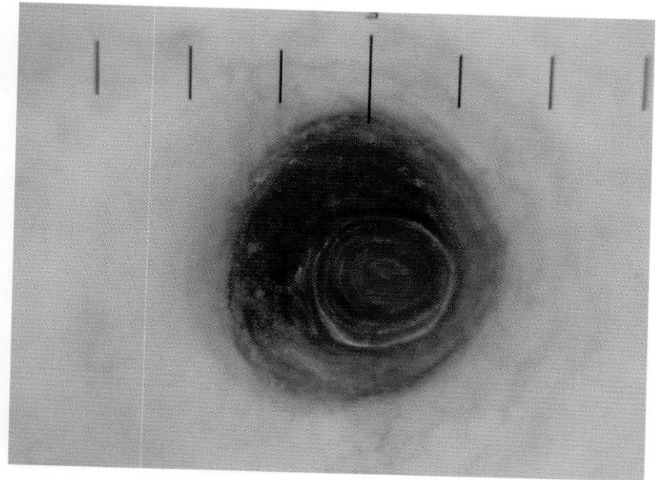

A dark brown hyperkeratotic lesion on the back of a 40-year-old woman: dermoscopy shows laminated keratin rings in keeping with a macrocomedone that was easily expressed.

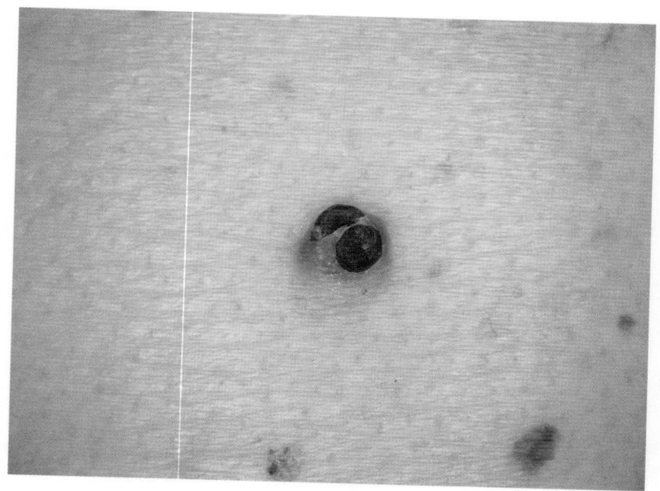

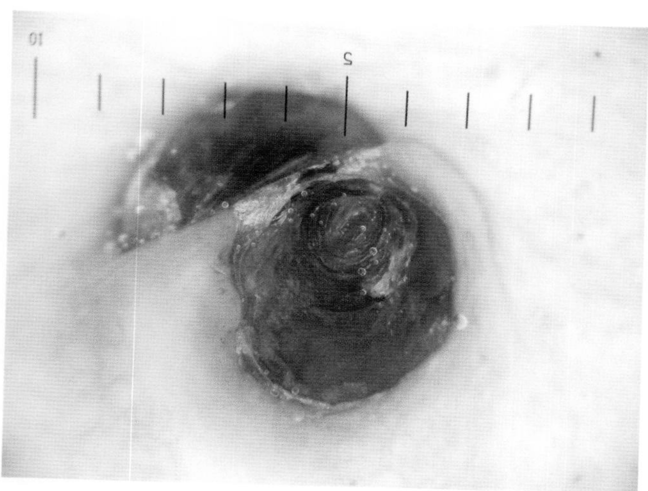

A keratotic papule on the upper back of a 50-year-old woman: dermoscopy shows two foci of pigmentation with concentric keratin rings in this bilobed macrocomedone.

Gentle expression with a comedone extractor is diagnostic.

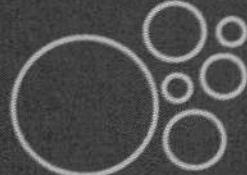

Solar lentigo – fingerprint pattern

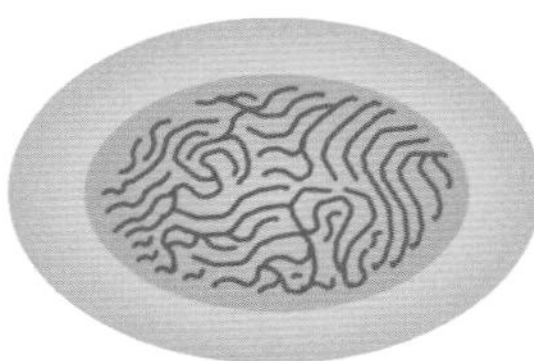

Solar lentigines may show a pattern of pigmentation with parallel lines and circles that have been described as a fingerprint pattern. These lines flow around follicular apertures and may merge to form a reticular pattern.

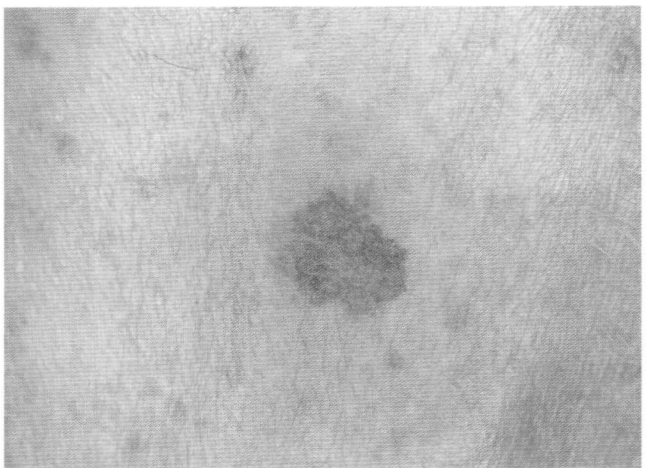

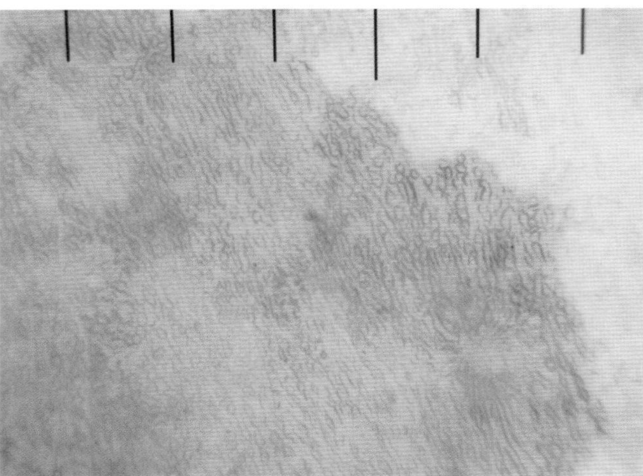

A pigmented macule on the dorsum of the hand on a 70-year-old woman: dermoscopy shows parallel lines forming a fine reticular network. The border is sharp but not moth-eaten. This is the fingerprint pattern of solar lentigo.

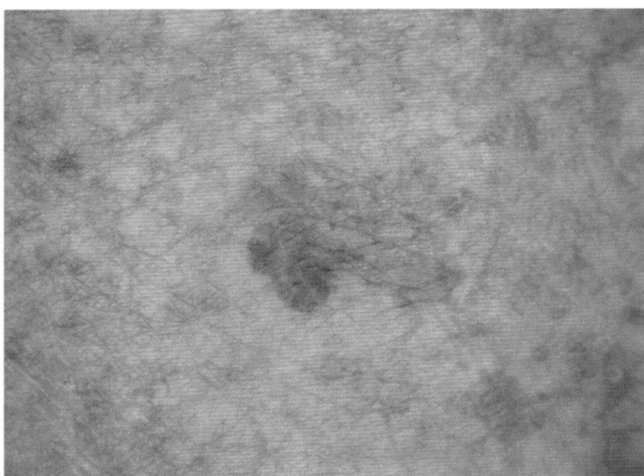

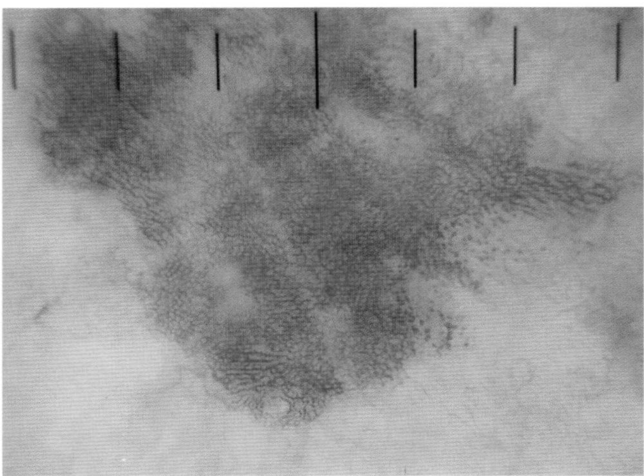

An angulated tan macule on the upper chest of a 60-year-old woman: dermoscopy shows a well-demarcated peripheral border plus fingerprint pattern with linear parallel lines of varying lengths blending into a reticular pattern in this solar lentigo.

Solar lentigines are dynamic and clinical and dermoscopic features may change and evolve with time.

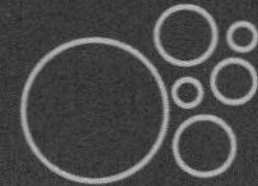

Solar lentigo – homogeneous pattern

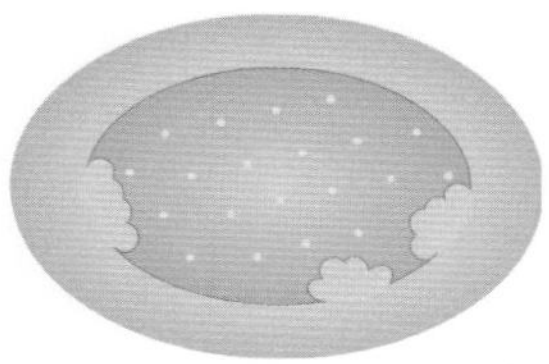

Solar lentigines may show a dominant pattern of homogeneous pigmentation. Additional features of a sharply demarcated and moth-eaten border and regular hypopigmented follicular apertures help to confirm the diagnosis. In dark lesions with ill-defined borders, there may be diagnostic concern as they can mimic melanocytic lesions.

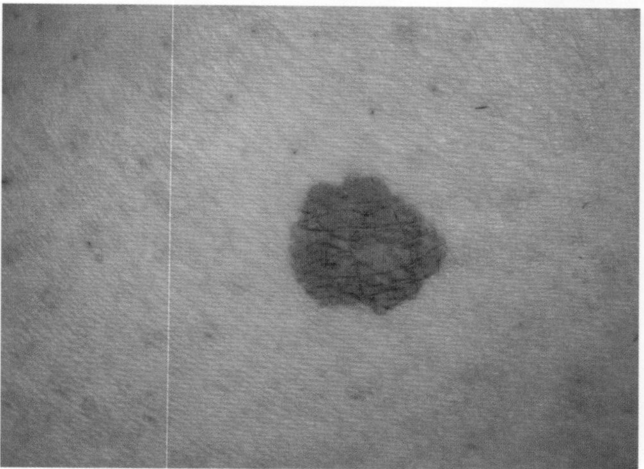

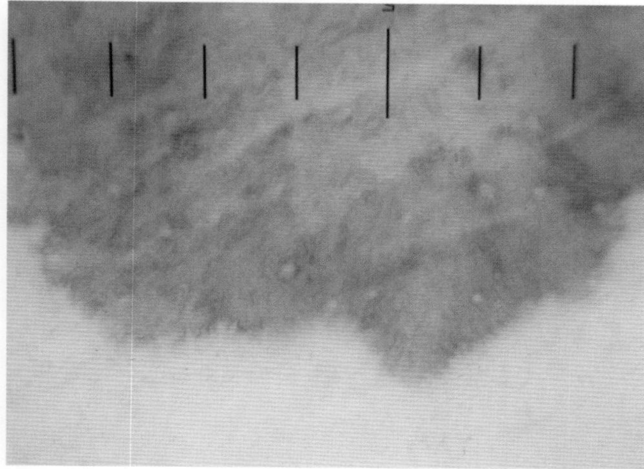

A tan macule on the lower leg of a 50-year-old woman: dermoscopy shows homogeneous tan pigmentation, follicular apertures and a well-demarcated peripheral border typical of solar lentigo.

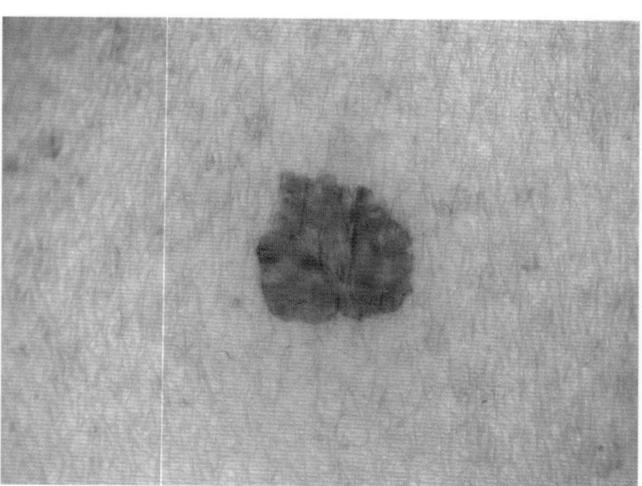

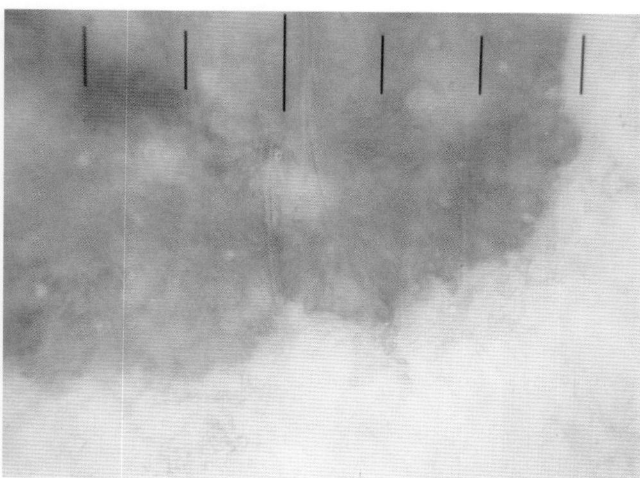

A tan macule on the arm of a 60-year-old woman: dermoscopy shows a well-demarcated moth-eaten peripheral border, homogeneous pigmentation with skin surface markings and regular follicular apertures in this solar lentigo.

Solar lentigines are typically multiple; therefore, look for similar lesions – consider a diagnostic biopsy if a lesion looks particularly different or distinct..

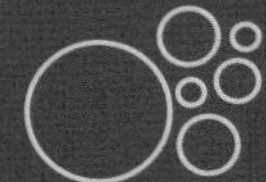

Solar lentigo – reticular pattern

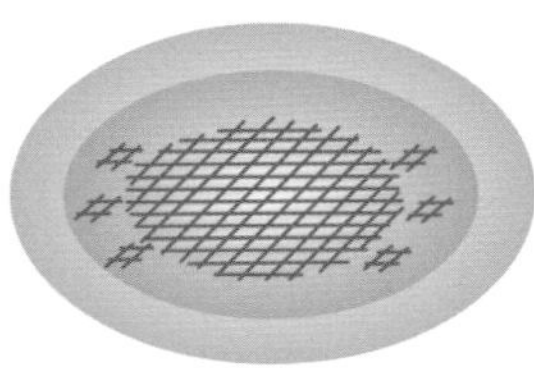

Solar lentigines may show a dominant pattern of reticular pigmentation, particularly across the trunk and back, giving a pigment network pattern. The reticular pigmented lines are thin and uniformly pigmented. The lines may show 'double lines' of pigmentation with dermoscopy and the peripheral margin is often less well-defined. In particularly hyperpigmented lesions with thick lines, they may be challenging to distinguish from naevi or lentigo maligna.

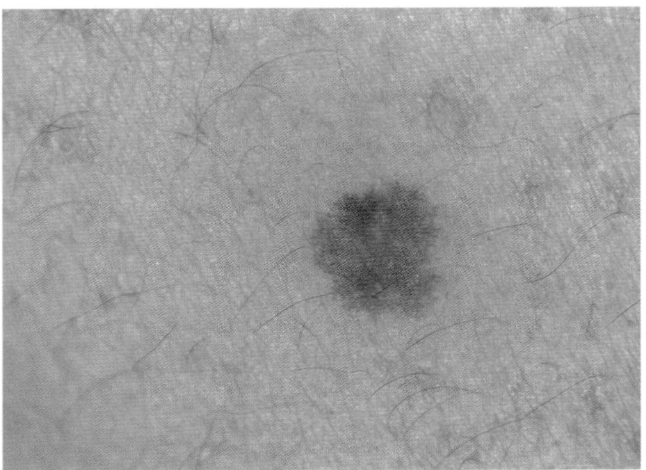

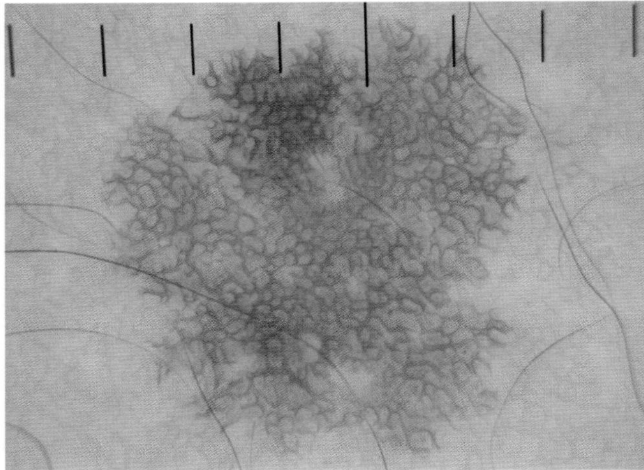

A tan macule on the upper back of a 50-year-old man: dermoscopy shows uniform reticular pigmentation with double lines in this solar lentigo.

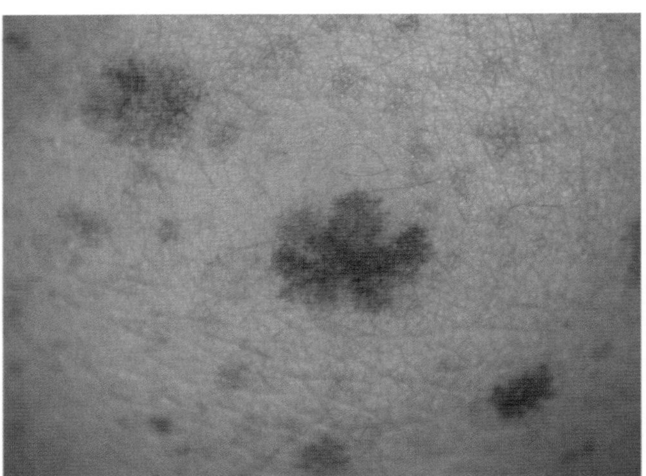

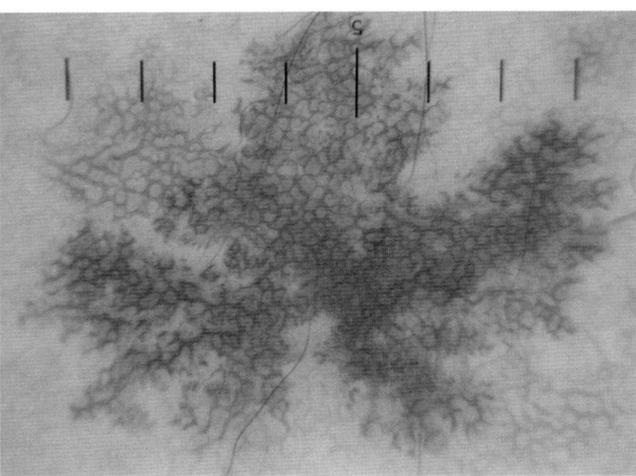

Multiple tan macules across the upper back of a 60-year-old man: dermoscopy shows uniform reticular pigmentation and double lines in this solar lentigo.

Lallas, A. et al. The dermoscopic inverse approach significantly improves the accuracy of human readers for lentigo maligna diagnosis. *J Am Acad Dermatol*. 2021;84(2):381–389.

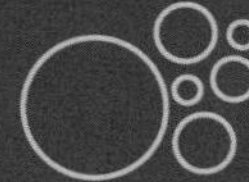

Solar lentigo – hyperpigmented 'ink spot'

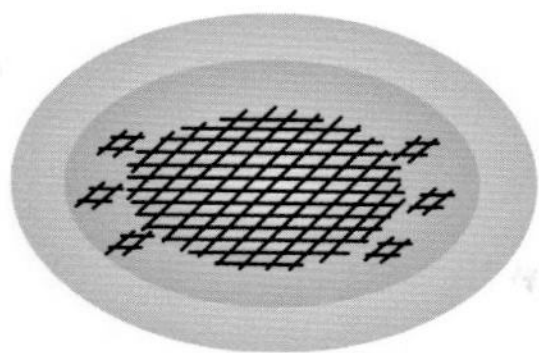

Solar lentigines with hyperpigmentation may be referred to as 'ink spot' lentigos. They occur on sun-exposed sites and are frequently multiple. The reticular pattern is clearly visible, both clinically and on dermoscopy. The reticular pigmented lines are thin and uniformly pigmented. If the lesion is solitary, the pigmentation is increased and the thickness of the lines are variable. There may be diagnostic concern and histopathology should be considered as they can mimic melanoma.

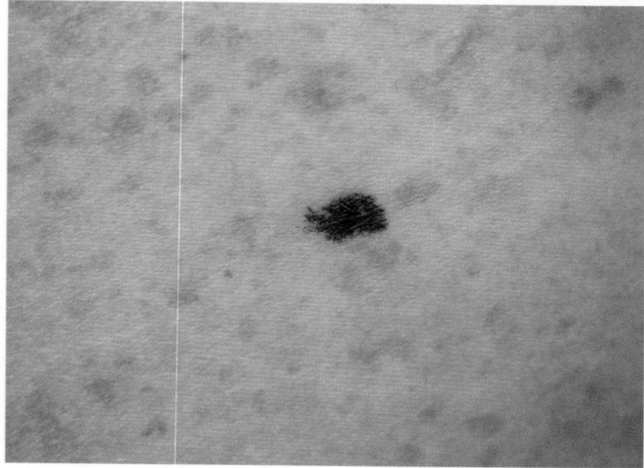

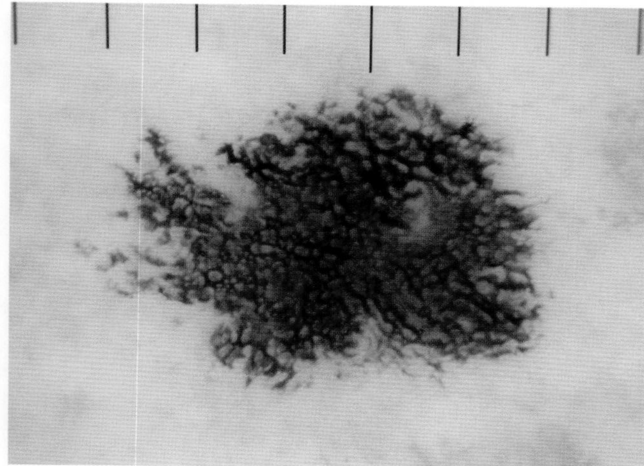

A dark macule on the upper back of a 50-year-old man: dermoscopy shows uniform reticular dark brown pigmentation in this hyperpigmented 'ink spot' lentigo.

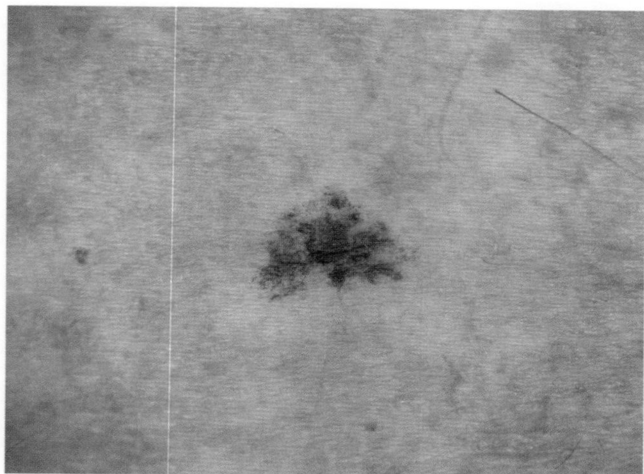

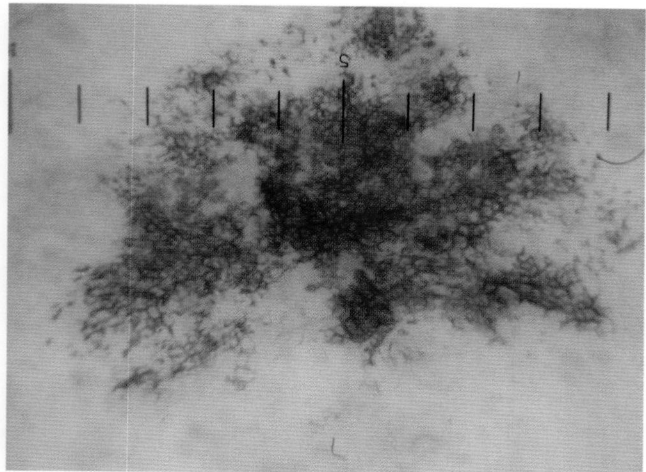

Multiple hyperpigmented macules across the upper back of a 70-year-old man with high UV exposure: dermoscopy shows uniform reticular pigmentation in this hyperpigmented 'ink spot' lentigo.

Langley, R. In vivo confocal scanning laser microscopy of benign lentigines: comparison to conventional histology and in vivo characteristics of lentigo maligna. *J Am Acad Dermatol*. 2006;55(1):88–97.

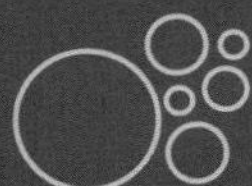

Solar lentigo – evolving seborrhoeic keratosis

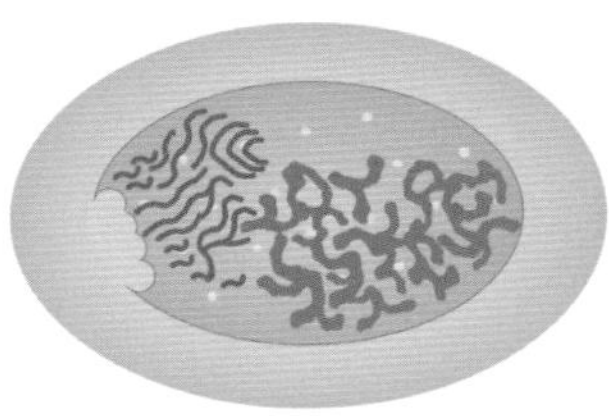

Solar lentigines and flat seborrhoeic keratoses may share clinical and histopathological features and therefore it is not uncommon for a solar lentigo to show additional dermoscopic features of an evolving seborrhoeic keratosis.

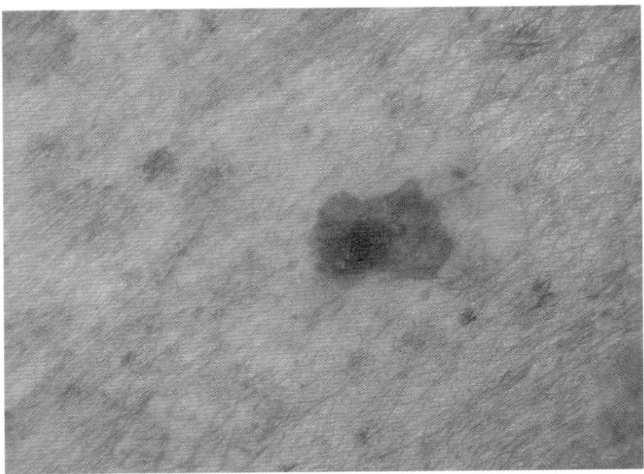

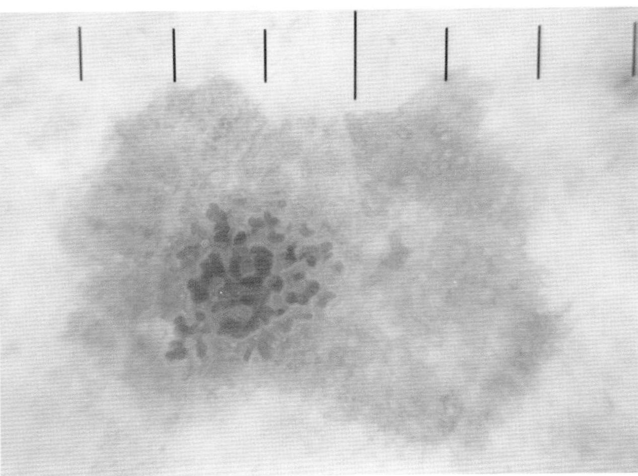

An angulated tan macule on the upper back of a 60-year-old woman: dermoscopy shows a well-demarcated moth-eaten border, reticular and homogeneous pigmentation and a focus of a cerebriform pattern in this solar lentigo with evolving seborrhoeic keratosis.

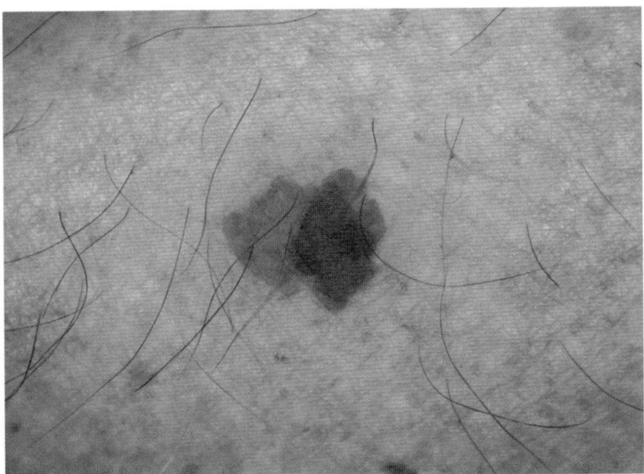

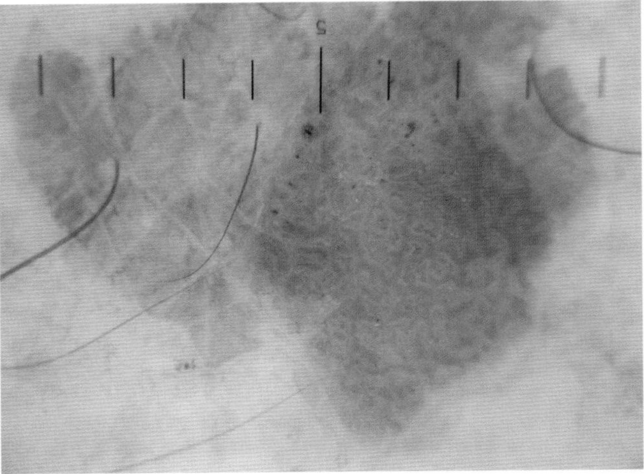

An angulated tan macule on the forearm of a 60-year-old man: dermoscopy shows a well-demarcated peripheral border, follicular openings and a zone with a ceribriform pattern in this solar lentigo with evolving seborrhoeic keratosis.

Although solar lentigines can sometimes be difficult to differentiate from lentigo maligna, they are not precursor lesions.

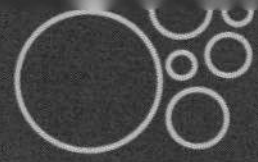

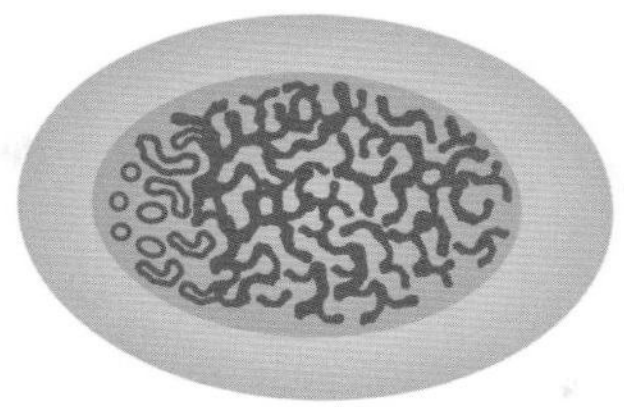

The cerebriform pattern is a common and easily recognised pattern for a seborrhoeic keratosis. The 'fat fingers' or 'sulci and gyri' are thick digitate linear, curvilinear branched or oval structures with variable amounts of keratin in between. This pattern may be subtle in early, evolving seborrhoeic keratoses and become more pronounced with time.

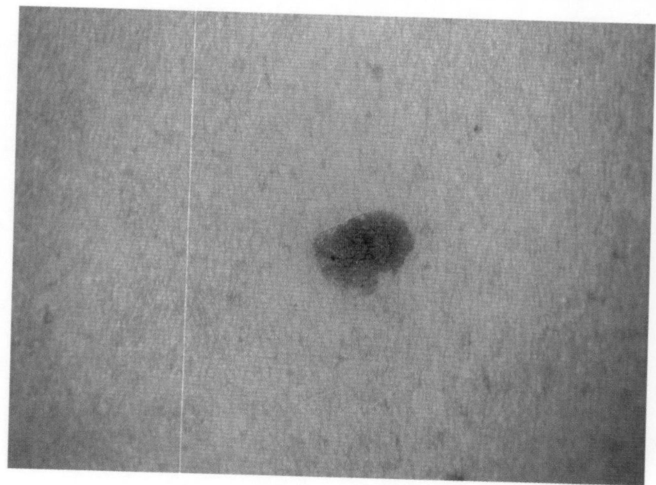

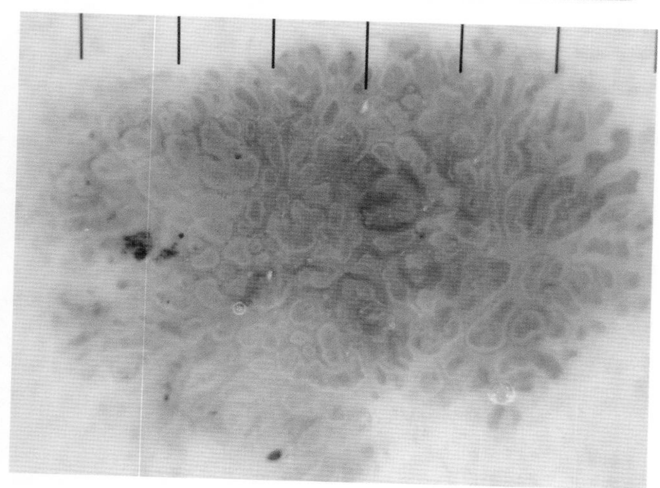

A brown warty keratotic plaque on the upper back of a 30-year-old woman: dermoscopy shows a uniform cerebriform pattern with 'fat fingers' in this seborrhoeic keratosis.

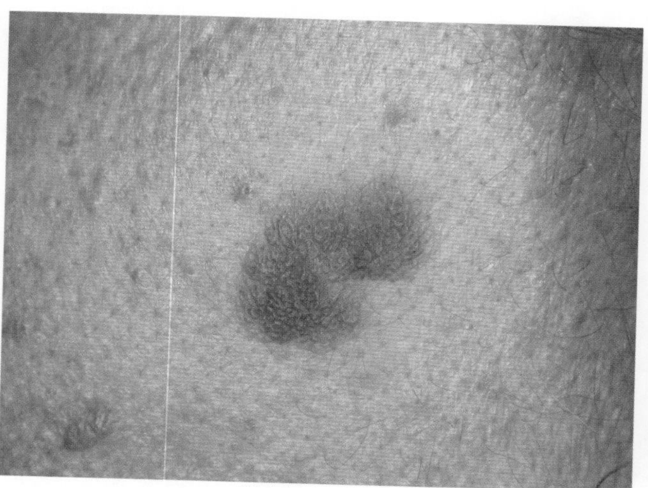

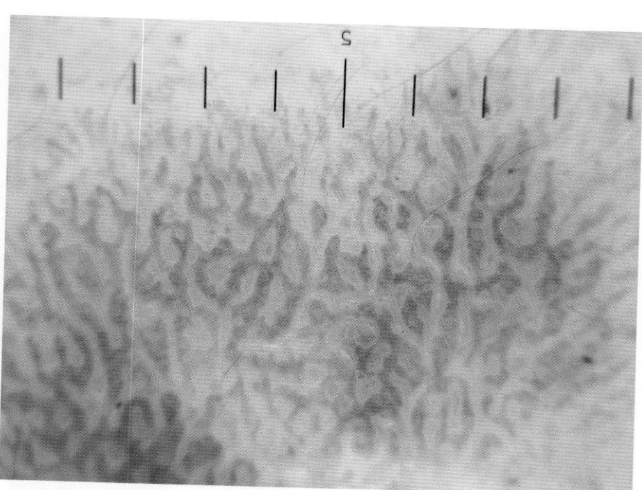

A brown warty plaque on the zygoma of a 70-year-old female: dermoscopy shows a uniform cerebriform pattern and multiple 'fat fingers' in this seborrhoeic keratosis.

Kopf, A.W., et al. 'Fat fingers': a clue in the dermoscopic diagnosis of seborrhoeic keratoses. *J Am Acad Dermatol.* 2006;55(6):1089–1091.

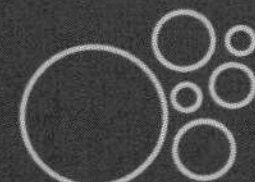

Seborrhoeic keratosis – homogeneous pattern

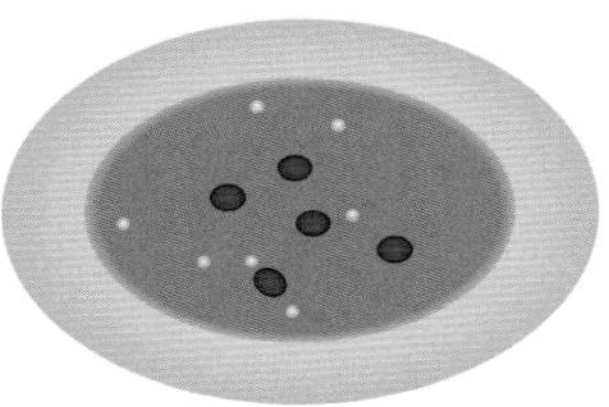

The background colour of pigmented seborrhoeic keratosis is typically a uniform light brown colour. Early seborrhoeic keratoses with increased homogeneous pigmentation and a relative lack of additional keratinising structures can mimic melanocytic lesions. On dermoscopy, these keratinising structures, although small, may be more clearly seen to confirm the diagnosis.

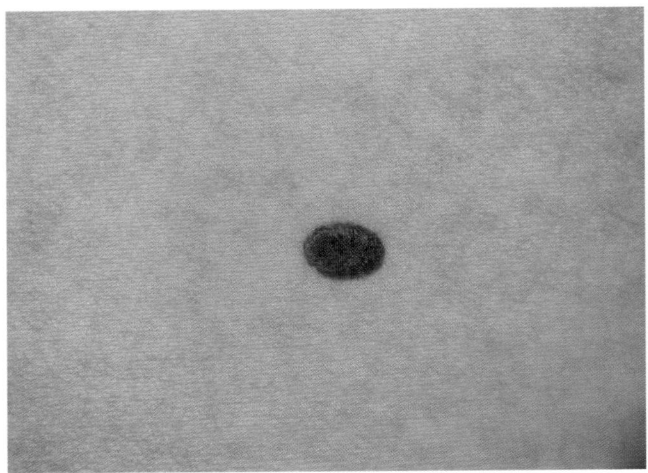

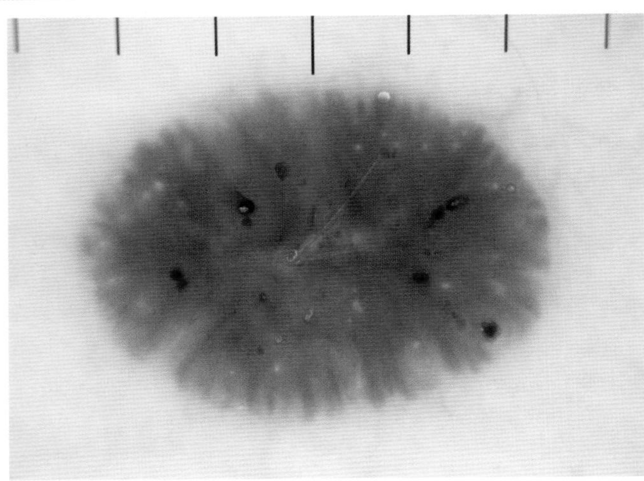

A brown warty plaque on the upper back of a 30-year-old man: dermoscopy shows a uniform homogeneous brown colour with additional brown comedo-like openings and white milia-like cysts in this seborrhoeic keratosis.

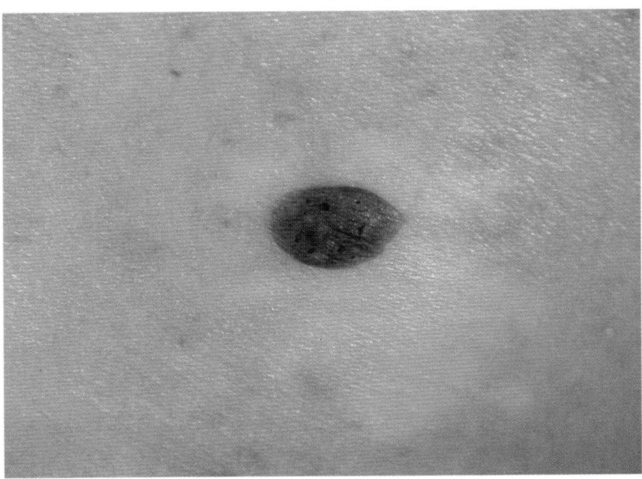

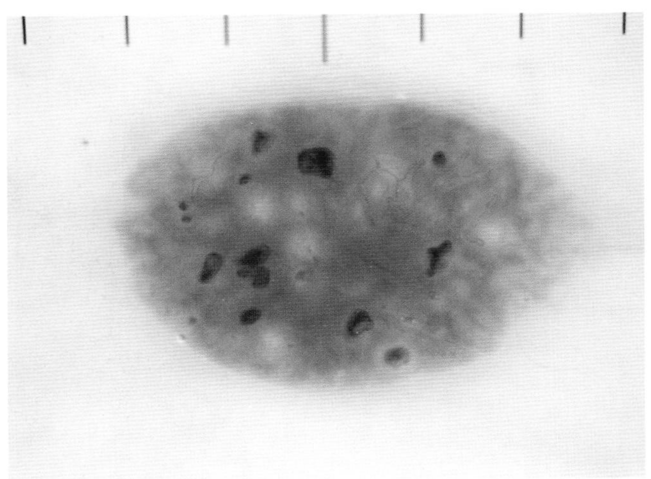

A brown warty plaque on the back of a 70-year-old female: dermoscopy shows a homogeneous and cerebriform pattern, with multiple brown comedo-like openings and white milia-like cysts in this seborrhoeic keratosis.

Examine all skin lesions with dermoscopy. Milia-like cysts are seen less well with polarised dermoscopy so best to toggle between the modes to identify clearly.

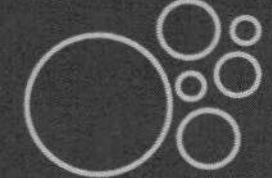

Seborrhoeic keratosis – keratotic pattern

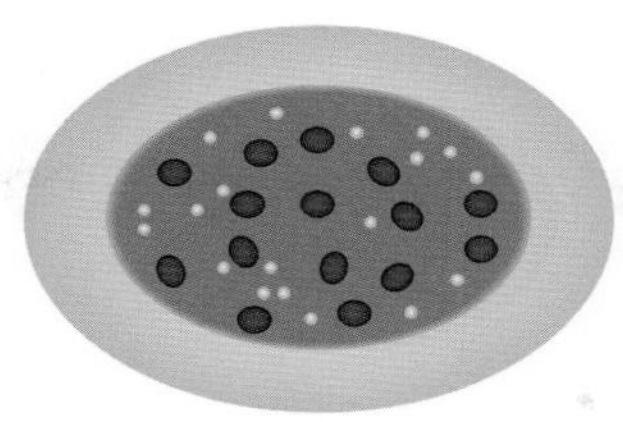

Seborrhoeic keratoses commonly exhibit a keratotic pattern with an excess of keratin structures within the epidermis (milia-like cysts) and penetrating through the surface of the epidermis (comedo-like openings). Milia-like cysts are small white round structures that light up when switching to non-polarised dermoscopy. Comedo-like openings are crater-like polymorphous structures filled with white, yellow, brown or black keratin plugs. They are often surrounded by a pale halo.

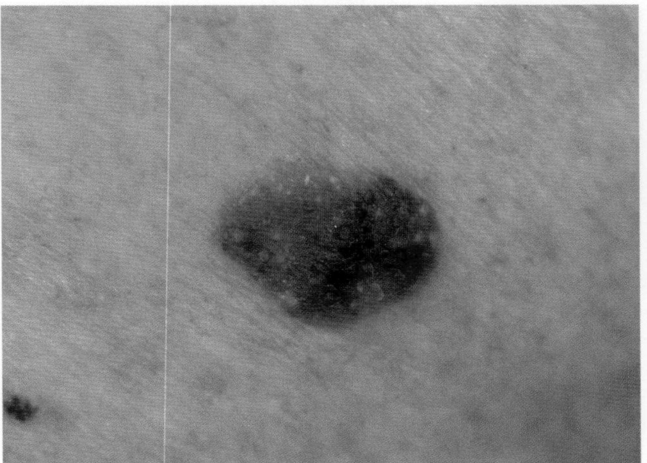

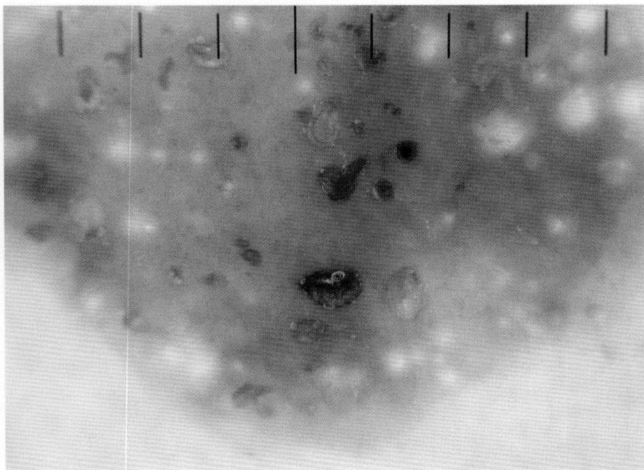

A keratotic plaque on the upper back of a 40-year-old man: dermoscopy shows multiple milia-like cysts and comedo-like openings in this typical seborrhoeic keratosis.

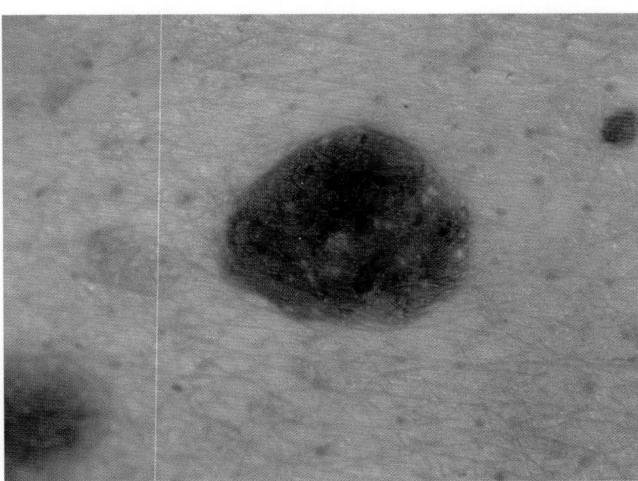

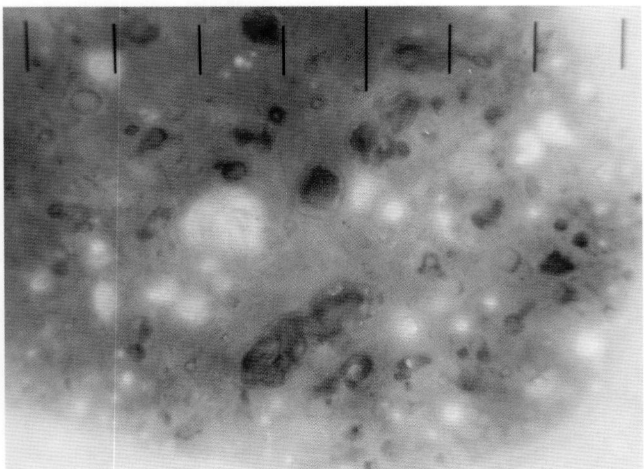

A keratotic plaque on the upper back of a 60-year-old man: dermoscopy shows multiple milia-like cysts and comedo-like openings in this typical seborrhoeic keratosis.

In hyperkeratotic seborrhoeic keratoses, the underlying features may be obscured by the plaques of keratin.

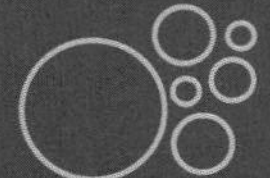

Seborrhoeic keratosis – hyperpigmented

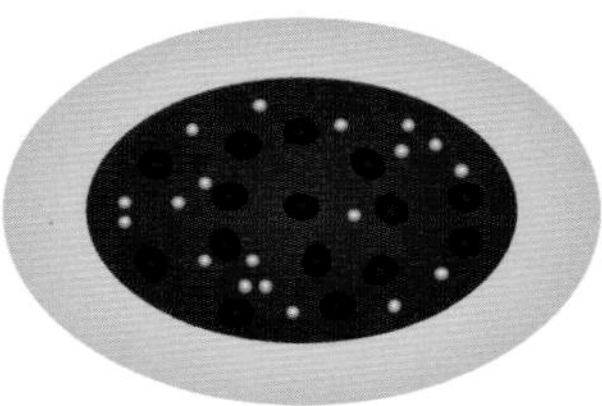

Hyperpigmented seborrhoeic keratoses are not uncommon. Typically, they occur as the predominant pattern in patients with dark skin. When solitary, particularly in patients with lighter skin, they can cause clinical concern. The typical dermoscopic features of seborrhoeic keratoses may be obscured due to increased pigmentation, therefore creating a clinicodermoscopic overlap with melanocytic lesions.

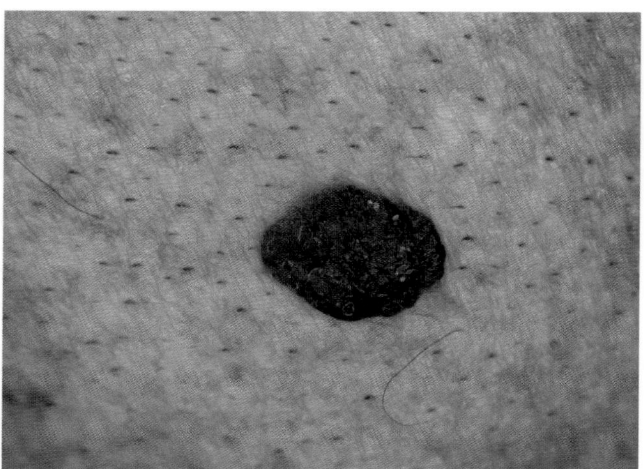

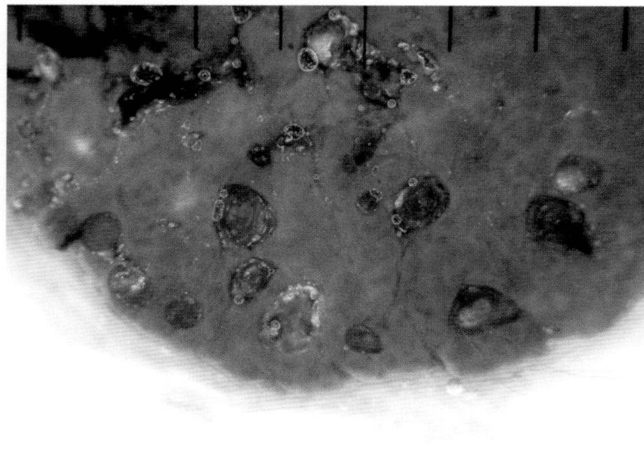

A dark warty plaque on the cheek of a 70-year-old man: dermoscopy shows background hyperpigmentation with comedo-like openings and milia-like cysts in this hyperpigmented seborrhoeic keratosis.

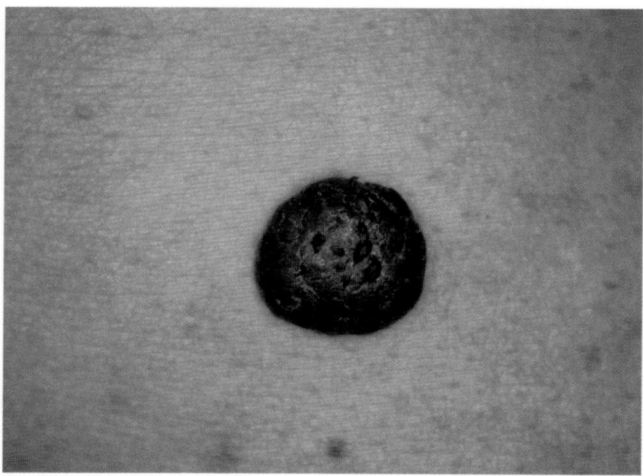

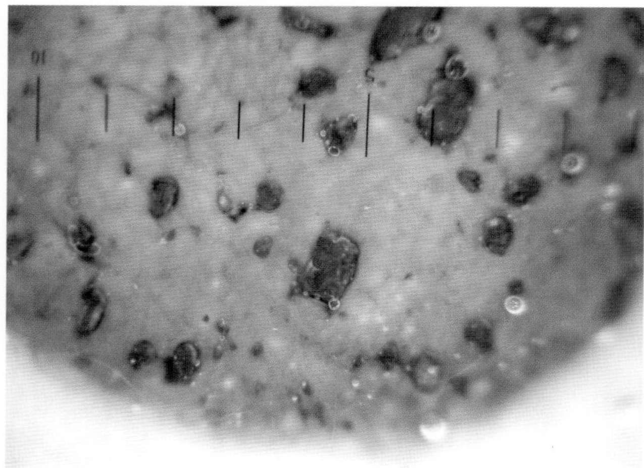

A hyperpigmented nodule on the back of a 40-year-old woman: dermoscopy shows greyish background pigmentation, multiple milia-like cysts and hyperpigmented comedo-like openings in this hyperpigmented seborrhoeic keratosis.

Consider verrucous melanoma specifically in this setting if the morphology is atypical.

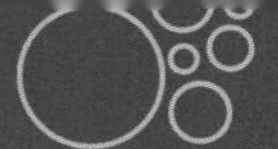

Seborrhoeic keratosis – hypopigmented

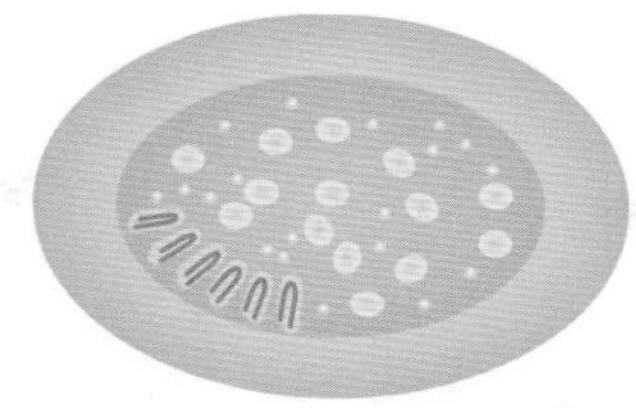

Hypopigmented seborrhoeic keratoses are more common in patients with light skin. The dermoscopic structures may be subtle and careful examination is required. It is not uncommon for vascular structures to predominate as haemoglobin would be the dominant chromophore in the skin. Irritated or traumatised seborrhoeic keratoses have a prominent yet ordered vascular pattern with looped or hairpin vessels and may mimic squamous cell carcinoma.

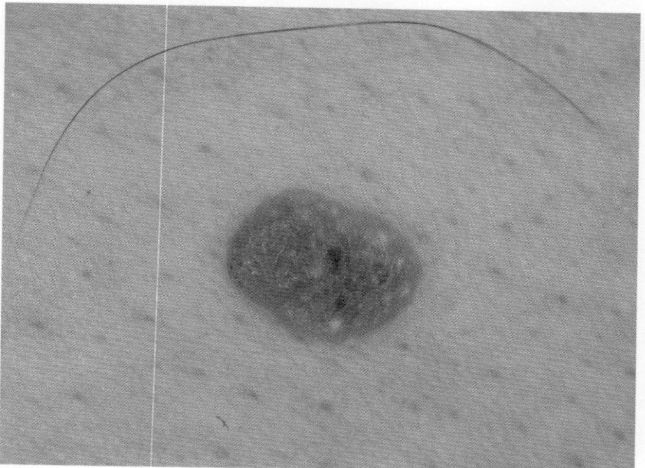

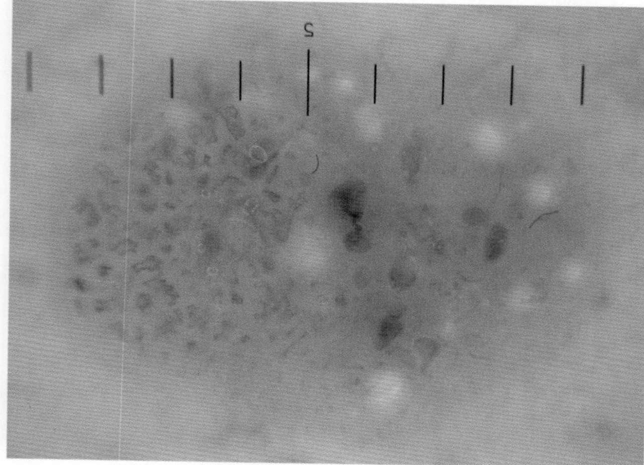

A pink and tan keratotic plaque on the neck of a 30-year-old man: dermoscopy shows one eccentric pole with looped or hairpin vessels and another with milia-like cysts and comedo-like openings in this hypopigmented irritated seborrhoeic keratosis.

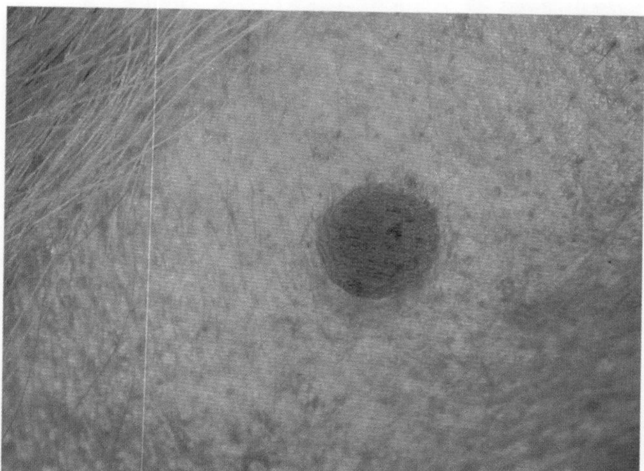

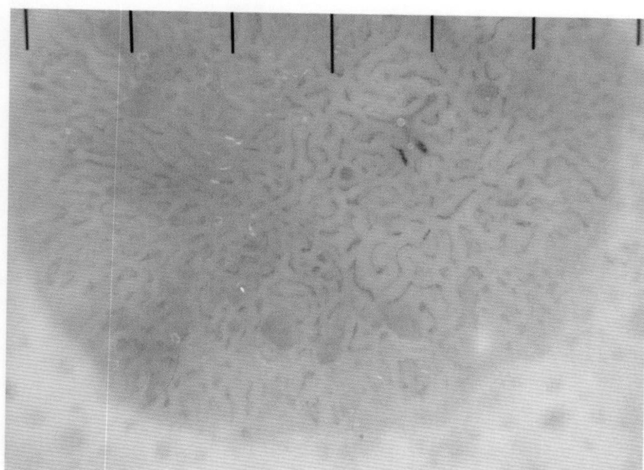

A pink plaque on the temple of a 40-year-old man: dermoscopy shows looped or hairpin vessels following a cerebriform background pattern resembling a maze in this hypopigmented seborrhoeic keratosis.

Squillace, L. et al. Unusual dermoscopic patterns of seborrhoeic keratosis. *Dermatology*. 2016;232:198–202.

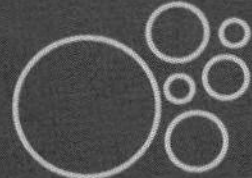

Seborrhoeic keratosis – irritated

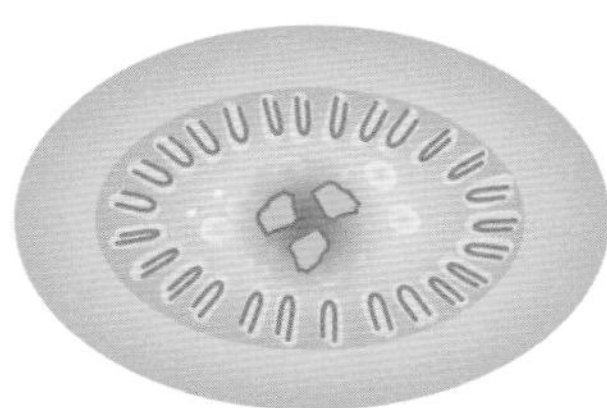

When seborrhoeic keratoses become irritated and inflamed, the vascular pattern increases and additional features including prominent looped or hairpin vessels, erosions and orange-brown crusts may develop. The background features of seborrhoeic keratosis may therefore become obscured and the clinical and dermoscopy overlap with squamous cell carcinoma. Consider a diagnostic biopsy if any diagnostic doubt remains.

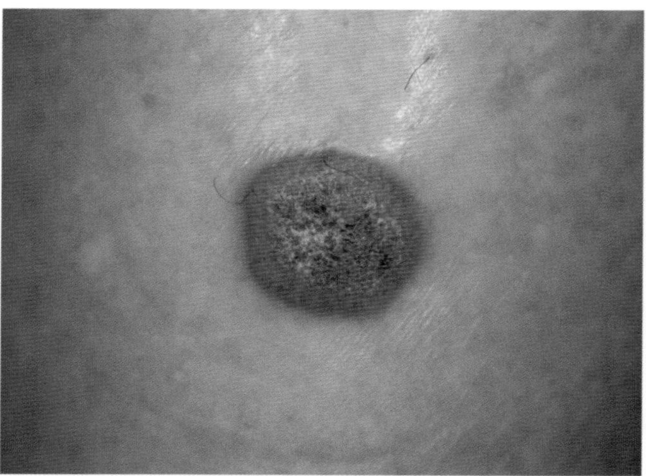

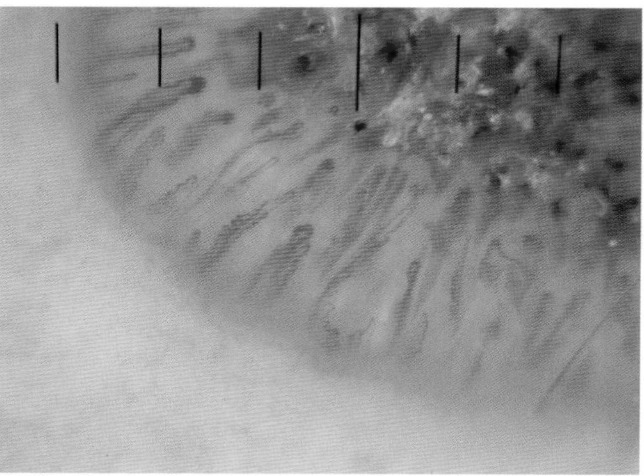

An inflamed plaque on the lower leg of a 60-year-old woman: dermoscopy shows concentrically distributed looped/hairpin vessels with central crusts and purple dots (thrombosis) in this histopathologically confirmed seborrhoeic keratosis.

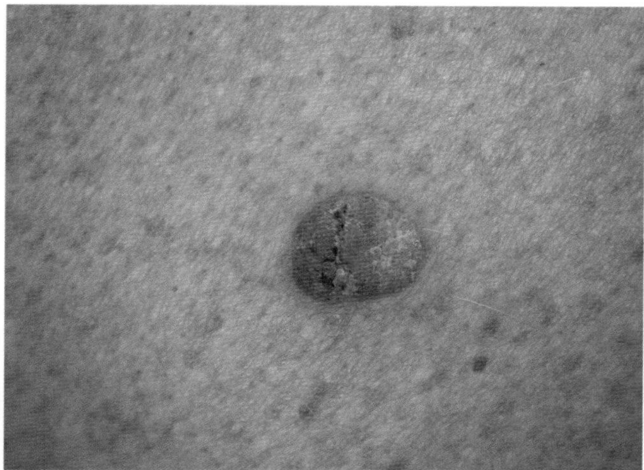

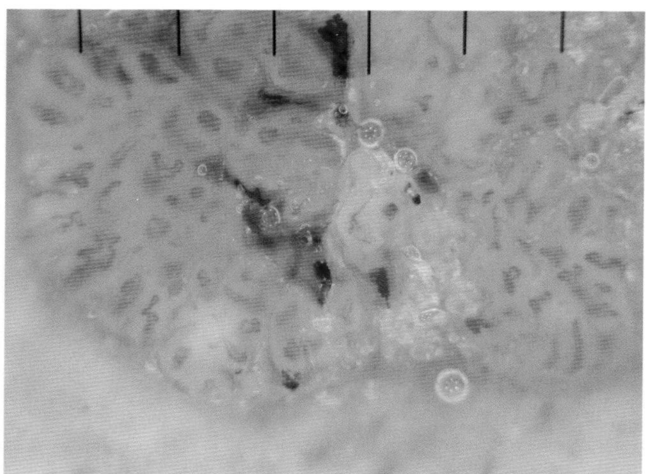

A pink keratotic plaque on the back of a 60-year-old woman: dermoscopy shows widespread looped/hairpin vessels, haemorrhages, blotches and crusts in this histopathologically confirmed inflamed seborrhoeic keratosis.

Consider a biopsy if any diagnostic concern remains following a detailed history, clinical and dermoscopic examination.

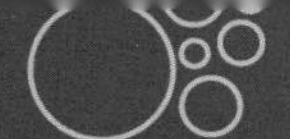

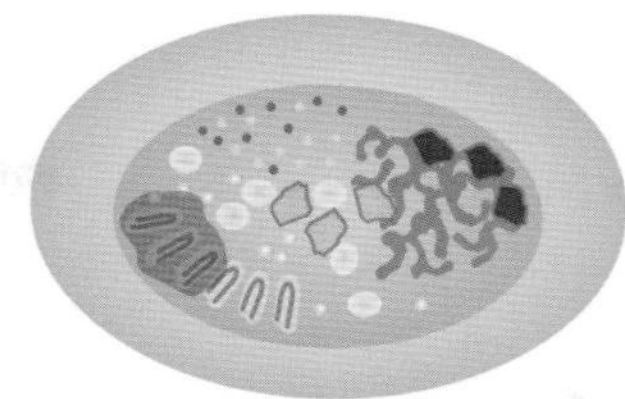

It is not uncommon for a seborrhoeic keratoses to become traumatized. This may cause concern to patients and the clinician as clinical features within the original skin lesion may be compromised. Dermoscopy can help to identify any residual elements of the baseline skin lesion.

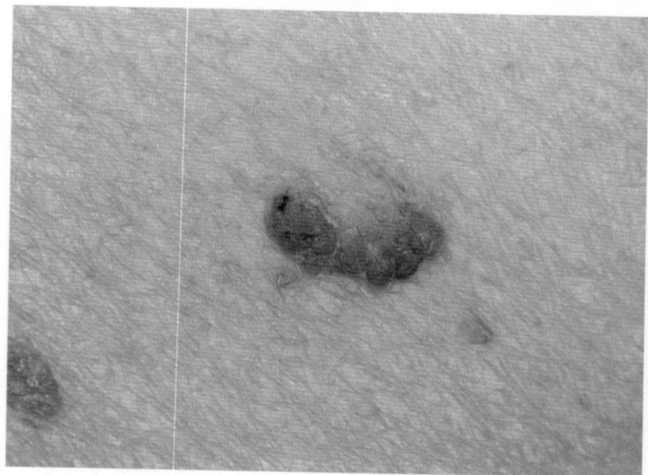

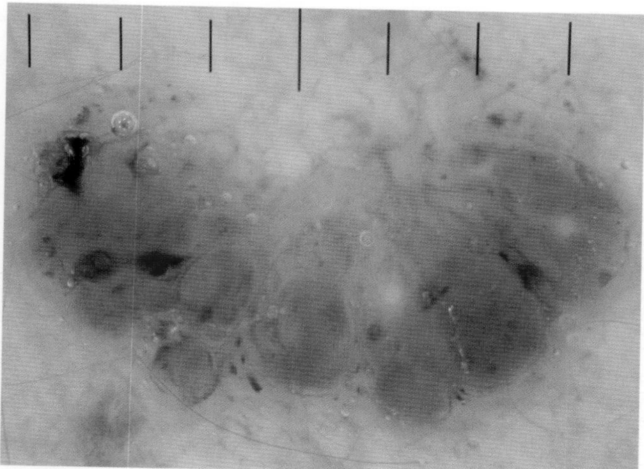

An arcuate keratotic plaque on the back with a history of trauma on a 40-year-old woman: dermoscopy shows haemorrhagic erosions, residual homogenous tan pigmentation, milia-like cysts and grey granular dots in this seborrhoeic keratosis.

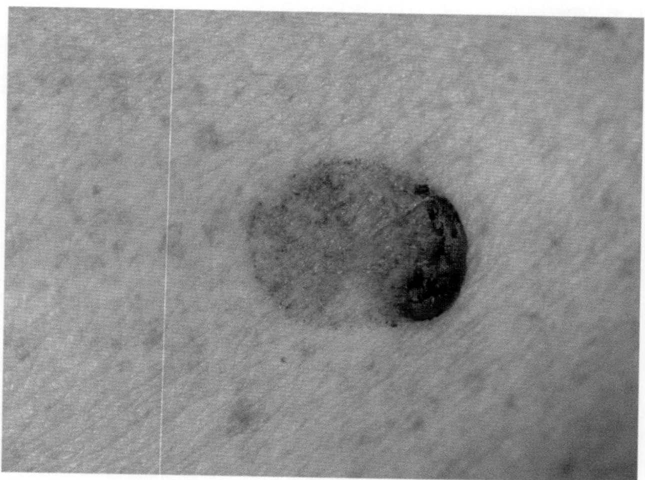

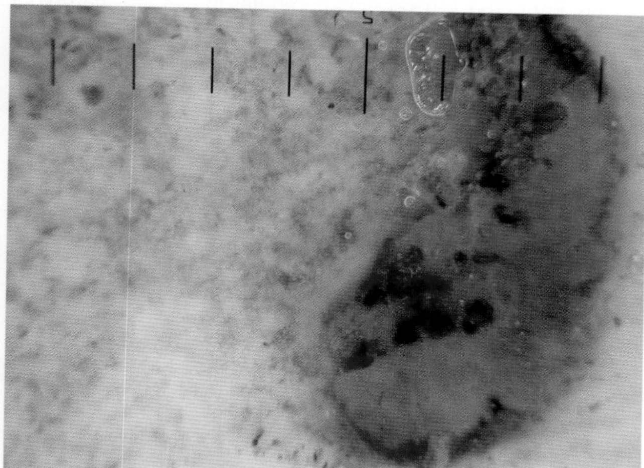

A keratotic remnant at the margin of a grey macule, with a history of trauma on the shoulder of a 70-year-old man: dermoscopy shows extensive grey granular dots (peppering), ulceration and haemorrhage with remnants of a seborrhoeic keratosis.

In traumatised seborrhoeic keratoses, the underlying features may be compromised – consider a biopsy if any diagnostic doubt remains.

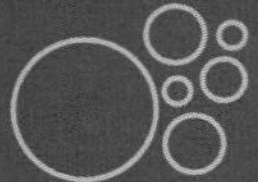

Seborrhoeic keratosis – clonal

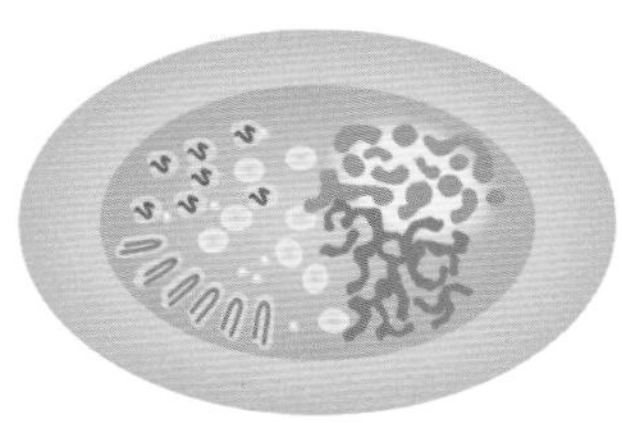

Clonal seborrhoeic keratoses are an uncommon subtype of seborrhoeic keratosis that may cause diagnostic concern due to suspicious clinical features that may mimic keratinocyte dysplasia, atypical melanocytic lesions, inflammatory and infective conditions. They are often solitary and typically occur on the lower leg. Dermoscopy may show the typical features of seborrhoeic keratoses but also polymorphous vessels, negative network and brown globules.

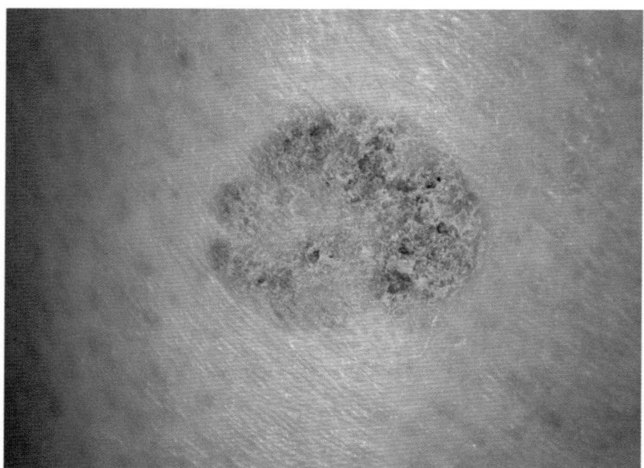

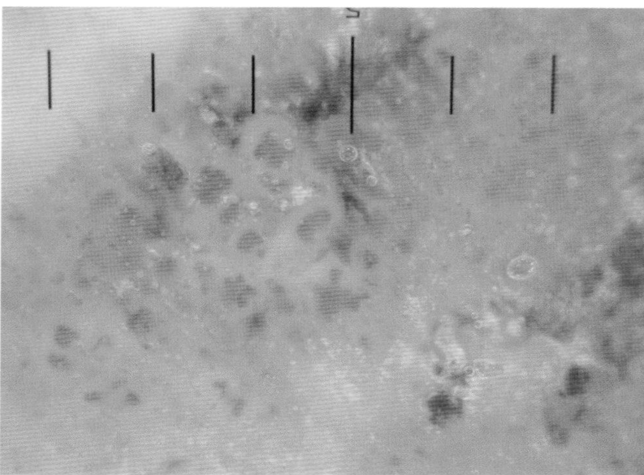

A suspicious pink-brown scaly plaque on the lower leg of a 70-year-old woman: dermoscopy shows irregular coiled or glomerular vessels, erythema and keratin aggregates in this histopathologically confirmed clonal seborrhoeic keratosis.

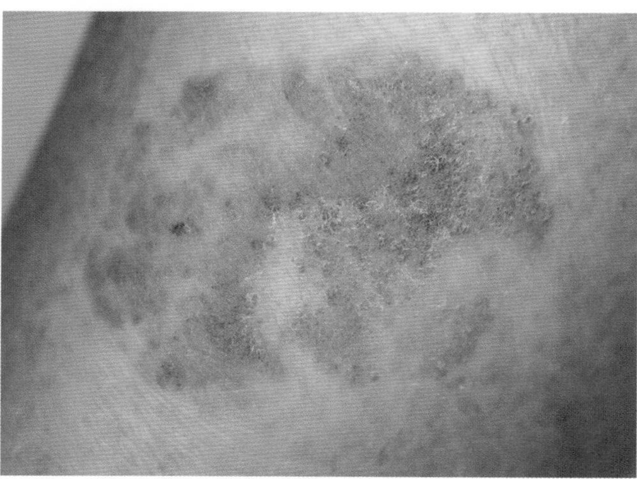

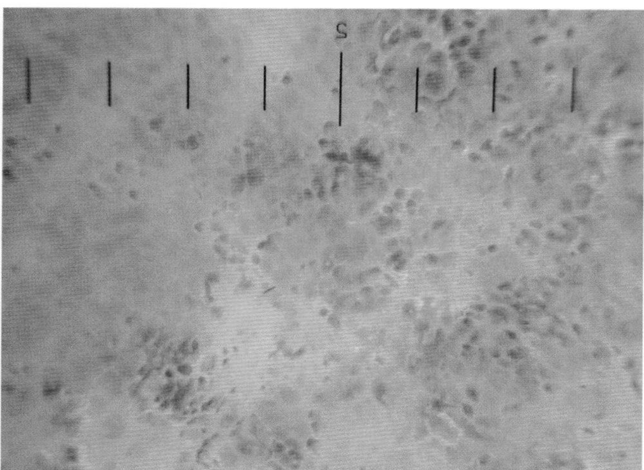

A large pink, brown warty plaque on the lower leg of a 60-year-old woman: dermoscopy shows erythema and multiple brown globules with negative network in this histopathologically confirmed clonal seborrhoeic keratosis.

Longo, C., et al. Clonal seborrhoeic keratosis: dermoscopic and confocal microscopy characterization. *J Eur Acad Dermatol Venereol*. 2014;28(10):1397–1400.

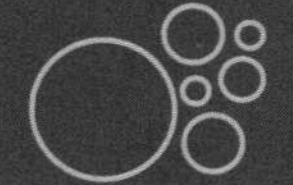

Clear cell acanthoma

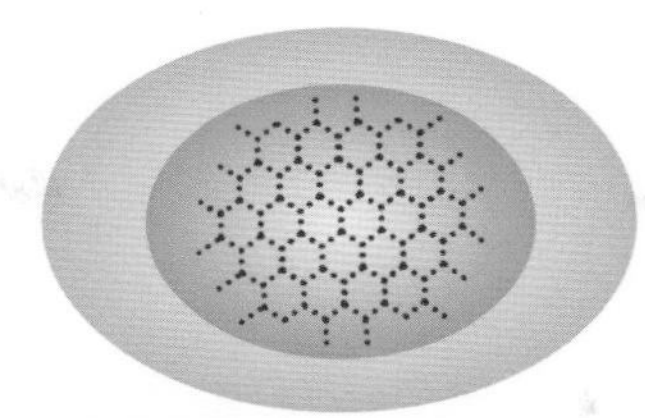

A clear cell acanthoma is a benign skin tumour and a variant of a seborrhoeic keratosis. They clinically present as an asymptomatic, solitary, slowly enlarging, red or red-brown, dome-shaped papule on the lower limbs. They may, rarely, be multiple. They have a distinct vascular morphology seen on dermoscopy with dotted and coiled or glomerular vessels that are regularly arranged, reported as a 'string or pearls' pattern.

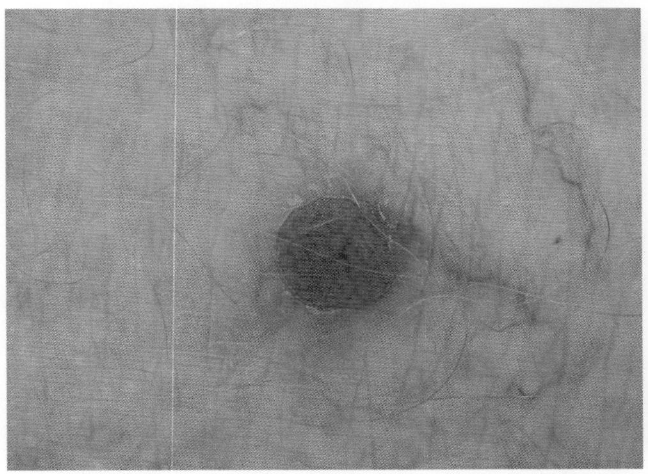

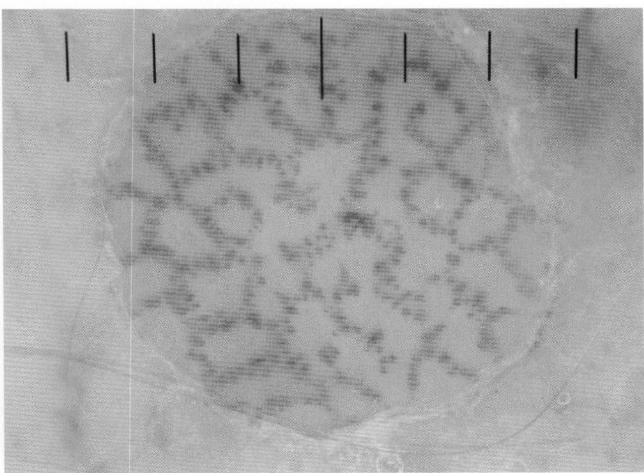

A solitary pink papule on the lower leg of an 80-year-old male: dermoscopy shows regularly arranged dotted and coiled/glomerular vessels in a 'string of pearls' pattern on a pink homogeneous background in this clear cell acanthoma.

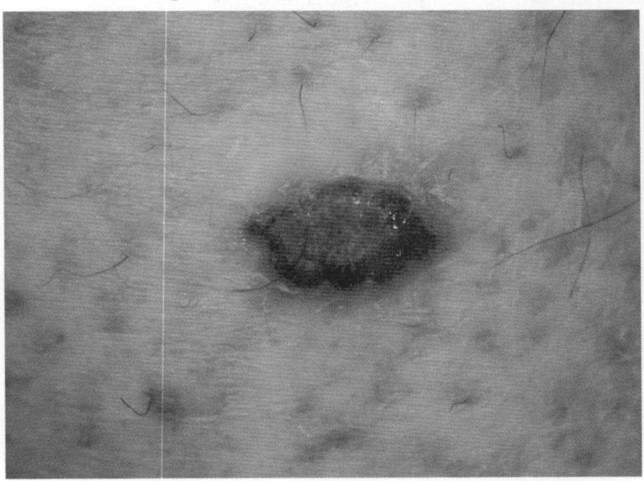

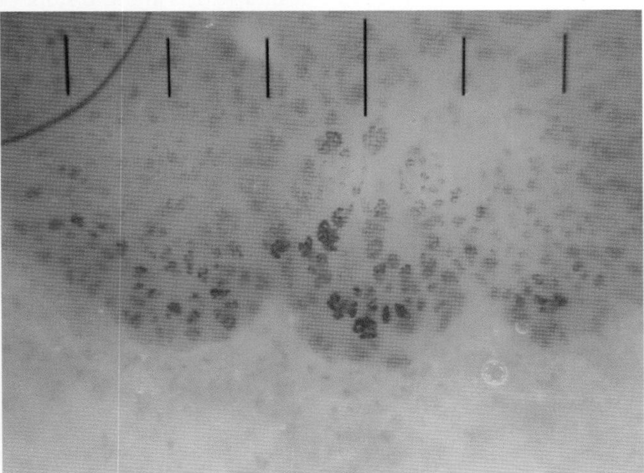

A vascular plaque on the lower leg of a 60-year-old female: dermoscopy shows dotted and coiled/glomerular vessels in a looped 'string of pearls' pattern on a pink homogeneous background in this histopathologically confirmed clear cell acanthoma.

Lyons, G. et al. Dermoscopic features of clear cell acanthomas: five new cases and a review of existing published cases. *Aust J Dermatol* 2015;56(3):206–11.

Benign lichenoid keratosis – inflammatory phase

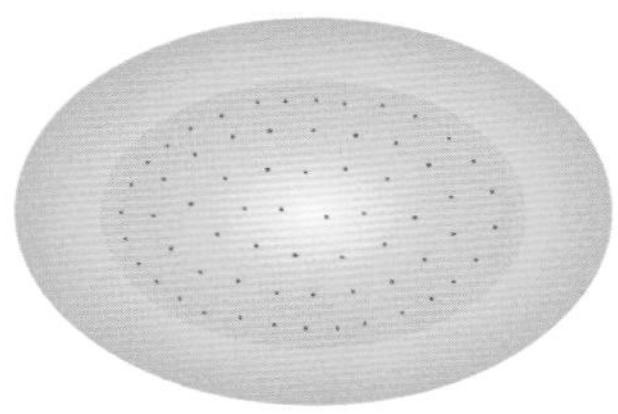

Benign epidermal skin lesions, typically solar lentigines or flat seborrhoeic keratoses may be affected by a host-induced lichenoid inflammatory response leading to short-lived changes in appearance. Importantly, during the inflammatory phase, the peripheral margin is typically very well-defined and residual features of the pre-existing skin lesion may not be visible. Dermoscopic features are often minimal with a uniform pink colour, and non-specific vascular dilatation.

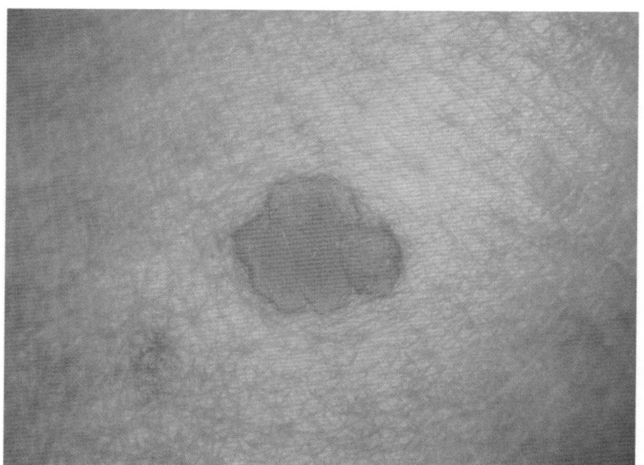

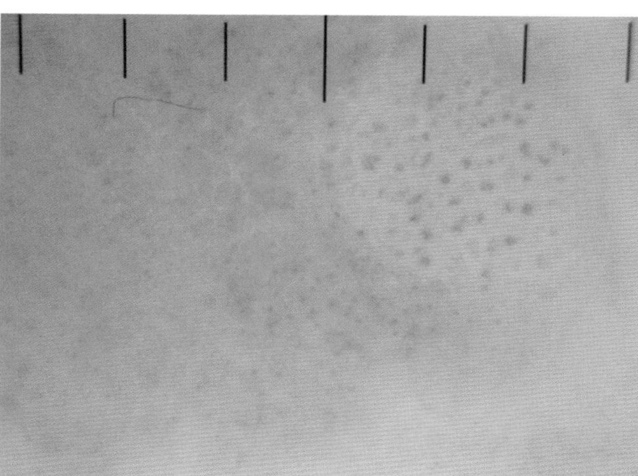

A new onset solitary pink plaque, with a clear peripheral margin, on the arm of a 40-year-old woman: dermoscopy shows a uniform pink colour with eccentric dotted vessels in this histopathologically confirmed benign lichenoid keratosis.

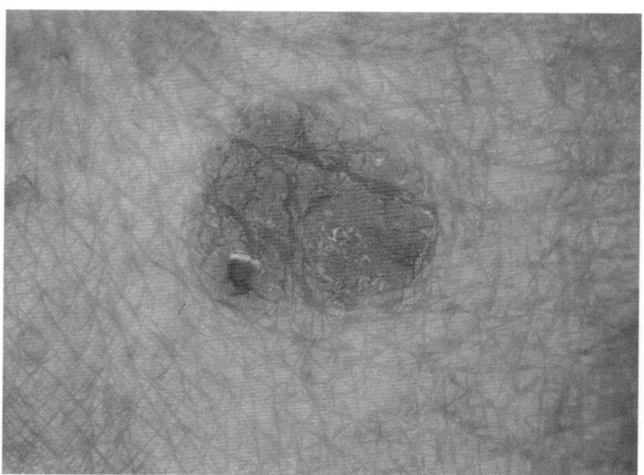

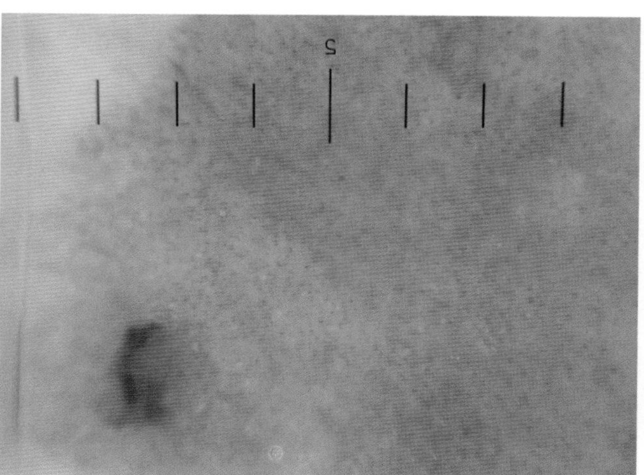

A 60 year-old woman with an excoriated pruritic and inflammed plaque on the dorsum of the hand: dermoscopy shows uniform erythema with dotted vessels in keeping with lichenoid inflammation in a solar lentigo.

Gori, A. et al. Clinical and dermoscopic features of lichenoid keratosis: A retrospective case study. *J Cutan Med Surg* 2018: 22(6):561–66

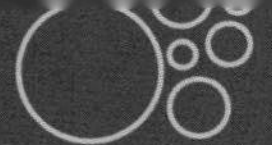

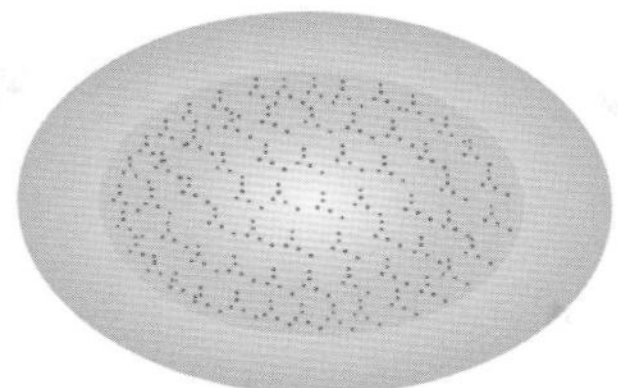

Following the inflammatory phase epidermal pigment descends into the dermis, leading to diffuse grey granular pigmentation. Frequently there is no evidence of the pre-existing skin lesion. On dermoscopy the grey dots are uniform in distribution across the lesion and also around follicles with a well-demarcated border. This appearance is described as 'peppering'.

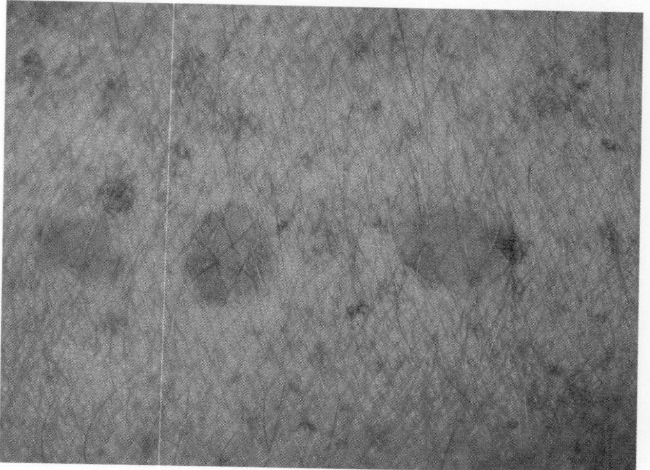

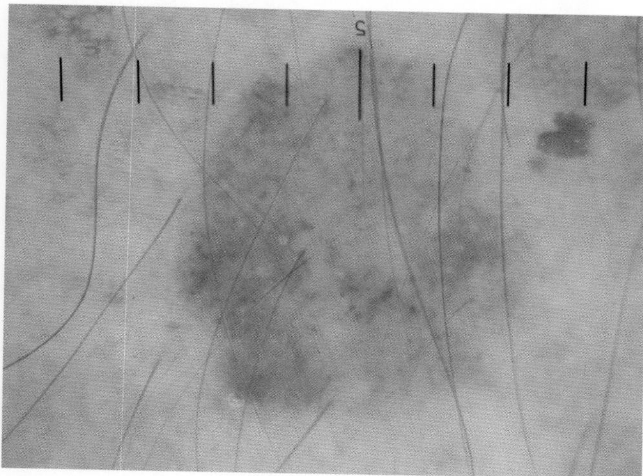

A pair of pigmented macules on the arm of a 50-year-old man: dermoscopy shows uniform grey granular peppering in this benign lichenoid keratosis arising from a solar lentigo.

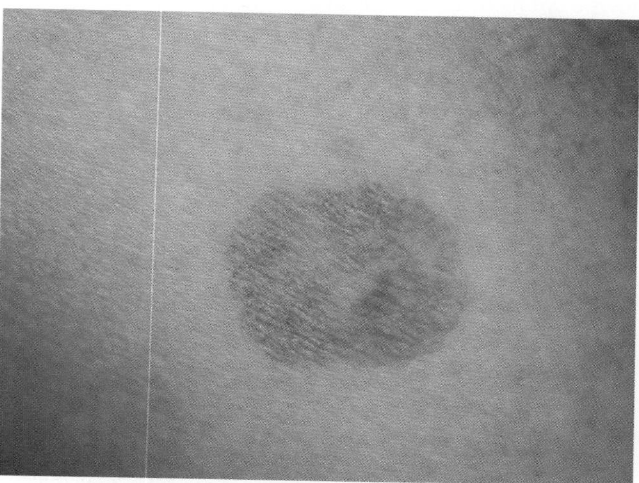

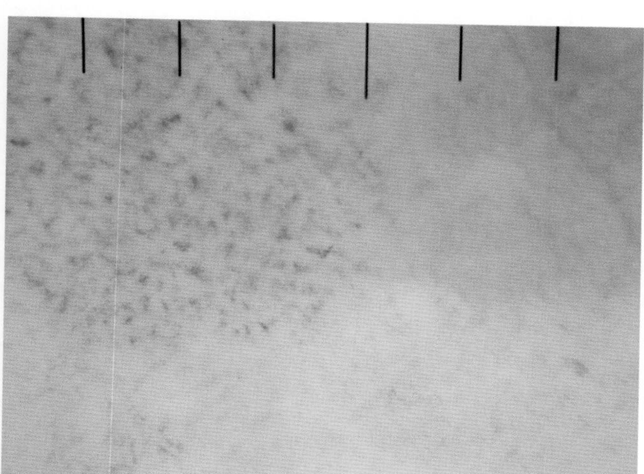

A two-tone grey-tan macule on the shoulder of a 60-year-old woman: dermoscopy shows remnants of a solar lentigo with a clearly defined zone of uniform grey peppering in this benign lichenoid keratosis arising in a solar lentigo.

Zaballos, P. et al. Studying regression of seborrhoeic keratosis in lichenoid keratosis with sequential dermoscopy imaging. *Dermatology*. 2010;220(2):103–109.

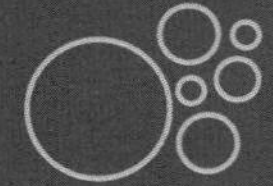

Dermatofibroma

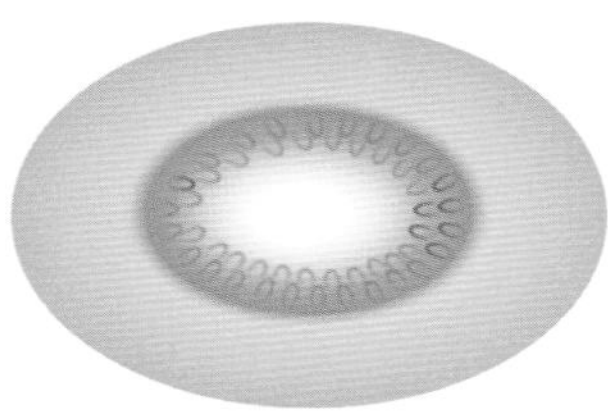

A dermatofibroma is a benign proliferation of dermal collagen. The cause is unknown, but they may be induced by an insect bite or an ingrown hair. They typically occur on exposed anatomical sites as slightly pigmented, firm dermal papulonodules which dimple on compression. Dermoscopic features include a peripheral pigment network and a central scar-like area. Dotted vessels may be seen within the annular structures of the network. Early dermatofibromas may mimic melanocytic lesions.

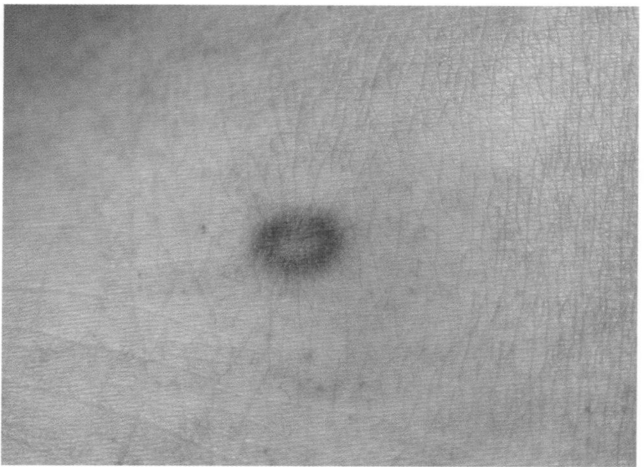

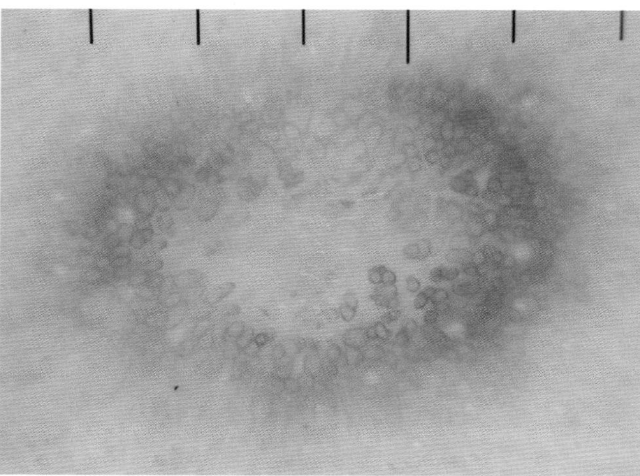

A tan plaque on the ankle of a 40-year-old woman: dermoscopy shows a symmetrical lesion with a central scar-like area and a peripheral pigment network in this dermatofibroma.

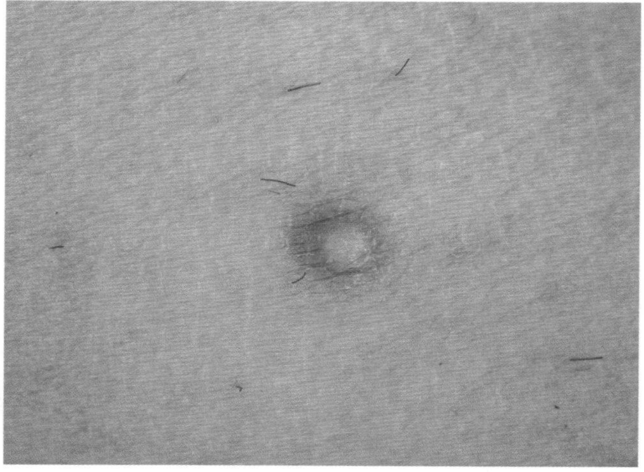

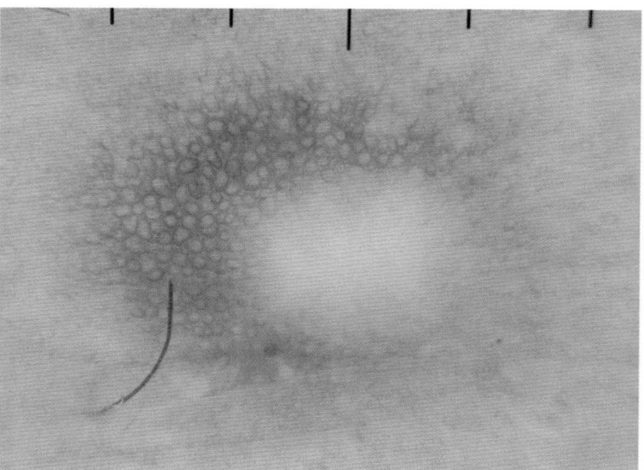

A solitary tan papule on the lower leg of a 30-year-old woman: dermoscopy shows a central scar-like area and a peripheral light brown pigment network in this dermatofibroma.

Puig, S. et al Dermoscopy of dermatofibroma. *Arch Dermatol.* 2005;141(1):122.

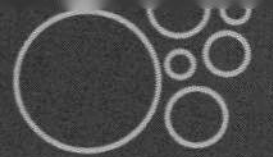

Dermatofibroma – hypopigmented

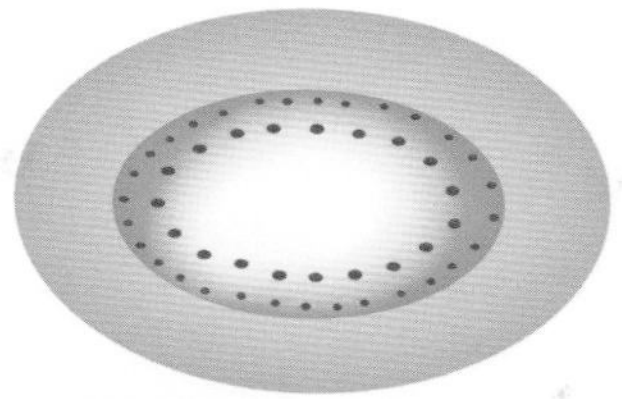

Dermatofibromas in patients with light skin may present as a solitary pink papule or nodule with dotted vessels on dermoscopy. The differential diagnosis is extensive and includes amelanotic melanoma and desmoplastic tumours. Histopathology should be considered if any index of suspicion remains following the history, clinical and dermoscopic examination.

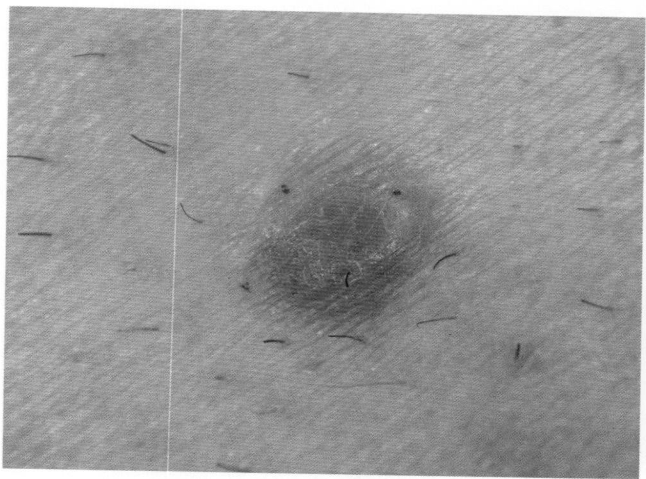

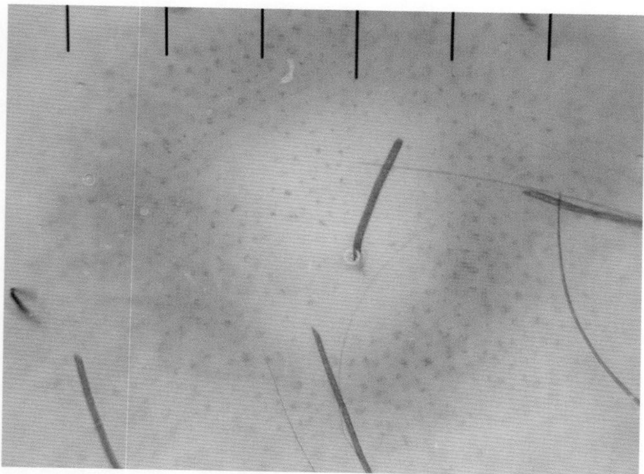

A solitary firm pink nodule/plaque on the lower leg of a 30-year-old woman: dermoscopy shows a background pale and pink structureless area with multiple dotted vessels in this histopathologically confirmed dermatofibroma.

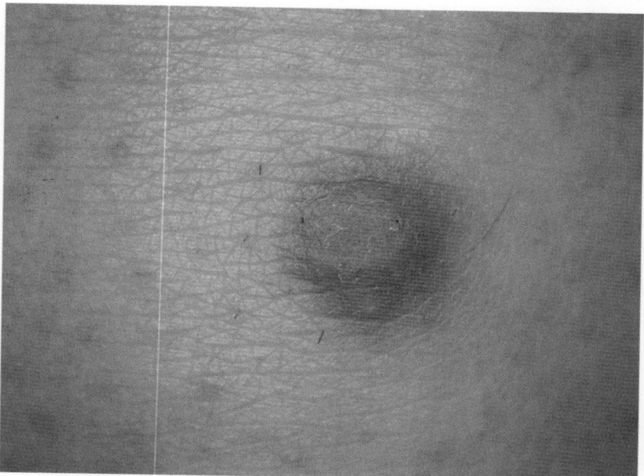

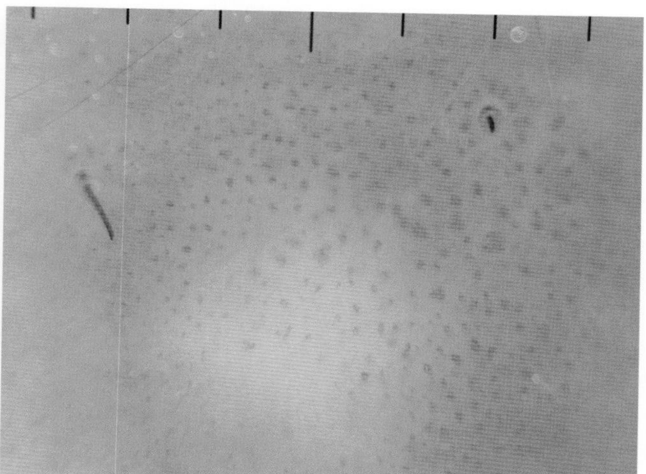

A solitary firm pink nodule on the lower leg of a 40-year-old woman: dermoscopy shows a background pale and pink structureless area with multiple dotted vessels in this histopathologically confirmed dermatofibroma.

Zaballos, P. et al. Dermoscopy of dermatofibromas: a prospective morphological study of 412 cases. *Arch Dermatol.* 2008;144(1):75–83.

Dermatofibroma – hyperpigmented

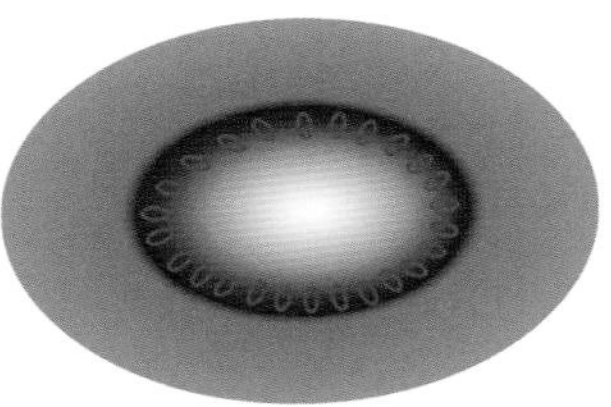

In dark skin, the pigmented features within a dermatofibroma are accentuated and the vascular features may be difficult to see or absent. When scarring develops the interface between the central scar and adjacent pigmented skin may help illustrate additional dermoscopic features including granular hyperpigmentation, follicular pigmentation and pigmented globules and black dots on the surface of the acanthotic epidermis.

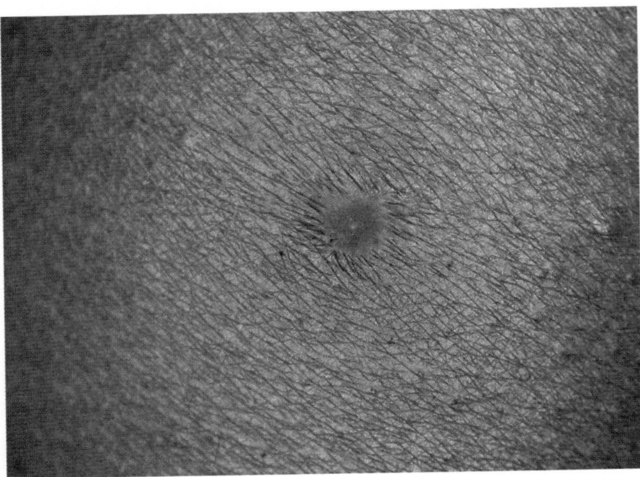

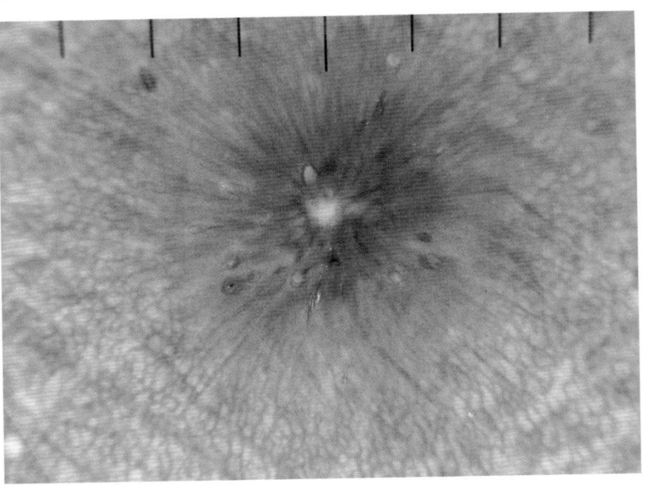

A pigmented plaque on the ankle of a 40-year-old woman: dermoscopy shows a symmetrical lesion with a small central scar-like focus, radiating granular hyperpigmentation and follicular circles in this dermatofibroma.

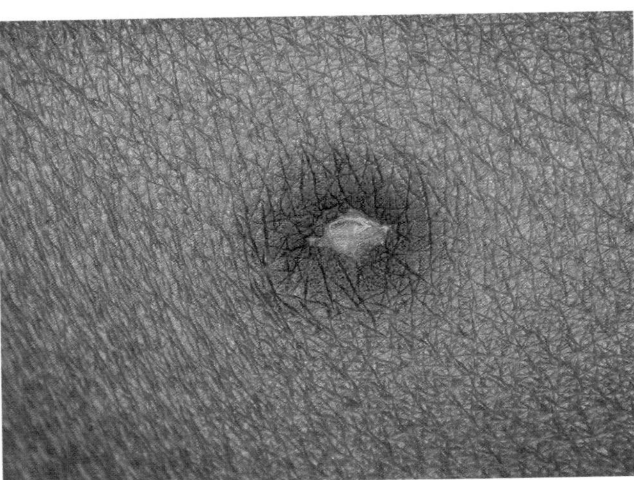

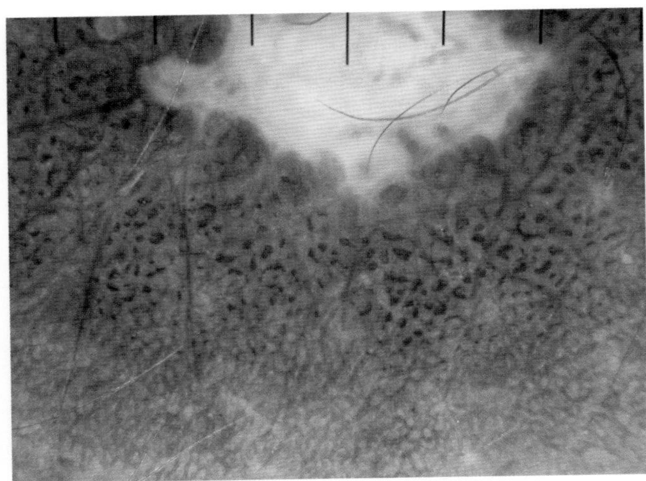

A scarred dermal plaque on the back of a 40-year-old woman: dermoscopy shows a central whitish-pink scar-like area and a clear demarcation to brown pigmented aggregates with black dots blending peripherally to normal skin in this dermatofibroma.

Clinical examination, history, and consideration of anatomical location are all features in addition to dermoscopy that help confirm a diagnosis of dermatofibroma in dark skin. Consider a biopsy if any diagnostic doubt remains

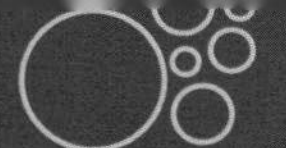

Dermatofibroma – atypical

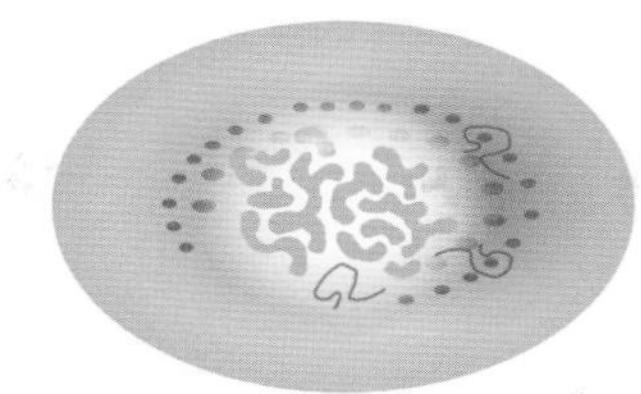

The differential diagnosis of dermatofibromas with an atypical pattern is extensive and includes a number of benign and malignant skin tumours. Common variants include cellular and aneurysmal dermatofibromas. However, as the clinical and dermoscopic features overlap with malignant lesions, histopathology is advised to confirm the diagnosis.

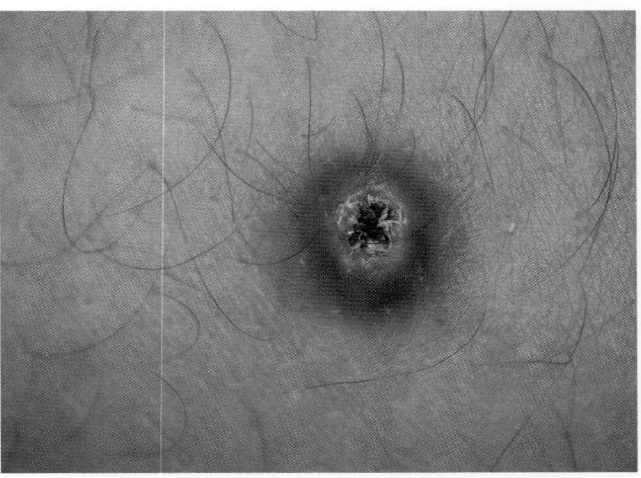

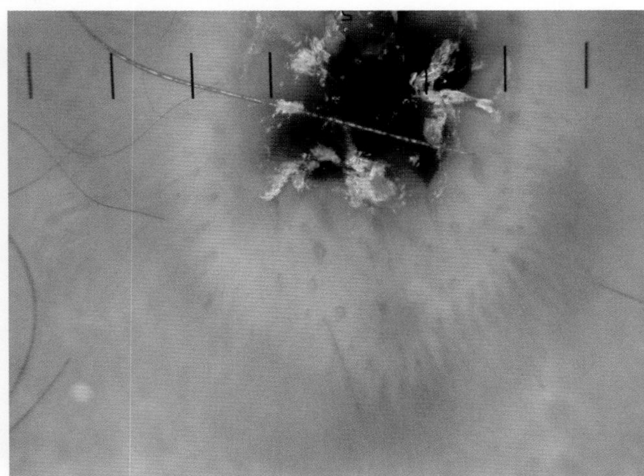

A firm ulcerated on the leg of a 50-year-old man: dermoscopy shows a purple background colour with radial hairpin vessels and central ulceration in this histopathologically confirmed aneurysmal dermatofibroma.

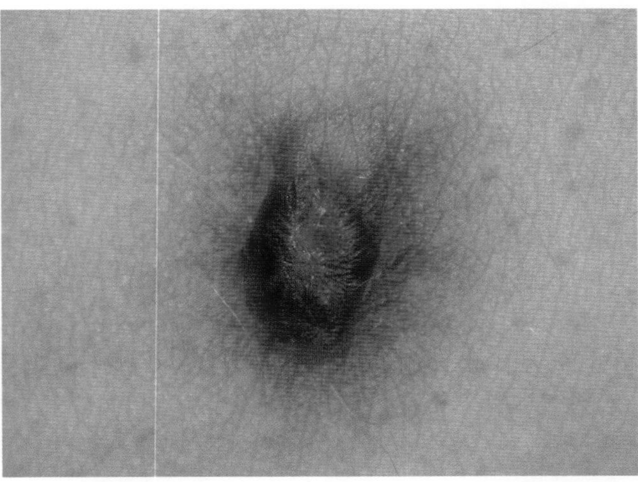

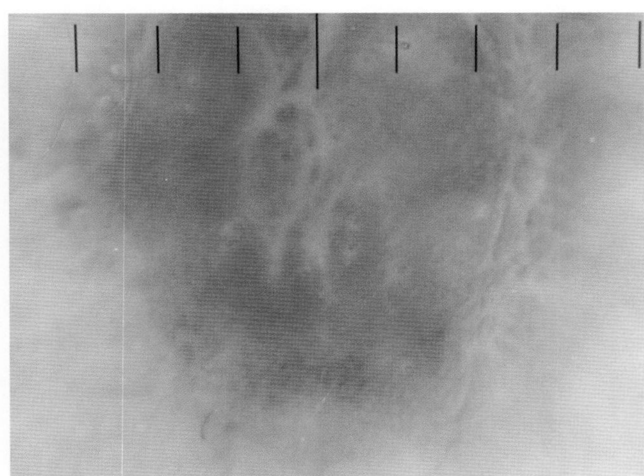

A suspicious indurated pigmented plaque on the lower leg of a 40-year-old woman: dermoscopy shows multiple colours and a negative network in this histopathologically confirmed dermatofibroma.

Consider excision for all non-typical dermatofibromas in order to avoid missing nodular melanoma.

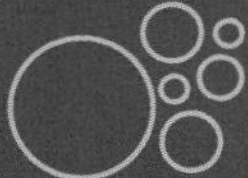

Dermatofibrosarcoma protuberans

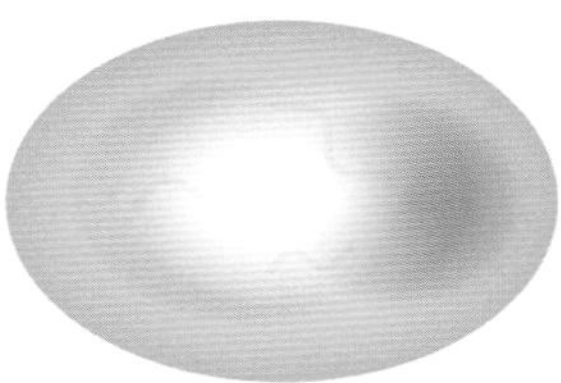

Dermatofibrosarcoma protuberans (DFSP) is a rare malignant tumour that may present a diagnostic challenge as it tends to lack epidermal features. Dermoscopy is of limited value as the features seen are non-specific, often multicomponent and include irregular tan pigmentation, shiny white structures, structureless areas and irregular vessels. Histopathology is required to confirm the diagnosis.

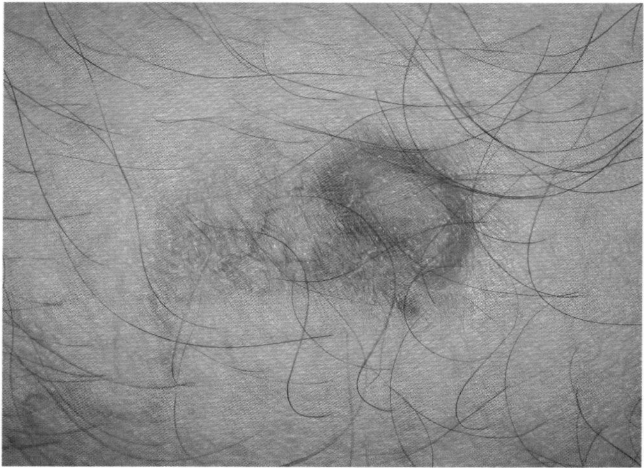

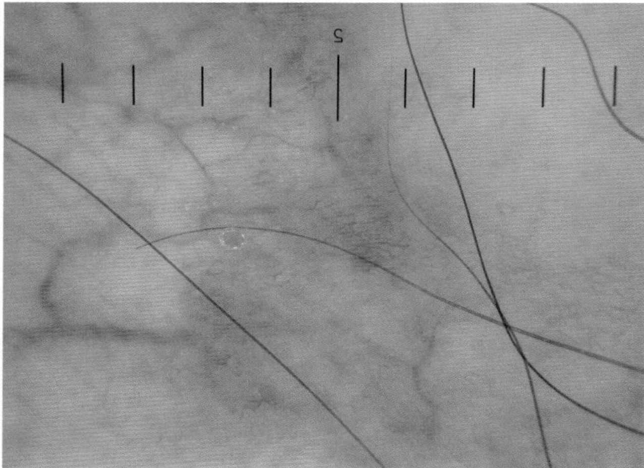

A solitary, firm and ill-defined, skin-coloured plaque on the lower abdomen of a 60-year-old man: dermoscopy shows structureless areas and irregular vessels of varying depth in this histopathologically confirmed DFSP.

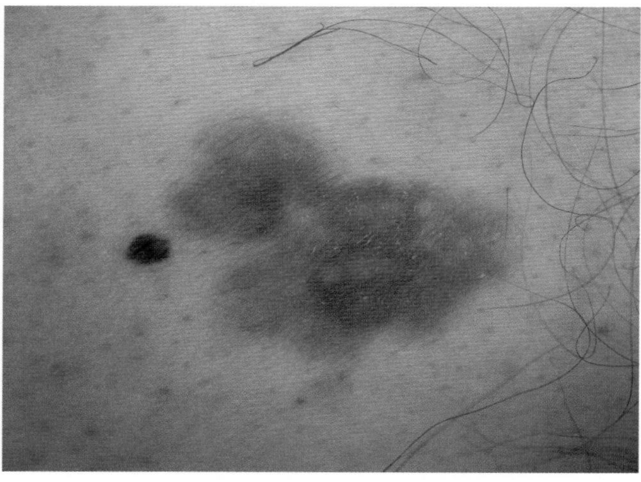

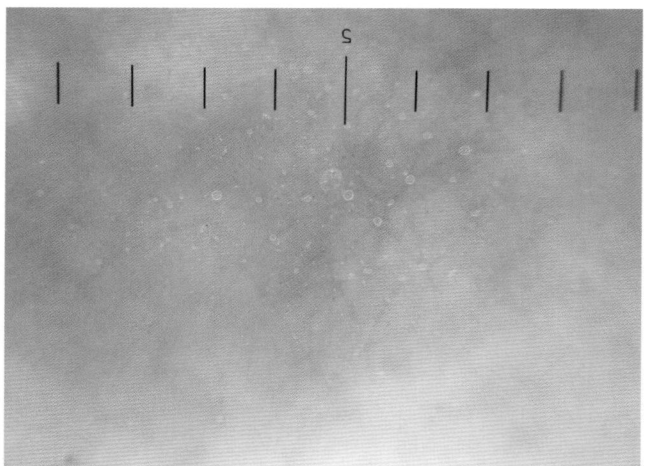

A solitary irregular ill-defined, brown-pink, nodular plaque on the lower back of a 50-year-old man: dermoscopy shows uniform structureless areas with no diagnostic features in this histopathologically confirmed DFSP.

Bernard, J. et al. Dermoscopy of dermatofibrosarcoma protuberans: a study of 15 cases. *Br J Dermatol*. 2013;169(1):85–90.

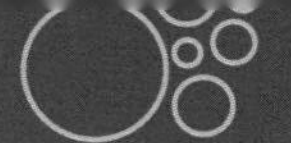

Neurofibromas

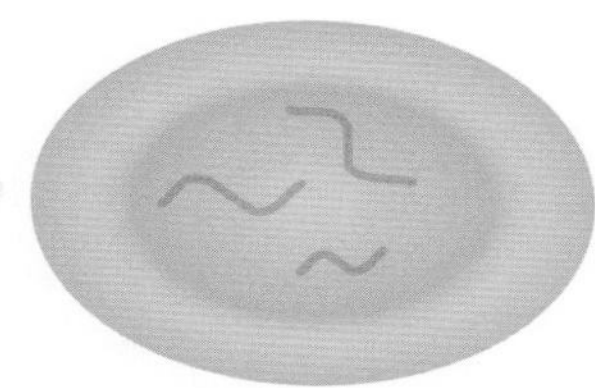

A neurofibroma is a benign tumour of the nerve sheath. They may occur sporadically as a single lesion or multiple as part of neurofibromatosis. They are soft skin-coloured fully compressible papules/nodules that have non-specific dermoscopic features including structureless areas, light peripheral pigmentation and poorly focused linear vessels. Solitary neurofibromas may require histopathology to confirm the diagnosis.

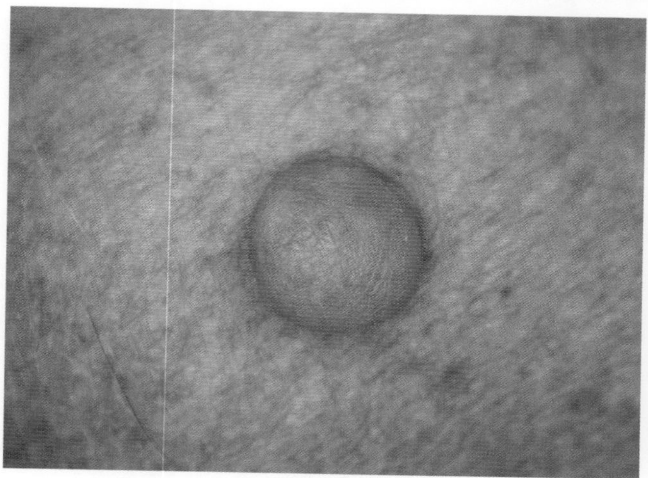

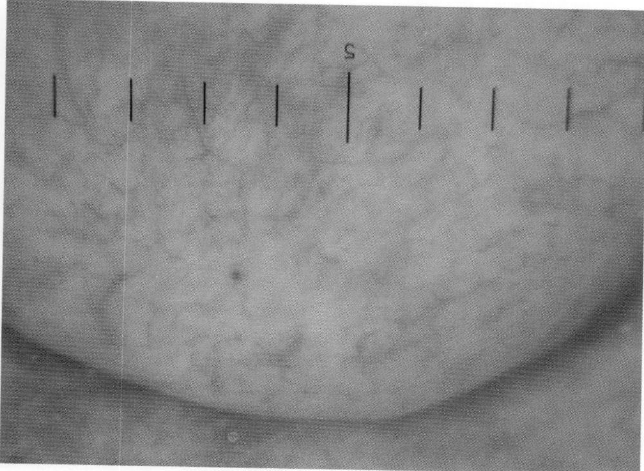

A solitary soft exophytic papule on the mid-back of a 70-year-old man: dermoscopy shows structureless areas and poorly focused linear vessels in this histopathologically confirmed neurofibroma.

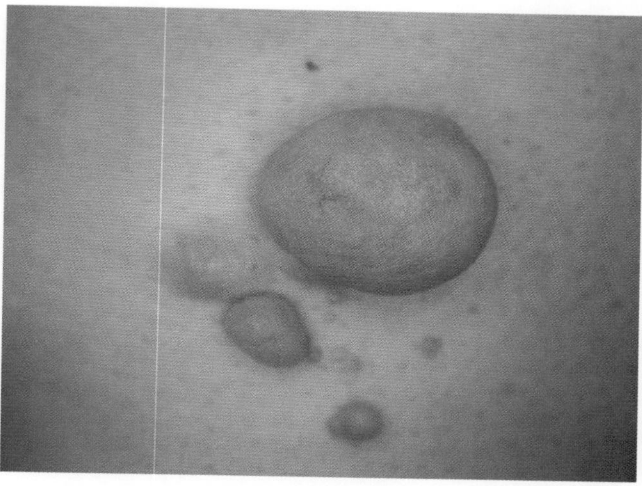

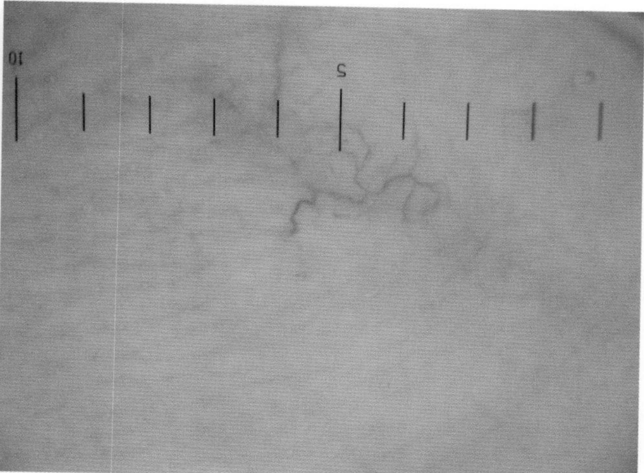

A segmental plaque of multiple soft exophytic papules on the flank of a 60-year-old woman with known segmental neurofibromatosis: dermoscopy shows only underlying background vessels in one of the clinically diagnosed neurofibromas.

Duman, N. and Elmas, M. Dermoscopy of cutaneous neurofibromas associated with neurofibromatosis Type 1. *J Am Acad Dermatol*. 2015;73(3):529–531.

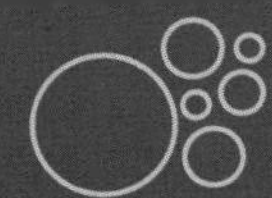

Porokeratosis

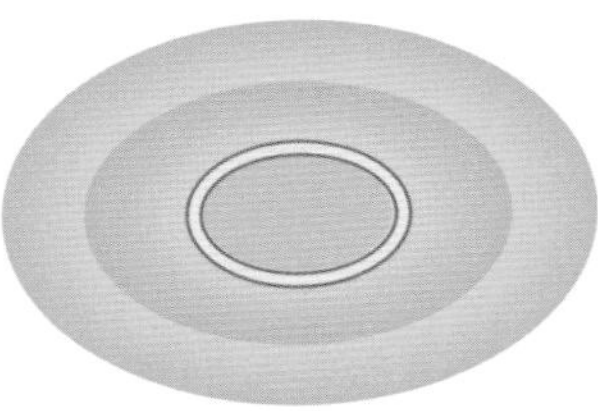

Porokeratosis is a disorder of keratinisation characterised by a single (porokeratosis of Mibelli) or multiple (disseminated superficial actinic porokeratosis, DSAP) annular atrophic plaque with a keratotic rim. The typical keratin rim corresponds to the cornoid lamella on histopathology, which is seen as a double-edged line on dermoscopy. Varying vessel types, shiny white structures and light brown pigmentation can sometimes be seen in the atrophic centre.

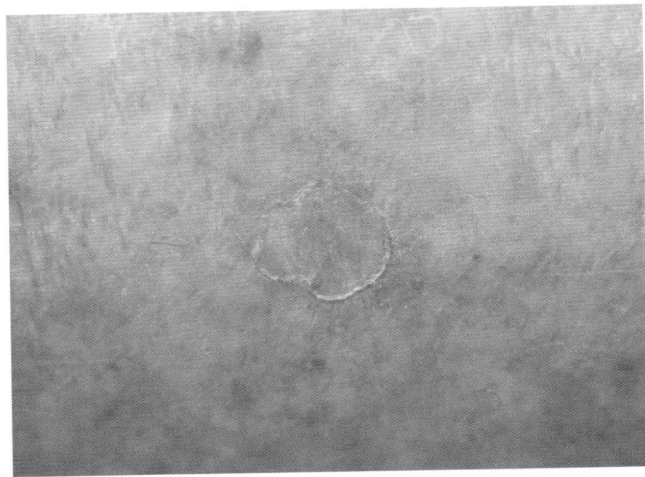

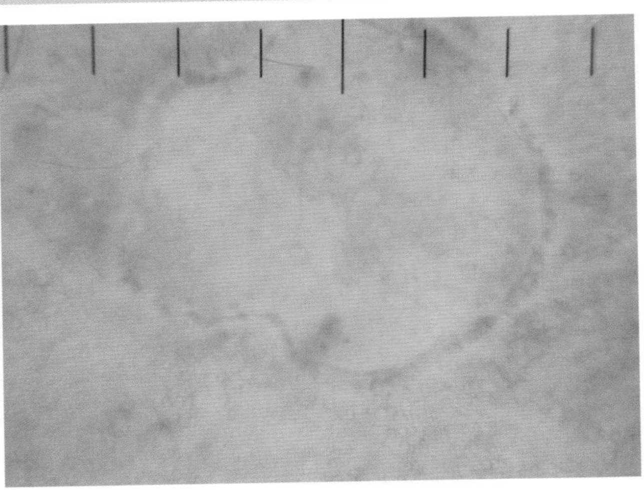

Multiple discrete scaly macules on the lower legs and forearms in a 60-year-old woman with known DSAP: dermoscopy shows the characteristic keratin rim corresponding to the histopathological cornoid lamella.

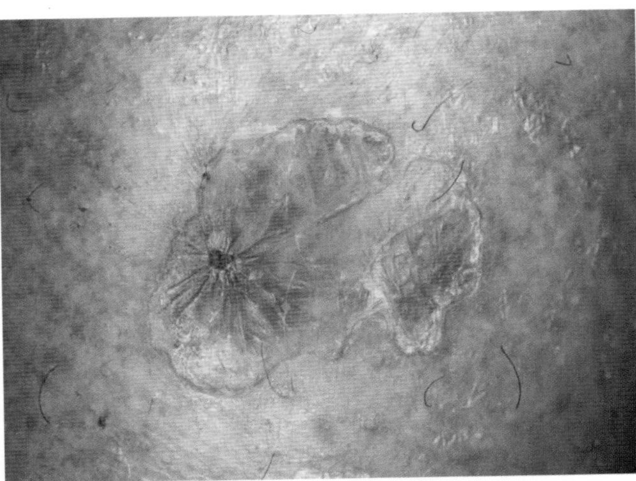

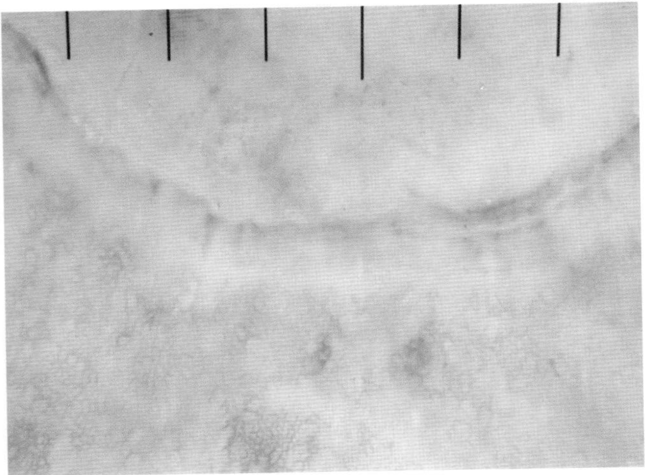

A large atrophic plaque of porokeratosis of Mibelli on the lower leg of a 55-year-old female: dermoscopy shows the characteristic keratin rim, photodamaged background skin and mild erythema as well as tiny dotted vessels within the keratin rim.

Zaar, O. et al. Dermoscopy of porokeratosis: results from a multicentre study of the International Dermoscopy Society. *J Eur Acad Dermatol Venereol*. 2021;35(10):2091–2096.

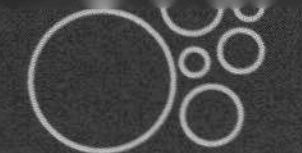

Porokeratosis cases

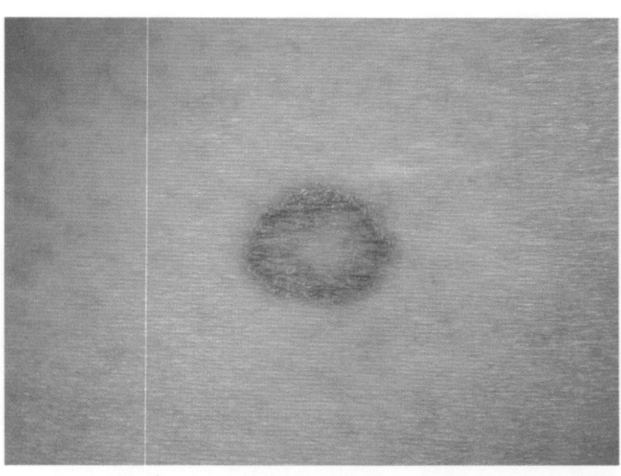

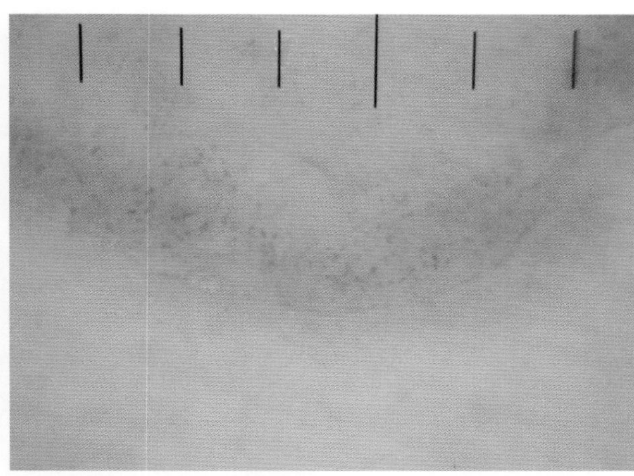

A pink and tan macule on the upper thigh of a 70-year-old woman: dermoscopy shows a clearly demarcated peripheral keratin rim and central tiny dotted and coiled/glomerular vessels in this case of porokeratosis

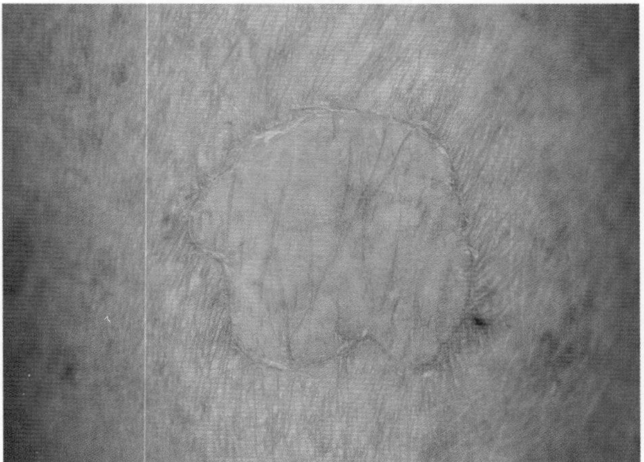

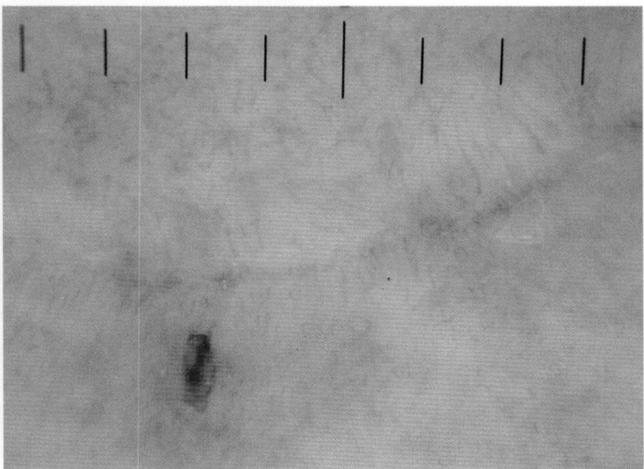

An inflamed plaque on the upper arm of a 60-year-old woman: dermoscopy shows multiple looped/hairpin and linear vessels at the peripheral margin and loss of pigmentation centrally.

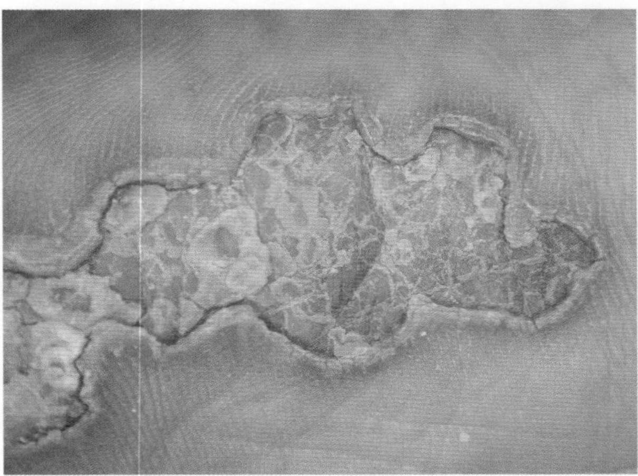

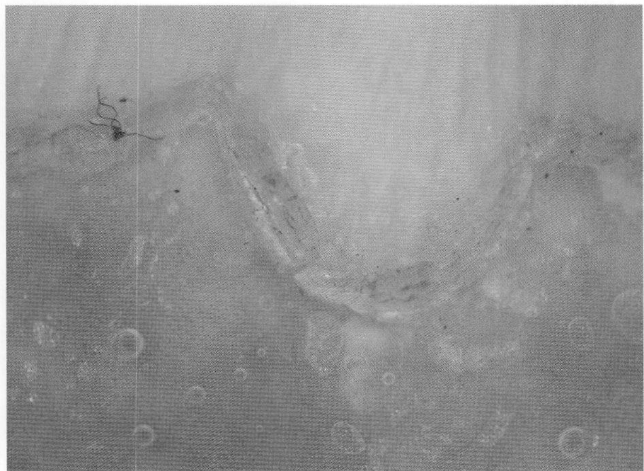

A lifelong case of giant porokeratosis of Mibelli on the foot extending onto the sole: dermoscopy shows erythema centrally and a peripheral hyperkeratotic margin.

Although typically affecting sun-damaged skin, porokeratosis can also develop in non photo-damaged skin. When inflamed it may cause diagnostic doubt as the keratin rim may be less visible.

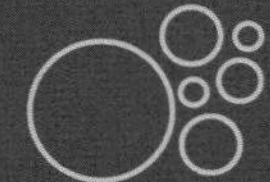

Epidermal naevus

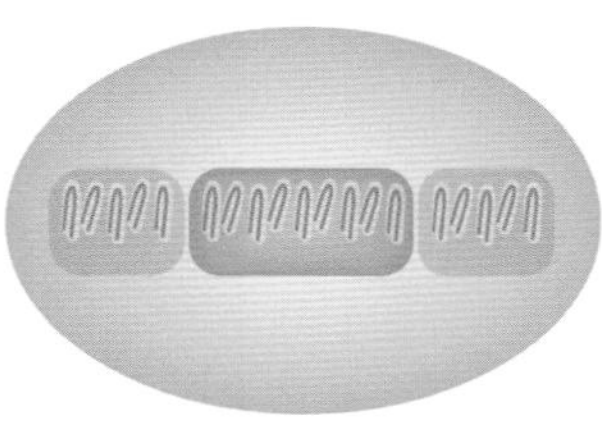

Epidermal naevi are benign cutaneous malformations caused by post-zygotic mosaicism affecting keratinocytes from the ectoderm. They develop in childhood, which helps to differentiate them from other dermatoses. The diagnosis is based on clinical presentation, which may be variable. They typically mimic both seborrhoeic keratoses and viral warts. An inflammatory variant is the inflammatory linear verrucous epidermal naevus (ILVEN).

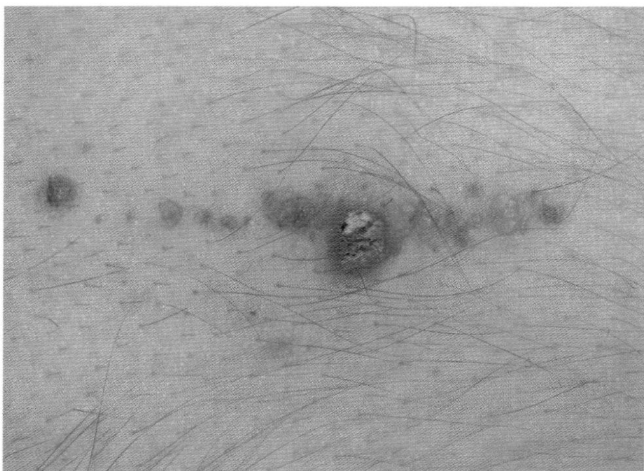

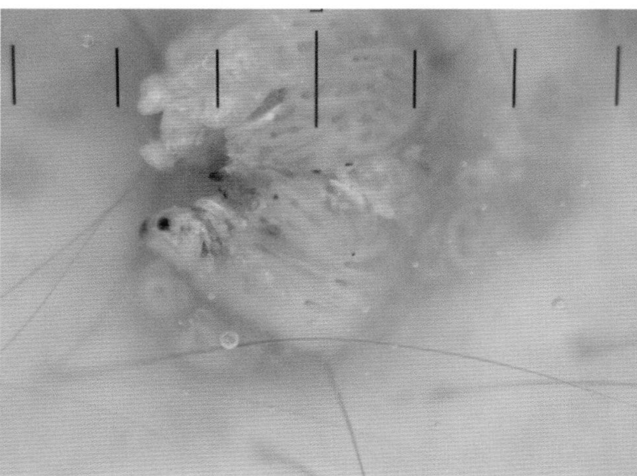

A linear warty plaque on the nape of the neck of a 20-year-old man unresponsive to treatment for viral warts: dermoscopy shows looped/hairpin vessels with black dots within keratin spires in keeping with ILVEN.

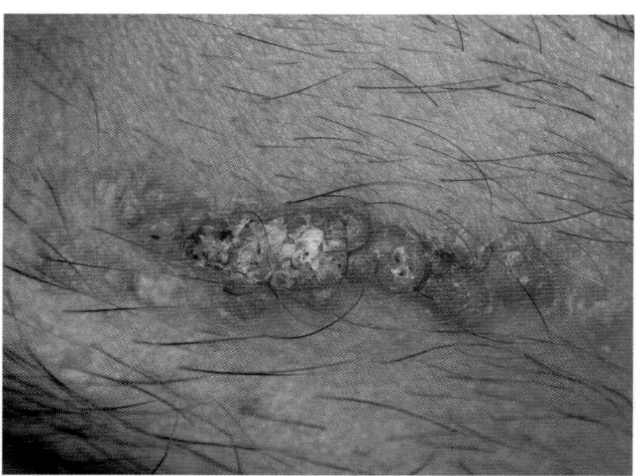

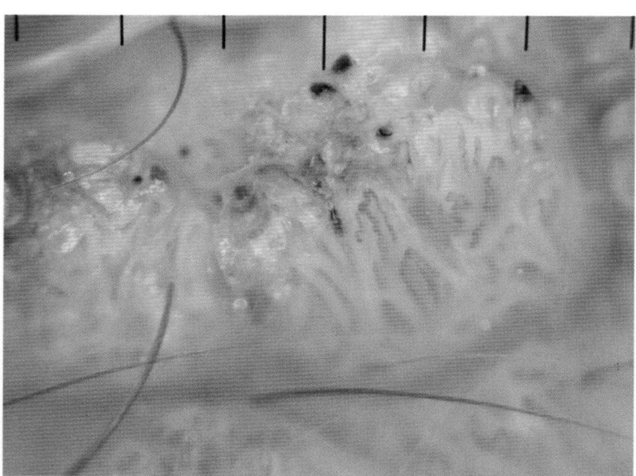

A linear inflamed warty lifelong plaque on the forehead of a 30-year-old man: dermoscopy shows looped vessels within filiform hyperkeratotic spires with white halos in another case of ILVEN.

Verzi, A. et al. Verrucous epidermal nevus: dermoscopy, reflectance confocal microscopy, and histopathological correlation. *Dermatol Pract Concept*. 2019;9(3):230–231.

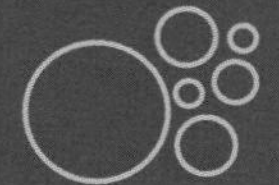

Epidermal naevus cases

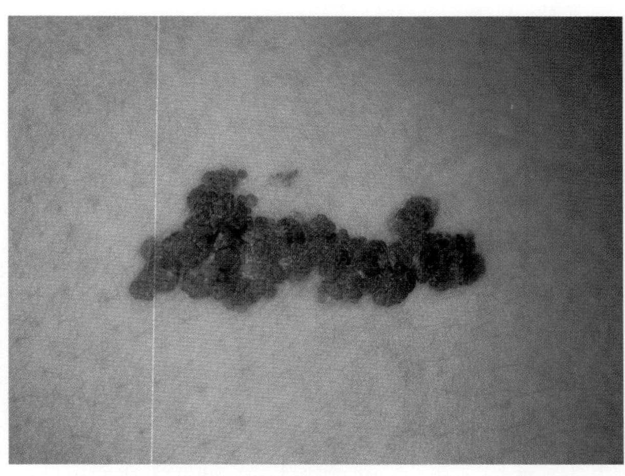

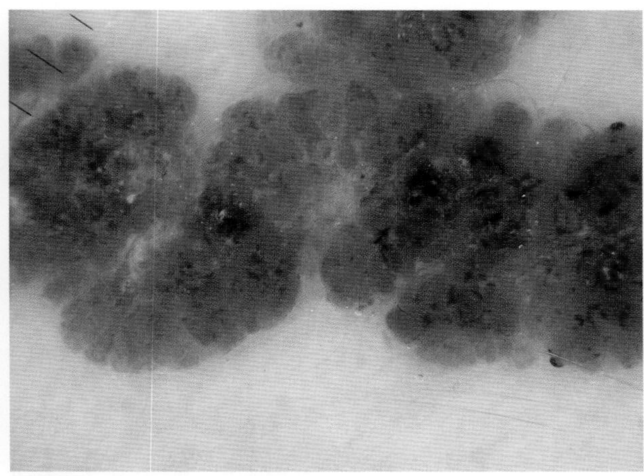

A longstanding variably pigmented warty linear plaque on the lower back of a 20-year-old woman: dermoscopy shows clearly demarcated brown keratin aggregates in keeping with an epidermal naevus.

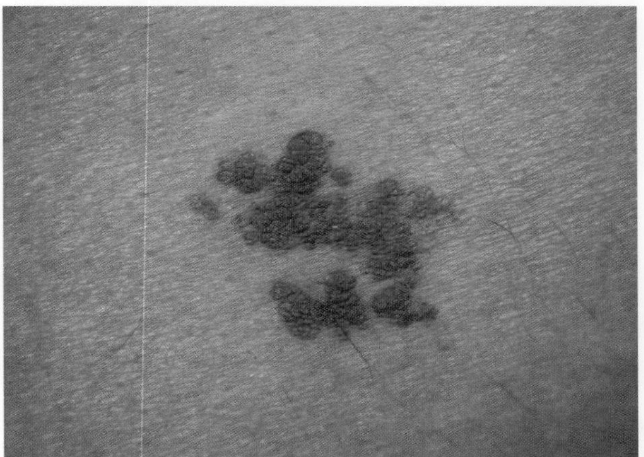

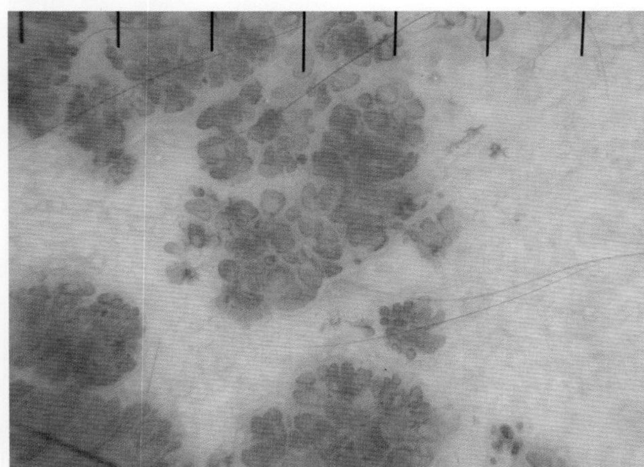

A multifocal warty plaque on the back of a 30-year-old-man: dermoscopy shows multiple brown annular globules coalescing to cerebriform structures (inferiorly) in this epidermal naevus.

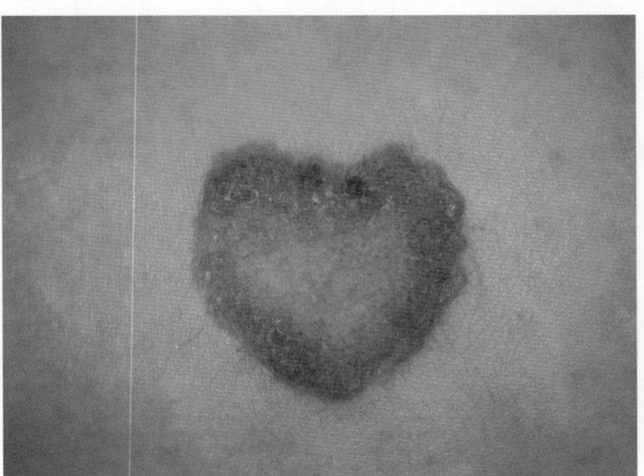

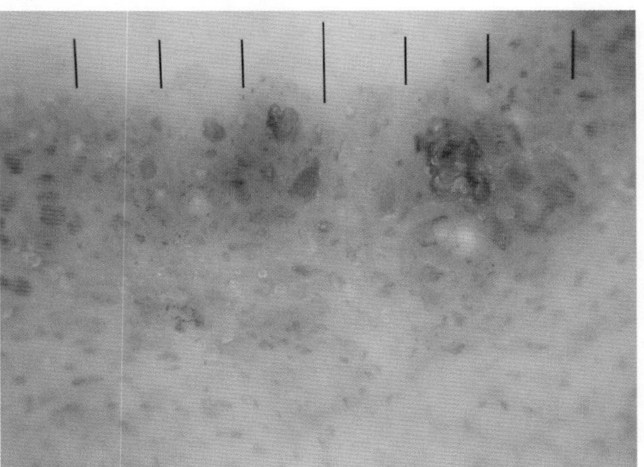

A heart-shaped (cordate) pink warty plaque on the leg of a 40-year-old woman: dermoscopy shows peripheral linear and coiled/glomerular vessels and yellow-brown keratin aggregates in this histopathologically confirmed epidermal naevus.

Typically features of a seborrheic keratosis may be present in an epidermal naevus. A biopsy may be required to confirm a diagnosis in atypical presentations.

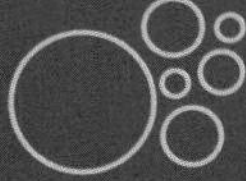

Cutaneous T-cell lymphoma

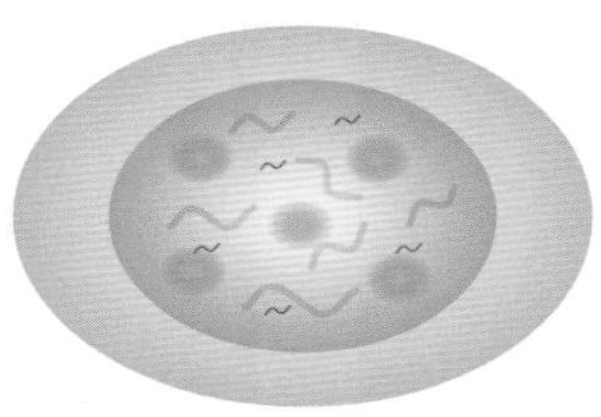

Cutaneous T-cell lymphoma (CTCL) has many presentations and these share clinical features with a range of inflammatory, infective and neoplastic dermatoses. Dermoscopy is non-specific and not reliable for this entity, hence diagnosis should always be confirmed with initial histopathology and then further investigations as required.

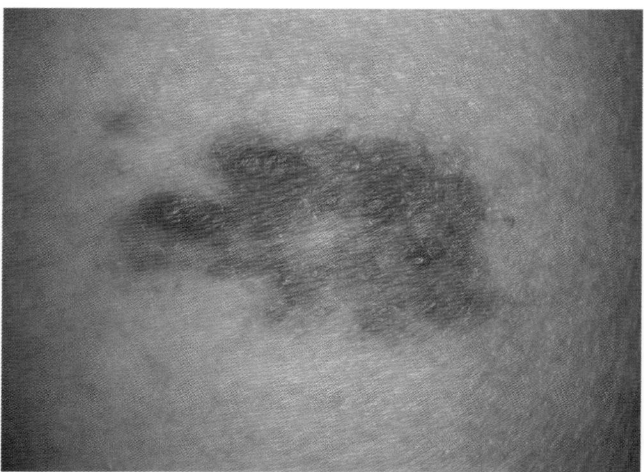

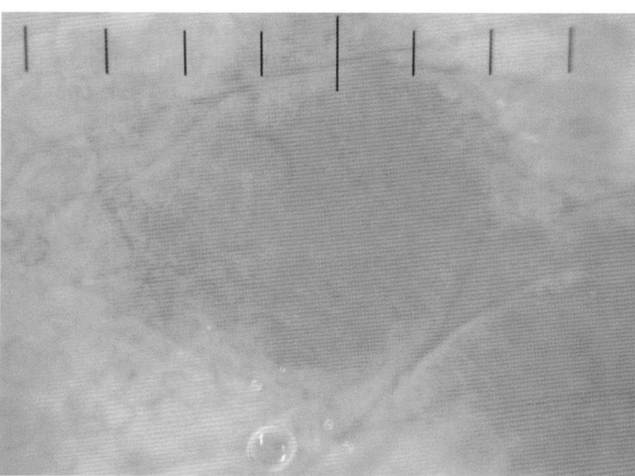

An erythematous multifocal plaque on the flank of a 60-year-old woman: dermoscopy shows structureless erythematous areas and poorly focussed short linear vessels in this histopathologically confirmed CTCL (anaplastic large cell lymphoma).

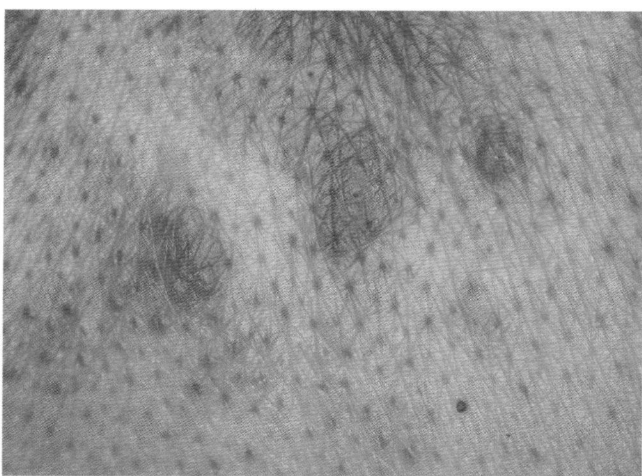

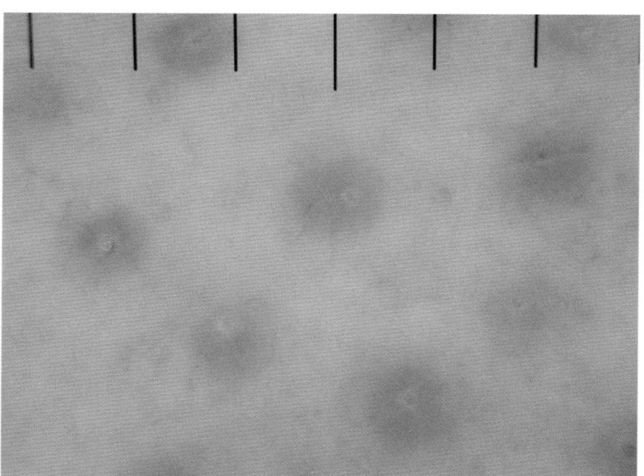

Coalescing erythematous papules on the back of a 50-year-old woman: dermoscopy shows perifollicular patchy structureless erythema confirmed histopathologically as CTCL (mycosis fungoides).

Lallas, A. et al. Dermoscopy of early stage mycosis fungoides. *J Eur Acad Dermatol. Venereol*. 2013;27(5):617–621.

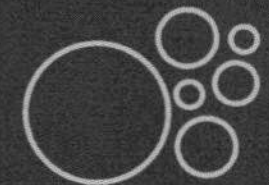

Pseudolymphoma

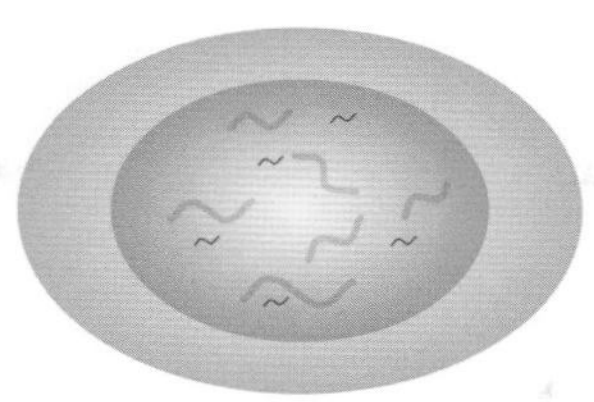

Cutaneous pseudolymphomas are a group of conditions that result in a benign reactive lymphocytic proliferation that mimics cutaneous lymphoma. There are many causes, including insect bite reactions, viral infections, drug reactions (e.g. vaccination) or tattoo reactions. Diagnosis is made by careful history and evaluation of clinical features in addition to histopathology. Dermoscopic features are not specific but may help to exclude other diagnoses.

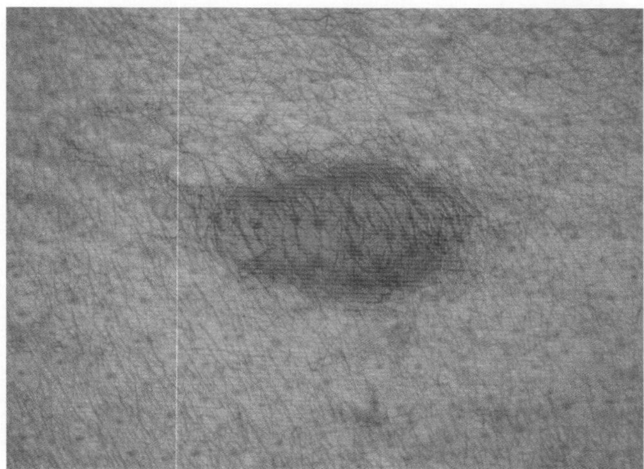

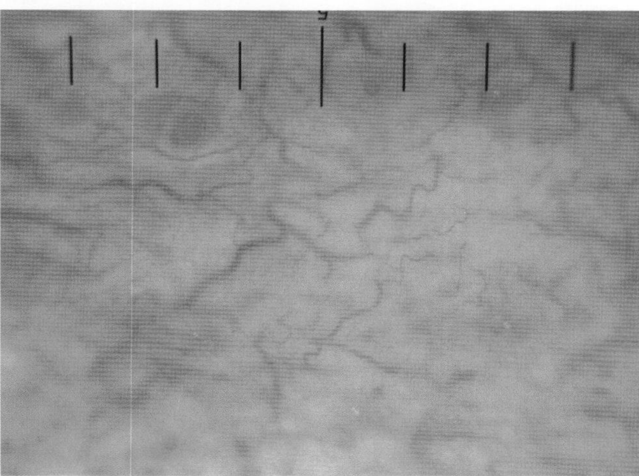

A solitary pink plaque on the upper chest of a 50-year-old man: dermoscopy shows erythema, broad poorly focused telangiectasia and follicular hyperkeratosis with an ill-defined margin in this histopathologically confirmed pseudolymphoma.

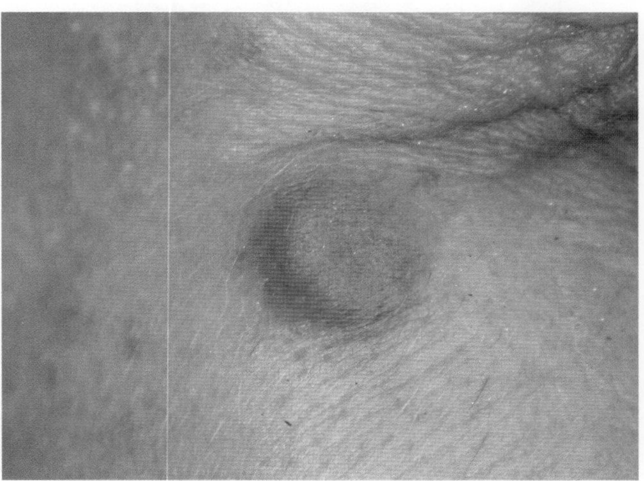

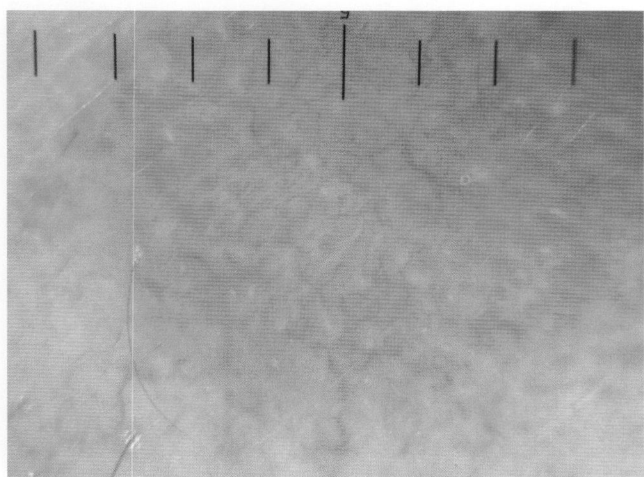

A solitary pink plaque on the lateral canthus of a 30-year-old woman: dermoscopy shows erythema and multifocal short linear vessels with an ill-defined peripheral margin in this histopathologically confirmed pseudolymphoma.

Bambonato, C. et al. Dermoscopy of lymphomas and pseudolymphomas. *Dermatol Clin*. 2018;36(4):377–388.

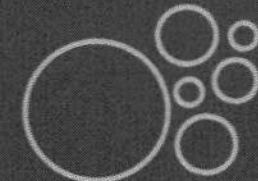

Eccrine poroma

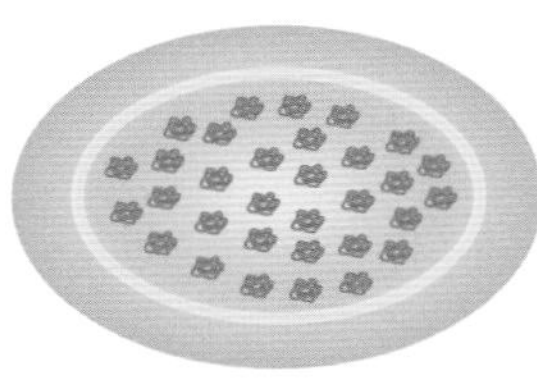

Eccrine poromas are uncommon solitary benign tumours frequently occurring on acral sites. They mimic other solitary pink skin tumours; hence histopathology is mandatory.

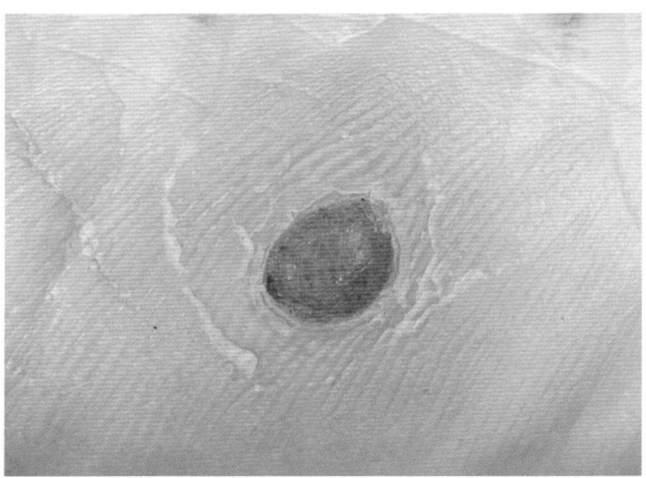

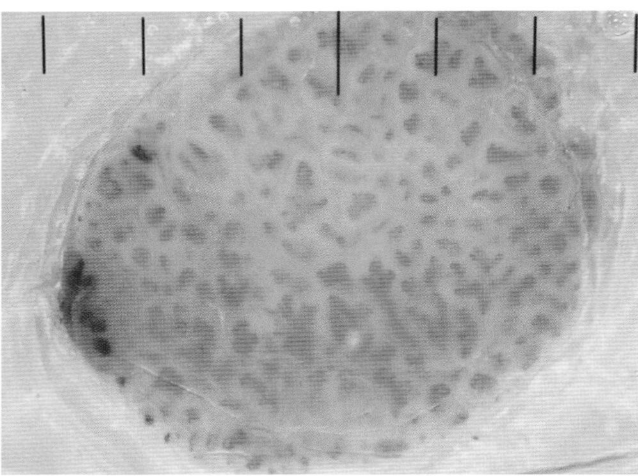

A well-circumscribed pink nodule on the sole of a 40-year-old woman: dermoscopy shows a peripheral keratin collarette and multiple glomerular vessels uniformly distributed across this histopathologically confirmed eccrine poroma.

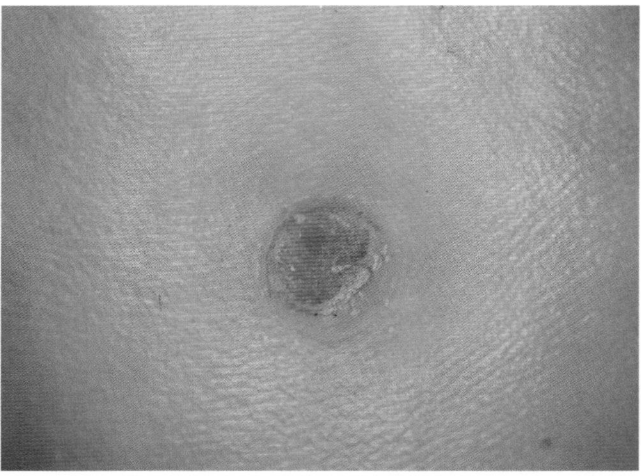

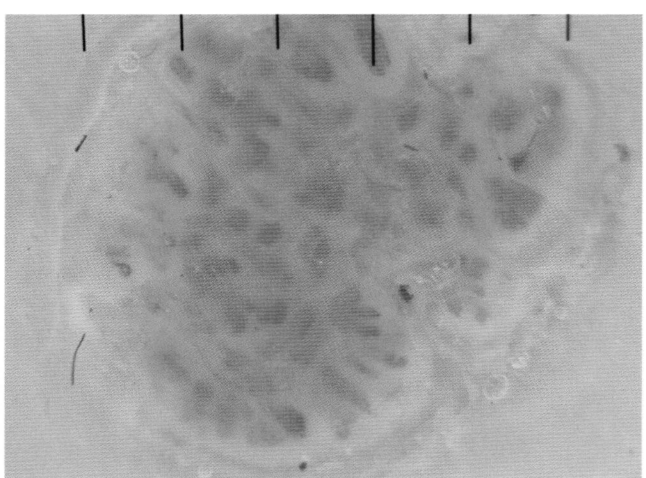

A well-circumscribed pink and keratotic papule on the sole of a 50-year-old man: dermoscopy shows a peripheral keratin collarette plus looped and glomerular vessels uniformly distributed across this histopathologically confirmed eccrine poroma.

Ferrari, A. et al. Eccrine poroma, a clinico-dermoscopic study of seven cases. *Acta Dermatol Venereol*. 2009:89(2):160–164.

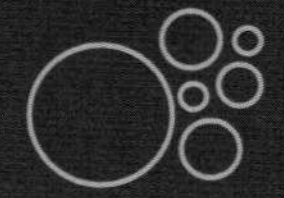

5 Basal cell carcinoma

Superficial basal cell carcinoma – pink 142
Superficial basal cell carcinoma – pink cases 143
Superficial basal cell carcinoma – pigmented 144
Superficial basal cell carcinoma – pigmented cases 145
Nodular basal cell carcinoma – pink and small 146
Nodular basal cell carcinoma – pink and small cases 147
Nodular basal cell carcinoma – pigmented and small 148
Nodular basal cell carcinoma – pigmented and small cases 149
Nodular basal cell carcinoma – pink and large 150
Nodular basal cell carcinoma – pink and large cases 151
Morphoeic/infiltrative basal cell carcinoma 152
Morphoeic/infiltrative basal cell carcinoma cases 153
Hypopigmented basal cell carcinoma 154
Hyperpigmented basal cell carcinoma 155
Seborrhoeic keratosis-like basal cell carcinoma 156
Fibroepithelioma of Pinkus 157

Diagnostic Dermoscopy: The Illustrated Guide, Second Edition. Jonathan Bowling.

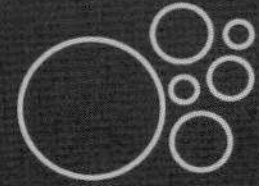

Superficial basal cell carcinoma – pink

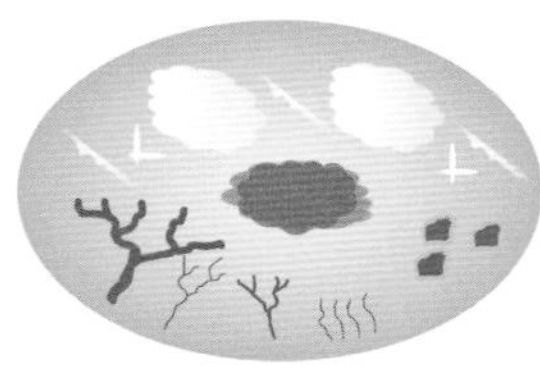

Superficial basal cell carcinoma (BCC) may present as a relatively asymptomatic pink patch on the skin. In time they may develop erosions or ulcerate. They may mimic inflammatory, infective and neoplastic dermatoses. The dermoscopic features include a pink background, arborising vessels, short fine telangiectasias, shiny white blotches and strands and erosions.

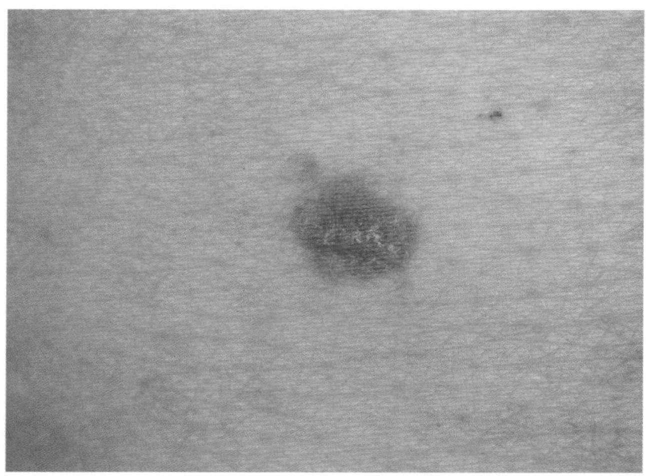

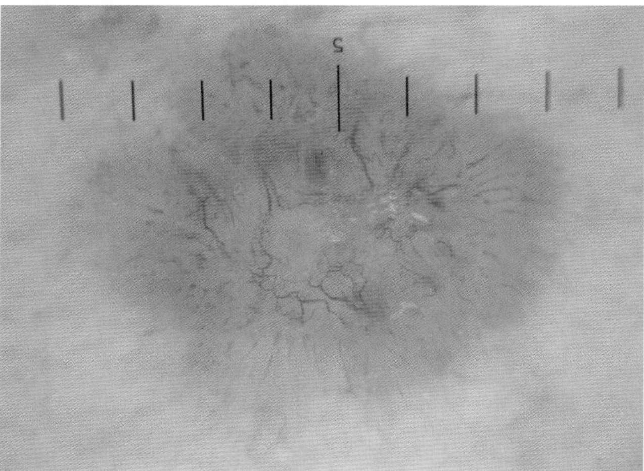

A pink plaque on the lower back of a 50-year-old woman: dermoscopy shows a solitary erosion, multiple sharply focused linear arborising vessels centrally and peripheral short fine telangiectasias in this superficial BCC.

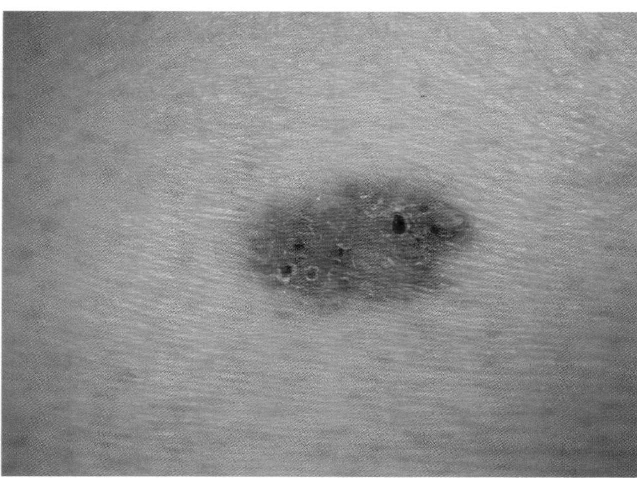

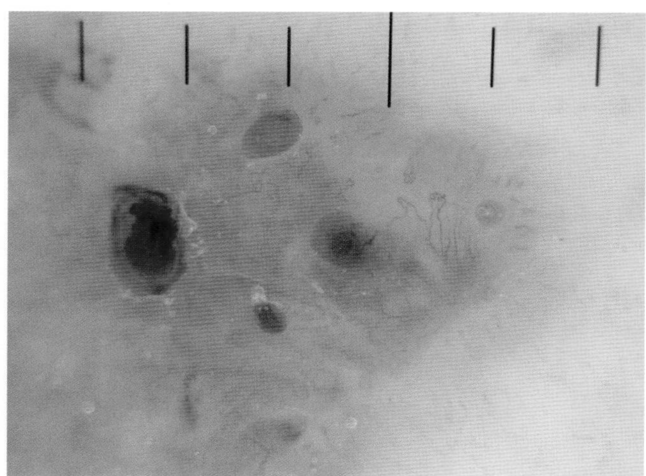

A pink plaque on the upper arm of a 60-year-old woman: dermoscopy shows erythema, a pink structureless background, multiple erosions, linear arborising vessels and peripheral short fine telangiectasias in this superficial BCC.

Reiter, O. et al. Dermoscopic features of basal cell carcinoma and its subtypes: A systematic review. *J Am Acad Dermatol.* 2021;85:653–664.

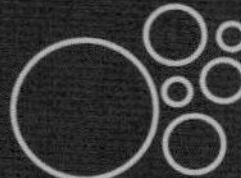

Superficial basal cell carcinoma – pink cases

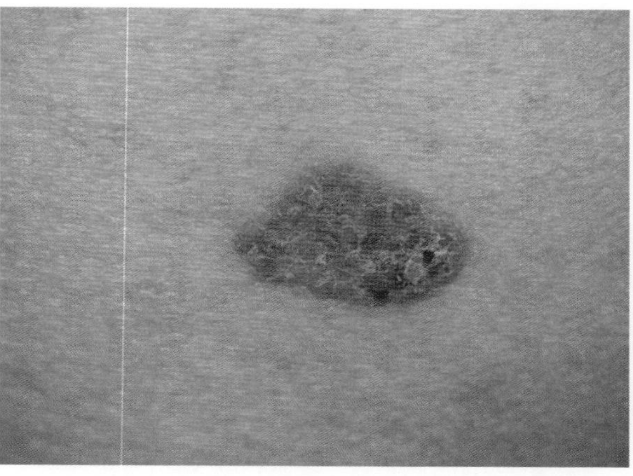

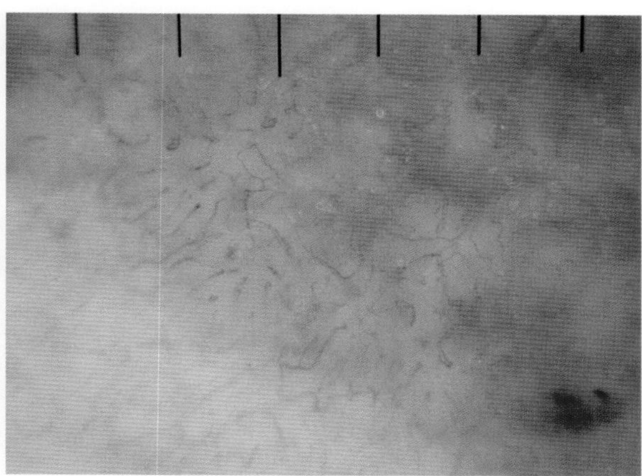

A pink scaly plaque on the lower back of a 50-year-old woman: dermoscopy shows peripheral short fine telangiectasias, linear arborising vessels, erythema and pink structureless areas in this superficial BCC.

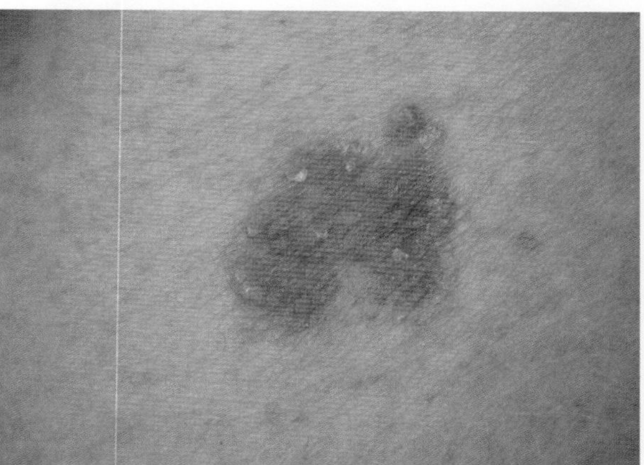

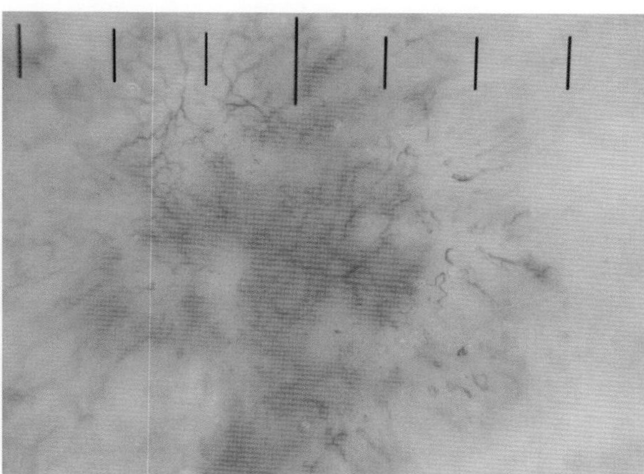

A pink plaque on the upper arm of a 50-year-old woman: dermoscopy shows peripheral short fine telangiectasias, linear arborising blood vessels, erythema and pink structureless areas in this superficial BCC.

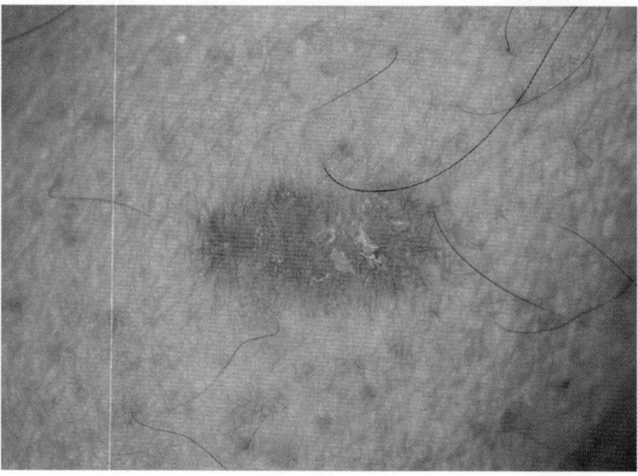

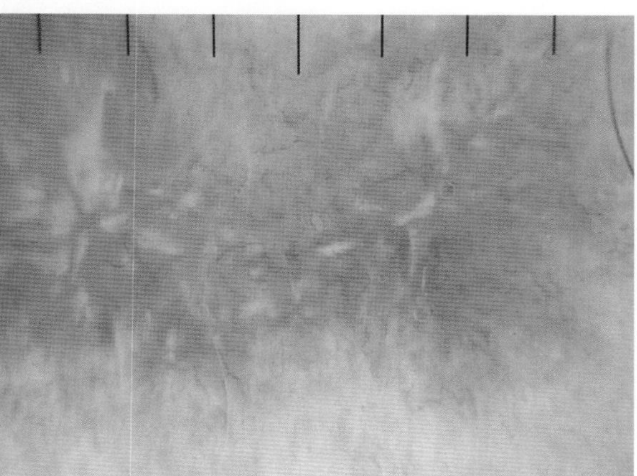

A pink scaly plaque on the upper thigh of a 60-year-old man: polarised dermoscopy shows shiny white blotches and strands, short fine telangiectasias, erythema and pink structureless areas in this superficial BCC.

Subtle non-pigmented sBCCs will become more prominent and easier to identify on dermoscopy with a short rub using an alcohol wipe. A novel clinical sign to aid in the diagnosis of superficial basal cell carcinoma.

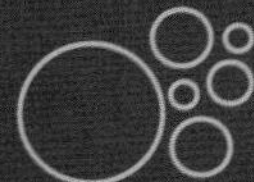

Superficial basal cell carcinoma – pigmented

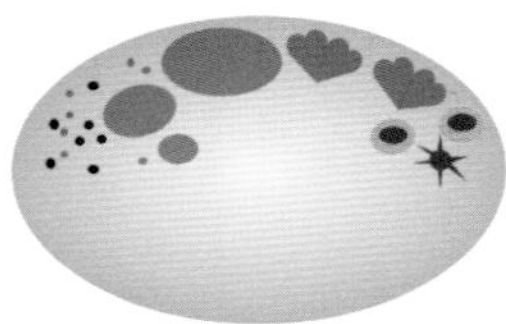

Pigmented superficial BCCs may present as a relatively asymptomatic brown/pink patch/macule on the skin. They can mimic seborrhoeic keratoses and melanocytic lesions. Small foci of pigment can be confirmed dermoscopically as a pigmented structure indicative of a BCC. The pigmented structures reflect melanin incorporation with in tumour aggregates; their concentration and depth give rise to the variable colours and shapes.

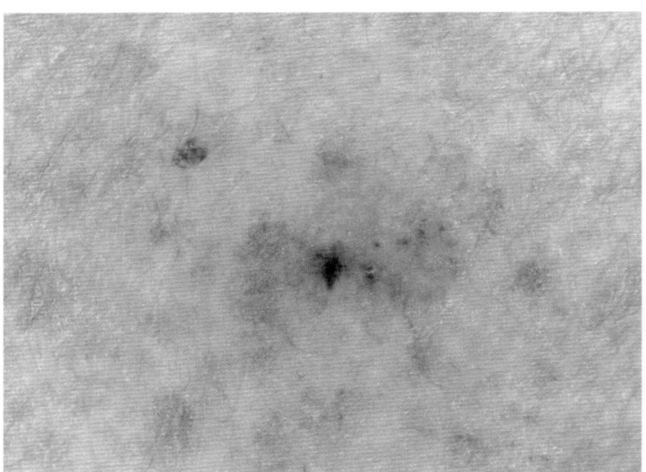

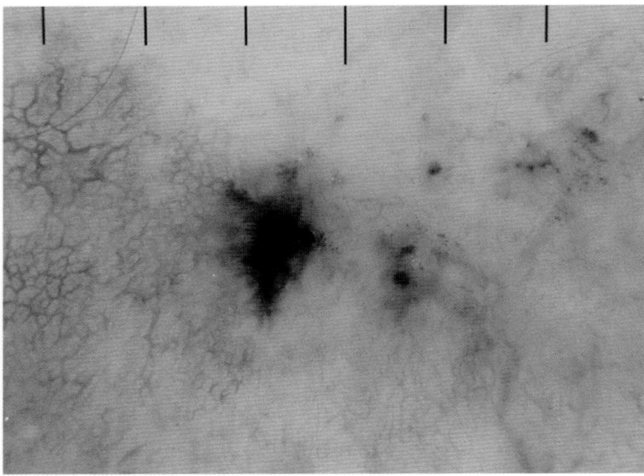

A partially pigmented plaque on the back of a 60-year-old man: dermoscopy shows a focus of hyperpigmentation, multiple foci of blue-grey dots surrounded by tan pigmentation (concentric structures) in this superficial pigmented BCC.

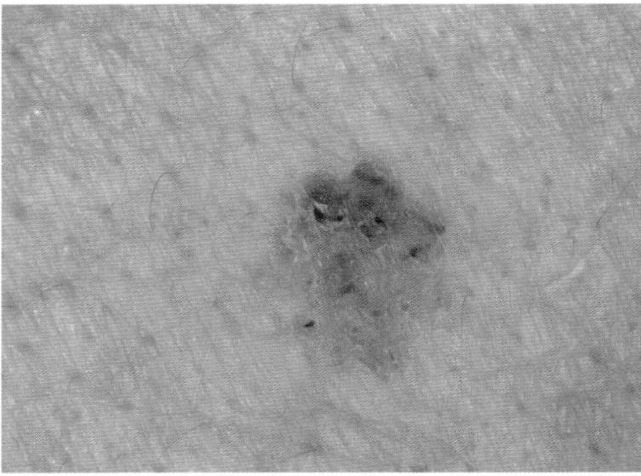

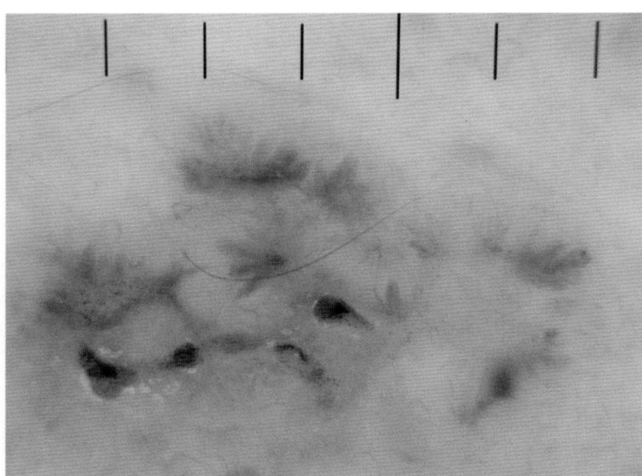

An irregular brown scaly plaque on the upper back of a 70-year-old man: dermoscopy shows multiple pigmented erosions with granular brown pigmentation and peripheral leaf-like structures in this superficial pigmented BCC.

Lallas, A. et al. The presence of pigmented structures can diminish the response rate of BCC to treatments such as photodynamic therapy. The dermatoscopic universe of basal cell carcinoma. *Dermatol Pract Concept*. 2014;4(3):11–24.

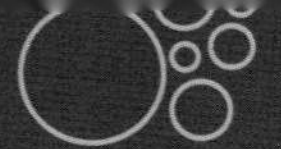

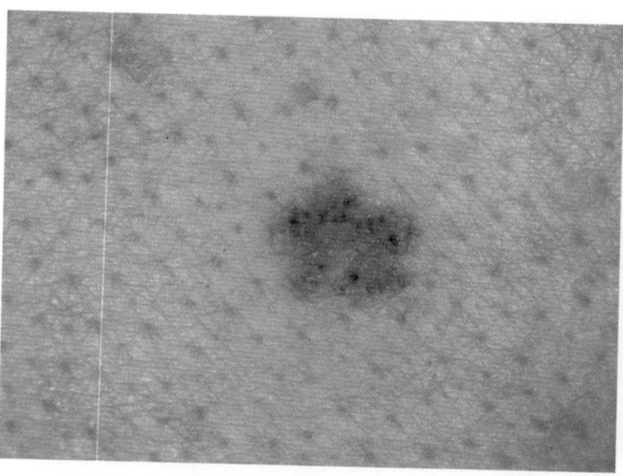

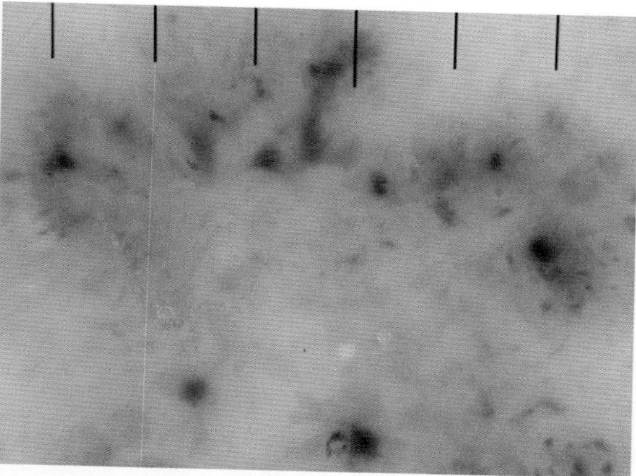

A tan macule with focal pigmentation on the back of a 40-year-old woman: dermoscopy shows central pink structureless areas, peripheral leaf-like areas, blue ovoid nests and tan pigmentation in this superficial pigmented BCC.

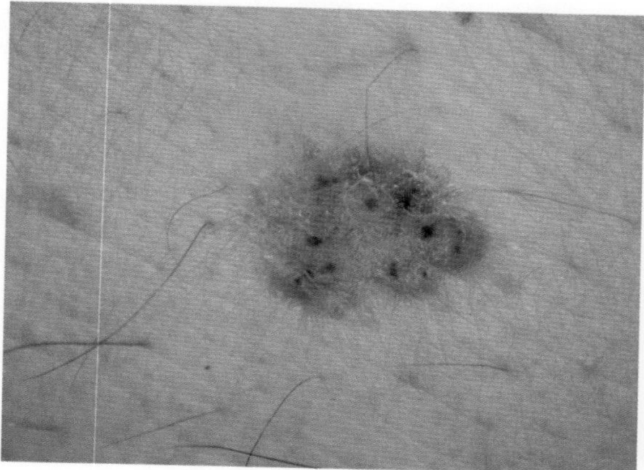

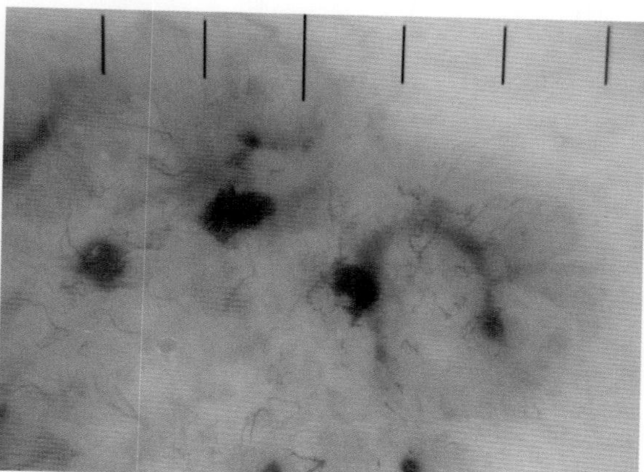

A pink plaque with focal areas of pigment on the lower back of a 60-year-old man: dermoscopy shows short fine telangiectasias, erythema, blue-grey ovoid nests and peripheral tan pigmentation in this pigmented BCC.

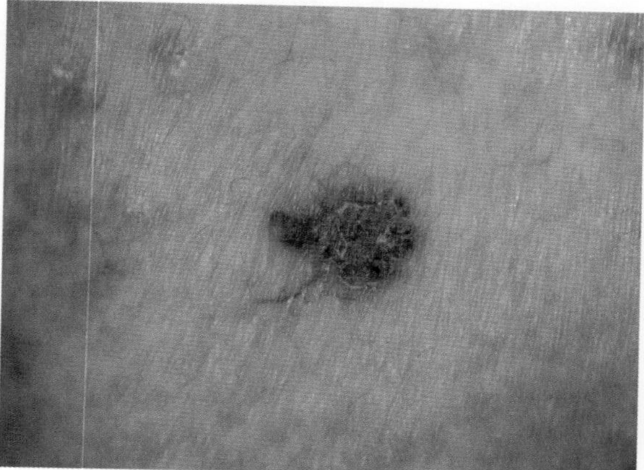

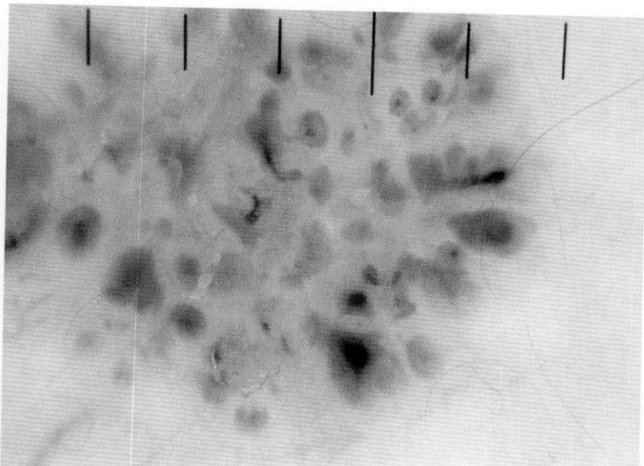

A pink and pigmented scaly macule on the upper back of a 70-year-old woman: dermoscopy shows short fine telangiectasias and multiple concentric structures of varying size in this pigmented superficial BCC.

Multiple brown and grey pigmented structures such as leaf-like areas and concentric structures are more common in pigmented superficial BCCs than in nodular BCCs.

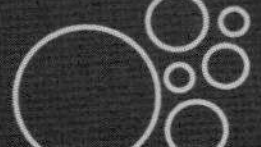

Nodular basal cell carcinoma – pink and small

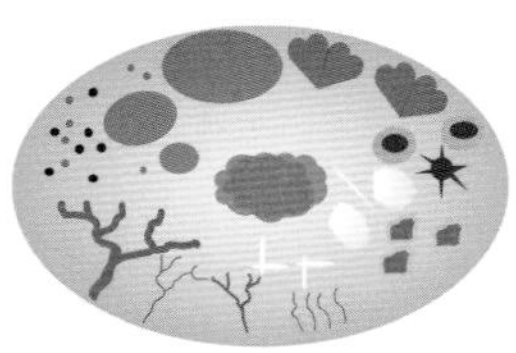

Nodular BCCs vary in pigmentation ranging from predominantly non-pigmented to those with a dominance of blue pigmented structures. They typically present as a clearly demarcated papule or nodule. Using dermoscopy to assess BCCs preoperatively may allow a more conservative surgical margin to be taken whilst not adversely affecting complete excision rates.

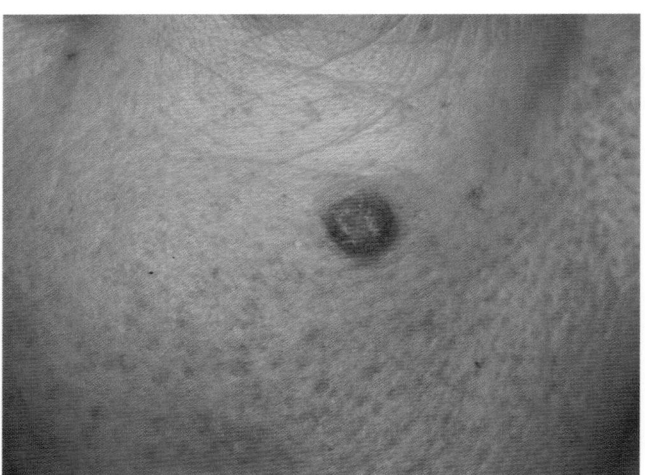

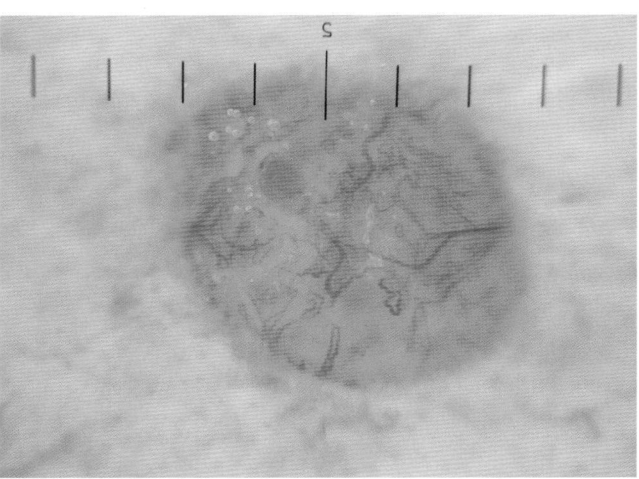

A well-defined pink nodule on the medial cheek of a 40-year-old woman: dermoscopy shows linear arborising vessels, an erosion and a pink structureless background in this nodular BCC completely excised with a 2 mm margin.

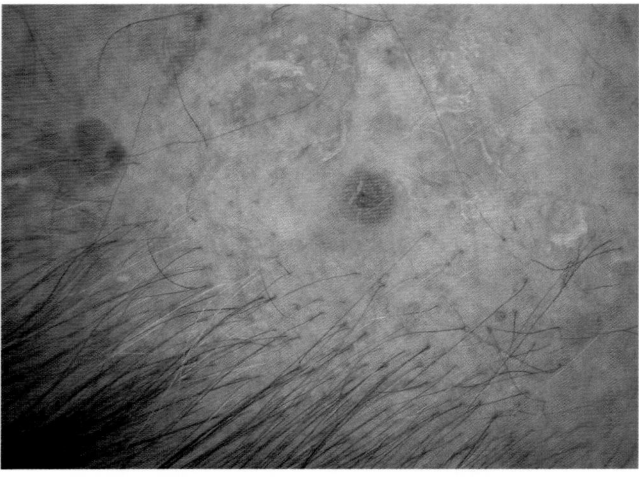

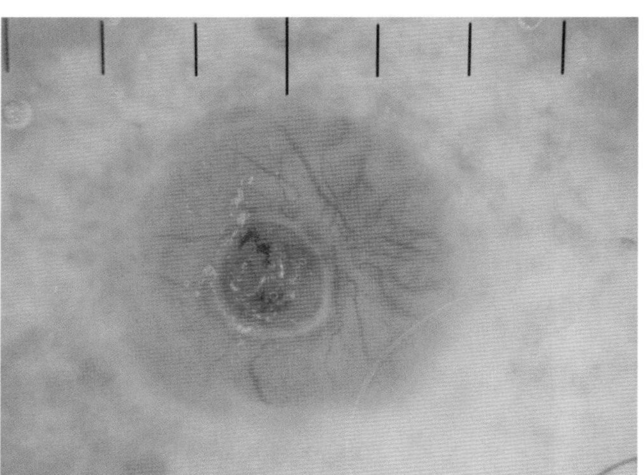

A well-defined ulcerated pink papule on the scalp of a 70-year-old man: dermoscopy shows central ulceration and linear arborising vessels on a pink structureless background in this nodular BCC completely excised with a 2 mm margin.

Caresana, G. and Giardini, R. Dermoscopy-guided surgery in basal cell carcinoma. *J Eur Acad Dermatol Venereol.* 2010;24(12):1395–1399.

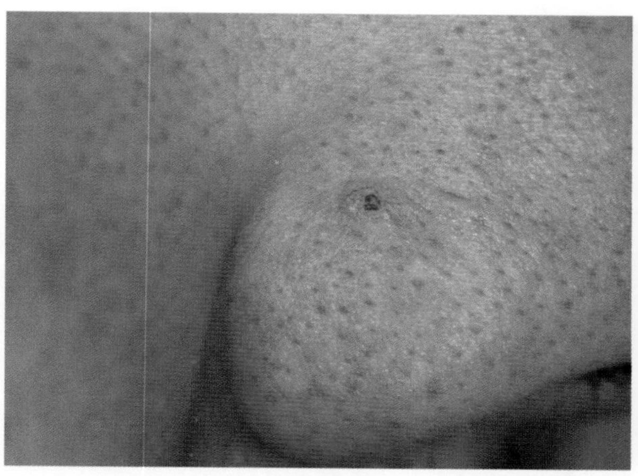
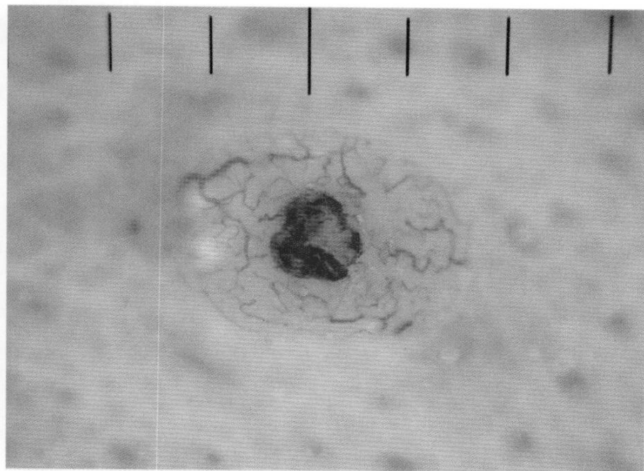

An erosion on the nasal ala of a 30-year-old man: dermoscopy shows a demarcated zone of arborising vessels with central ulceration in this small nodular BCC completely excised with a 2 mm margin.

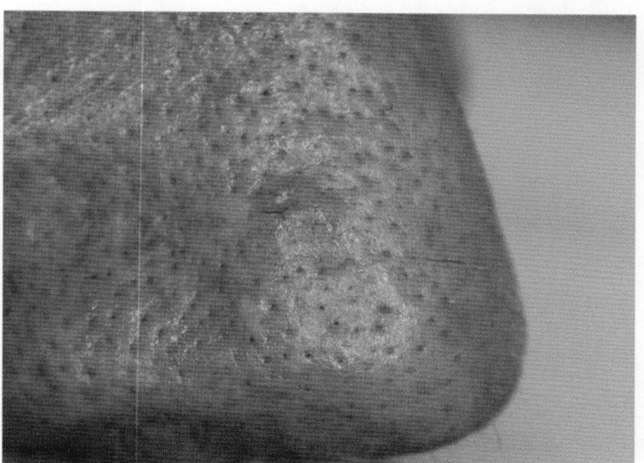
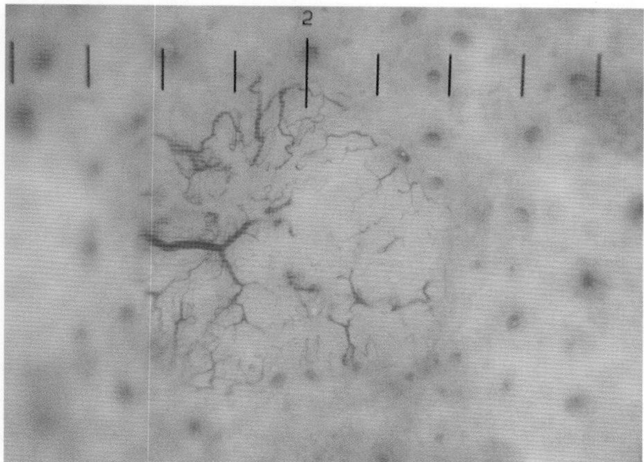

A pink papule on the nasal supratip of a 50-year-old man: dermoscopy shows a defined zone of linear arborising vessels and pink structureless background in this nodular BCC completely excised with a 2 mm margin.

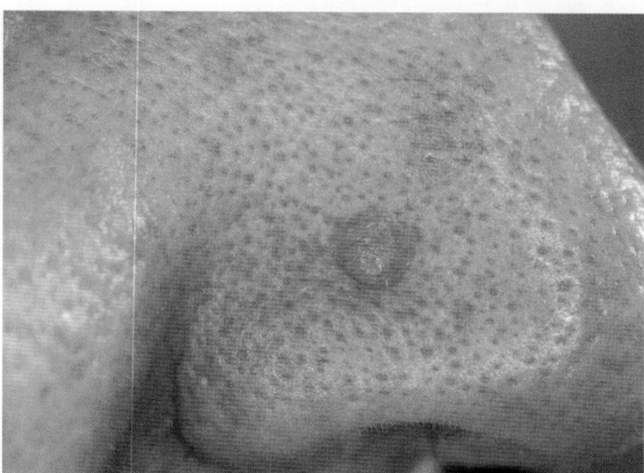
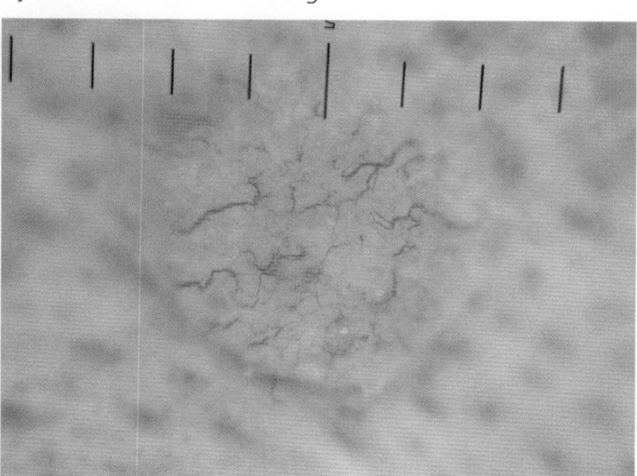

A pink telangiectatic plaque on the nose of a 60-year-old man: dermoscopy shows a clearly demarcated zone of linear arborising vessels, with pink structureless areas in this nodular BCC completely excised with a 2 mm margin.

Only consider adapting a narrow tumour excision margin if the margin of the BCC is clearly defined on dermoscopy and the morphology is in keeping with a nodular subtype.

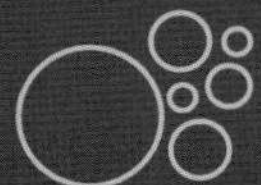

Nodular basal cell carcinoma – pigmented and small

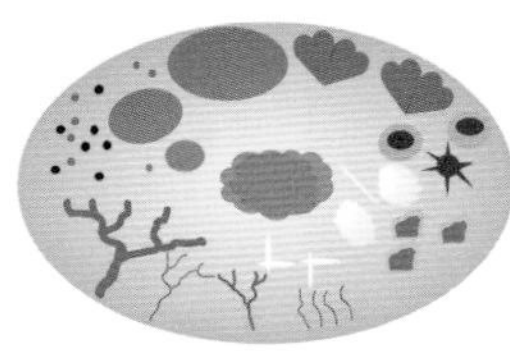

Nodular BCCs may present with a dominance of pigmented structures. Typical vascular features may be obscured as the concentration of pigmented structures increases, making these lesions more suspicious clinically, mimicking melanocytic lesions. The presence of ulceration and/or shiny white blotches and strands may guide the diagnosis. They may present as a clearly demarcated papule or nodule, which dermoscopy may show a clear border between the tumour and background skin.

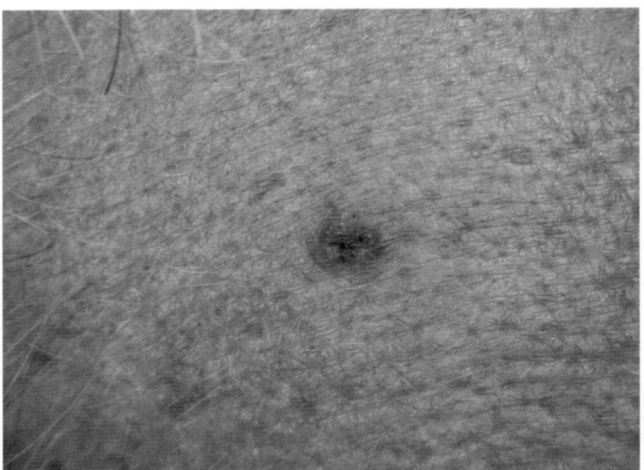

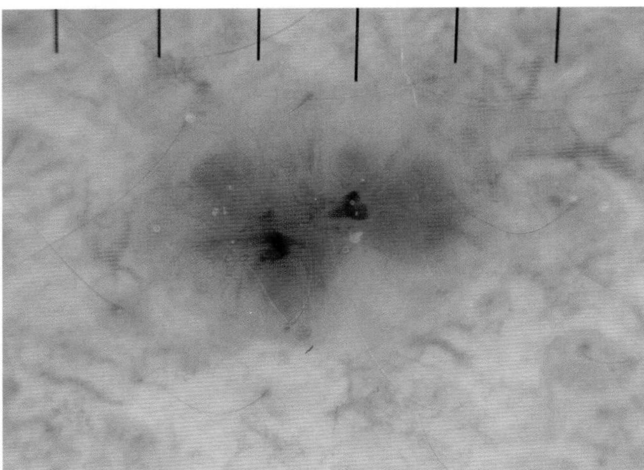

A pigmented plaque on the temple of a 70-year-old man: dermoscopy shows blue-grey ovoid nests, central erosions and linear arborising vessels in this pigmented nodular BCC completely excised with a 2 mm margin.

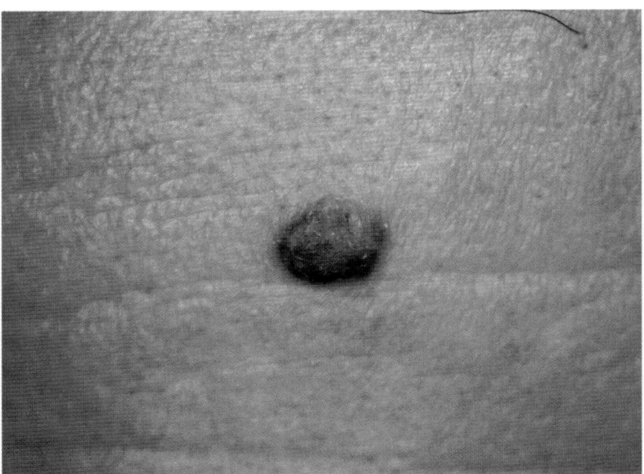

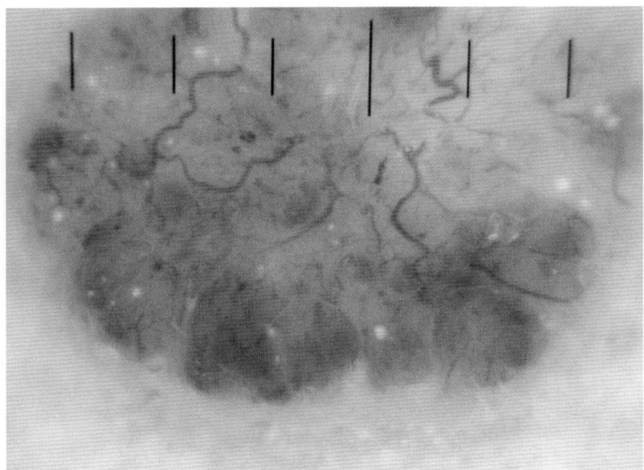

A pigmented plaque on the forehead of a 40-year-old man: dermoscopy shows multiple blue-grey ovoid nests, brown granular pigmentation, yellow-whitish globules, and linear arborising vessels in this pigmented nodular BCC.

Ito, T. et al. Narrow-margin excision is a safe, reliable treatment for well-defined, primary pigmented basal cell carcinoma: an analysis of 288 lesions in Japan. *J Eur Acad Dermatol Venereol*. 2015;29(9):1828–1831.

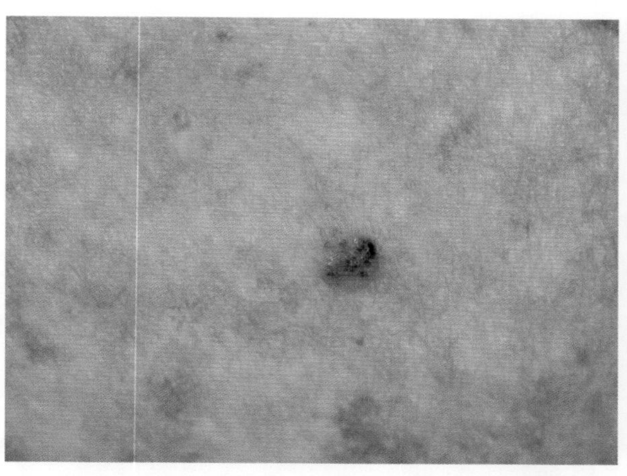

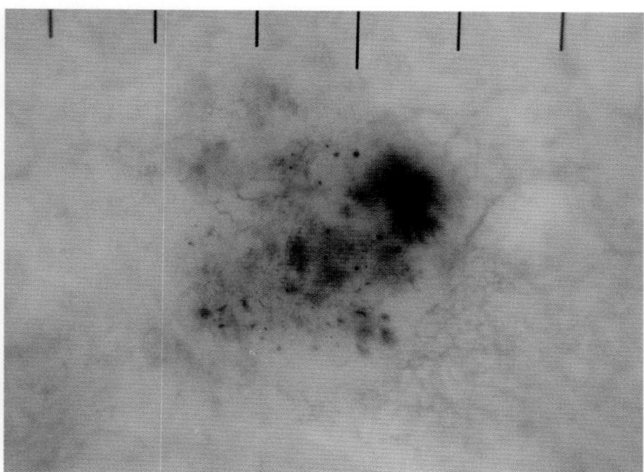

A small pigmented macule on the upper arm of a 60-year-old woman: dermoscopy shows a few arborising vessels and multiple blue-grey globules, dots and granules in this pigmented nodular BCC.

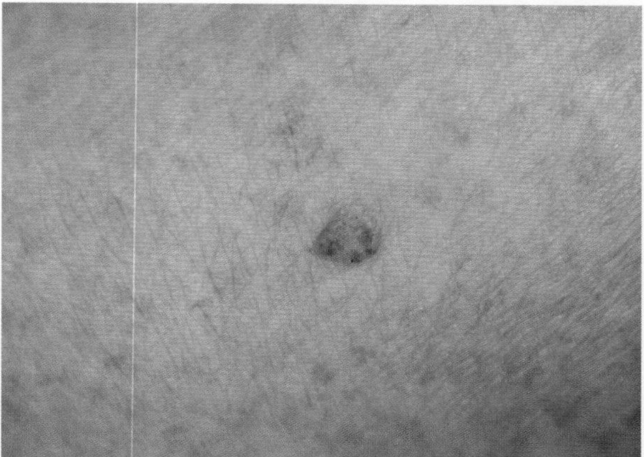

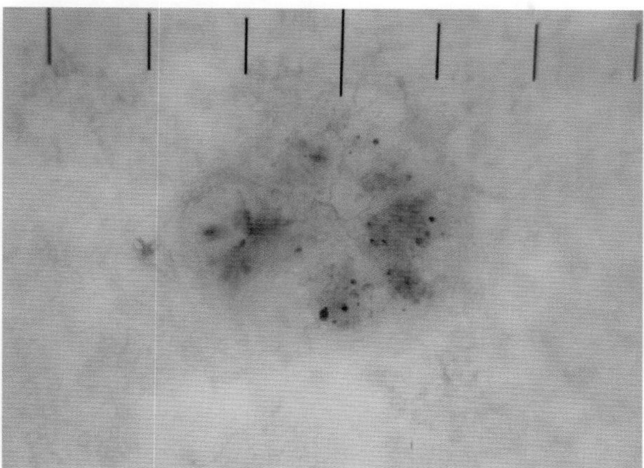

A pigmented plaque on the upper back of a 60-year-old man: dermoscopy shows multiple blue-grey dots and globules in this nodular BCC mimicking a melanocytic lesion.

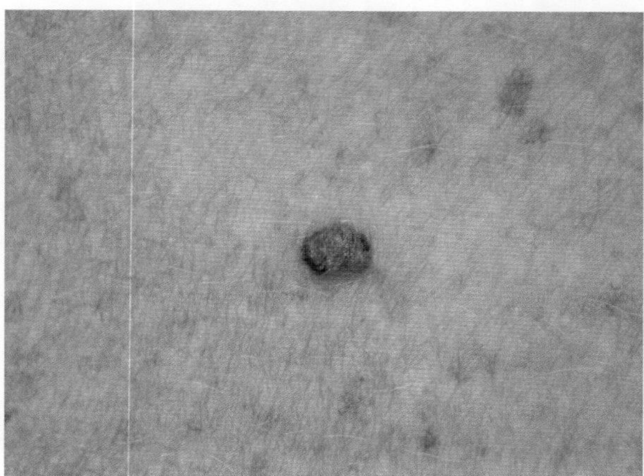

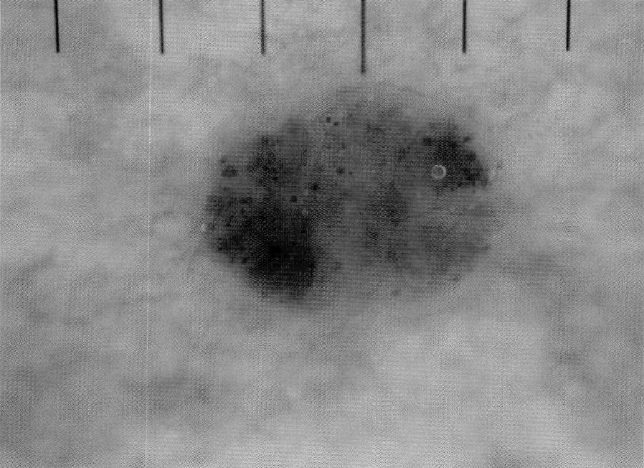

A small brown papule on the upper arm of a 60-year-old woman: dermoscopy shows blue-grey dots and globules and arborising vessels in this clearly demarcated nodular BCC mimicking a melanocytic lesion.

Small pigmented BCC may mimic melanocytic lesions. Careful dermoscopic analysis is required to reach the correct diagnosis as they may alarm the novice.

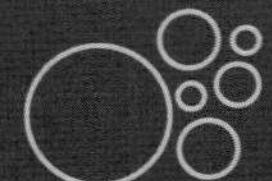

Nodular basal cell carcinoma – pink and large

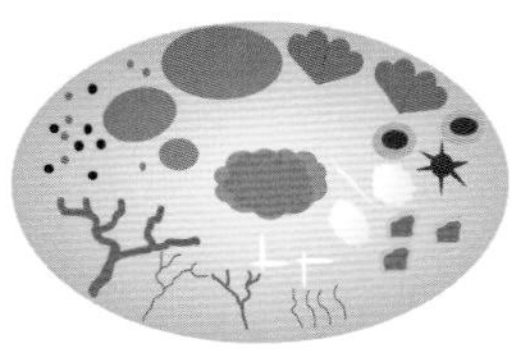

Larger nodular BCCs typically have clinical features that make diagnosis straightforward. Telangiectatic pearly papules, nodules or plaques with or without ulceration are typical clinical features. On dermoscopy, the additional features of shiny white blotches and strands can be seen with polarised dermoscopy as well as a clearer view of arborising vessels, erosions, ulceration, typical pigmented structures and the peripheral margin of the tumour.

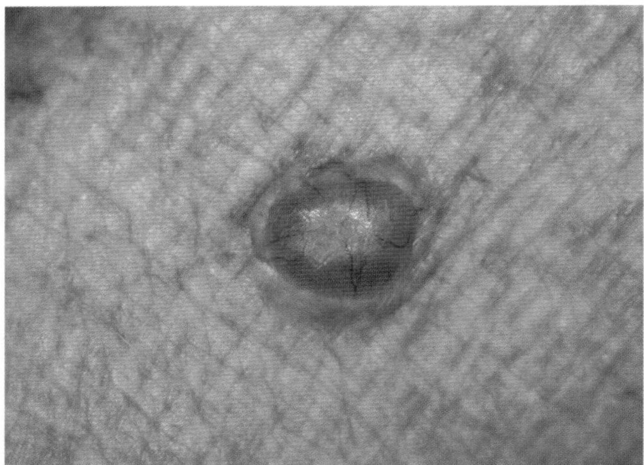

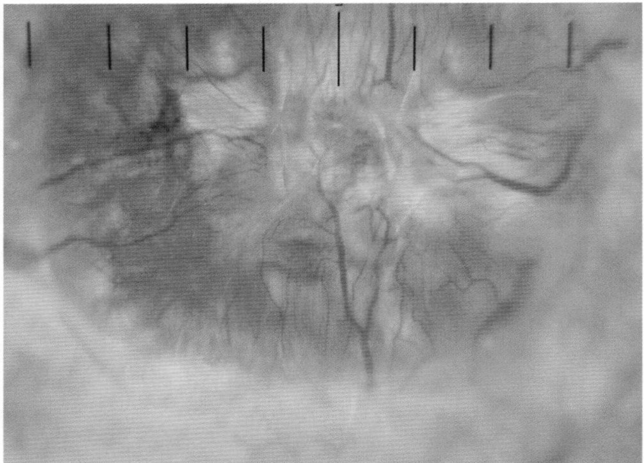

A well-defined pink nodule on the medial upper arm of a 90-year-old woman: polarised dermoscopy shows linear arborising vessels and multiple shiny white blotches and strands in this nodular BCC.

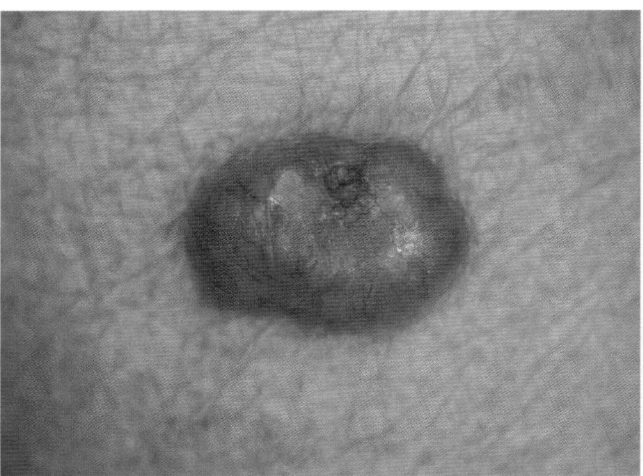

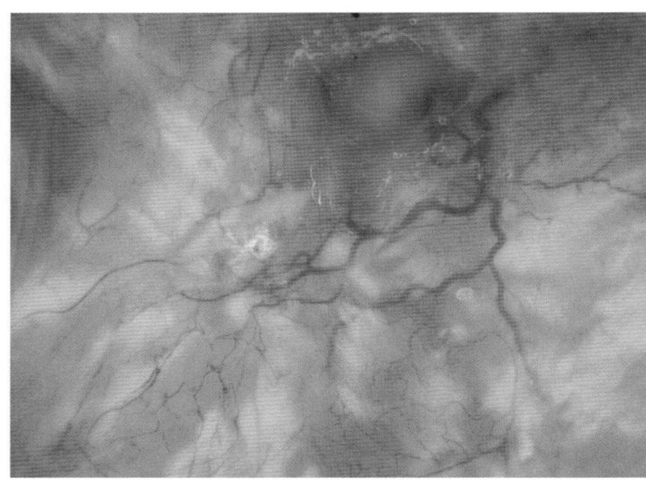

A well-defined pink nodule with focal ulceration on the back of a 70-year-old woman: polarised dermoscopy shows multiple shiny white blotches and strands, linear arborising vessels and ulceration in this nodular BCC.

Ishizaki, S. et al. The contribution of dermoscopy to early excision of basal cell carcinoma: A study on the tumor sizes acquired between 1998 and 2013. *J Dermatol Sci*. 2016;84(3):360.

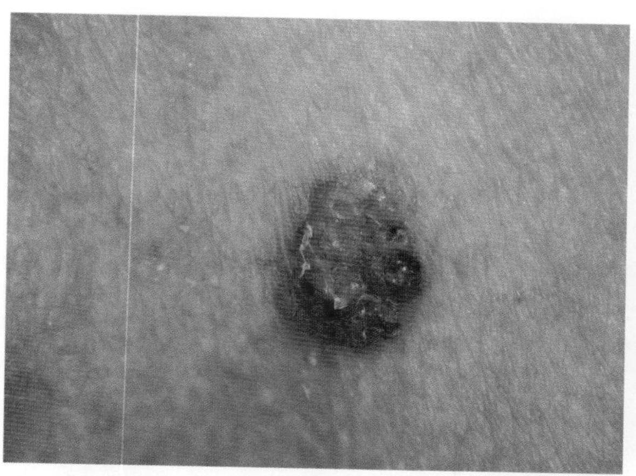
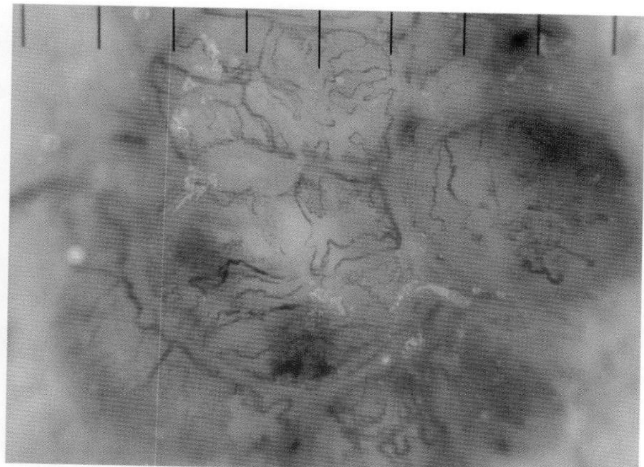

A well-defined pearly, telangiectatic nodule on the upper arm of a 70-year-old woman: dermoscopy shows arborising vessels, pink structureless areas and peripheral blue-grey globules in this nodular BCC.

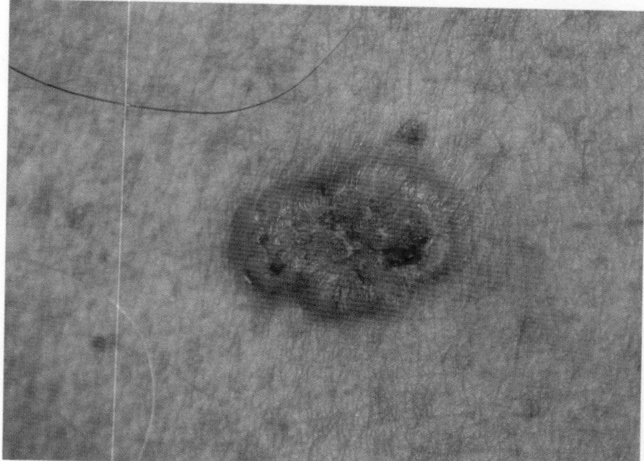
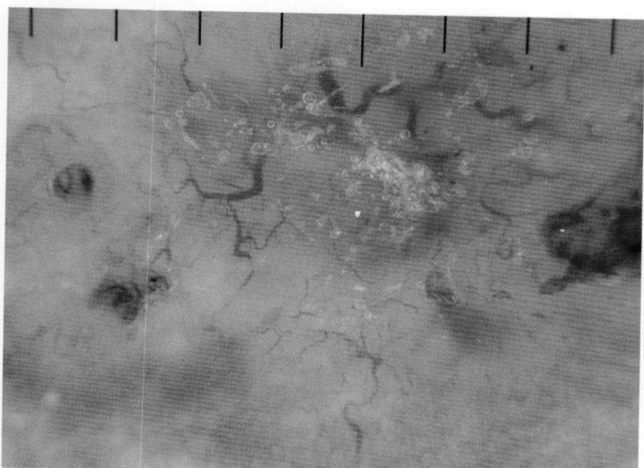

A well-defined pearly, telangiectatic, ulcerated plaque on the chest of a 70-year-old man: dermoscopy shows arborising vessels, erosions, ulceration, and a blue-grey ovoid nest at 4 o' clock in this nodular BCC.

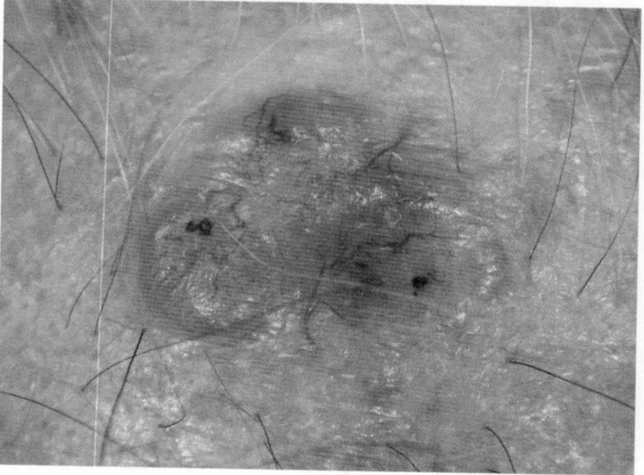
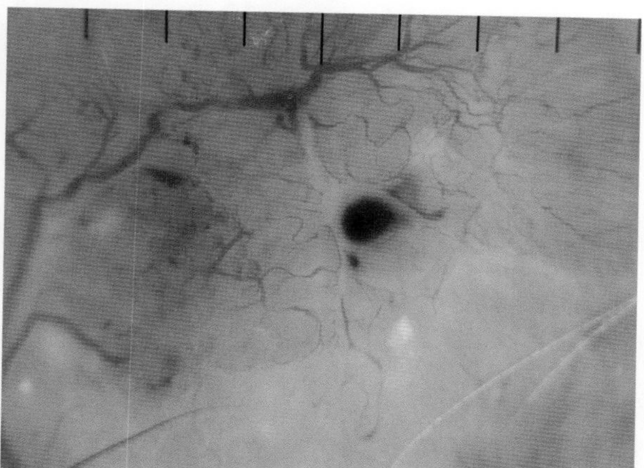

A pearly telangiectatic plaque on the scalp of a 70-year-old man: dermoscopy shows arborising vessels within pink structureless areas, grey-brown granular pigmentation and a solitary blue-grey ovoid nest in this nodular BCC.

BCCs are defined best by their colour and vasculature. Diagnosis is enhanced with polarising dermoscopy. Larger BCCs share the same features as small BCCs, but over a larger surface area.

Morphoeic/infiltrative basal cell carcinoma

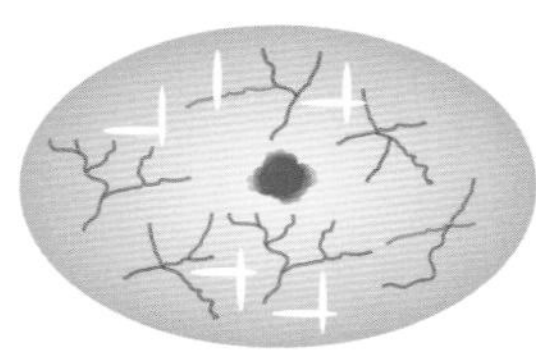

Morphoeic/infiltrative BCCs may present clinically as a scar-like plaque with less epidermal features than nodular or superficial BCCs. Consequentially, they tend to have fewer dermoscopic features, with typically only linear arborising vessels. The transition between normal skin and tumour is typically ill-defined. Pre-surgical diagnostic accuracy of infiltrative BCCs is enhanced by combining clinical and dermoscopic examination.

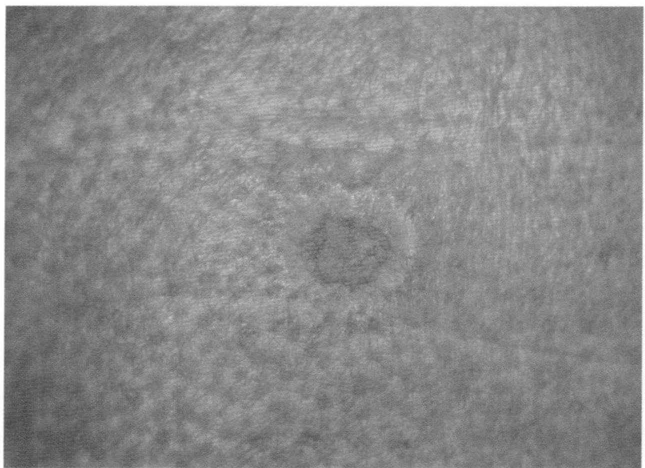

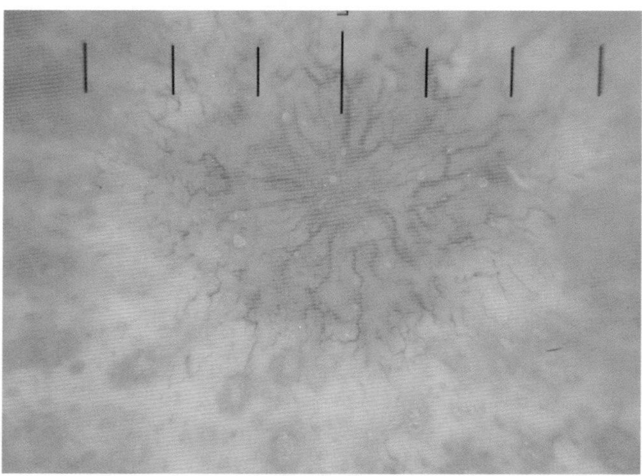

A sclerotic plaque on the forehead of a 70-year-old man: dermoscopy shows multiple foci of linear arborising vessels and background peripheral pale sclerotic stroma with ill-defined margins in this infiltrative BCC.

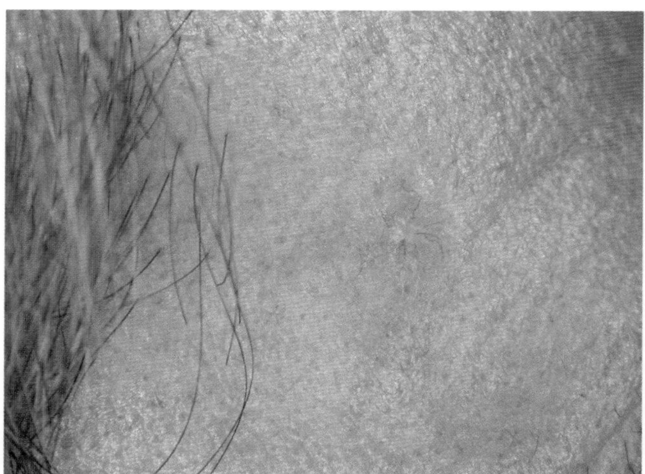

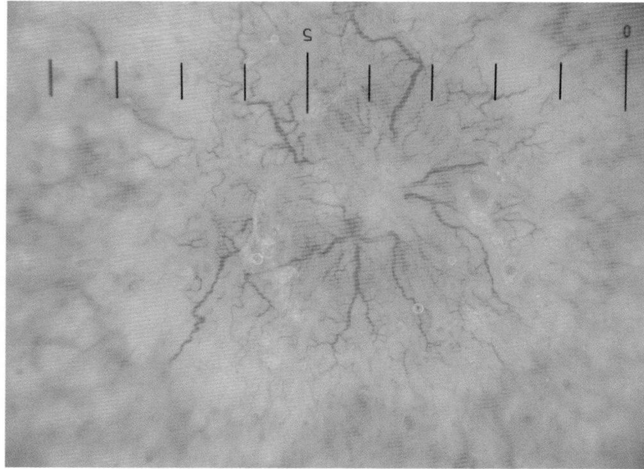

A sclerotic telangiectatic plaque on the temple of a 70-year-old man: dermoscopy shows multiple sharply focused linear arborising vessels and background pale sclerotic stroma in this infiltrative BCC.

Pampena, R. et al. Clinical and Dermoscopic Factors for the Identification of Aggressive Histologic Subtypes of Basal Cell Carcinoma. *Front Oncol*. 2021;10:630458.

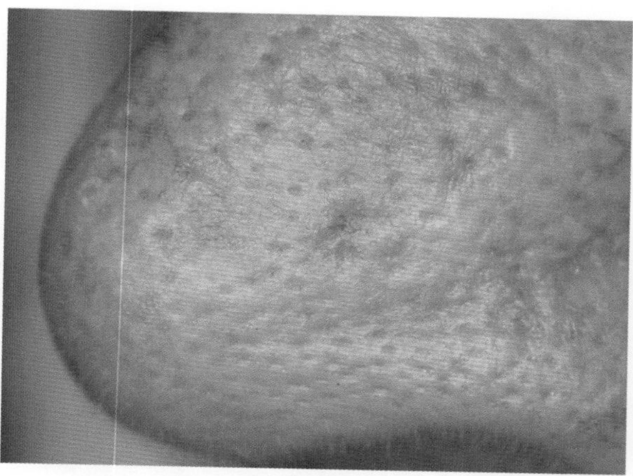

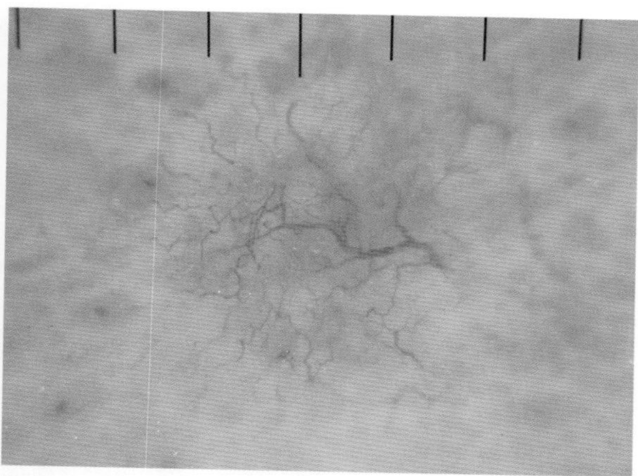

An ill-defined sclerotic and telangiectatic plaque on the lateral nasal tip of a 60-year-old man: dermoscopy shows arborising vessels centrally with an ill-defined peripheral margin in this infiltrative BCC treated with Mohs surgery.

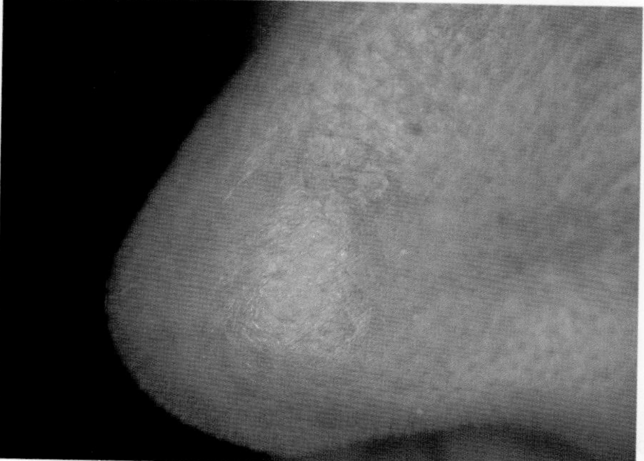

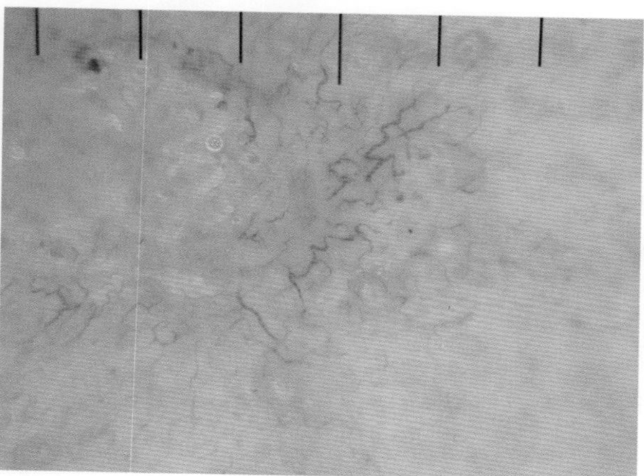

An ill-defined sclerotic plaque on the nasal side wall of a 25-year-old woman: dermoscopy shows a pink structureless area and linear arborising vessels with an ill-defined margin in this infiltrative BCC treated with Mohs surgery.

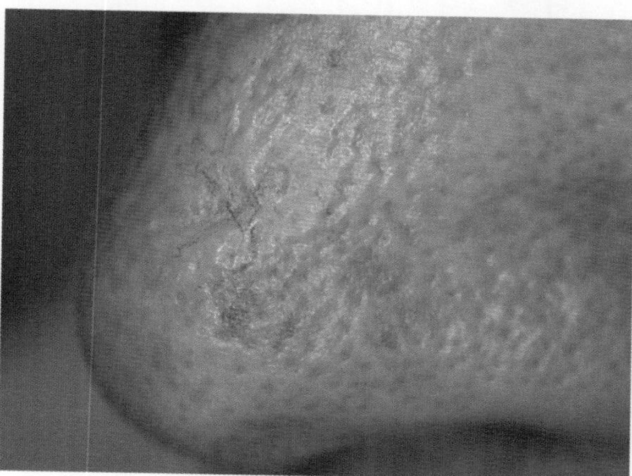

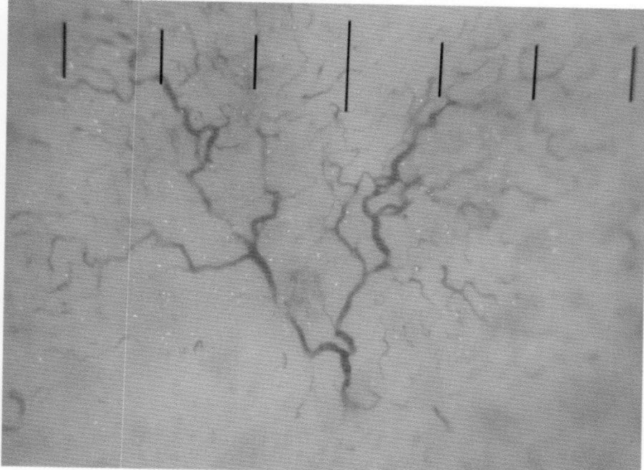

A sclerotic plaque on the supra-nasal tip of a 50-year-old woman: dermoscopy shows arborising vessels with an ill-defined peripheral margin and pale background in this infiltrative BCC treated with Mohs surgery.

Consider taking a preoperative biopsy to confirm the histopathological subtype for ill-defined infiltrative BCCs since Mohs surgery may be required.

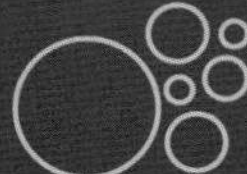

Hypopigmented basal cell carcinoma

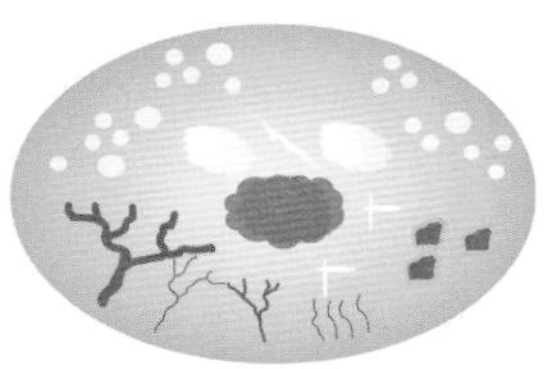

BCCs may present clinically as skin-coloured papules that can mimic benign dermal naevi. On close inspection with dermoscopy, additional features of BCC are easily seen, including pigmented structures, linear arborising vessels and shiny white blotches and strands. Multiple aggregated yellow-white globules are a relatively novel feature described in higher risk BCCs such as morphoeic subtype. These represent dystrophic calcification and are not observed in superficial BCCs.

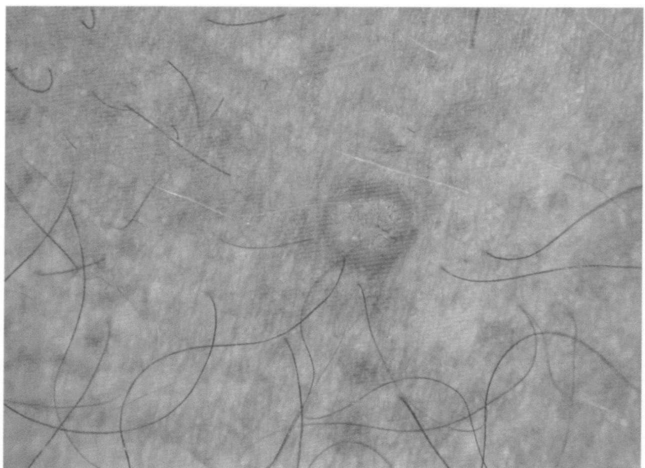

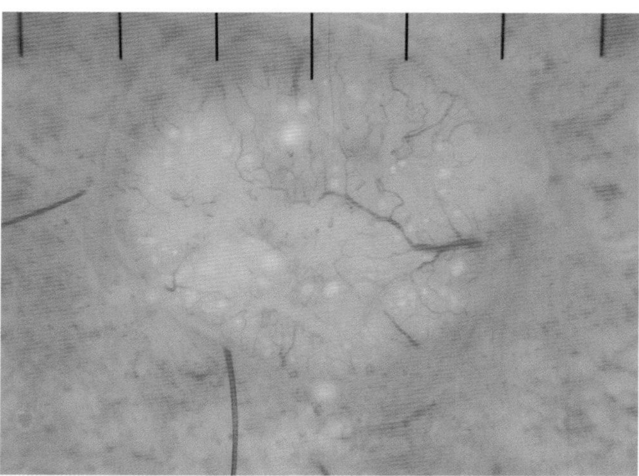

An asymptomatic skin-coloured papule on the chest of a 60-year-old man: dermoscopy shows linear arborising vessels and multiple aggregated yellow-white globules in this nodular BCC.

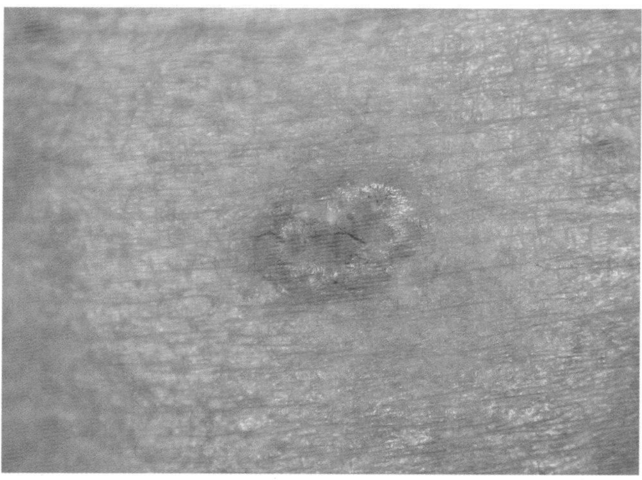

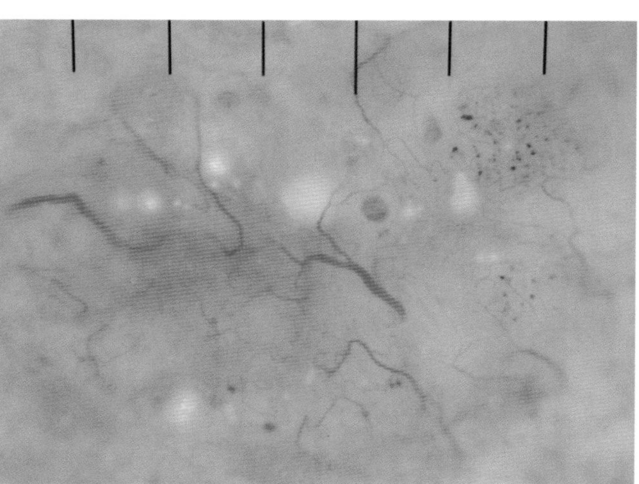

A pearly hypopigmented plaque on the forehead of a 70-year-old woman: dermoscopy shows additional features of multiple blue-grey dots and granules, linear arborising vessels and multiple aggregated yellow-white globules in this nodular BCC.

Navarrete-Dechent, C. et al. Association of Multiple Aggregated Yellow-White Globules With Nonpigmented Basal Cell Carcinoma. *JAMA Dermatol*. 2020;156(8):882–890.

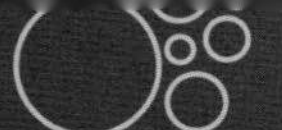

Hyperpigmented basal cell carcinoma

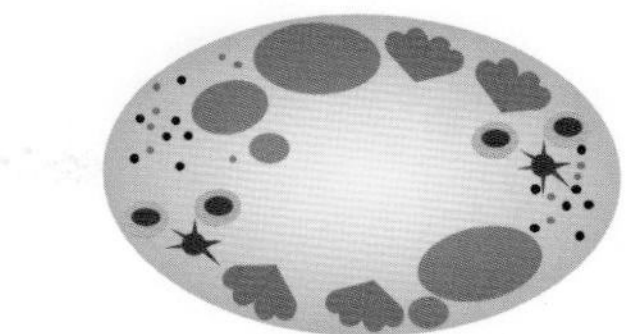

BCCs may present clinically as hyperpigmented tumours. In this scenario, the overlap in clinical features with an atypical melanocytic lesion can be high. Dermoscopy may or may not help in confirming the diagnosis and histopathology is mandatory to confirm the diagnosis.

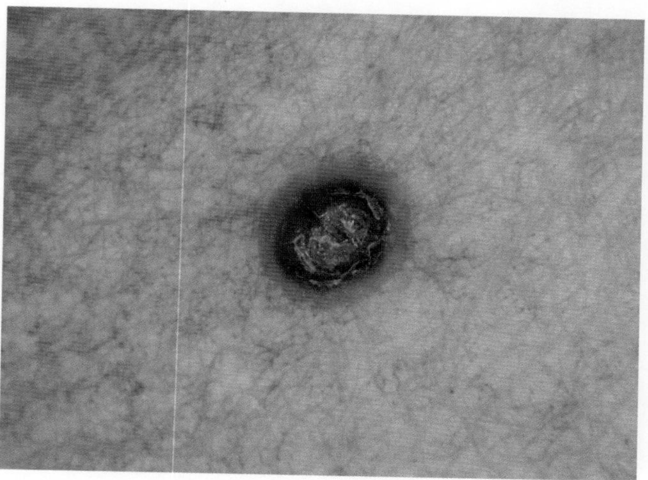

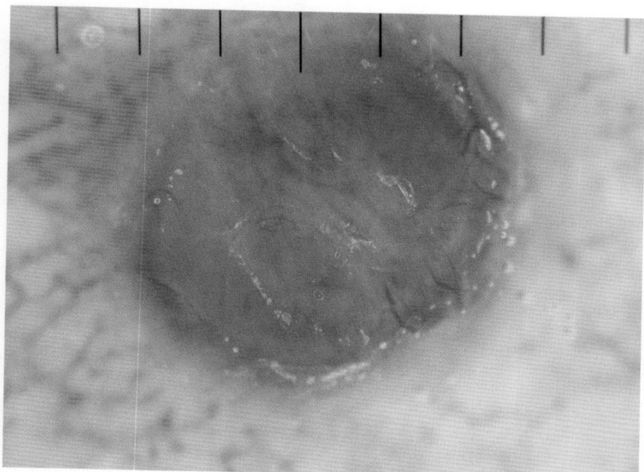

A suspicious, asymptomatic hyperpigmented tumour on the upper arm of a 60-year-old woman: dermoscopy shows homogeneous slate blue coloration with peripheral broad telangiectasias in this histopathologically confirmed nodular BCC.

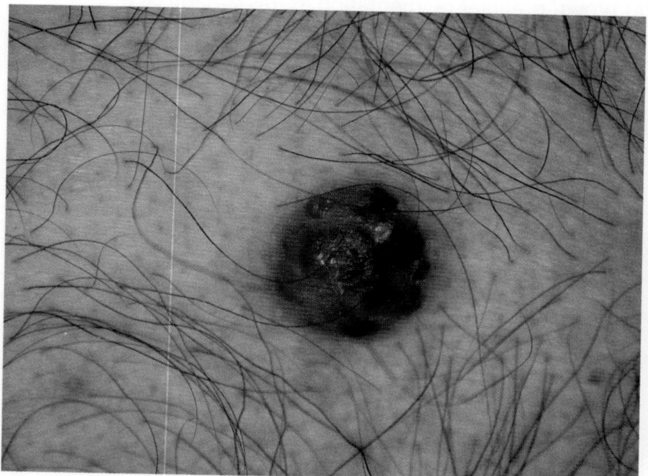

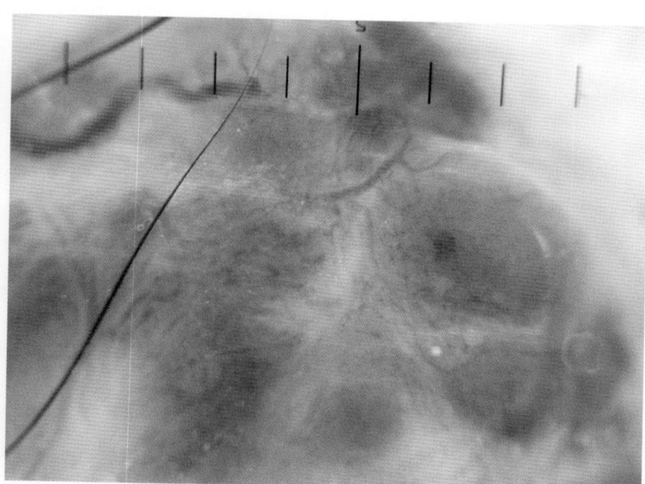

A hyperpigmented nodule mimicking nodular melanoma, on the chest of a 50-year-old man: dermoscopy shows broad arborising vessels and large blue-grey ovoid nests in this histopathologically confirmed nodular BCC.

Consider urgent excision of hyperpigmented BCCs to avoid any diagnostic delay, as clinical and dermoscopic features may overlap with nodular melanoma. These tumours are a challenge to diagnose without doubt.

Seborrhoeic keratosis-like basal cell carcinoma

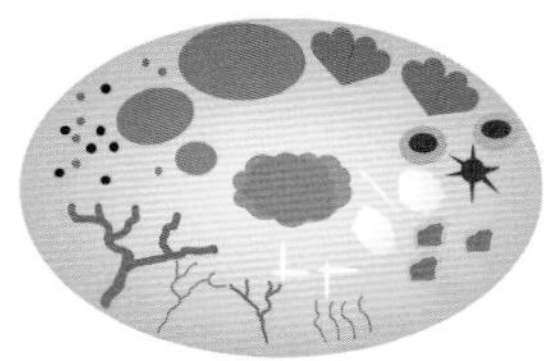

In patients with multiple seborrhoeic keratoses it is not unusual to find a small BCC hidden amongst the population of benign skin lesions. History is often lacking and the BCC is only found on careful examination of all skin lesions. In this scenario it typically presents as a pale shiny brown plaque mimicking the neighbouring seborrhoeic keratoses with features on dermoscopy favouring a BCC rather than a seborrhoeic keratosis.

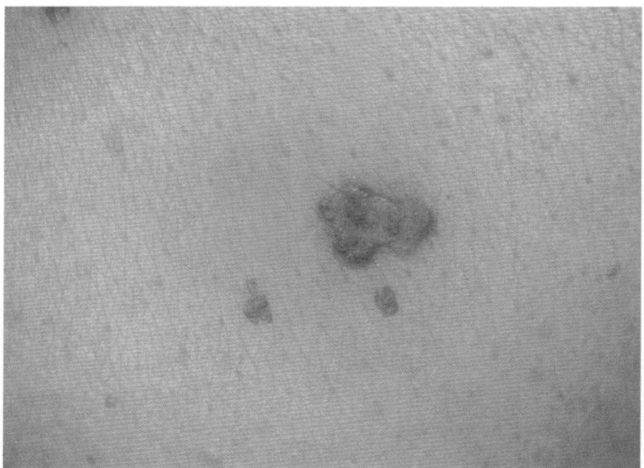

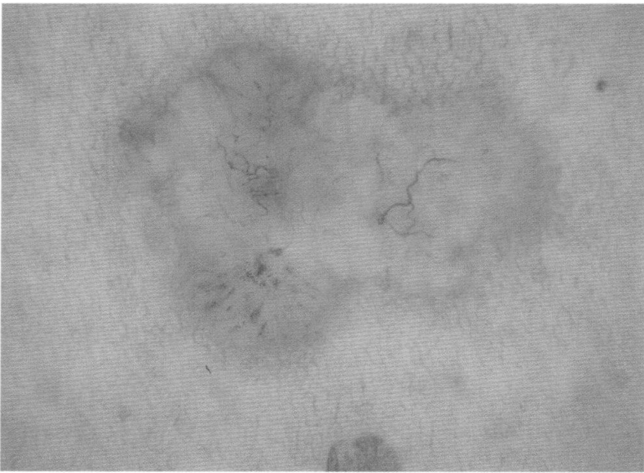

A well-defined pale brown plaque on the abdomen of a 50-year-old woman: dermoscopy shows linear arborising vessels, peripheral short fine telangiectasias, pale pink structureless areas and brown granular pigmentation in this superficial BCC.

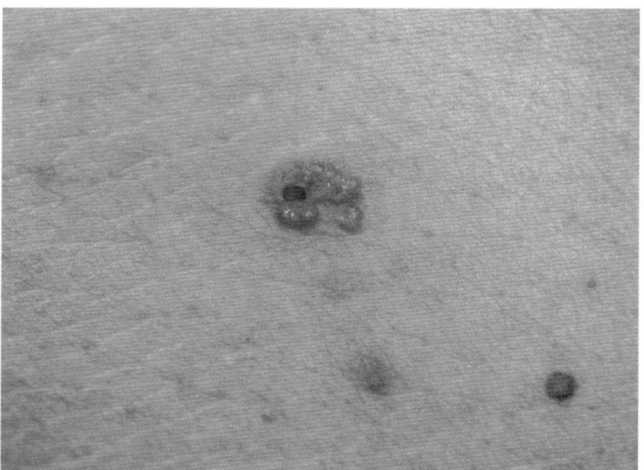

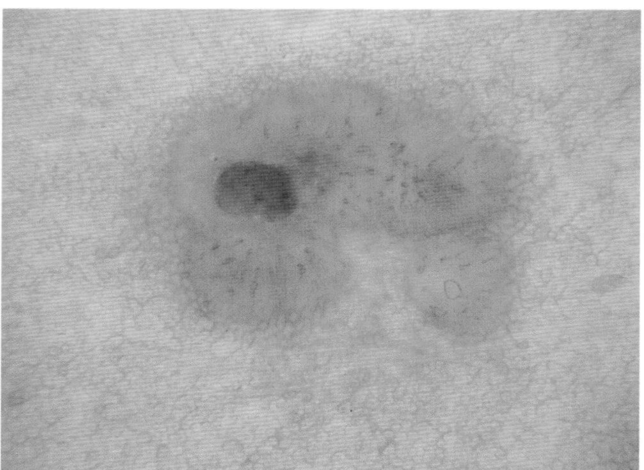

A well-defined pinkish brown plaque with a focal erosion on the lower back of a 70-year-old woman: dermoscopy shows a focal erosion, peripheral short fine telangiectasias and brown granular pigmentation in this BCC.

Takenouchi, T. Key points in dermoscopic diagnosis of basal cell carcinoma and seborrheic keratosis in Japanese. *J Dermatol.* 2011;38(1):59–65.

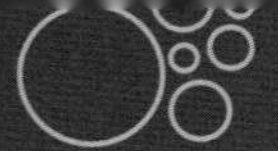

Fibroepithelioma of Pinkus

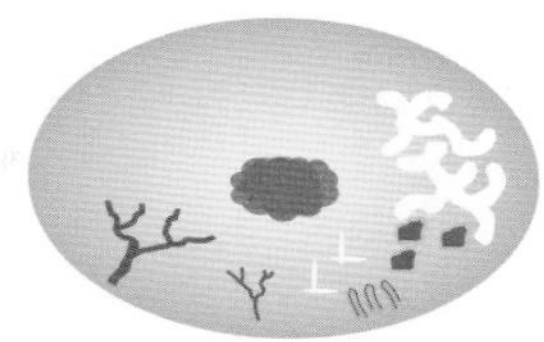

Fibroepithelioma of Pinkus is a rare subtype of BCC, which typically presents as a pink, light brown or skin-coloured papule or plaque on the trunk. It can resemble many skin lesions, including dermal nevus, pedunculated fibroma, acrochordon, seborrhoeic keratosis and melanoma. The dermoscopic features reported include polymorphous vessels, arborising vessels often surrounded by white lines, milia-like cysts, blue-grey dots and shiny white structures.

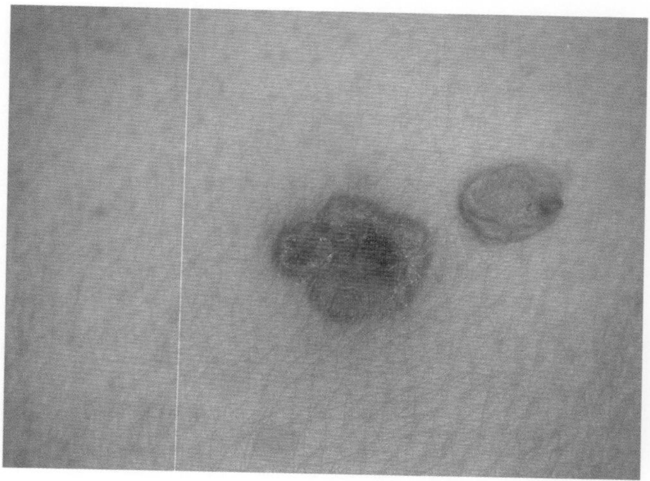

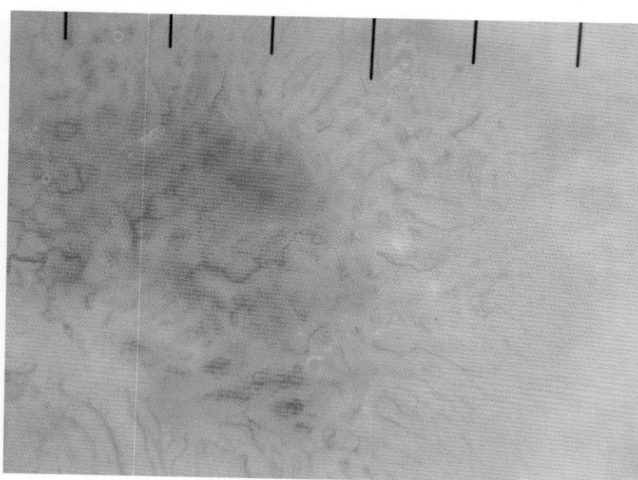

A well-defined pink plaque on the lower back of a 50-year-old woman: dermoscopy shows linear arborising vessels surrounded by white lines and erosions in this fibroepithelioma of Pinkus.

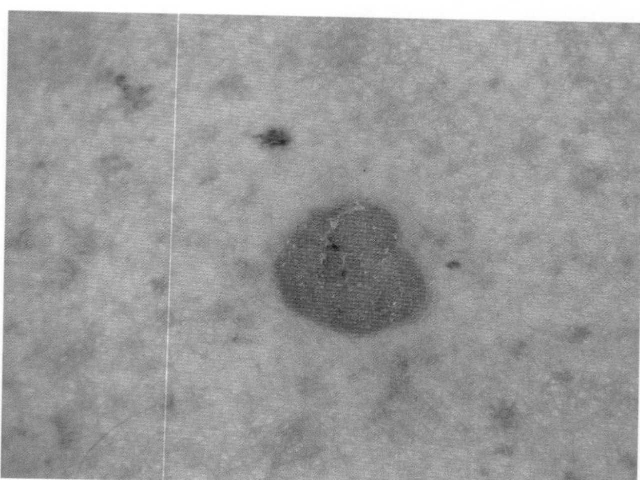

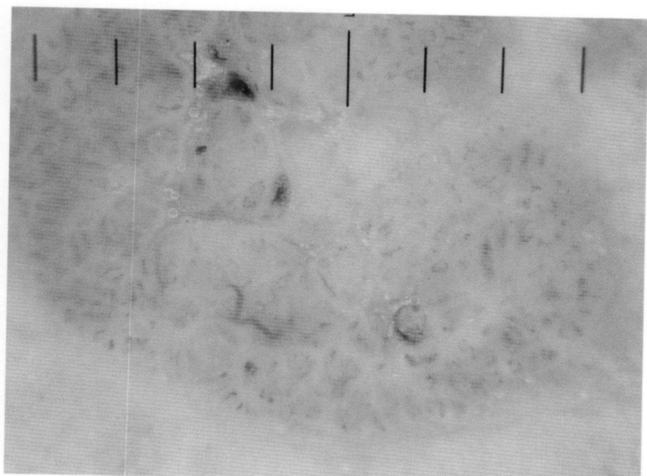

A well-defined pink nodule on the lower back of a 70-year-old man: dermoscopy shows polymorphous vessels surrounded by white lines and erosions in this fibroepithelioma of Pinkus.

Reggiani, C. et al. Fibroepithelioma of Pinkus: case reports and review of the literature. *Dermatology*. 2013;226(3):207–211.

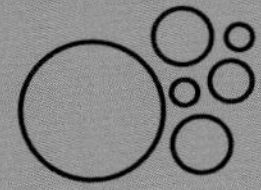

6 Keratinocyte dysplasia

Actinic keratosis grade I 159
Actinic keratosis grade II 160
Actinic keratosis grade III 161
Actinic keratosis – follicular hyperkeratosis 162
Bowen's disease – classical 163
Bowen's disease – hypertrophic 164
Bowen's disease – pigmented 165
Bowen's disease – digital 166
Squamous cell carcinoma – white circles 167
Squamous cell carcinoma – keratoacanthoma 168
Squamous cell carcinoma – moderately differentiated 169
Squamous cell carcinoma – ulcerated 170
Squamous cell carcinoma – poorly differentiated 171

Diagnostic Dermoscopy: The Illustrated Guide, Second Edition. Jonathan Bowling.

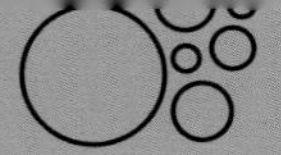

Actinic keratosis grade I

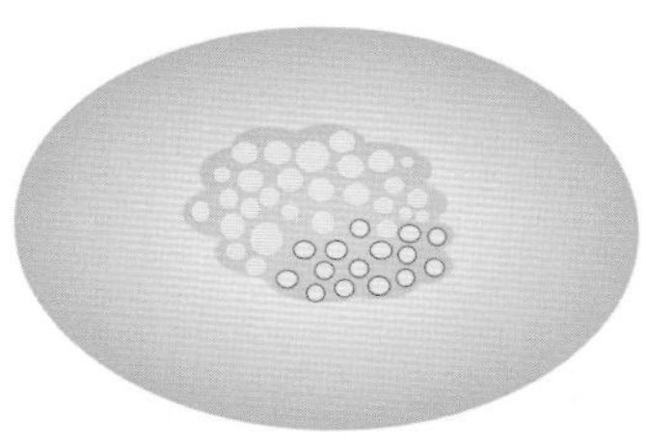

Actinic keratoses can present clinically in a number of ways depending upon the degree of keratinisation (thin or thick, focal or follicular), and additional features such as erythema and pigmentation. Thin grade I actinic keratoses are detectable as a roughened hyperkeratotic macule, which on dermoscopy shows increased keratinising features around follicles.

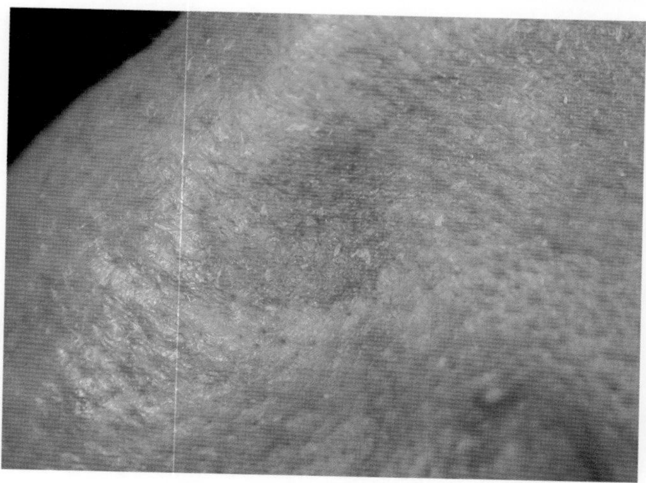

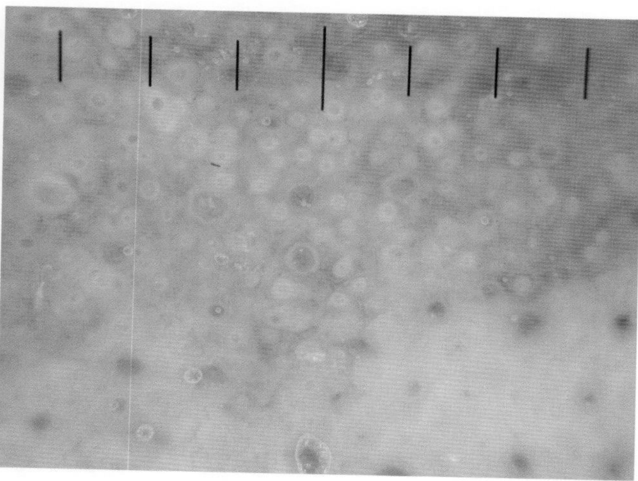

A keratotic macule on the nasal bridge of a 60-year-old woman: dermoscopy shows an increase in keratinising features around follicles with small white circles, keratin, brown granular pigmentation and a clear inferior border in this actinic keratosis.

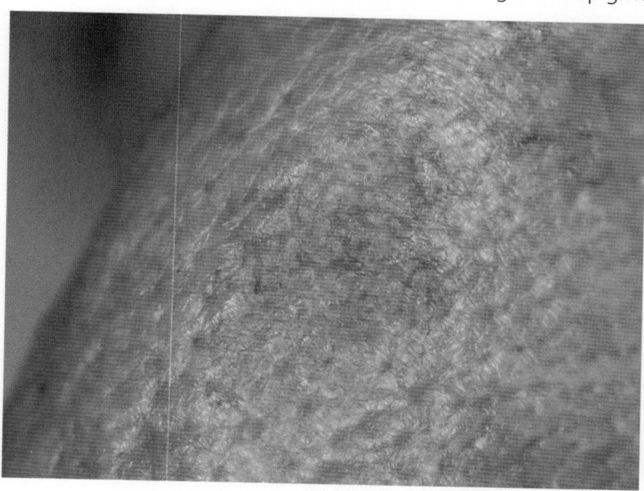

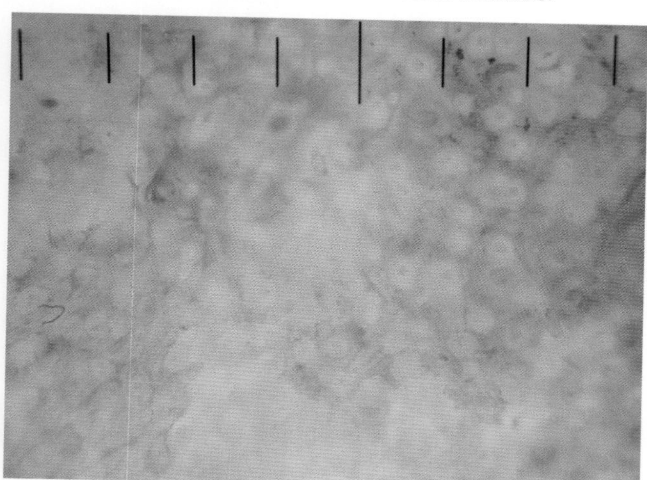

A keratotic macule on the nasal bridge of a 60-year-old man: dermoscopy shows follicular prominence with keratinising structures and brown granular pigmentation in this thin pigmented actinic keratosis.

Zalaudek, I. et al. Dermatoscopy of facial actinic keratosis, intraepidermal carcinoma, and invasive squamous cell carcinoma: a progression model. *J Am Acad Dermatol*. 2012;66(4):589–97.

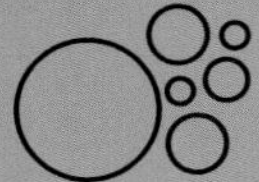

Actinic keratosis grade II

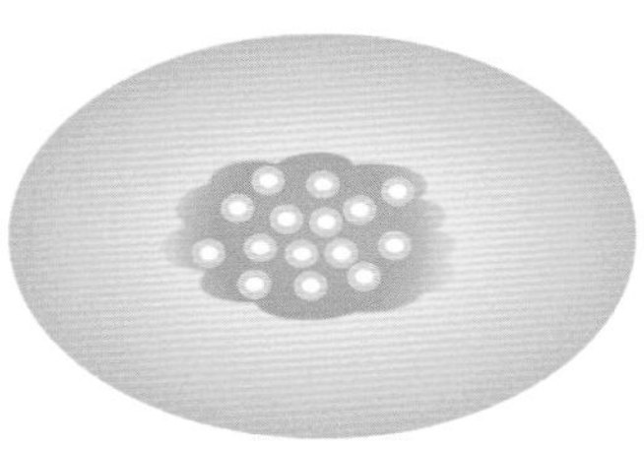

Actinic keratoses with erythema and follicular keratinisation show a composite appearance on dermoscopy, which has been described as a 'strawberry' pattern. This is characterized by a background red pseudonetwork consisting of hazy and out-of-focus interfollicular vessels, associated with prominent follicular openings surrounded by a white halo.

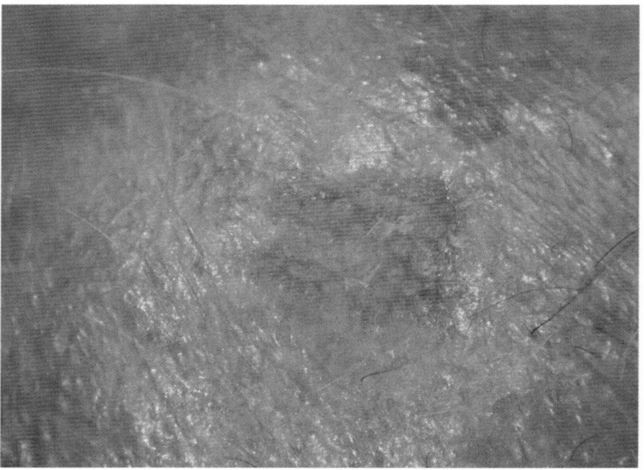

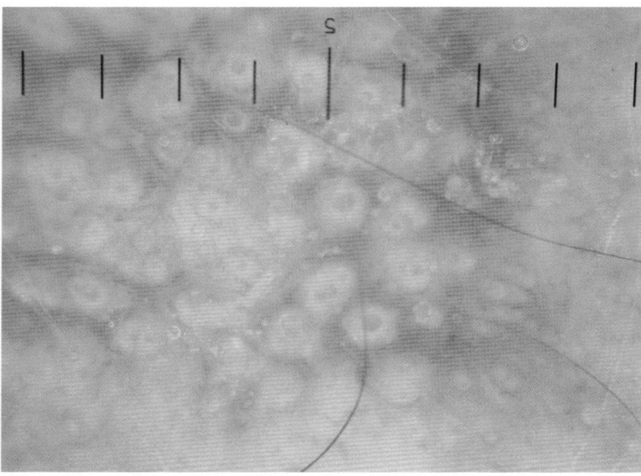

A pink hyperkeratotic plaque on the scalp of a 70-year-old man: dermoscopy shows background erythema with small, poorly focused vessels between the follicles surrounded by a white halo in this histopathologically confirmed actinic keratosis.

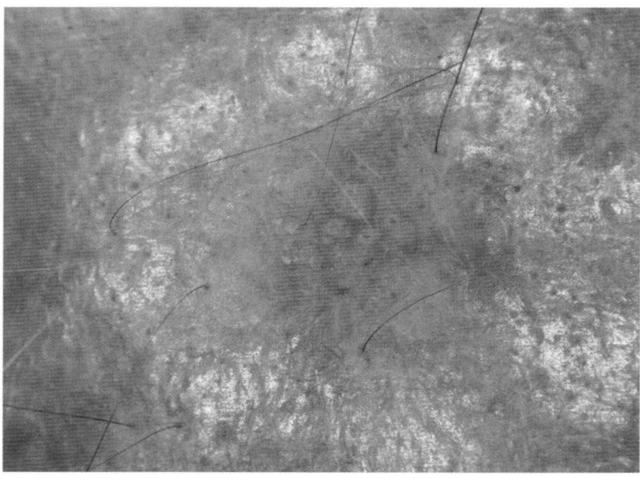

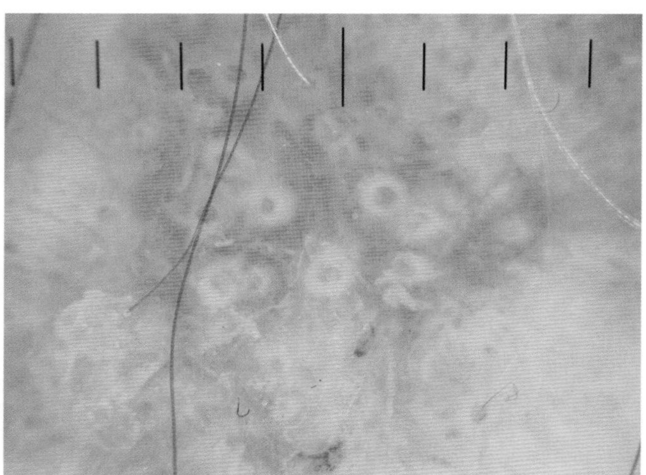

A further pink hyperkeratotic plaque on the scalp of the same 70-year-old man: dermoscopy shows similar features of background erythema with follicular openings surrounded by a white halo in this histopathologically confirmed actinic keratosis.

Zalaudek, I. et al. Dermoscopy of facial non-pigmented actinic keratosis. *Br J Dermatol*. 2006;155(5):951–956.

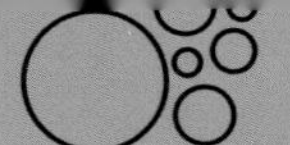

Actinic keratosis grade III

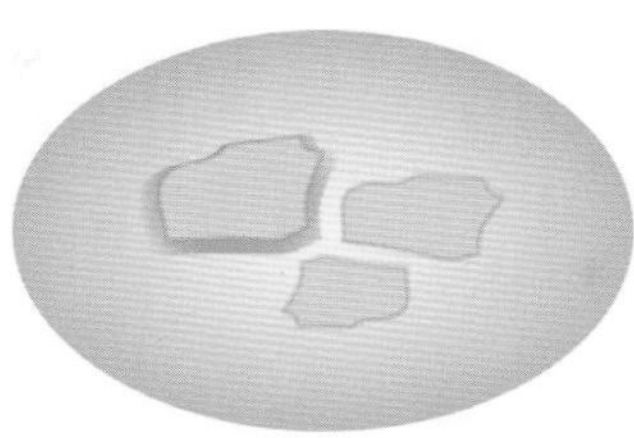

Actinic keratoses with prominent hyperkeratosis show relatively few dermoscopic features. The hyperkeratosis obscures any features hidden beneath the plaque. Clinical features such as pain and tenderness or the presence of induration are important additional symptoms/signs that may indicate invasive squamous cell carcinoma (SCC).

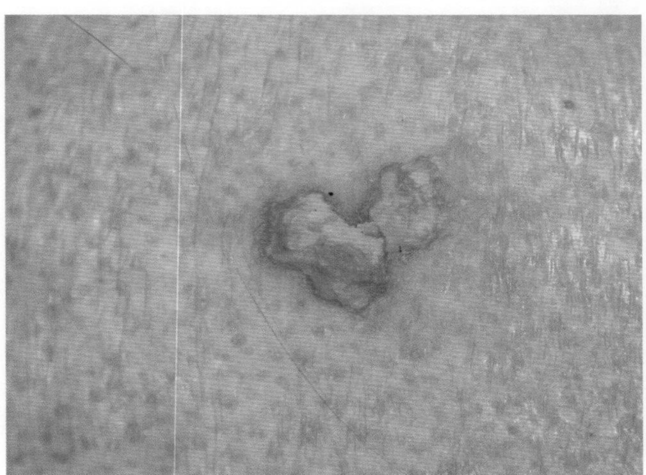

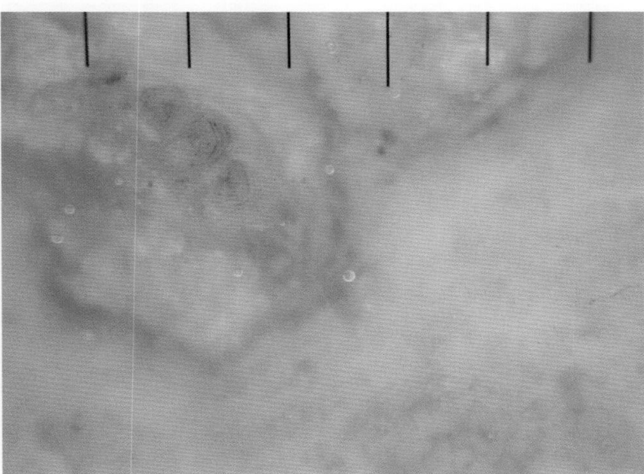

A focal asymptomatic hyperkeratotic plaque on the vertex of the scalp of a 75-year-old man: dermoscopy shows a yellow and white keratin crust, with no additional features and no erythema at the base in this hyperkeratotic actinic keratosis.

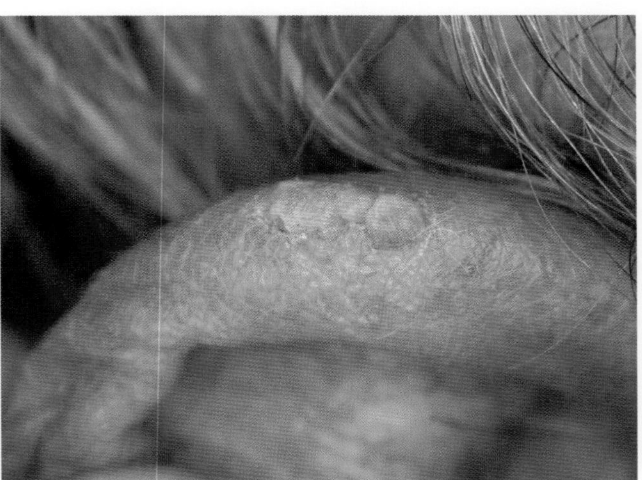

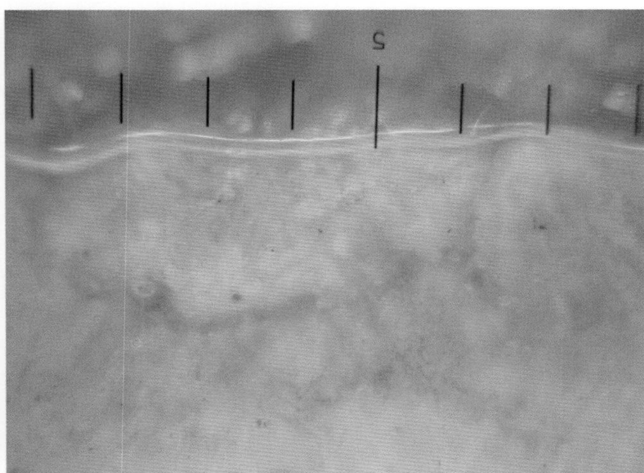

An asymptomatic linear hyperkeratotic plaque on the helical rim of an 80-year-old man: dermoscopy shows a yellow-white keratin crust, with no additional features and no erythema at the base in this hyperkeratotic actinic keratosis.

Reinehr, C.P.H. and Bakos, R.M. Actinic keratoses: review of clinical, dermoscopic and therapeutic aspects. *An Bras Dermatol.* 2019;94(6):637–657.

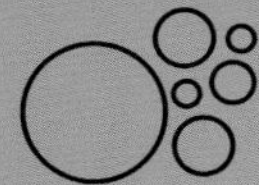

Actinic keratosis – follicular hyperkeratosis

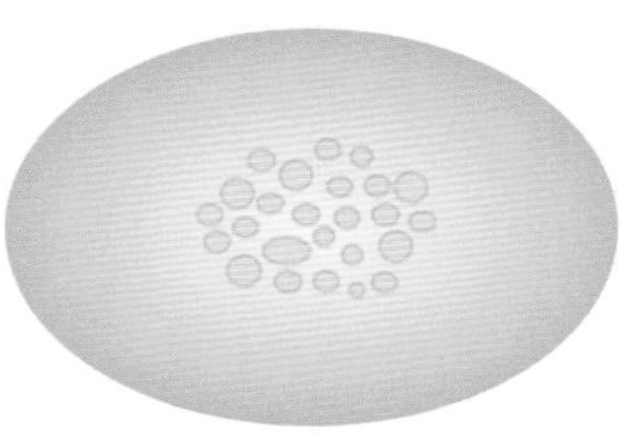

When actinic keratoses present with follicular involvement they have a distinct dermoscopic pattern of multiple focal hyperkeratotic aggregates. Additional features of pigmentation may or may not be present.

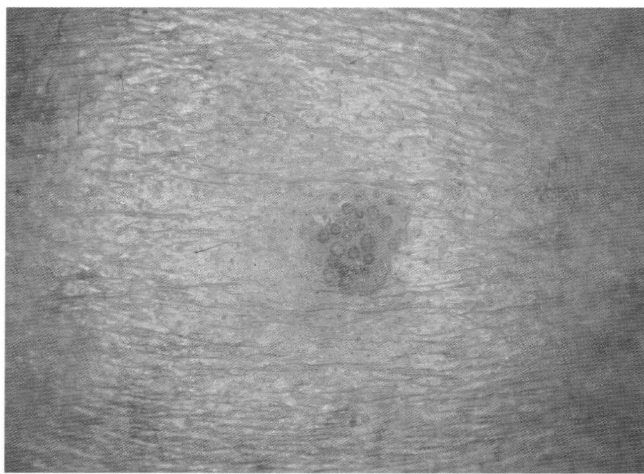

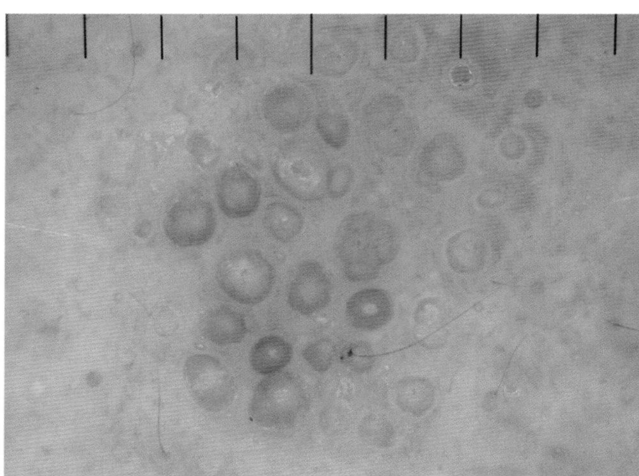

A solitary hyperkeratotic plaque on the anterior scalp of a 65-year-old man: dermoscopy shows multiple focal yellow keratotic aggregates surrounded by brown rings in this hypertrophic actinic keratosis.

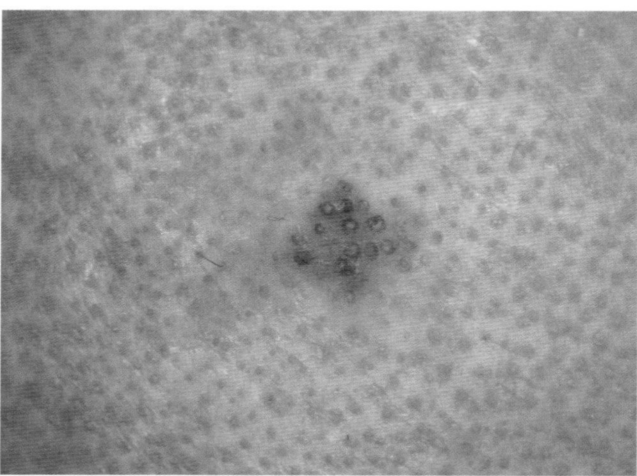

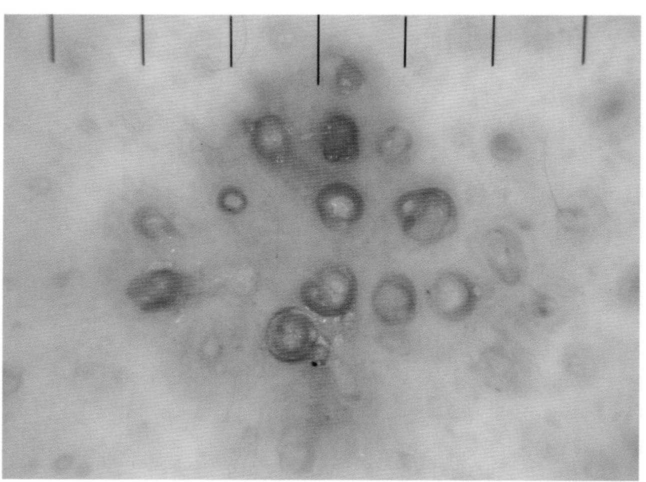

A hyperkeratotic plaque on the scalp of a 60-year-old man: dermoscopy shows multiple focal brown pigmented keratotic aggregates surrounded by brown rings in this pigmented hyperkeratotic actinic keratosis.

Consider a diagnostic biopsy of any actinic keratosis where clinical concern for SCC is present.

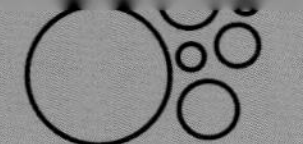

Bowen's disease – classical

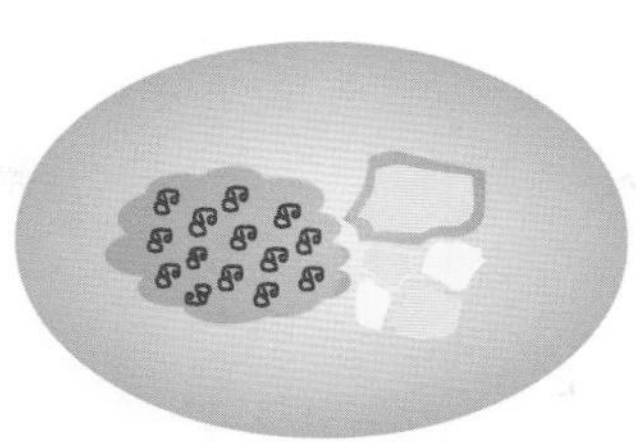

Bowen's disease, otherwise known as intraepidermal carcinoma or SCC in situ, is a common form of keratinocyte cancer precursor lesion most frequently found in the elderly. As with other keratinocyte cancers, a range of clinical and dermoscopic presentations can be observed.

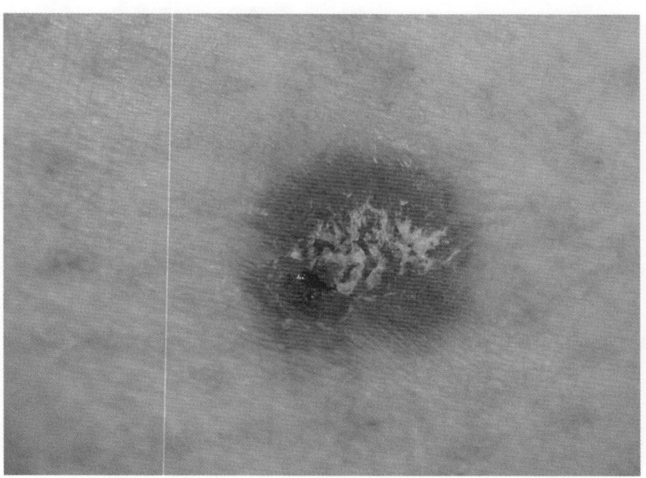

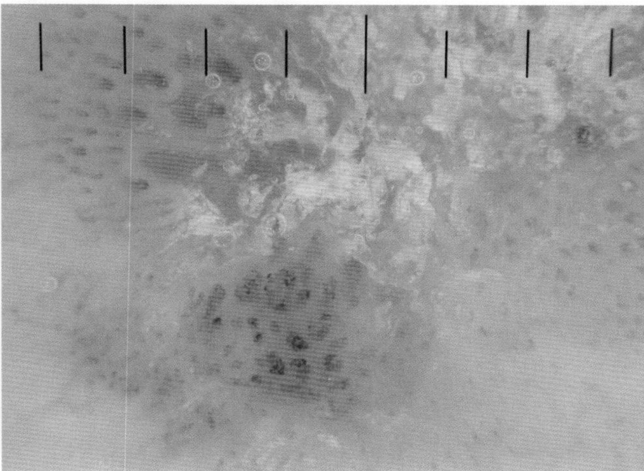

A 70-year-old woman with a long-standing scaly plaque on the leg: dermoscopy shows yellow and white hyperkeratosis as well as coiled or glomerular vessels in clusters in this histopathologically confirmed Bowen's disease.

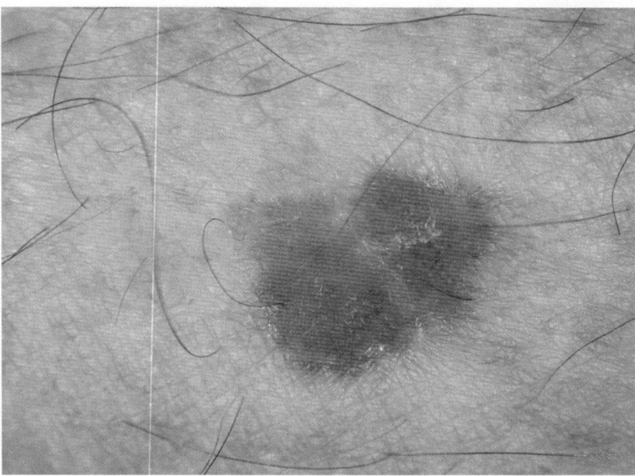

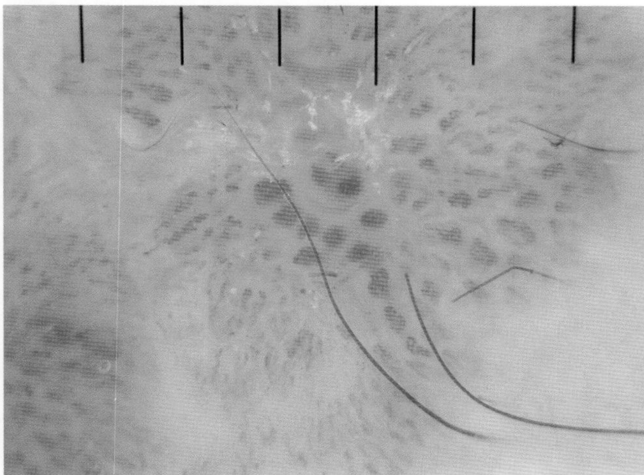

A 60-year-old man with a well-circumscribed erythematous plaque on the leg: dermoscopy shows erythema, predominantly coiled or glomerular vessels and hyperkeratosis in this histopathologically confirmed Bowen's disease.

The dotted or glomerular vessels in Bowen's disease will sometimes form linear arrays.

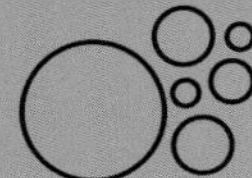

Bowen's disease – hypertrophic

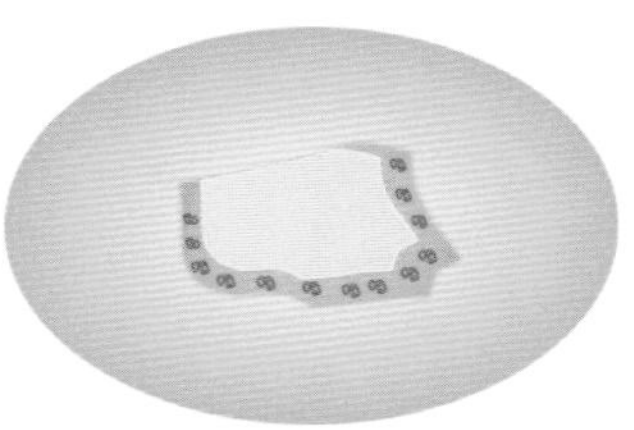

When Bowen's disease becomes hypertrophic, vascular features at the periphery may provide the best clues. Hypertrophic Bowen's disease may mimic SCC due to the induration and hence a histopathological confirmation of the diagnosis should be considered.

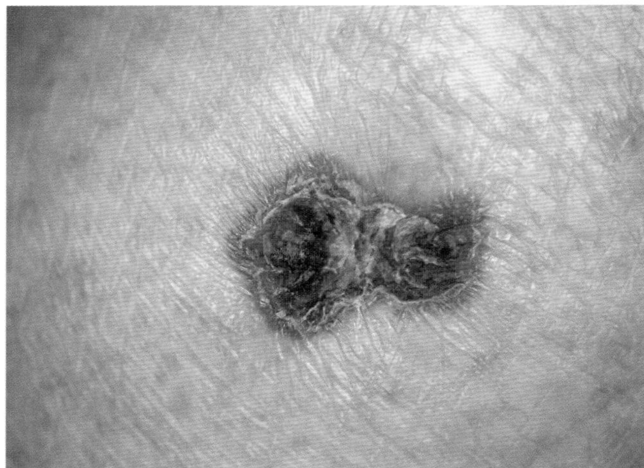

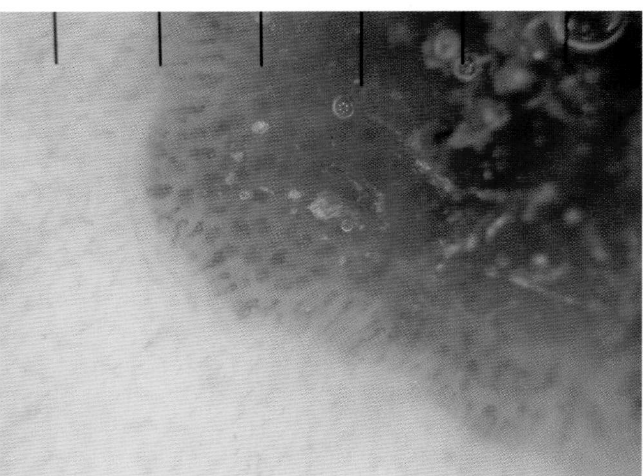

A solitary long-standing hyperkeratotic plaque on the lower leg of a 65-year-old man: dermoscopy shows central keratinisation with peripheral coiled or glomerular vessels in this histopathologically confirmed Bowen's disease.

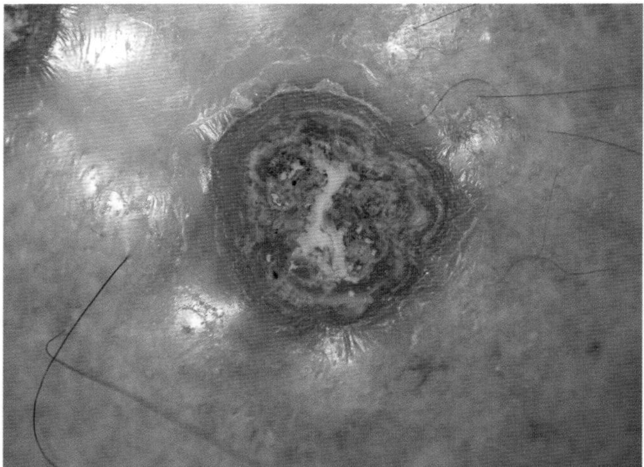

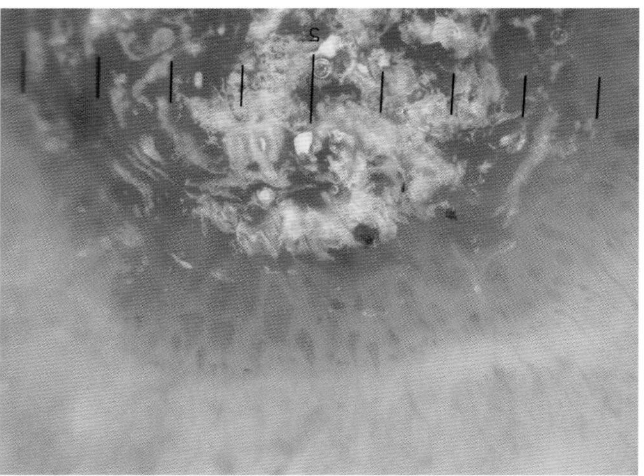

An indurated hyperkeratotic plaque with peripheral erythema on the scalp of an 85-year-old man: dermoscopy shows central hyperkeratosis with peripheral erythema and coiled or glomerular vessels, confirmed as Bowen's disease on histopathology.

Papageorgiou, C. et al. Accuracy of dermoscopic criteria for the differentiation between superficial basal cell carcinoma and Bowen's disease. *J Eur Acad Dermatol Venereol*. 2018;32(11):1914–1919.

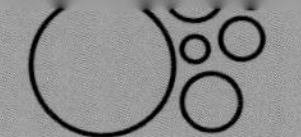

Bowen's disease – pigmented

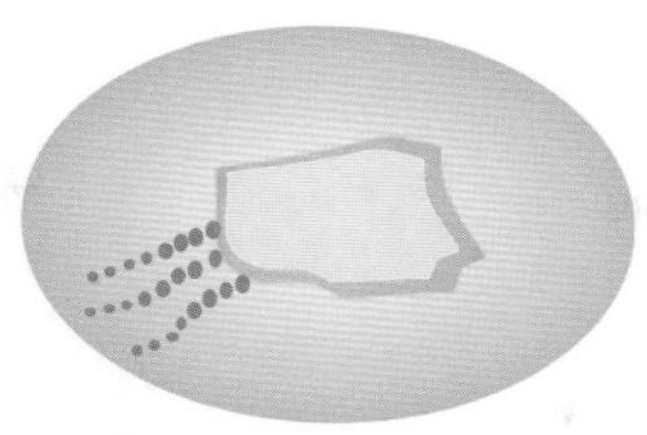

Pigmented Bowen's disease can provide a diagnostic challenge as many features may overlap with melanoma. Pigmented Bowen's disease is more frequently found in populations with long-term high UV exposure. Whilst only a fraction of them are pigmented, linear arrays of dotted or glomerular vessels and/or brown/grey dots are characteristic dermoscopic features. A diagnostic biopsy should be considered if any clinical and/or dermoscopic doubt exists.

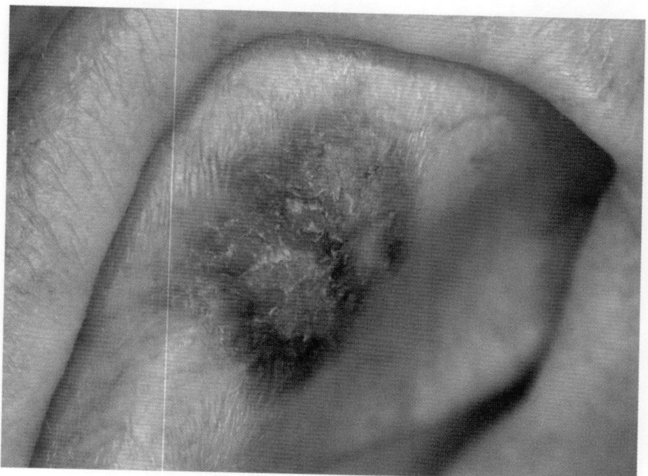

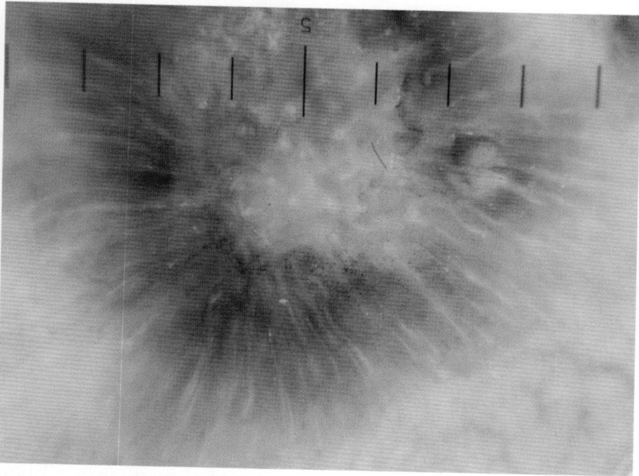

A suspicious hyperkeratotic variably pigmented plaque within the right ear of a 70-year-old man: dermoscopy shows central erythema with keratin and multiple brown dots in a linear array at the peripheral margin, confirmed as pigmented Bowen's disease.

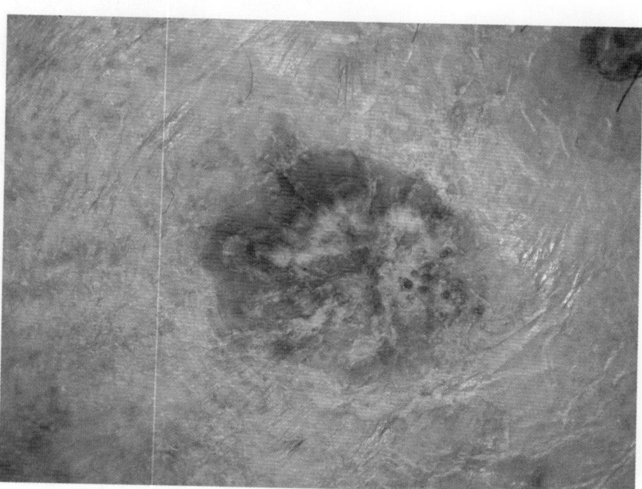

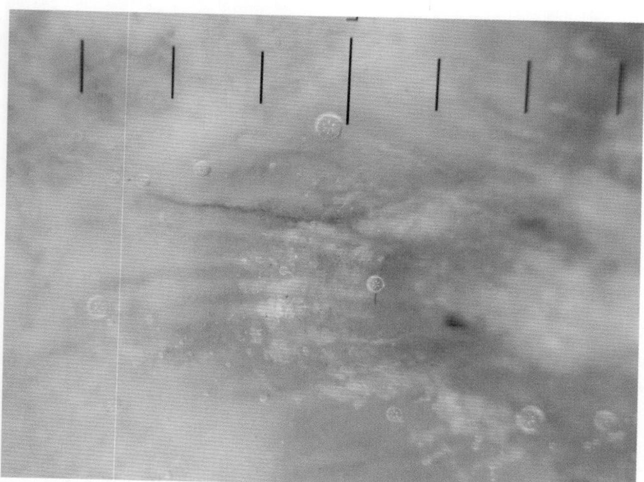

An 80-year-old man with a variably pigmented hyperkeratotic plaque on the vertex of his photodamaged scalp: dermoscopy shows hyperkeratosis and a linear focus of multiple brown dots radiating peripherally, confirmed as Bowen's disease.

Cameron, A. et al. Dermatoscopy of pigmented Bowen's disease. *J Am Acad Dermatol*. 2010;62(4):597–604.

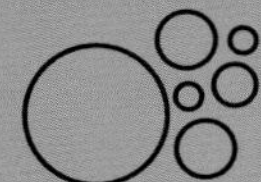

Bowen's disease – digital

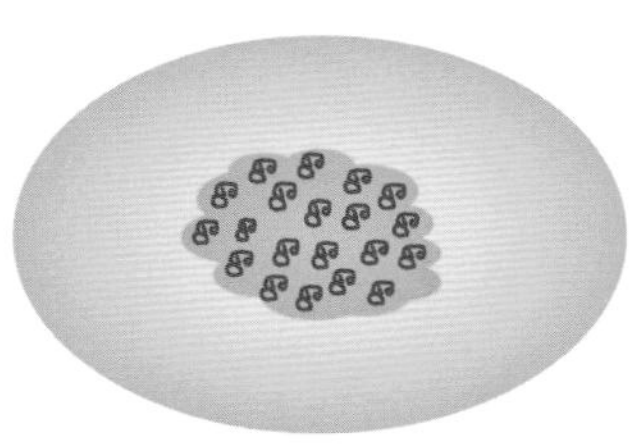

Bowen's disease may present as a solitary long-standing lesion on the dorsal aspect of a digit. The history is often that of a presumed inflammatory lesion failing to respond to topical steroids. Dermoscopic features include coiled or glomerular vessels, erosions, erythema and hyperkeratosis. A diagnostic biopsy should be considered if any clinical and/or dermoscopic doubt exists.

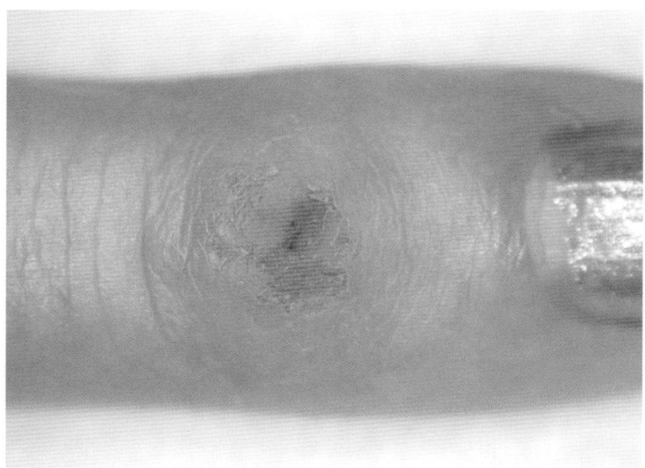

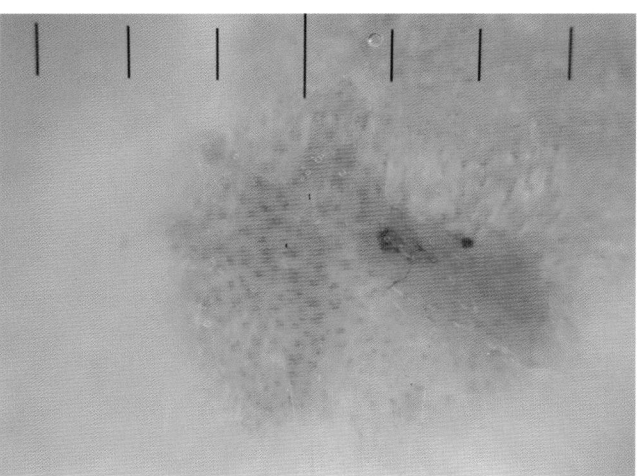

A 12-month history of a long-standing erythrosquamous plaque on the dorsum of the index finger of a 50-year-old woman: dermoscopy shows clustered coiled or glomerular vessels, erythema and micro-erosions, confirmed as Bowen's disease.

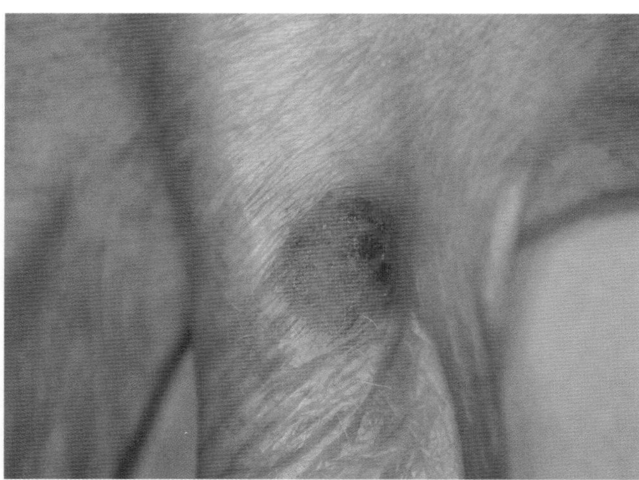

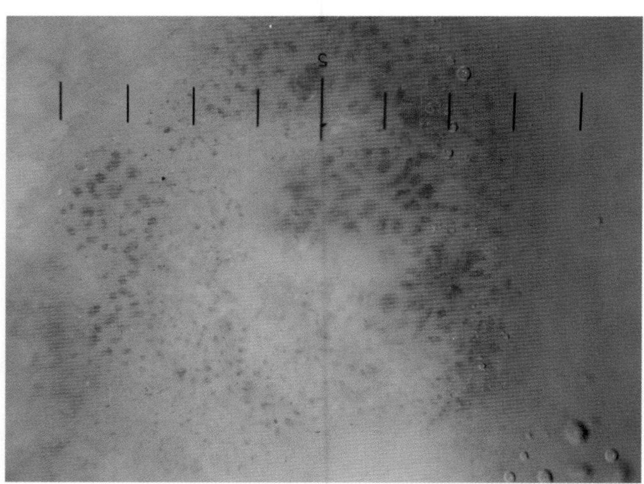

A 70-year-old woman with a long-standing plaque on the dorsum of her ring finger: dermoscopy of the lesion shows uniform coiled or glomerular vessels in this histopathologically confirmed Bowen's disease.

A clearly demarcated peripheral margin is a subtle dermoscopic clue favouring the diagnosis of digital Bowen's disease rather than an inflammatory process.

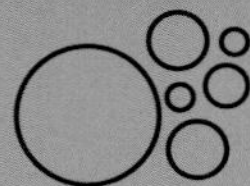

Squamous cell carcinoma – white circles

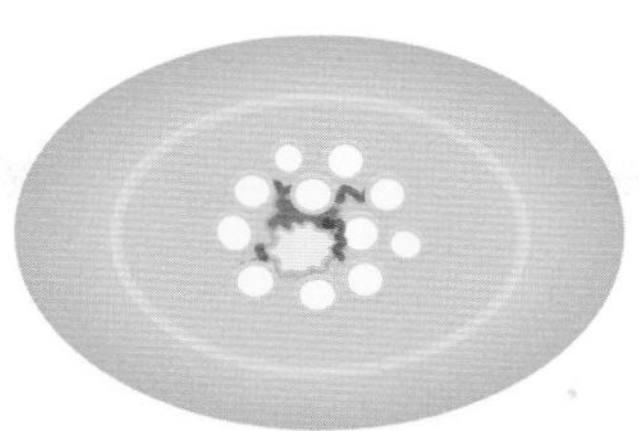

SCCs typically arise on photodamaged sites and may share features of actinic damage. As all skin tumours start small, any new plaque or papule on sites of photodamage should be examined closely for features in keeping with SCC. White circles, erosions and hairpin/looped or irregular vessels are subtle features that may be seen in early SCC. A paucity of overlying hyperkeratosis may indicate moderate differentiation.

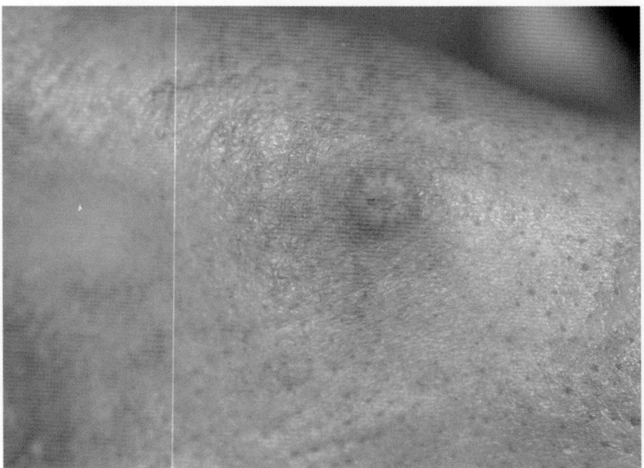

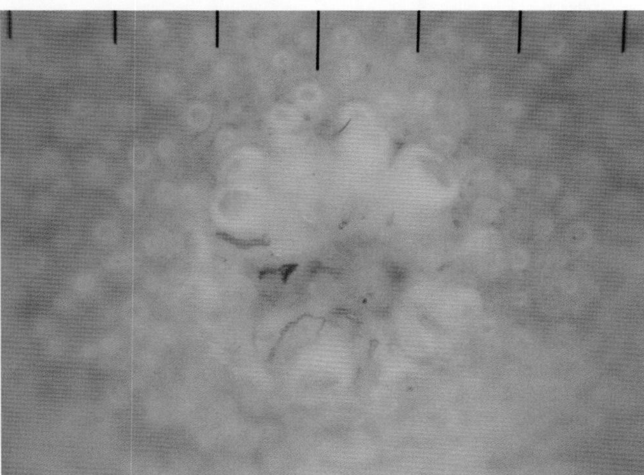

A 45-year-old man with a history of high UV exposure and a 6-week history of a new 3 mm papule on the nasal bridge: dermoscopy shows peripheral white circles and central erosion with linear-irregular vessels in this moderately differentiated SCC.

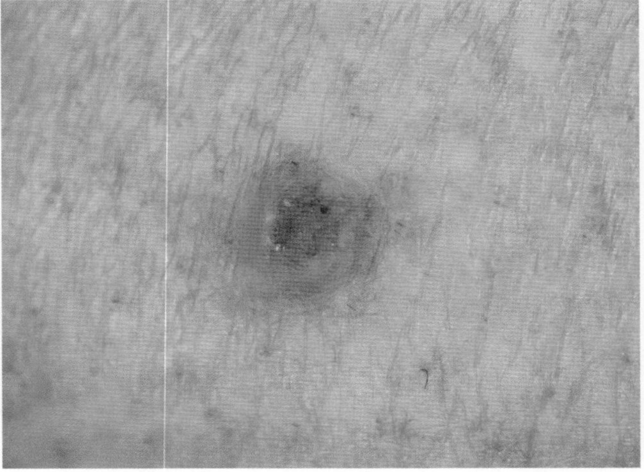

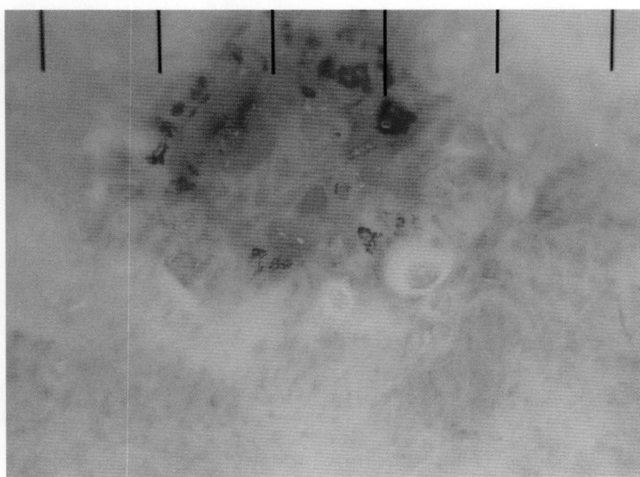

A 60-year-old female with a history of multiple BCCs with a new 5 mm ulcerated plaque on her shin: dermoscopy shows white circles and central erosion with linear-irregular and glomerular vessels. Histopathology confirmed a moderately differentiated SCC.

Lallas, A. et al. The clinical and dermoscopic features of invasive cutaneous squamous cell carcinoma depend on the histopathological grade of differentiation. *Br J Dermatol*. 2015;172(5):1308–15.

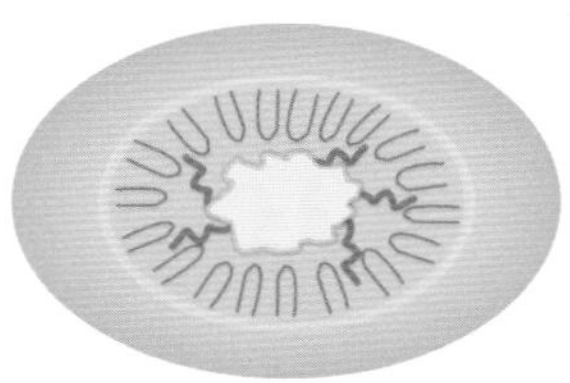

Keratoacanthomas share many clinical and dermoscopic features of well-differentiated SCCs.

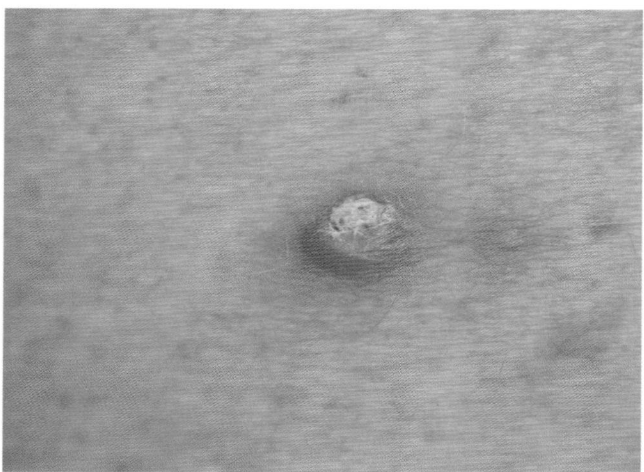

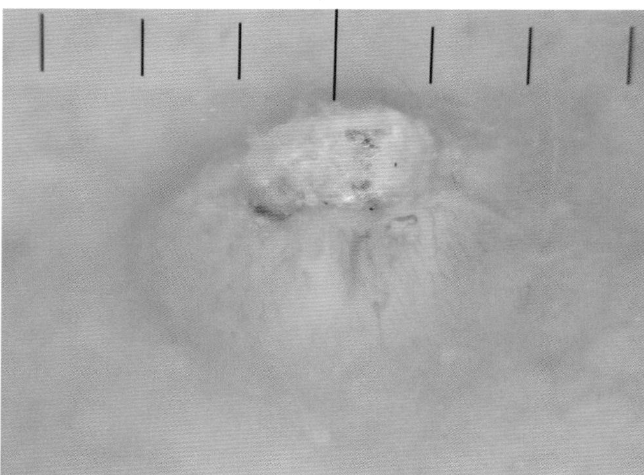

A 60-year-old female with a 4-week history of a domed hyperkeratotic nodule on the leg: dermoscopy shows central hyperkeratosis with peripheral looped or hairpin vessels radiating centrally. Keratoacanthoma was confirmed on histopathology.

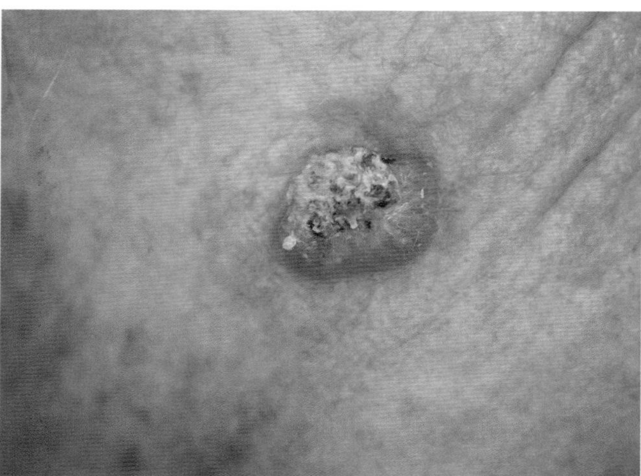

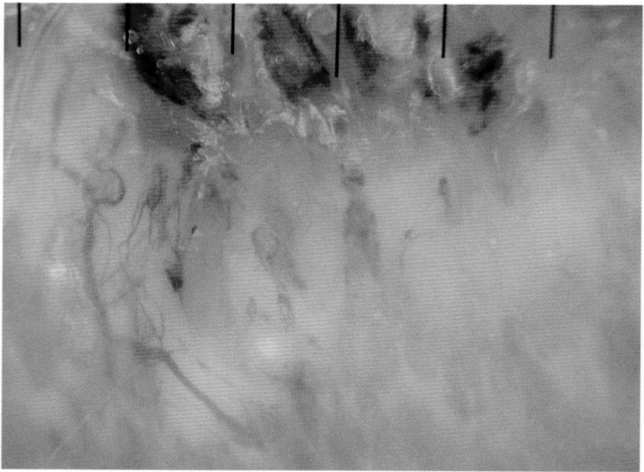

An 80-year-old woman with a 2-month history of an enlarging keratinising nodule on her zygoma: dermoscopy shows central keratinisation with peripheral ectatic and looped or hairpin vessels. Histopathology confirmed a keratoacanthoma.

Rosendahl, C. et al. Dermoscopy of squamous cell carcinoma and keratoacanthoma. *Arch Dermatol*. 2012;148(12):1386–1392.

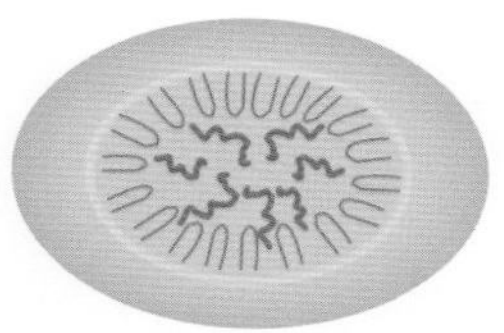

More poorly differentiated SCCs will show less keratinising structures and an increase in vascular structures. Ulceration and atypical vessels are non-discriminatory and may be the only clinical and dermoscopic feature found in a number of these tumours.

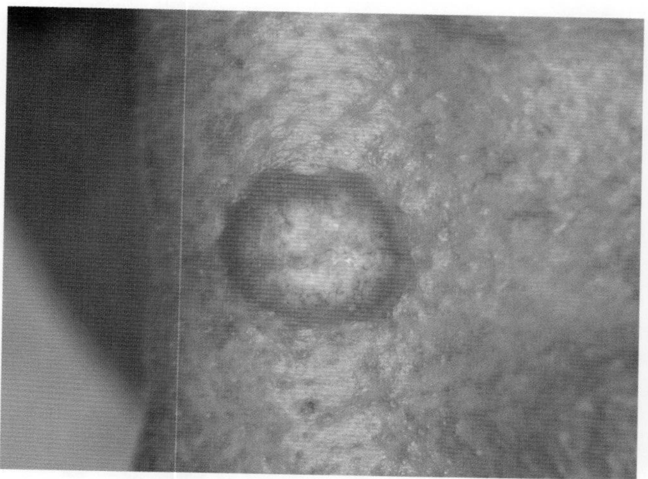

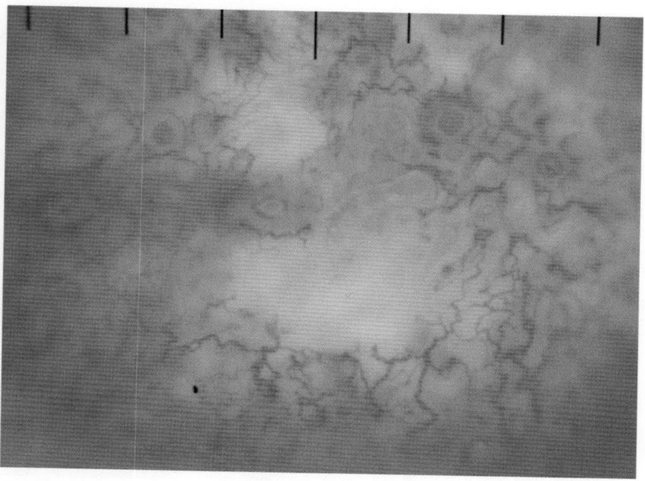

A 70-year-old female with a 4-week history of an enlarging nodule on the nasal bridge: dermoscopy shows irregular anastomising vessels and white circles with follicular keratinisation in this histopathologically confirmed moderately differentiated SCC.

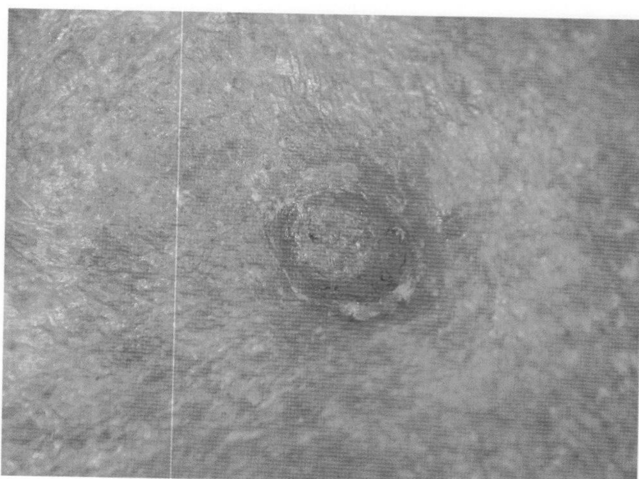

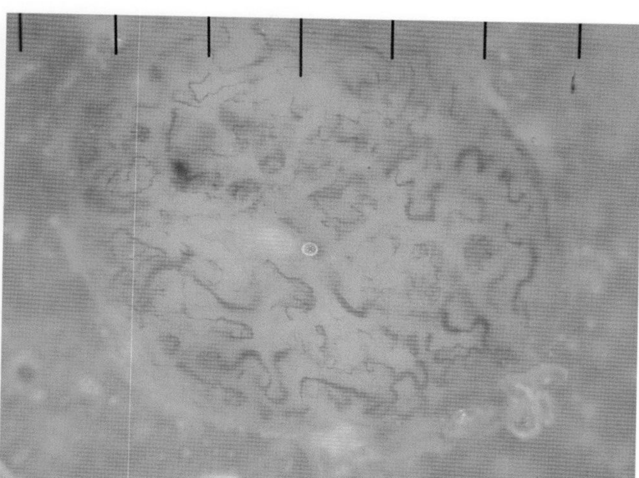

A 70-year-old man with a 3-week history of an enlarging nodule on the nasal side wall: dermoscopy shows erythema, dilated linear-irregular vessels without keratinization in this histopathologically confirmed moderately differentiated SCC.

A solitary enlarging pink papule or nodule with atypical vessels can be due to many skin cancers; only histopathology will confirm the diagnosis.

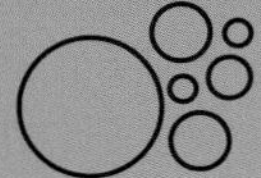

Squamous cell carcinoma – ulcerated

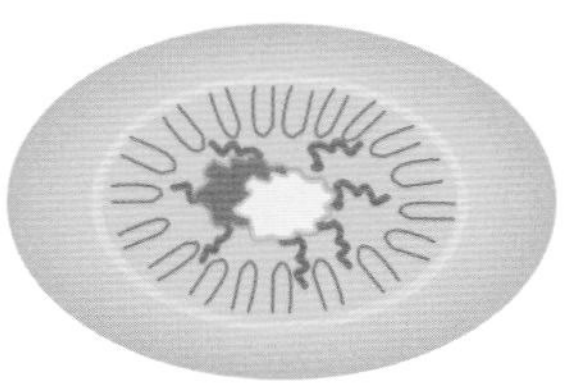

SCCs and keratoacanthomas share clinical and dermoscopic features; the diagnosis should always be confirmed with histopathology. Well-differentiated SCCs and keratoacanthomas will show more keratinising structures whereas poorly differentiated SCCs will tend to show fewer keratinising structures, more vascular features and possibly ulceration.

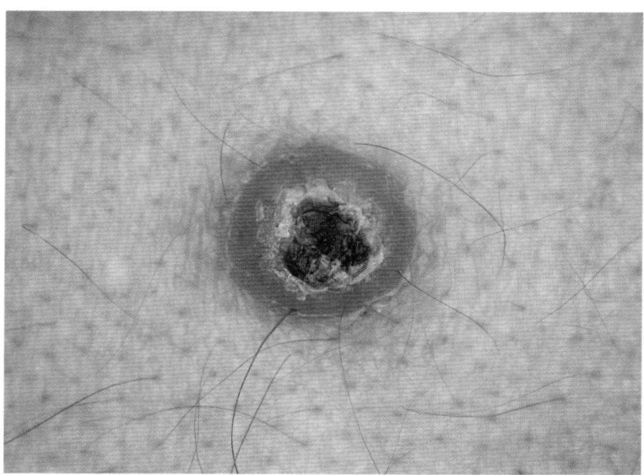

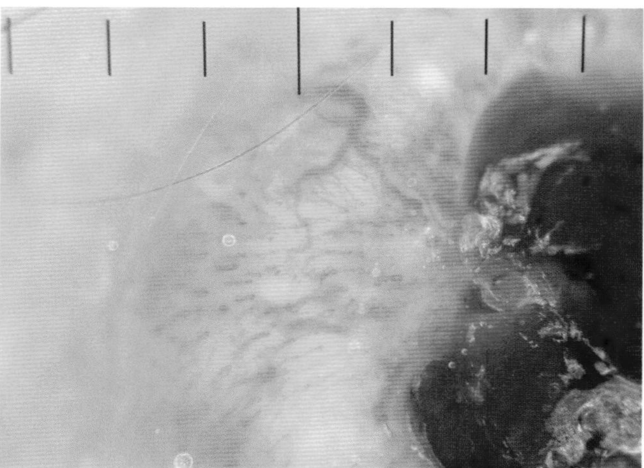

A 45-year-old man with a rapidly growing ulcerated nodule on the upper back: dermoscopy shows broad ectatic and looped or hairpin vessels radiating towards the central area of ulceration in this moderately differentiated SCC.

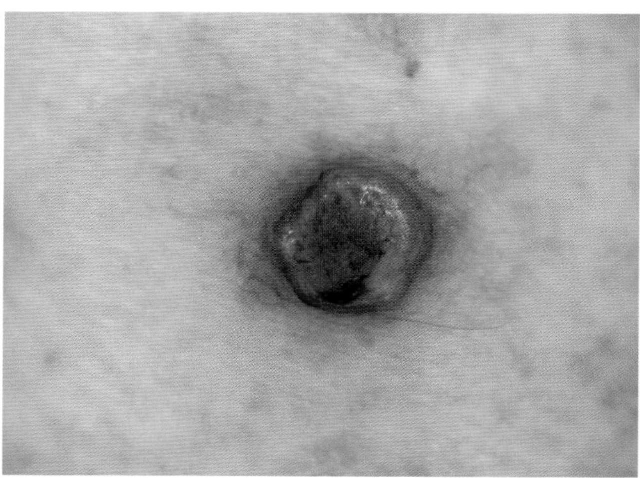

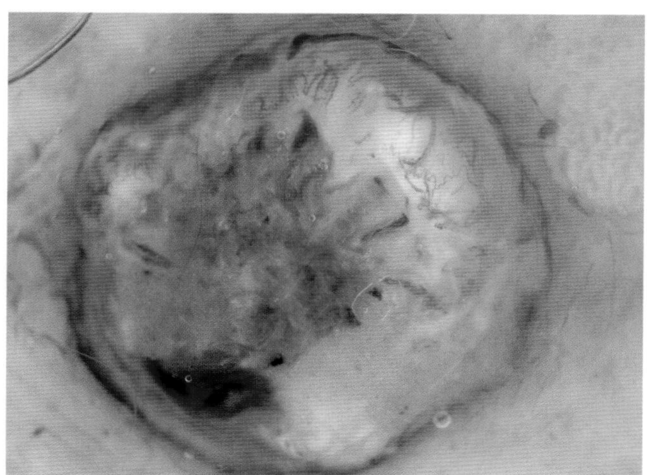

A 70-year-old woman with a hyperkeratotic nodule on the cheek: dermoscopy shows hyperkeratosis, ulceration, a combination of large, anastamosing, ectatic, looped or hairpin vessels in this moderately differentiated SCC.

Paoli J. Predicting adequate surgical margins for cutaneous squamous cell carcinoma with dermoscopy. *Br J Dermatol.* 2015;172(5):1186–7.

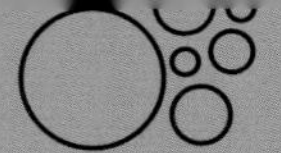

Squamous cell carcinoma – poorly differentiated

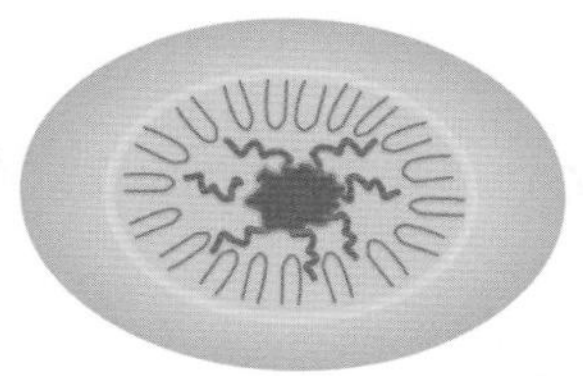

Poorly differentiated SCCs typically show minimal or no keratinising structures and hence ulceration is a common feature. Polymorphous vessels within an ulcerated area usually indicates a more aggressive tumour. In SCC, this would point towards a poorly differentiated subtype.

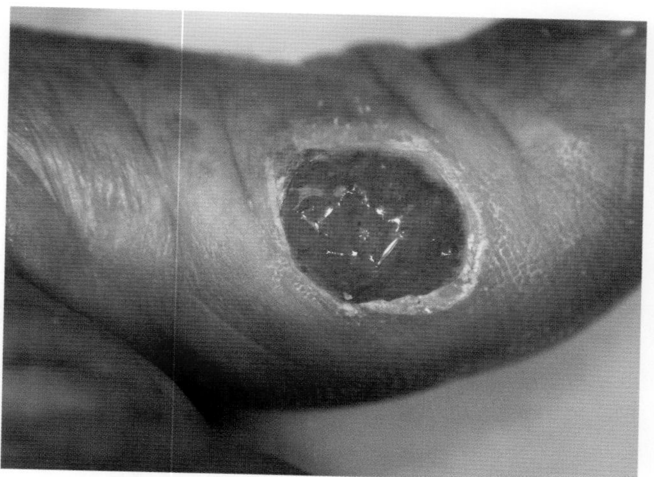

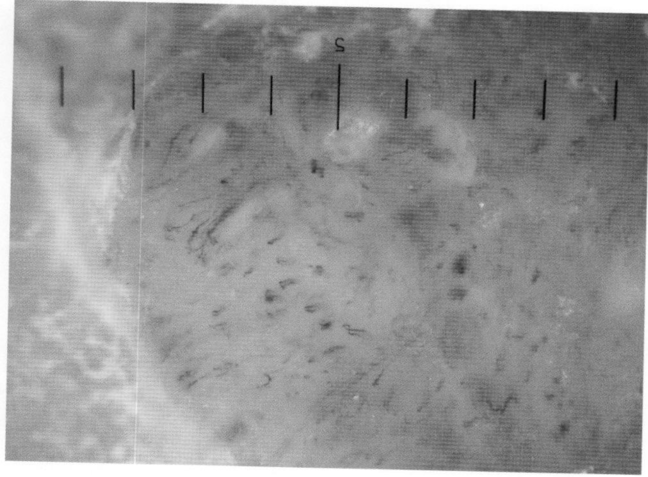

A 65-year-old man with a 3-month history of an ulcerated lesion on the left thumb: dermoscopy shows background erythema and widespread polymorphous vessels in this histopathologically confirmed poorly differentiated SCC.

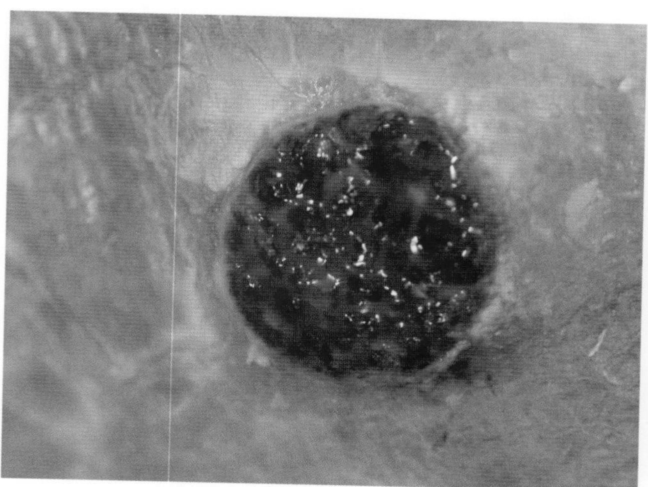

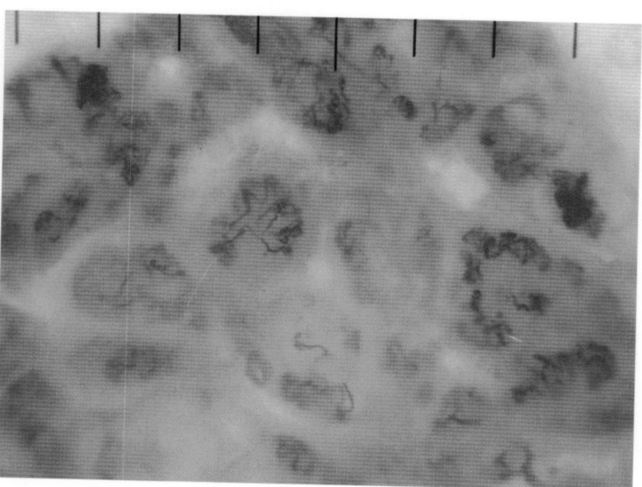

An 80-year-old woman with a 2-month history of a non-healing ulcer on the leg: dermoscopy shows erythema, ulceration and dilated linear-irregular and coiled or glomerular vessels in this histopathologically confirmed poorly differentiated SCC.

These tumours require more aggressive management sometimes multidisciplinary and more frequent follow-up.

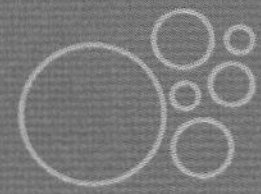

7.1 Acral melanocytic lesions

Acquired acral naevi	173
Acral parallel furrow pattern	174
Acral lattice pattern	175
Acral fibrillar pattern	176
Congenital acral naevus	177
Acral lentiginous melanoma	178
Acral lentiginous melanoma cases	179
ALM – brown-grey pigmentation	180
ALM – brown-grey pigmentation cases	181
Advanced acral lentiginous melanoma	182

Diagnostic Dermoscopy: The Illustrated Guide, Second Edition. Jonathan Bowling.

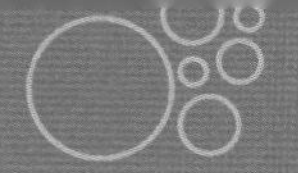

Acquired acral naevi

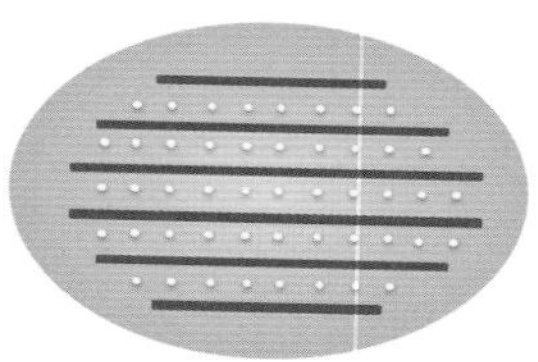

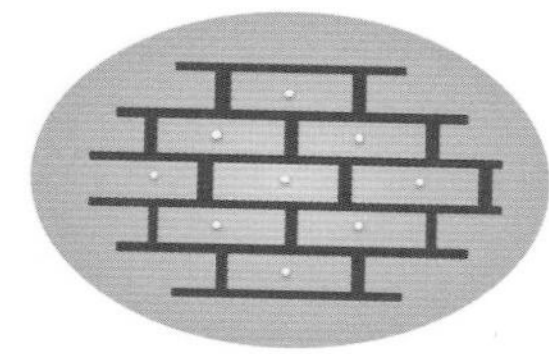

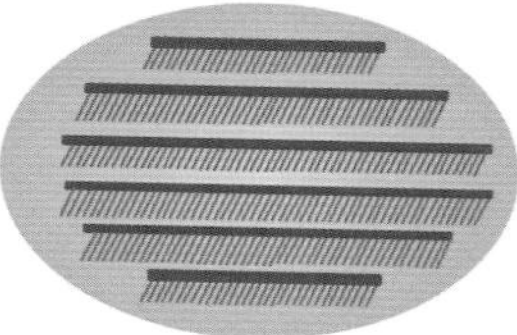

Acquired acral naevi tend to fall into three predominant pigment patterns depending upon their anatomical location.

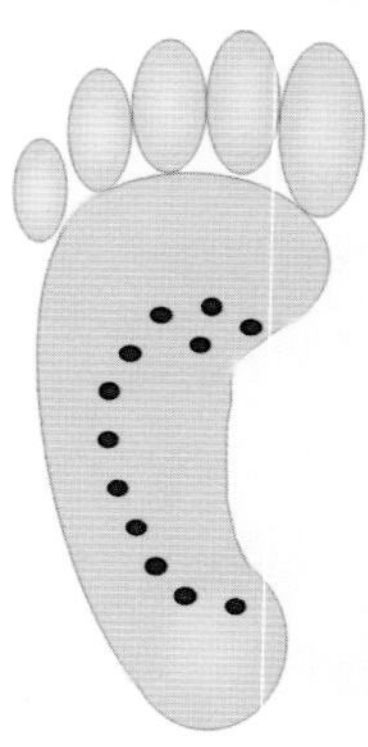

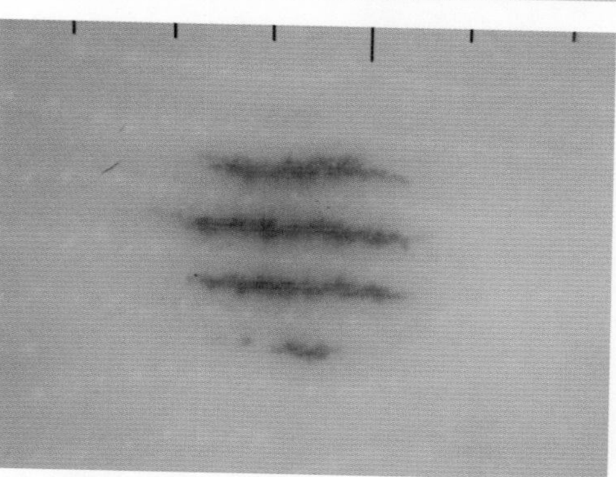

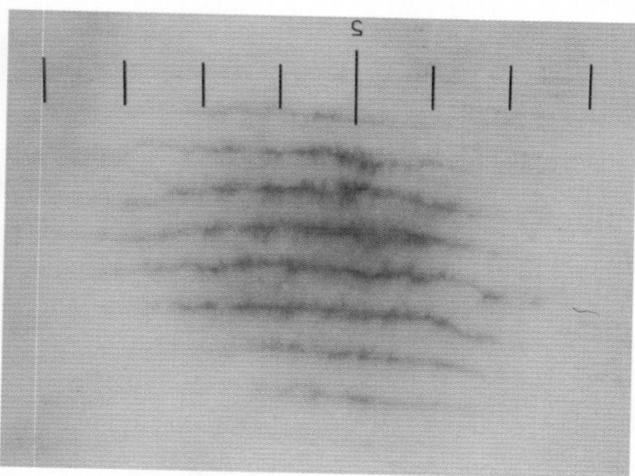

Parallel furrow pattern found just inside of the weight-bearing skin.

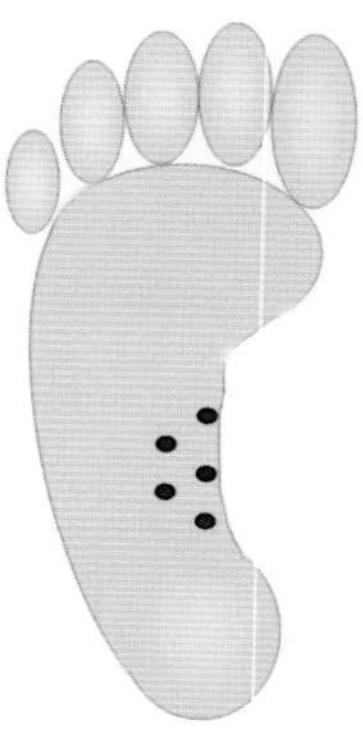

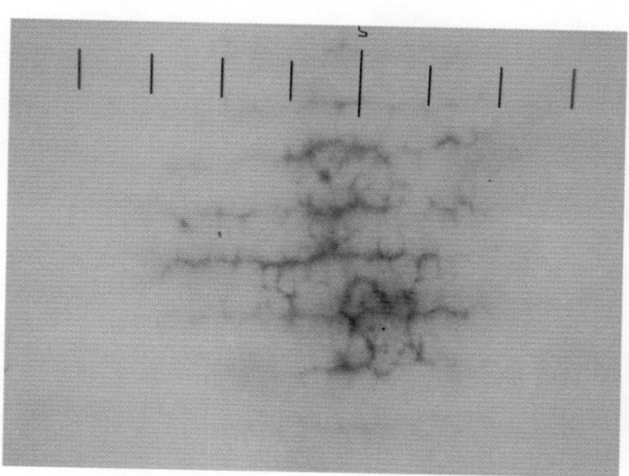

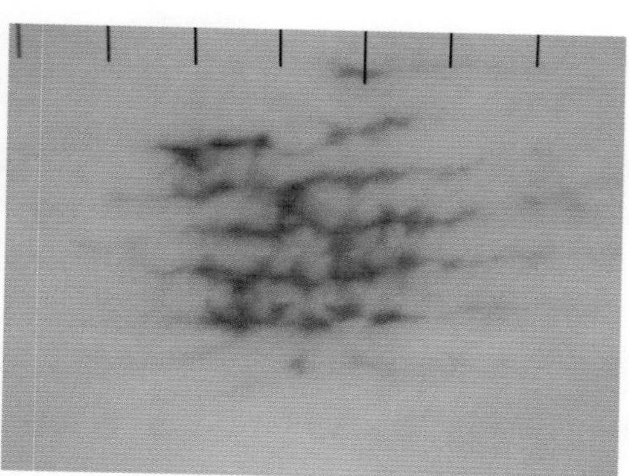

Lattice pattern found on the instep.

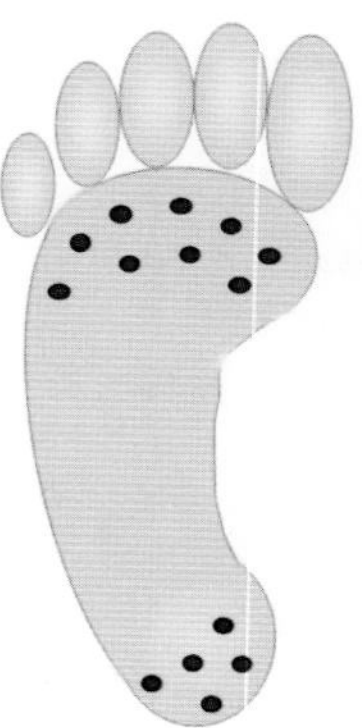

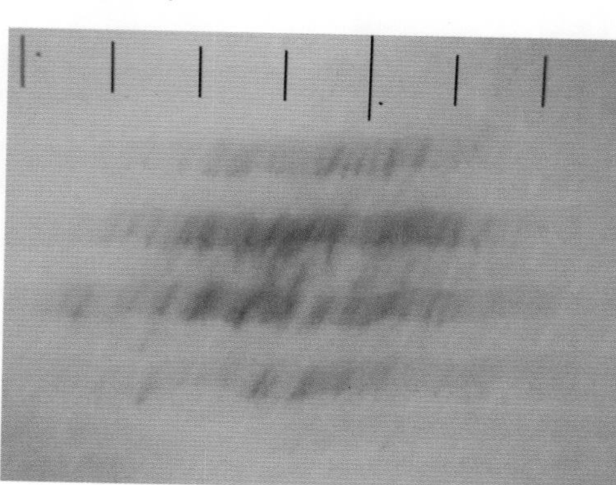

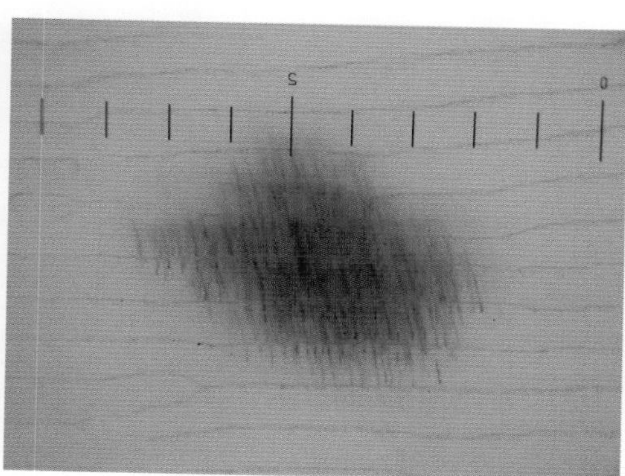

Fibrillar pattern found on weight-bearing skin.

Miyazaki, A. et al. Anatomical and dermoscopic patterns seen in melanocytic nevi on the soles: a retrospective study. *J Am Acad Dermatol*. 2005;53:230–236.

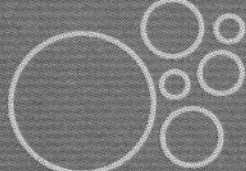

Acral parallel furrow pattern

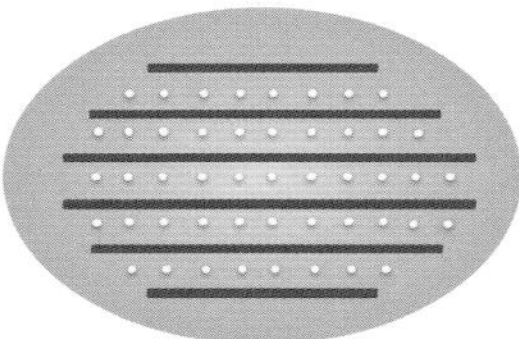

The parallel furrow pattern of pigmentation is the principal morphology seen in acral naevi. The lines of pigment are thin and originate in the furrow of the acral dermatoglyphics. The ridges of the dermatoglyphics are highlighted by the presence of white dots correlating to the eccrine gland openings. Dermatoglyphics is a word deriving from the Ancient Greek language for skin carving. This feature, which is shared with primates, enhances grip.

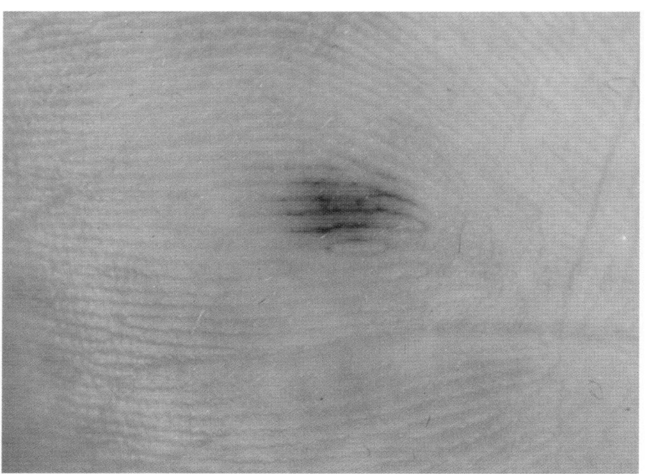

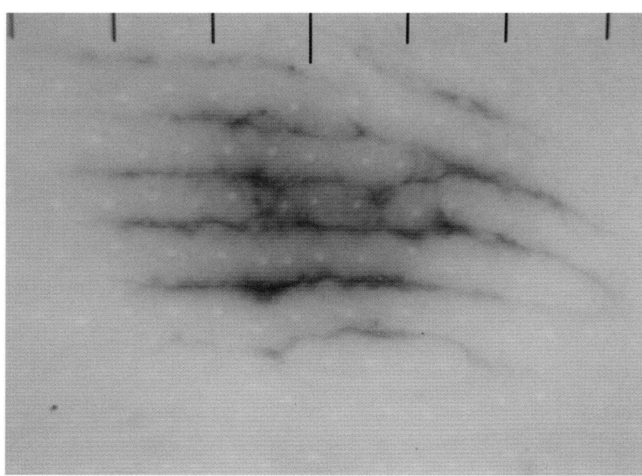

A 5 mm junctional naevus on the sole of a 30-year-old woman: dermoscopy shows the parallel furrow pattern of pigmentation with white dots of the acrosyringia along the ridges of the dermatoglyphics.

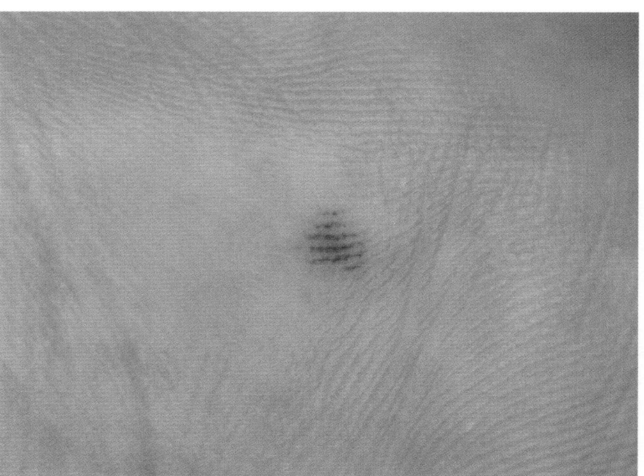

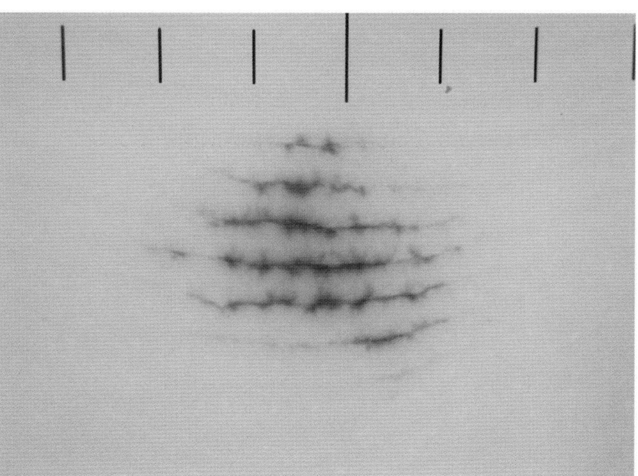

A 3 mm junctional naevus on the palm of a 20-year-old woman: dermoscopy shows the parallel furrow pattern with thin strands outlining the grooves in the dermatoglyphics.

The primary pattern of an acral naevus is often best seen at the margins of the lesion.

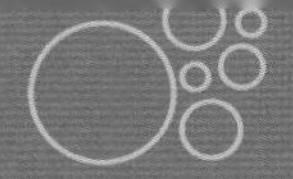

Acral lattice pattern

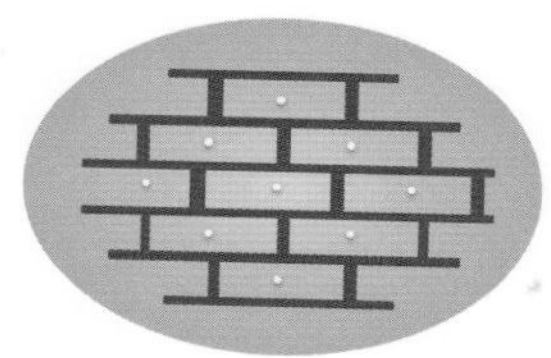

Lattice pigmentation is a variant of parallel pigmentation whereby the pigment links adjacent parallel furrow lines. On the soles, it typically signifies naevi located on the instep.

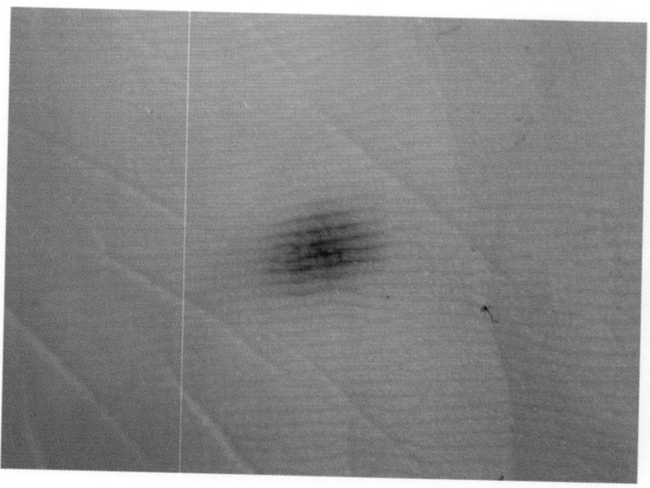

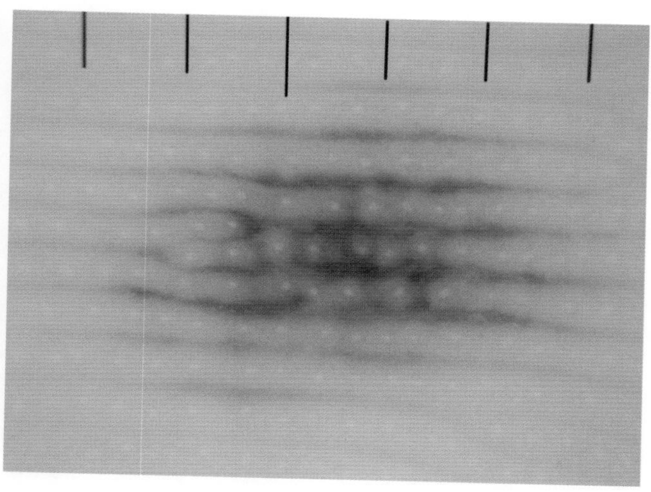

A 5 mm junctional naevus on the instep of a 20-year-old woman: dermoscopy shows a lattice-like pattern with white dots of the acrosyringia along the ridges of the dermatoglyphics.

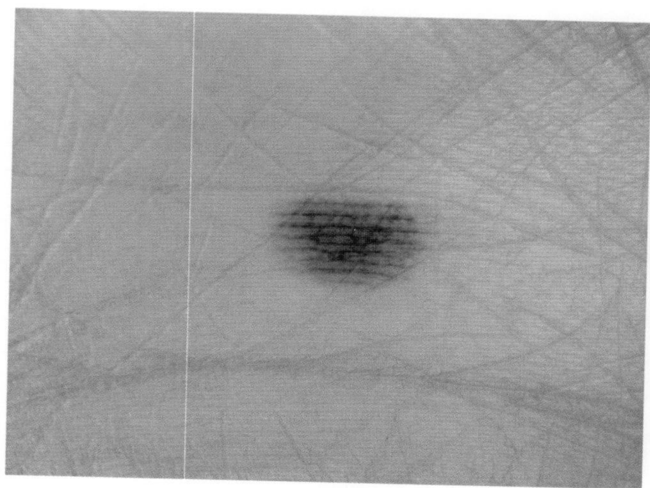

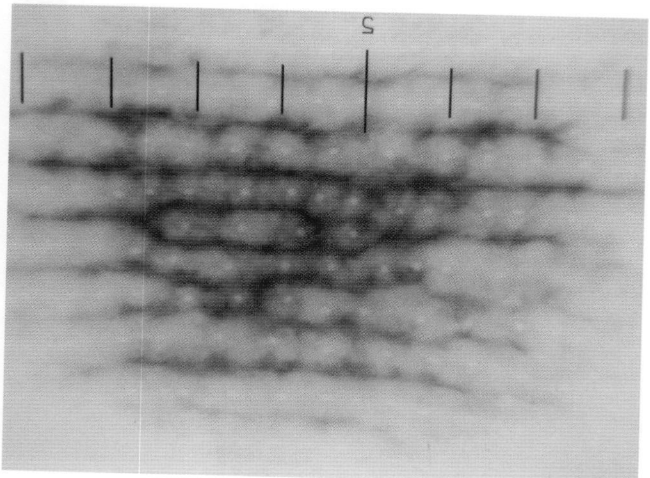

A 7 mm junctional naevus on the palm of a 15-year-old girl: dermoscopy shows a lattice-like pattern with subtle reticulation between the parallel furrow lines with white dots of the acrosyringia along the ridges of the palmar dermatoglyphics.

Saida T. Dermoscopic Patterns of Acral Melanocytic Nevi. *Arch Dermatol* 2007;143(11):1423–6.

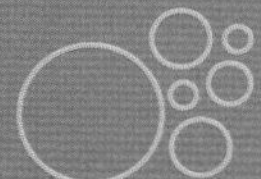

Acral fibrillar pattern

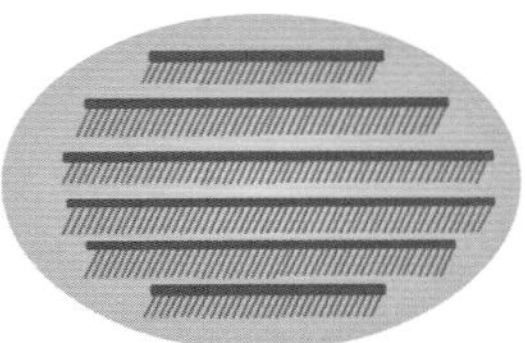

Fibrillar pigmentation is a variant of parallel pigmentation whereby the pigment produced migrates from the point of origin across the dermatoglyphics. The pigmented lines are uniform and thin and run perpendicular to the dermatoglyphics. This pattern is created by pressure effects and typically occurs on weight-bearing areas on the sole. Beware of the atypical fibrillar pattern which is a potential clue to melanoma.

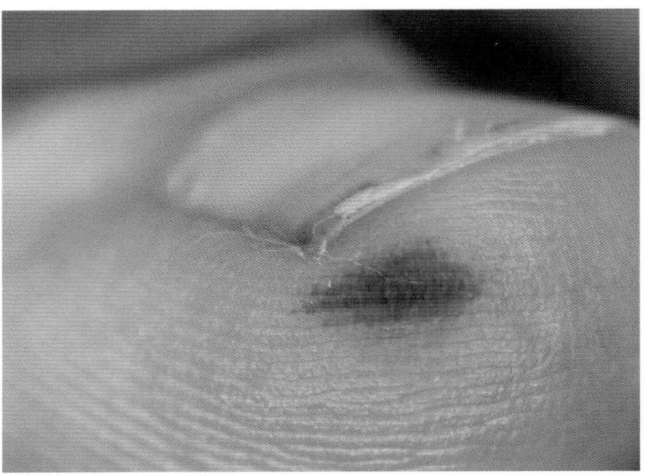

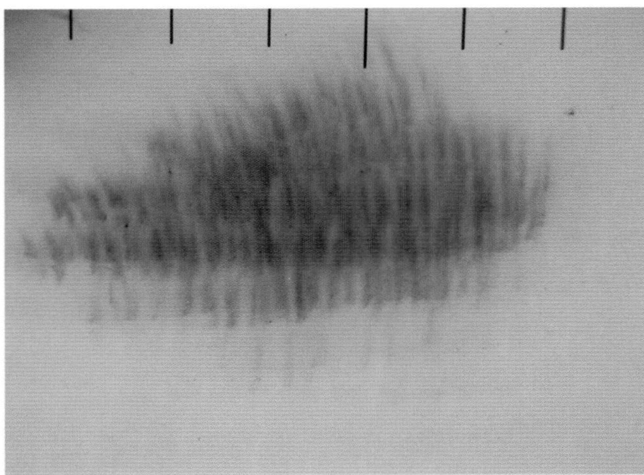

A 5 mm junctional naevus on the tip of the great toe of a 30-year-old woman: dermoscopy shows multiple uniform thin pigmented lines running perpendicular to the dermatoglyphics.

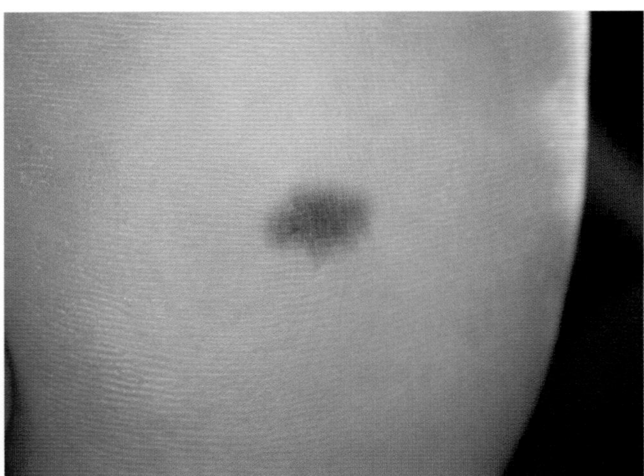

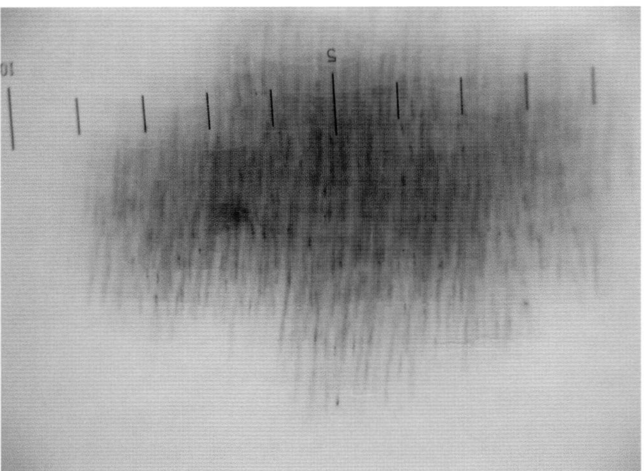

An 8 mm junctional naevus on the sole of a 20-year-old man: dermoscopy shows multiple thin parallel lines of pigmentation running perpendicular to the dermatoglyphics.

The fibrillar or filamentous pattern occurs on weight-bearing skin and can be restored to the furrow pattern by applying lateral pressure. Bowling J. Fibrillar pattern of an acquired plantar acral melanocytic naevus. *Clin Exp Dermatol*. 2007;32(1):103.

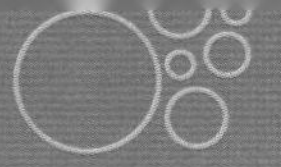

Congenital acral naevus

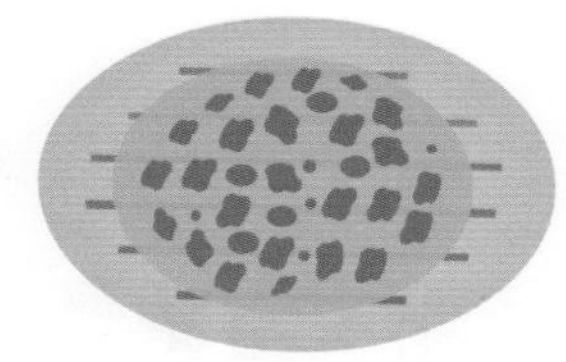

Congenital acral naevi will typically have a long history of a stable growth pattern. They may cause diagnostic concern due to clinical features of size, shape and pigmentation. Dermoscopy may show mixed patterns with central structureless, cobblestone or globular morphology, with variable pigmentation and more typical acral patterns at the peripheral margin. They may share dermoscopic features of melanoma and hence excision should be considered if any clinical concern arises.

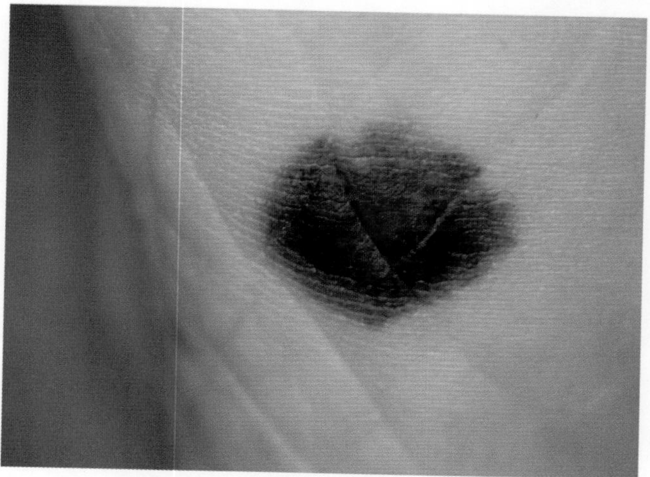

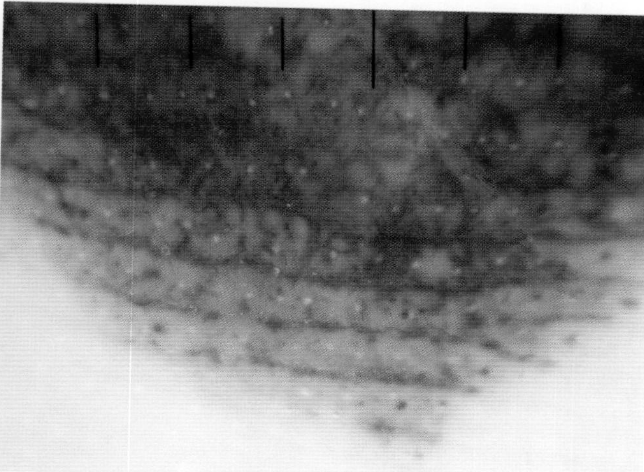

A lifelong hyperpigmented acral congenital naevus on the lateral sole: dermoscopy shows central structureless pigmentation and a parallel furrow pattern with globules at the peripheral margin.

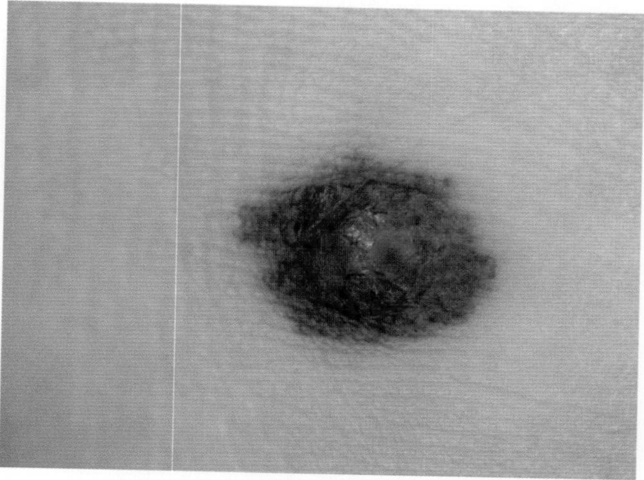

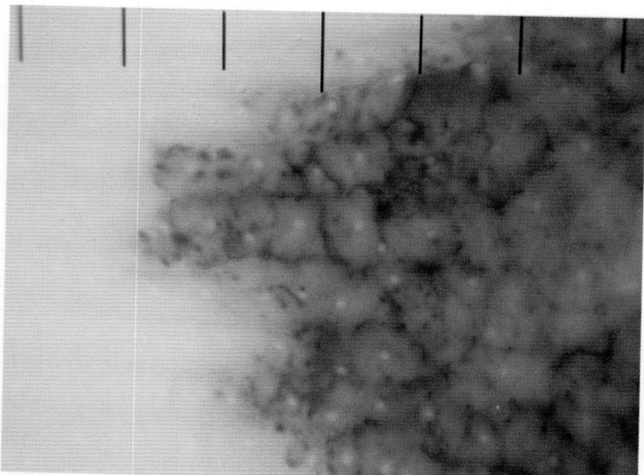

A longstanding pigmented acral congenital naevus on the sole: dermoscopy shows a lattice pattern and globules at the peripheral margin plus variable pigmentation and a structureless area centrally.

Roh D. Comparison of dermoscopic features between congenital and acquired acral melanocytic nevi in Korean patients. *J Eur Acad Dermatol Venereol*. 2020;34(5):1004–1009.

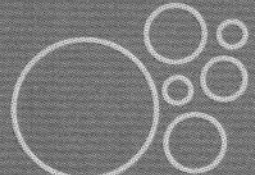

Acral lentiginous melanoma

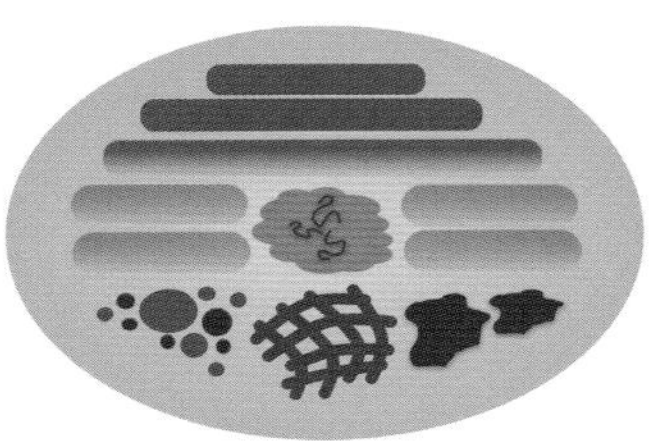

Acral lentiginous melanoma (ALM) may present in many forms. In early cases, it may present as a pigmented macule with a non-typical acral pattern, irregular pigmentation and/or globules. Wallace's line is the eponym pertaining to the transgredal zone of the palmoplantar surface delineating the junction with the remainder of the hand or foot. Melanocytic lesions in this zone can have unpredictable patterns.

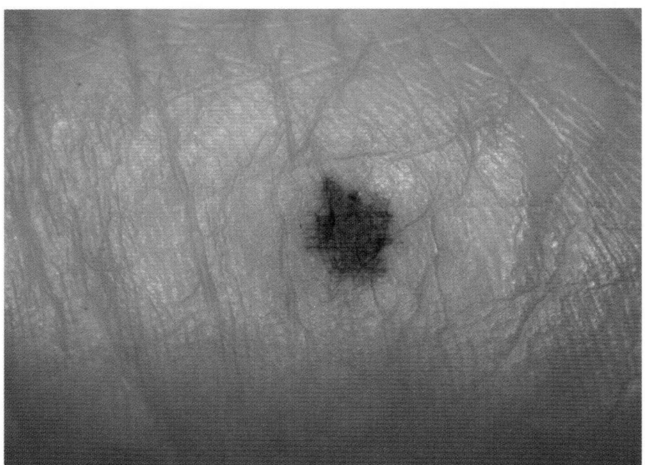

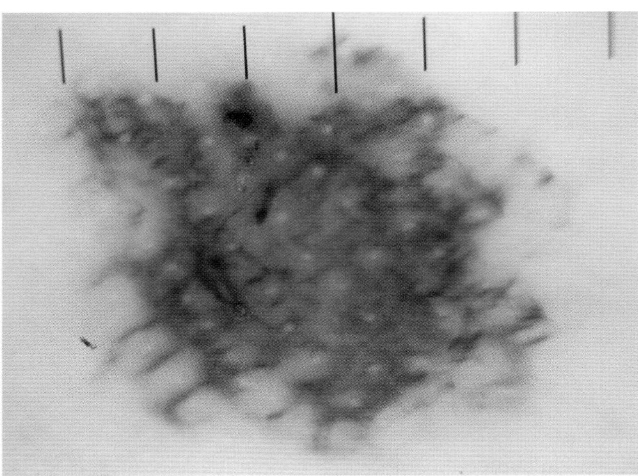

A 5 mm pigmented macule on the lateral sole of a 40-year-old woman: dermoscopy shows a chaotic and atypical reticular pattern with both grey hues and black globules with histopathology showing melanoma in situ (MIS).

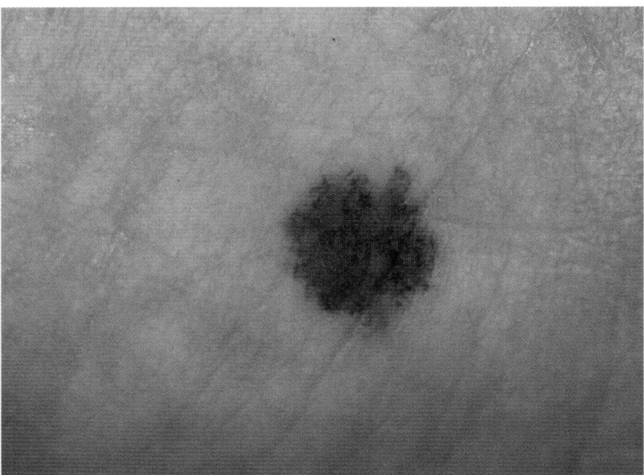

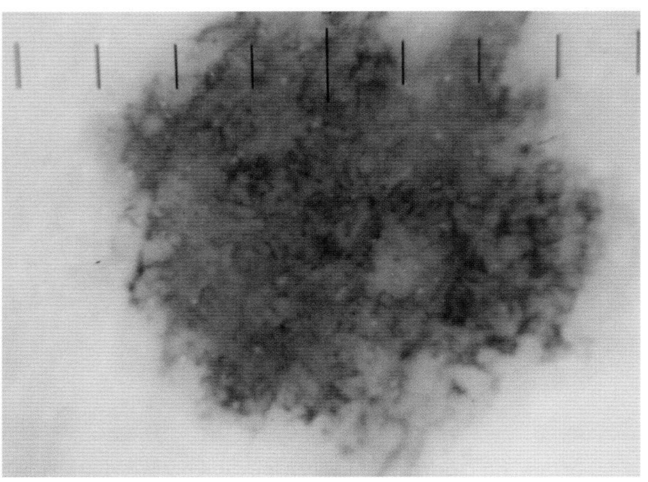

A 6 mm pigmented macule on the lateral sole of a 50-year-old woman: dermoscopy shows an atypical pigment network and irregular pigmented globules in this acral MIS.

Melanoma on acral sites may resemble melanoma on non-acral sites.

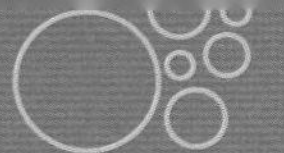

Acral lentiginous melanoma cases

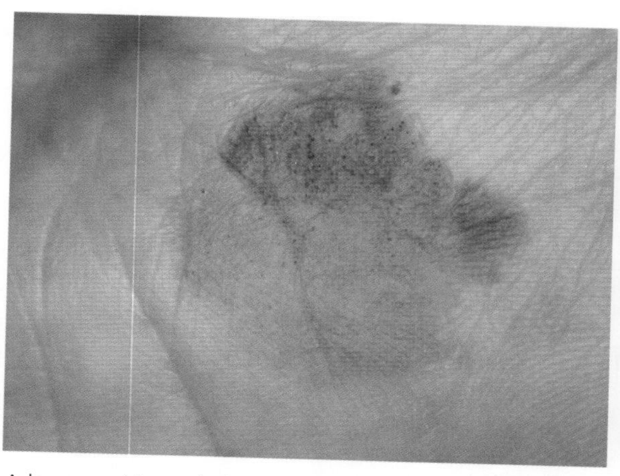

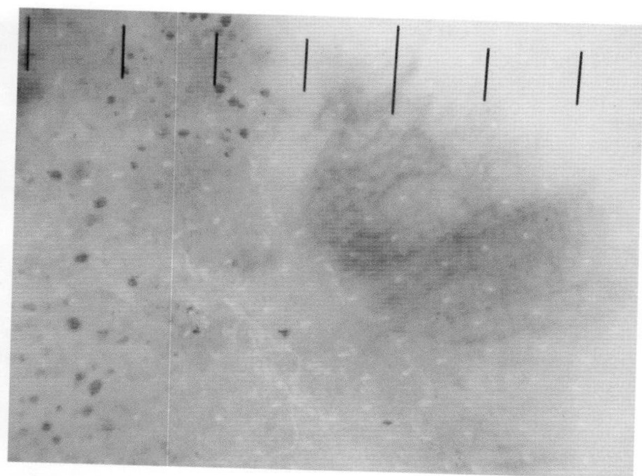

A large and irregularly shaped pigmented macule on the palm of a 40-year-old woman: dermoscopy shows multiple brown globules, erythema and eccentric brown granular pigmentation in this 0.3 mm thick ALM.

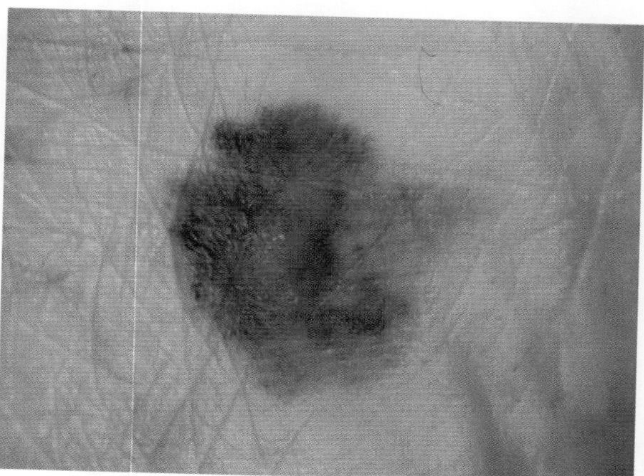

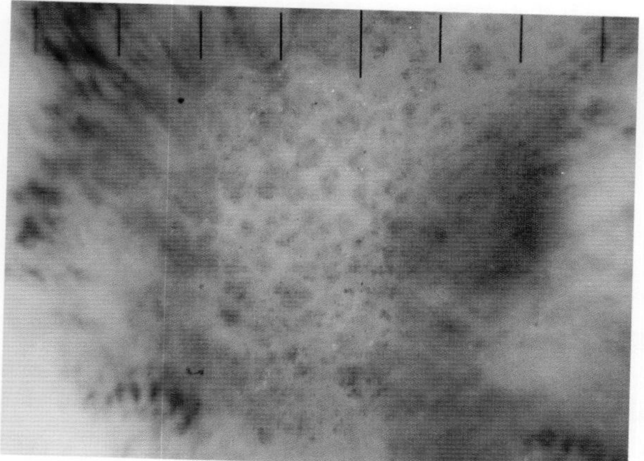

An irregularly pigmented plaque on the sole of a 75-year-old man: dermoscopy shows irregular brown granules, structureless areas and central atypical vessels in a negative network in this 0.6 mm thick ALM.

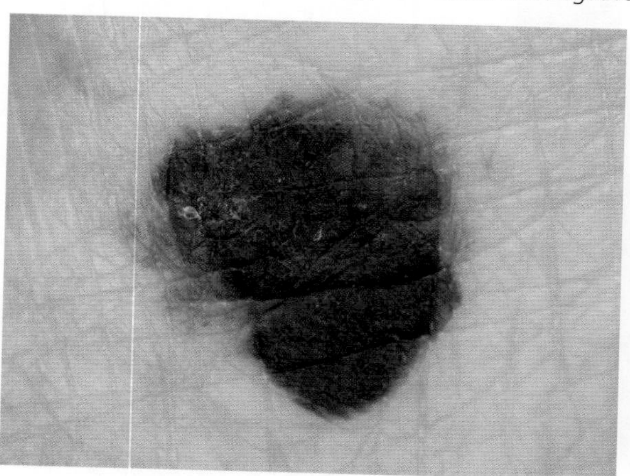

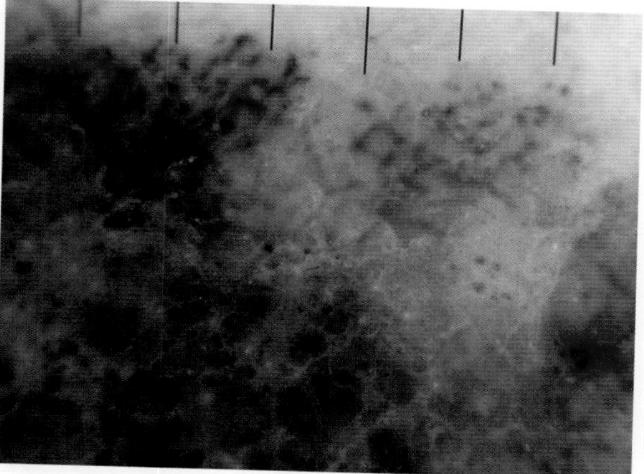

A hyperpigmented plaque on the instep of a 50-year-old woman: dermoscopy shows multiple colours, black dots, irregular dark blotches, globules, and streaks in this 0.9 mm thick ALM.

Lallas A. et al. The BRAAFF checklist: a new dermoscopic algorithm for diagnosing acral melanoma. *Br J Dermatol* 2015;172(4):1041–9.

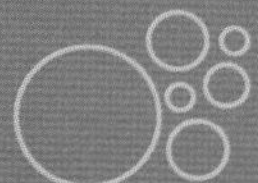

ALM – brown-grey pigmentation

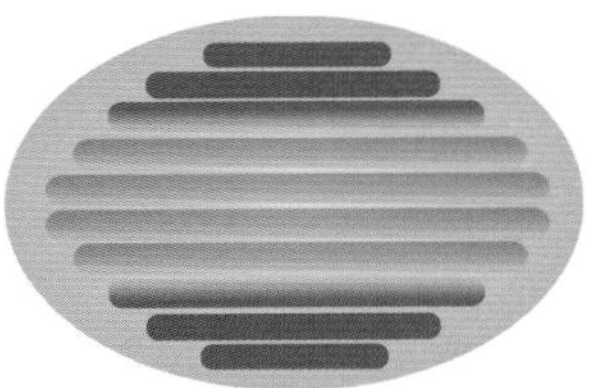

ALM may initially present in the in situ phase as an ill-defined brown-grey pigmented macule on the sole with indistinct clinical margins. Dermoscopic features include brown-grey granular pigmentation which may be ill-defined or preferentially located on the ridges of the dermatoglyphics, giving a parallel ridge pattern. This feature often extends beyond the more obvious focus of invasive disease when present.

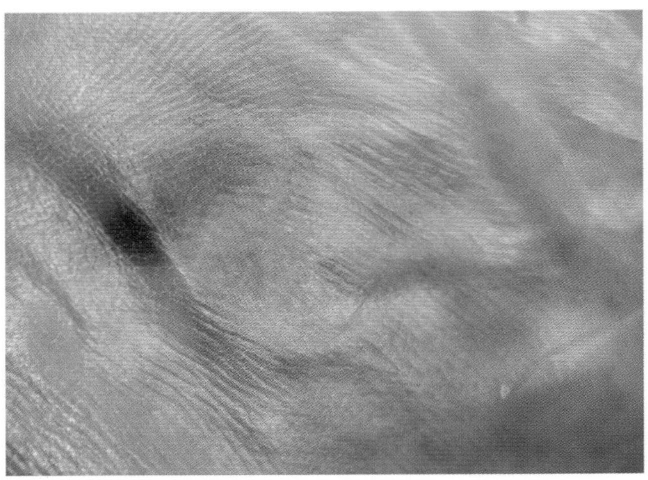

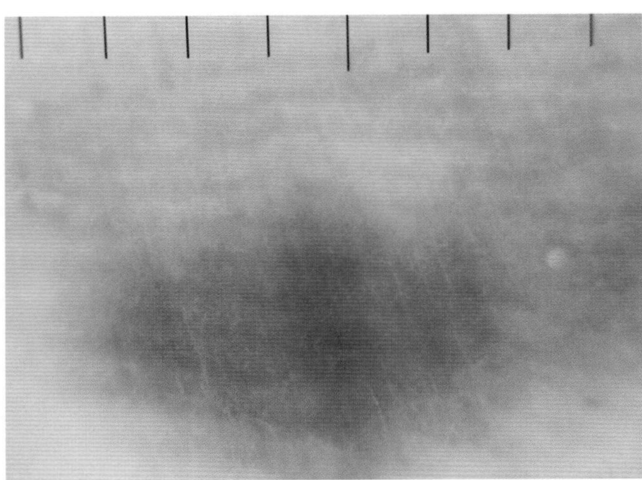

An ill-defined patch of pigmentation on the sole of an 80-year-old man: dermoscopy shows brown-grey granular pigmentation with increased density along the dermatoglyphic ridges confirmed as ALM in situ.

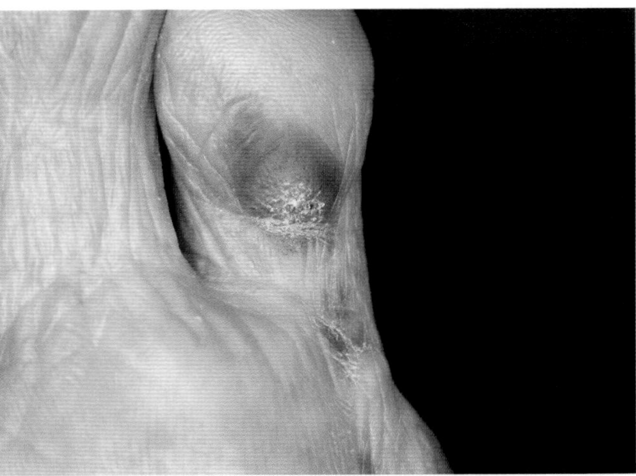

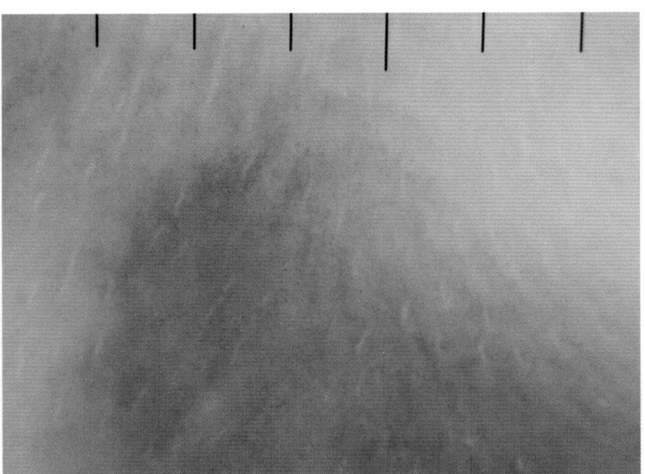

An ulcerated tumour of the toe of a 70-year-old man: dermoscopy of the non-ulcerated area shows ill-defined granular pigmentation and subtle parallel ridge pattern corresponding to the in situ component of this 1.8 mm thick ALM.

Parallel ridge pattern is pathognomonic of in situ acral lentiginous melanoma and may only be focal.

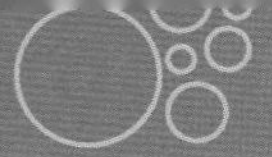

ALM – brown-grey pigmentation cases

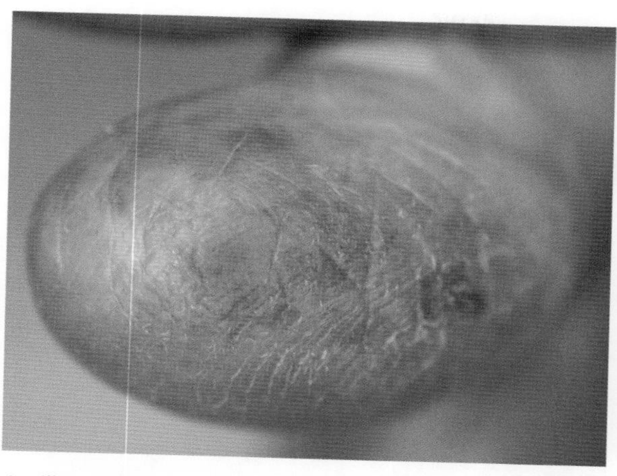

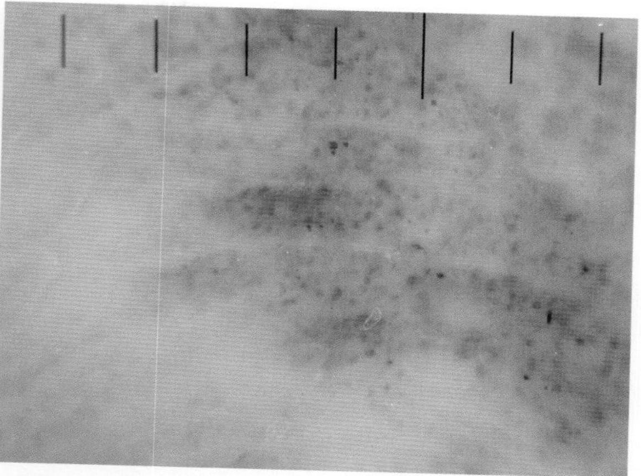

An ill-defined pigmented macule on the pulp of the fourth toe of a 70-year-old woman: dermoscopy shows parallel ridge pattern with granular grey and brown pigmentation in this ALM in situ.

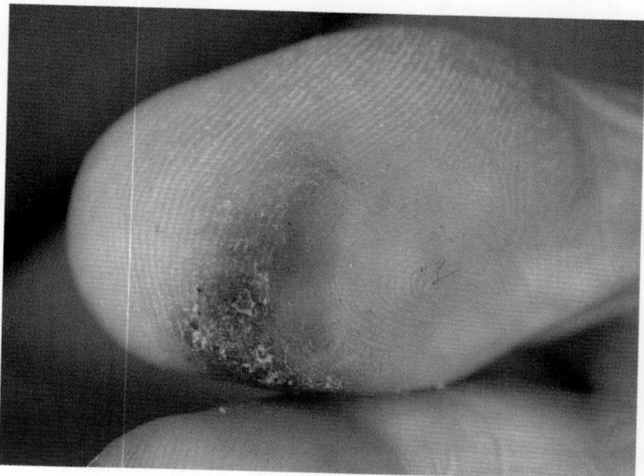

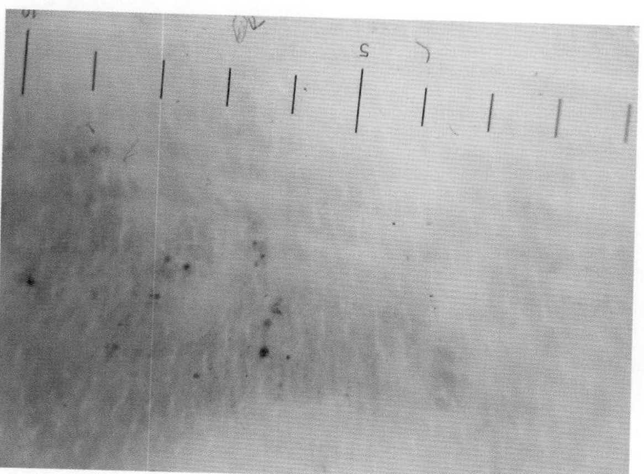

An irregularly pigmented patch on the great toe in a 60-year-old woman: dermoscopy on the peripheral pigmentation shows brown-grey granules in a parallel ridge pattern in the in situ component of this 0.6 mm thick ALM.

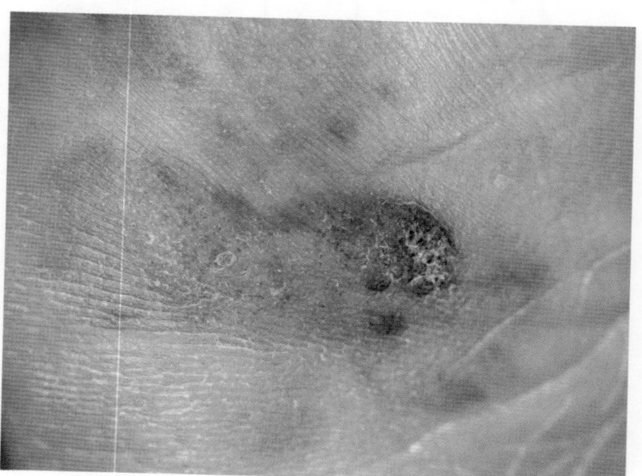

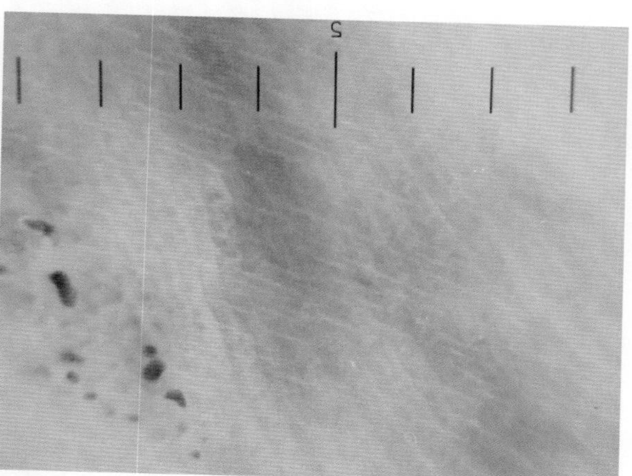

A large pigmented and hyperkeratotic patch on the sole of a 70-year-old man: dermoscopy of the macular component shows brown-grey granular pigmentation of the in situ zone in this 1.9 mm thick ALM.

Examine the peripheral margins of acral lentiginous melanomas to look for subtle clues to in situ disease.

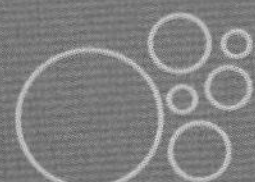

Advanced acral lentiginous melanoma

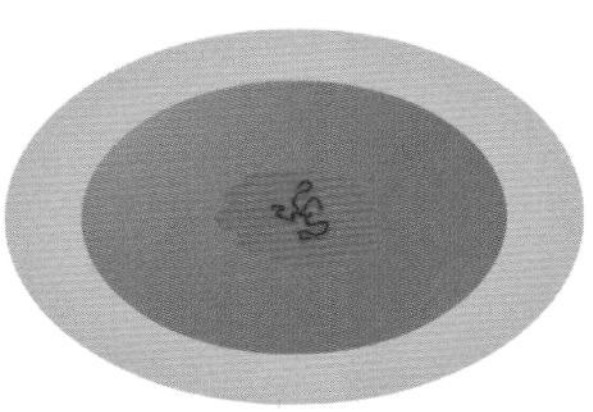

The late presentation of acral melanoma is unfortunately not an uncommon clinical scenario. These tumours may present in a number of ways, including as a thick tumour or as a large ulcer. Dermoscopy of the invasive component is often of limited value and a diagnostic biopsy may help differentiate these melanomas from other thick acral tumours.

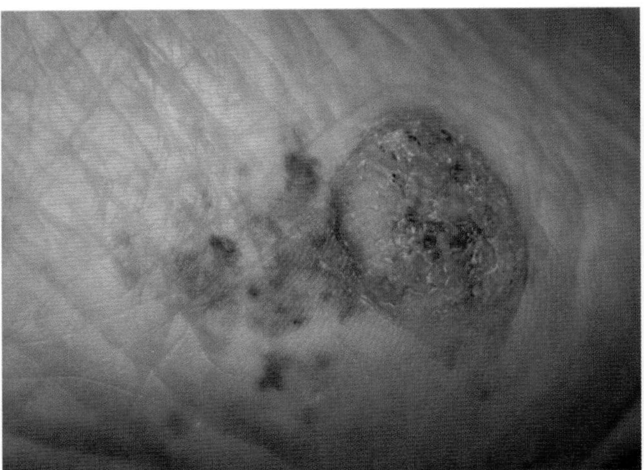

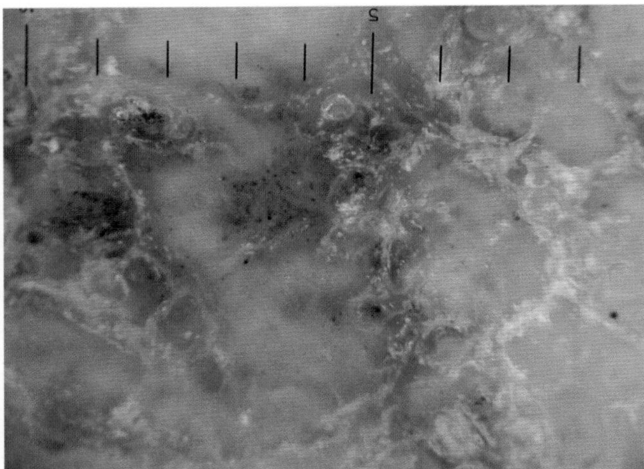

A large nodule on the instep of a 70-year-old man with obvious clinical peripheral in situ disease: dermoscopy of the invasive component shows black dots and blue-grey structureless areas and hyperkeratosis in this 4.6 mm thick ALM.

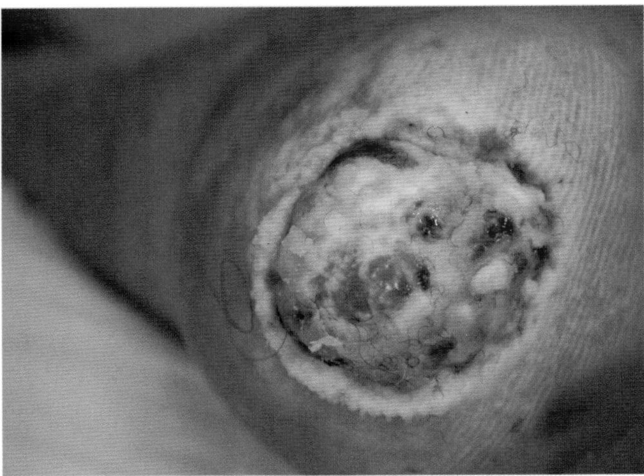

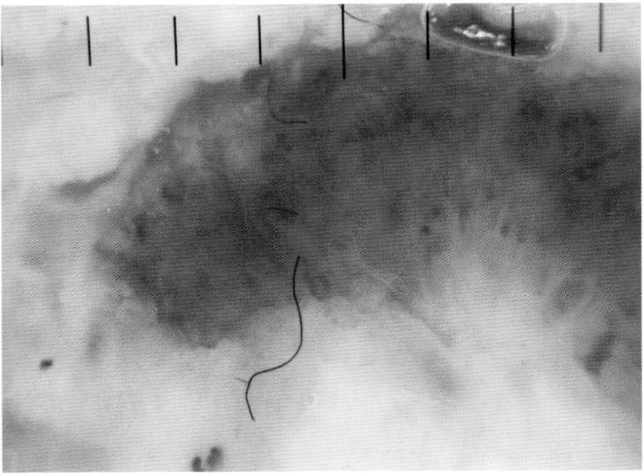

A large ulcer on the heel of a 90-year-old man: dermoscopy shows non-specific ulceration, milky red erythema and adherent debris in this 4.1 mm thick ALM.

Dermoscopy may be of limited benefit in thick tumours. Beware of atypical verrucous lesions that don't behave like a wart.

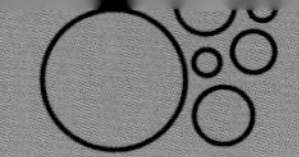

7.2 Onychoscopy

Nail matrix naevus 184
Nail apparatus melanoma in situ 185
Early invasive nail apparatus melanoma 186
Advanced nail apparatus melanoma – pigmented 187
Advanced nail apparatus melanoma – non-pigmented 188
Nail unit squamous cell carcinoma 189
Erythronychia 190
Onychopapilloma 191
Subungual haematoma 192
Subungual haematoma cases 193
Periungual warts 194
Onychomycosis 195
Chloronychia – green nails 196
Nail pigmentation – exogenous 197
Capillaroscopy 198

Diagnostic Dermoscopy: The Illustrated Guide, Second Edition. Jonathan Bowling.

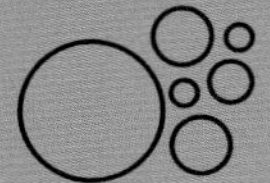

Nail matrix naevus

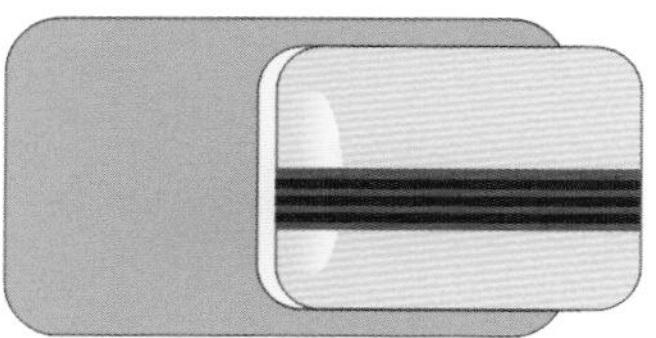

Nail matrix naevi produce a thin band of melanonychia. Naevi arising from the proximal matrix cause pigmentation to arise from beneath the proximal nail fold or proximal to the lunula. Naevi arising from the distal matrix will show clearing proximally. Free edge dermoscopy helps distinguish these variants with a proximally based naevus showing pigment primarily at the top of the nail plate and vice versa. If the naevus is not enlarging, the band of pigmentation is uniform in width along its entire length.

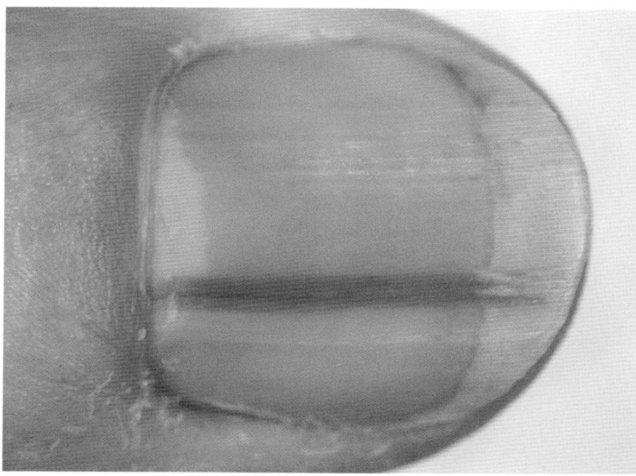

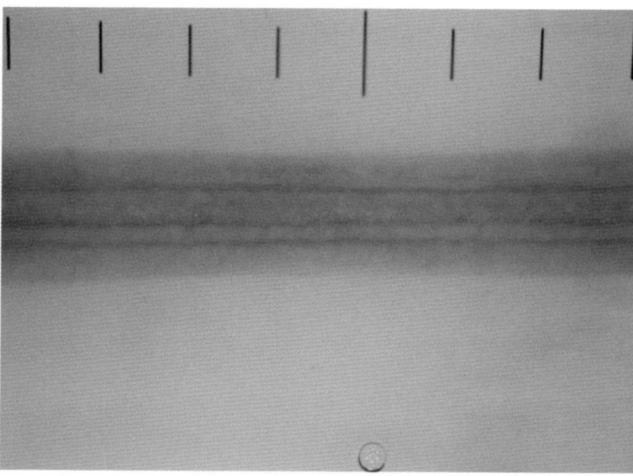

Longtitudinal melanonychia arising from the proximal matrix: dermoscopy shows uniform parallel lines of brown pigmentation without significant variation in pigment intensity in this nail matrix nevus.

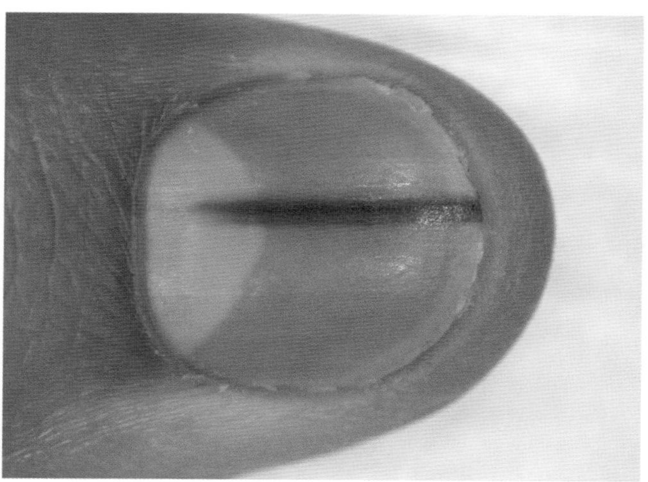

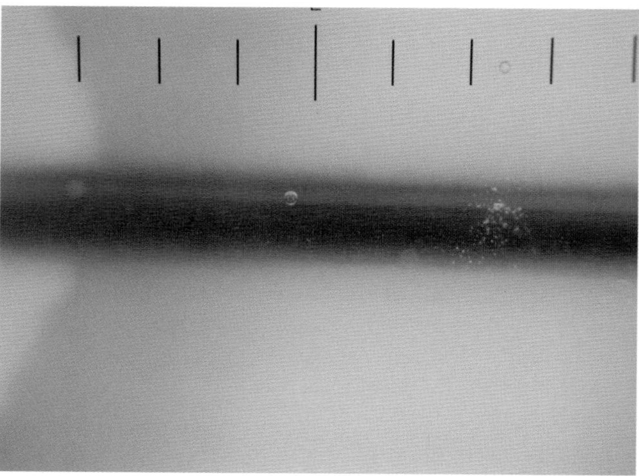

Longtitudinal melanonychia on the nail plate arising from the distal matrix: dermoscopy shows a uniform black band in a histopathologically confirmed nail matrix naevus.

Benati, E. et al. Clinical and dermoscopic clues to differentiate pigmented nail bands: an International Dermoscopy Society study. *J Eur Acad Dermatol Venereol*. 2017:31(4):732–736.

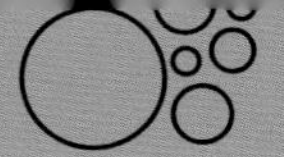

Nail apparatus melanoma in situ

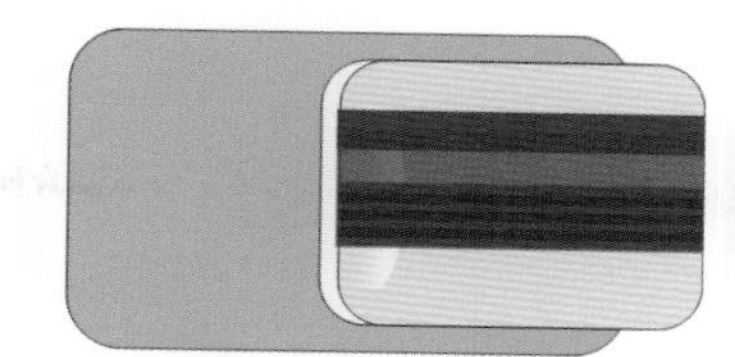

Melanoma in situ (MIS) of the nail apparatus produces a broad band of melanonychia and on dermoscopy parallel lines of pigmentation that vary in colour and width. The lines may sometimes lose their parallel arrangement in melanoma. The nail plate typically shows no thinning or dystrophy, which is a feature more typical of invasive melanoma. MIS can extend superficially to the adjacent nail fold skin causing irregular pigmentation (so called Hutchinson's sign).

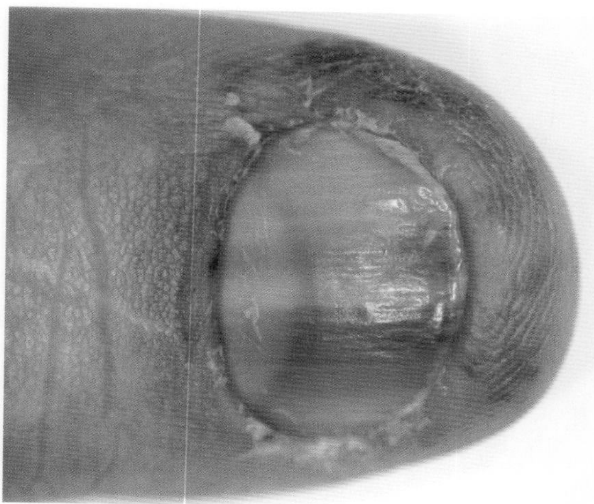

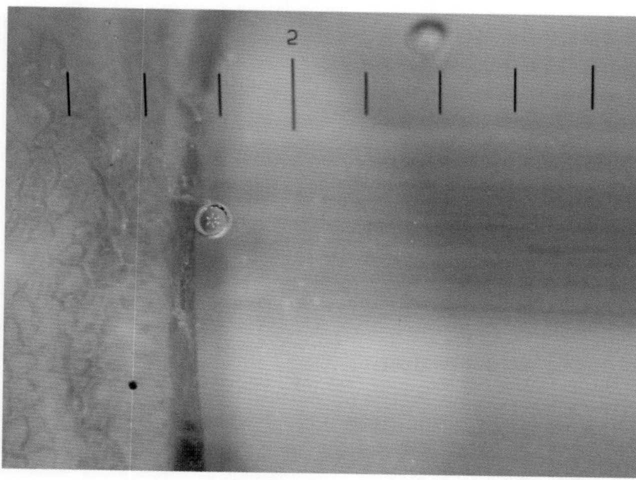

Variable pigmentation on the thumb without nail dystrophy: dermoscopy shows broad irregular bands of melanonychia and clear Hutchinson's sign with pigment extending onto the hyponychium in this MIS.

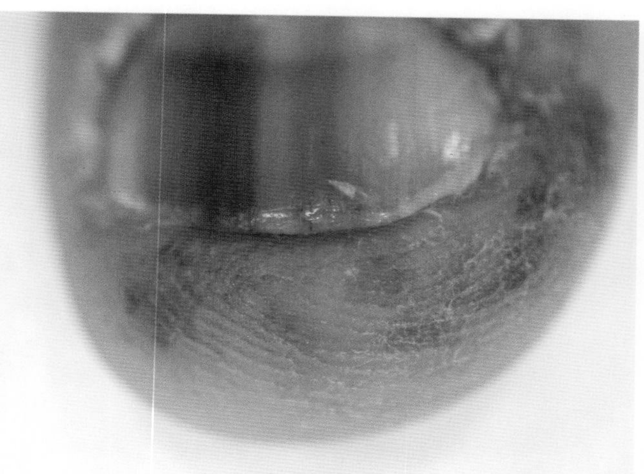

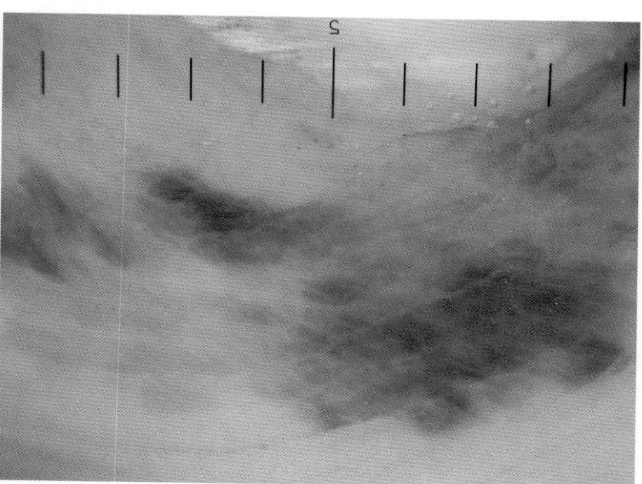

A clear view of a healthy nail plate with irregular parallel lines of pigmentation, irregular pigmentation extending onto the tip of the thumb and lateral nail folds: dermoscopy shows irregular pigmentation including the parallel ridge pattern.

As nail apparatus MIS evolves, its irregular pattern of lines varying in colour, width and spacing may resemble a barcode. Di Chiacchio, N.D. et al. Consensus on melanonychia nail plate dermoscopy. *An Bras Dermatol*. 2013;88(2):309–313.

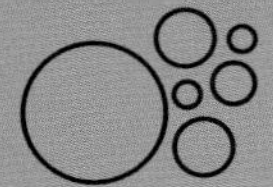

Early invasive nail apparatus melanoma

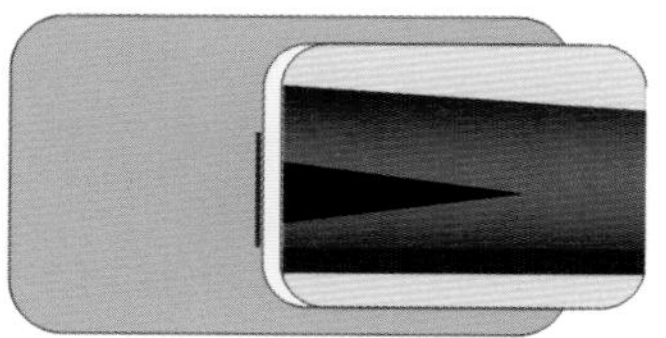

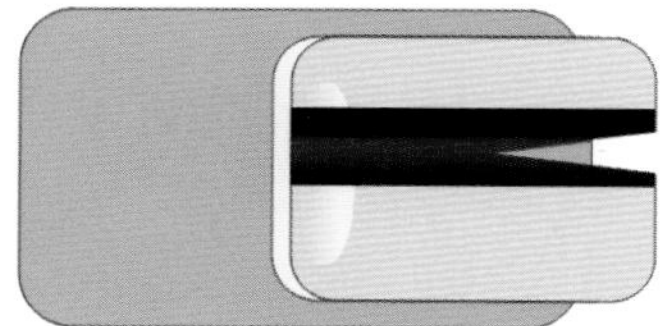

Early nail matrix melanoma presents as a band of irregularly pigmented melanonychia that becomes broader, more atypical and polychromatic over time. Additionally, a band that is broader proximally (the 'triangle sign') should raise suspicion for melanoma as it indicates growth. Nail dystrophy may steadily evolve as the tumour invades and destroys the nail matrix. Microscopic nail fold pigment only evident on dermoscopy is a clue to melanoma and known as micro-Hutchinson's sign.

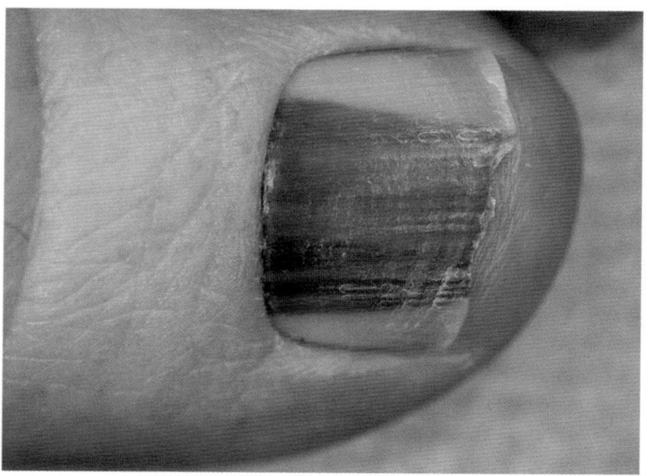

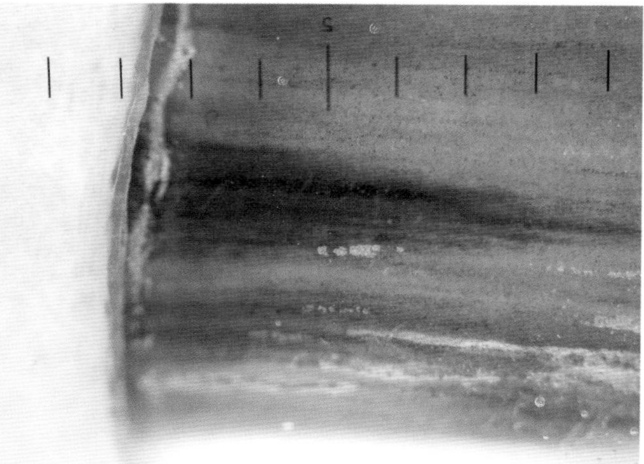

A 0.5 mm thick nail matrix melanoma with a broad triangulated and irregular band with distal nail fragility localised to the area of pigmentation: dermoscopy shows polychromasia and a triangular zone of hyperpigmentation proximally.

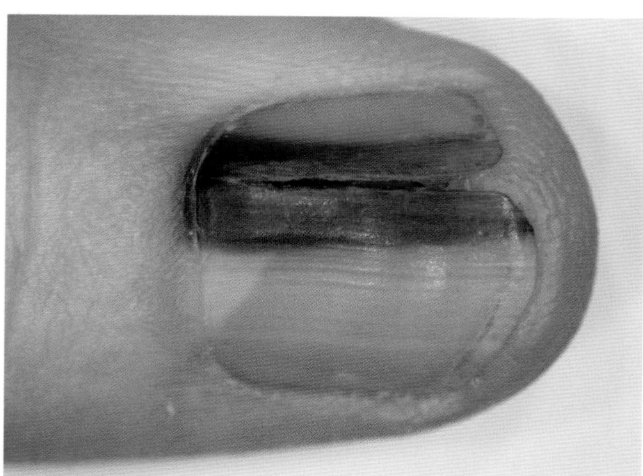

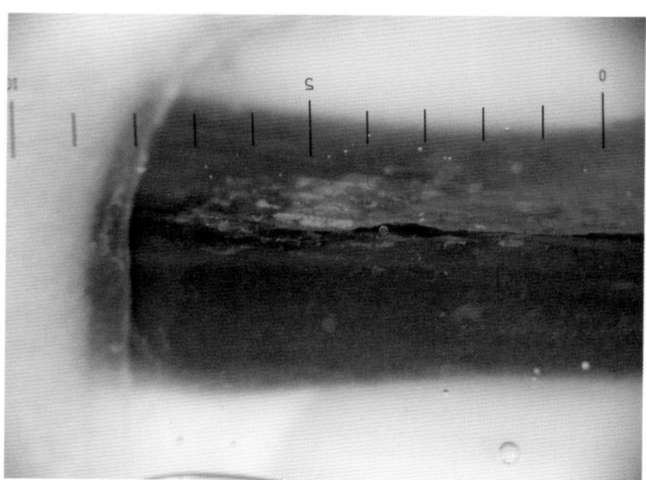

A 0.6 mm thick nail matrix melanoma with subtle broadening of the band of melanonychia proximally and nail dystrophy causing a longitudinal fissure: dermoscopy clearly shows broadening of the pigmentation proximally and blurred margins.

Phan, A. et al. Dermoscopic features of acral lentiginous melanoma in a large series of 110 cases in a white population. *Br J Dermatol*. 2010;162(4):765–771.

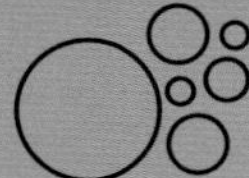

Advanced nail apparatus melanoma – pigmented

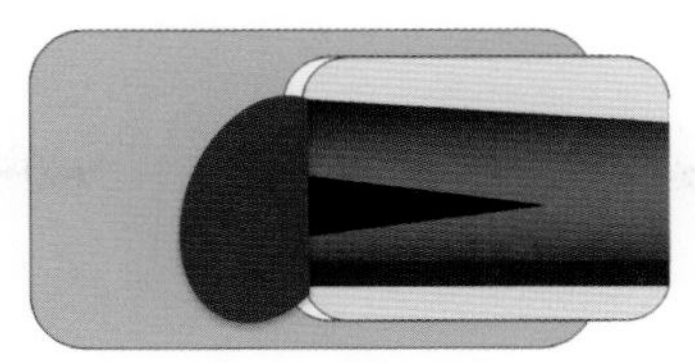

As a nail apparatus melanoma progresses, the nail unit becomes replaced with tumour, with loss of the nail plate. Factors that influence the clinical appearance include the duration of the tumour and related Breslow thickness. Once the nail is lost, dermoscopy is less useful for diagnosis.

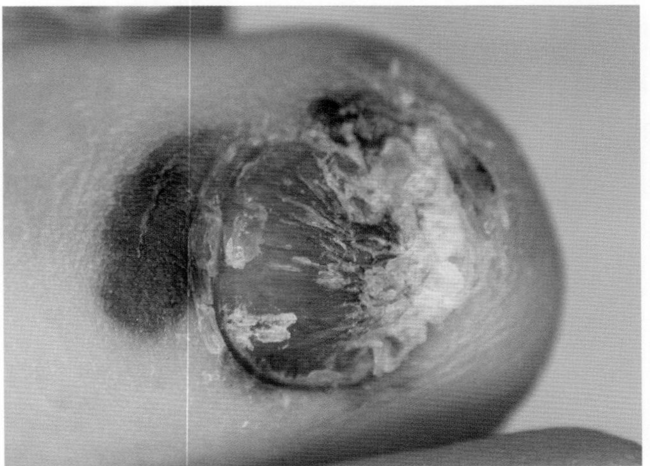

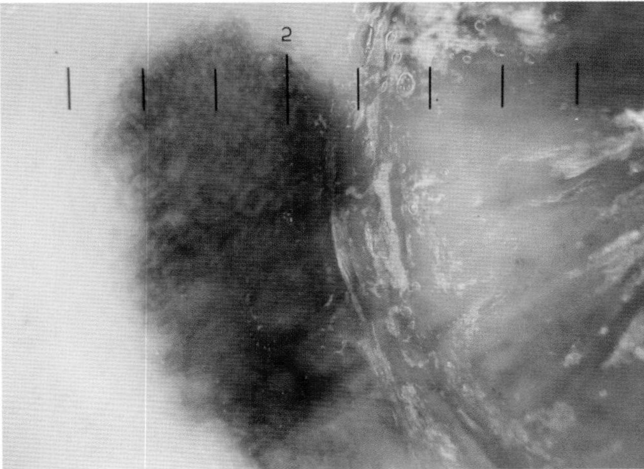

A 0.6 mm nail apparatus melanoma with nail plate loss and a positive Hutchinson's sign: dermoscopy of the proximal nail fold shows irregular pigmentation with atypical pigment network.

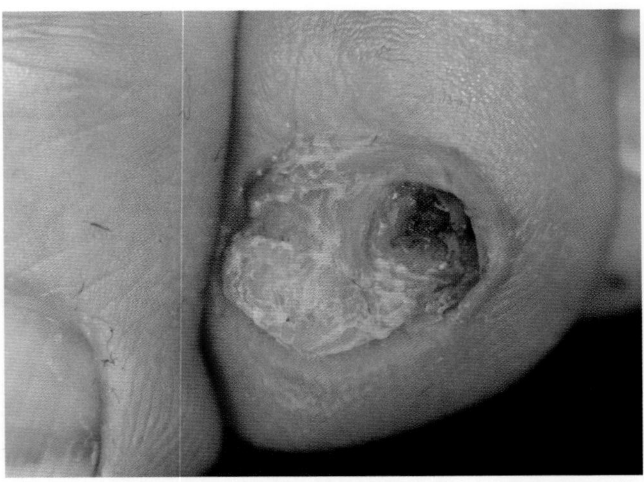

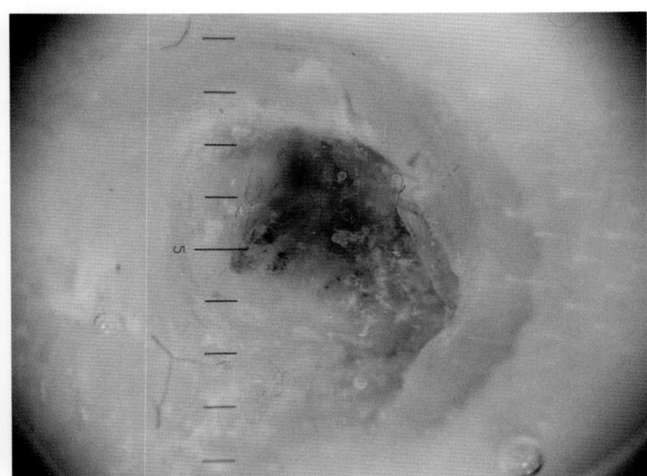

A 4.0 mm nail apparatus melanoma with nail plate dystrophy and a focal zone of hyperpigmentation thought initially to be fungal in nature: dermoscopy shows irregular hyperpigmentation and black dots.

Nail apparatus melanoma occurs primarily on the thumb or great toe in patients over 50 years. Consider the diagnosis when the band is over 3 mm or covers >40% of the nail plate's width. Up to 30% of cases will be amelanotic.

Advanced nail apparatus melanoma – non-pigmented

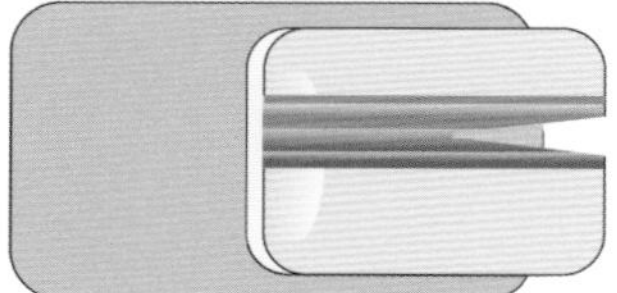

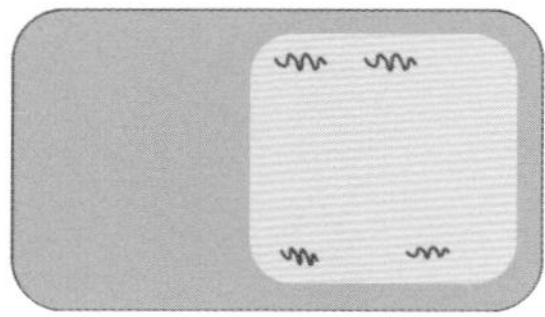

Advanced and hypopigmented nail apparatus melanomas may present with erythro-xanthonychia, onycholysis or fissuring of the nail. These melanomas typically lack dermoscopic detail and hence the diagnosis (albeit challenging) is predominantly made on clinical grounds confirmed with a biopsy for histopathology. Where there is an isolated nail dystrophy without a clear cause such as onychomycosis or trauma, consider taking a diagnostic nail matrix biopsy.

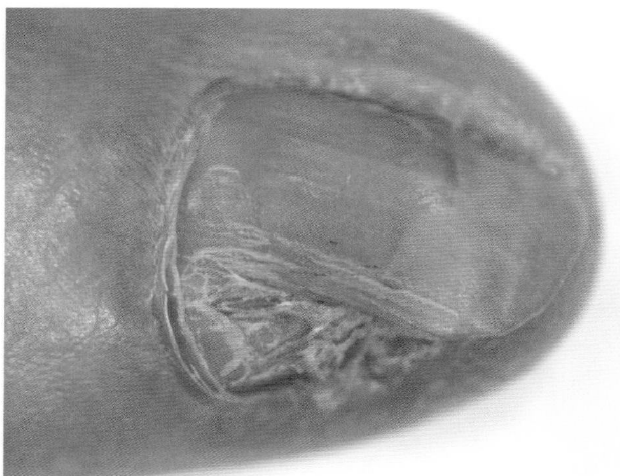

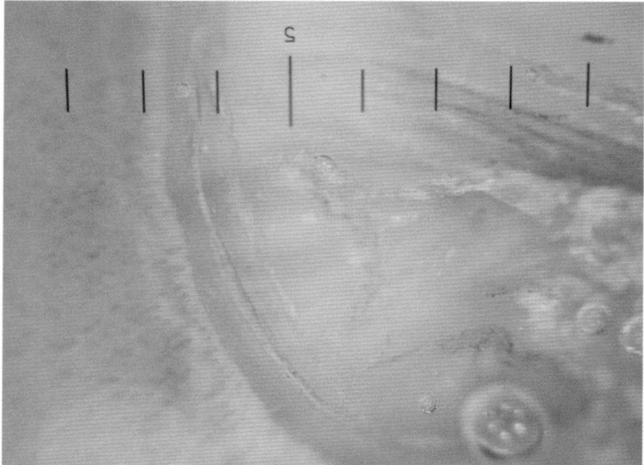

A 1.5 mm thick nail apparatus melanoma with onycholysis and focal nail plate erosion and dystrophy: dermoscopy provides little additional information, highlighting the importance of a diagnostic biopsy.

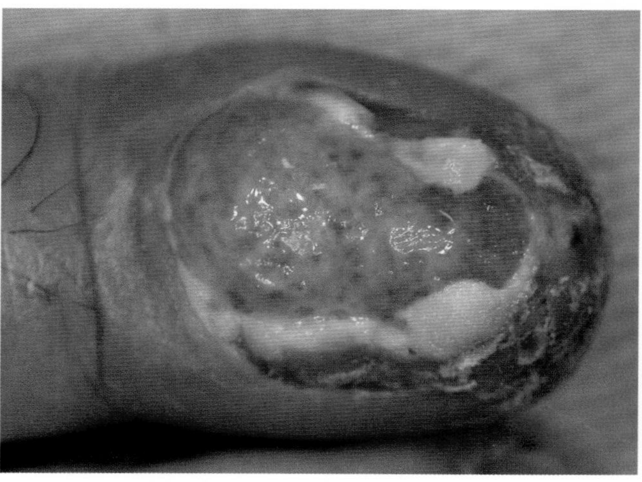

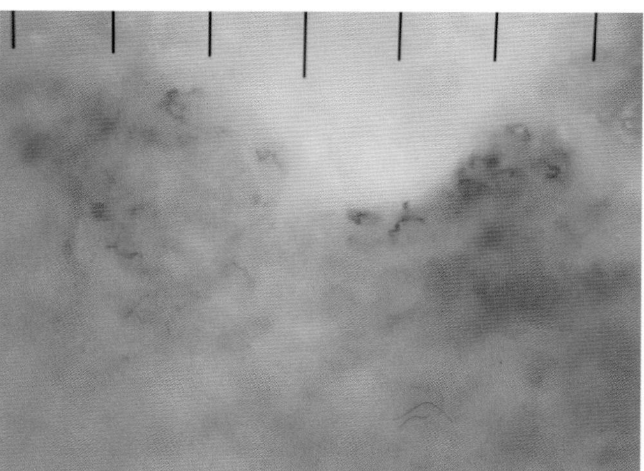

Total nail loss (anonychia) and ulceration in this 6.0 mm thick melanoma with involved lymph nodes at presentation: dermoscopy shows milky erythema and polymorphous vessels.

Ogata, D. et al. Nail apparatus melanoma in a Japanese population: a comparative study of surgical procedures and prognoses in a large series of 151 cases. *Eur J Dermatol*. 2017:27(6):620–626.

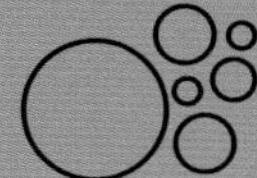

Nail apparatus squamous cell carcinoma

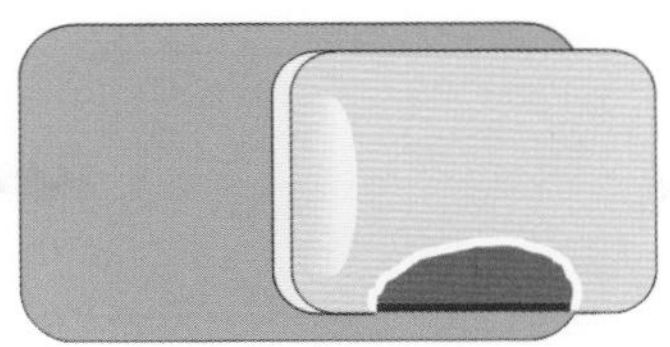

Squamous cell carcinoma (SCC) is the most common tumour of the nail apparatus yet frequently misdiagnosed. It may present with localised hyperkeratosis or onycholysis along with leuko-xanthonychia. The dermoscopic features are very broad so always consider a diagnostic biopsy for progressive lesions.

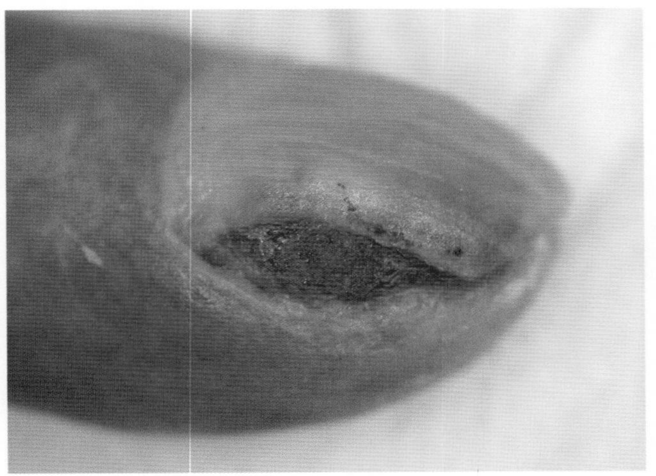

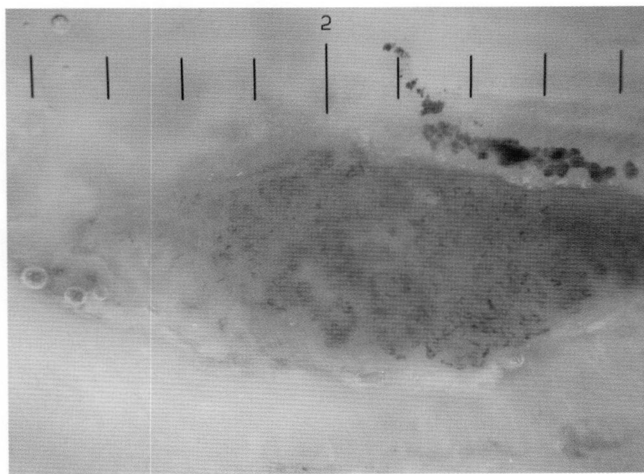

A solitary dystrophic nail with exudative tumour arising from beneath the lateral margin: dermoscopy shows atypical vessels and erythema in this moderately differentiated SCC.

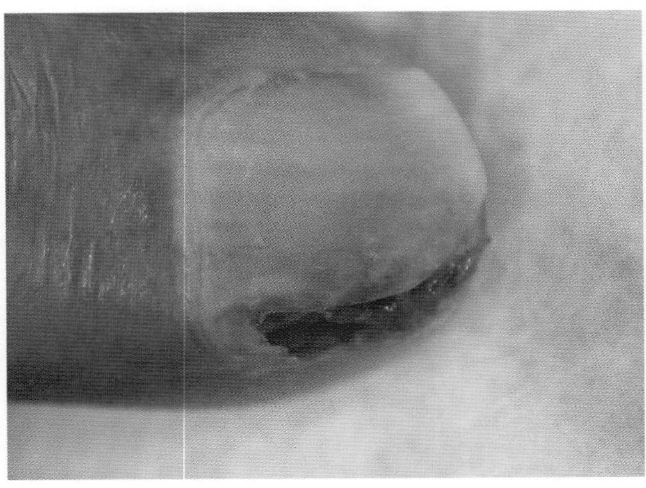

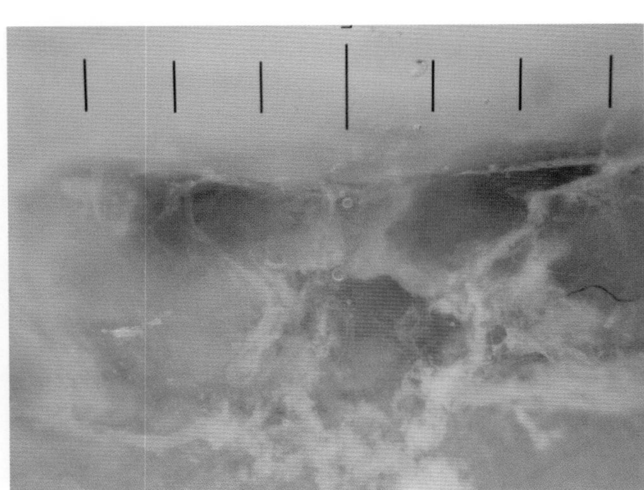

A solitary dystrophic nail with an exudative tumour affecting the lateral nail fold: dermoscopy shows ulceration and keratin debris in this moderately differentiated SCC.

Teysseire, S. et al. Dermoscopic features of subungual squamous cell carcinoma: A study of 44 cases. *Dermatology.* 2017; 233:184–191.

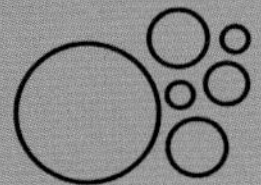

Erythronychia

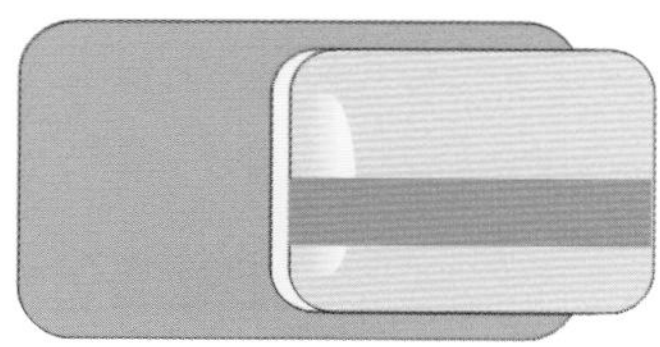

Erythronychia in a solitary nail should prompt the clinician to consider investigating to confirm or exclude an underlying neoplastic or dysplastic process. Erythronychia in multiple nails is less alarming and may be idiopathic or associated with inflammatory dermatoses.

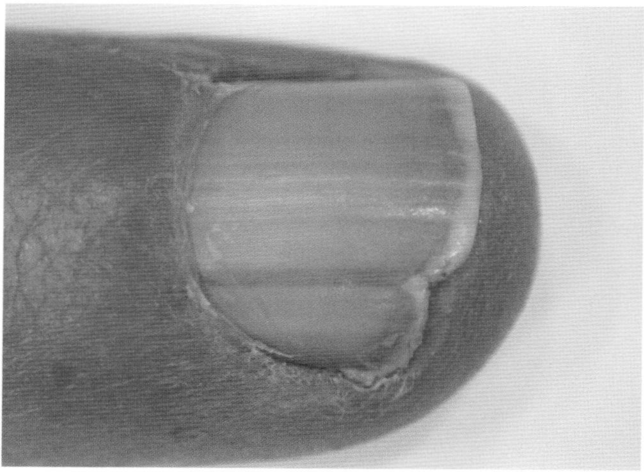

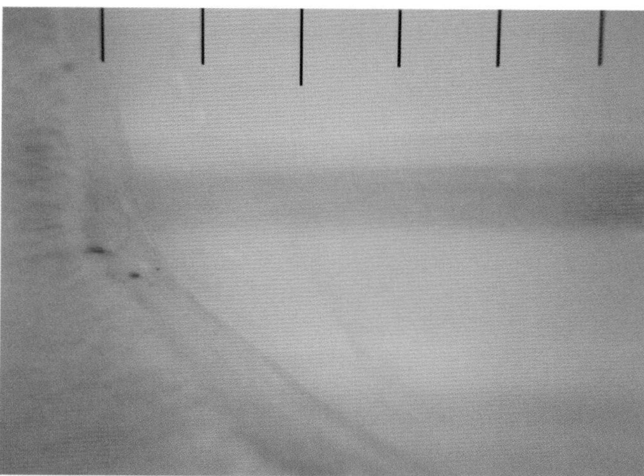

A thin band of erythronychia on multiple nails with distal notching at the free edge in a patient with Darier's disease: dermoscopy shows a thin uniform band of erythronychia.

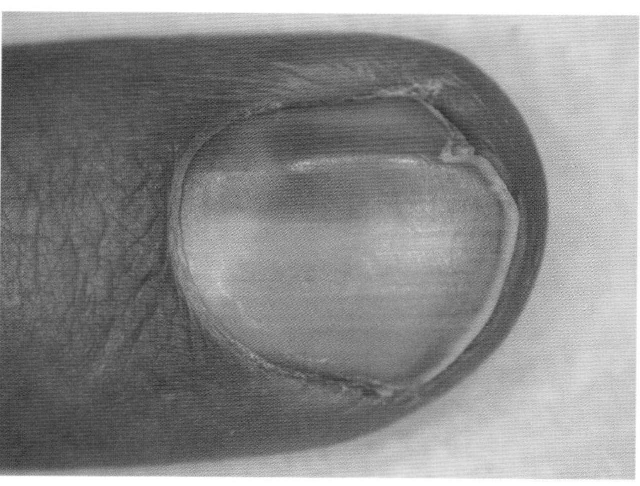

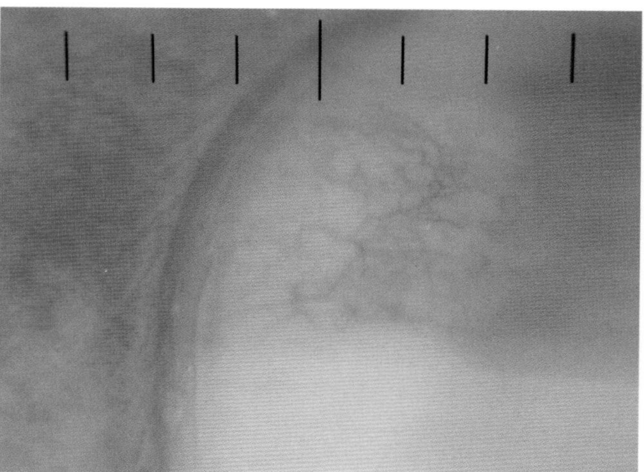

A broad band of erythronychia in a solitary nail with tenderness and distal notching: dermoscopy shows the underlying vascular component and accounts for the distal notching in a histopathologically confirmed glomus tumour (best confirmed via MRI).

The longtitudinal red and white striped nails of Darier's disease (an inheritable disorder of keratinisation) are sometimes referred to as "candy cane" nails. De Berker, D. et al. Erythronychia. *Dermatol Ther*. 2012;25(6):603–611.

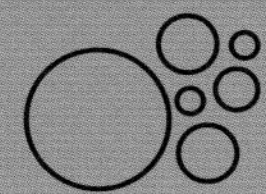

Onychopapilloma

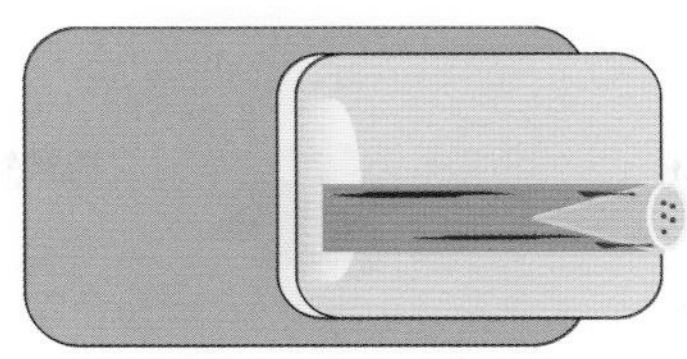

Onychopapilloma is an uncommon, benign tumour of the nail bed and distal matrix. It typically presents with a longitudinal band of erythronychia and splinter haemorrhages with focal distal subungual keratosis. The differential diagnosis includes glomus tumour, SCC in situ, Darier's disease and lichen planus.

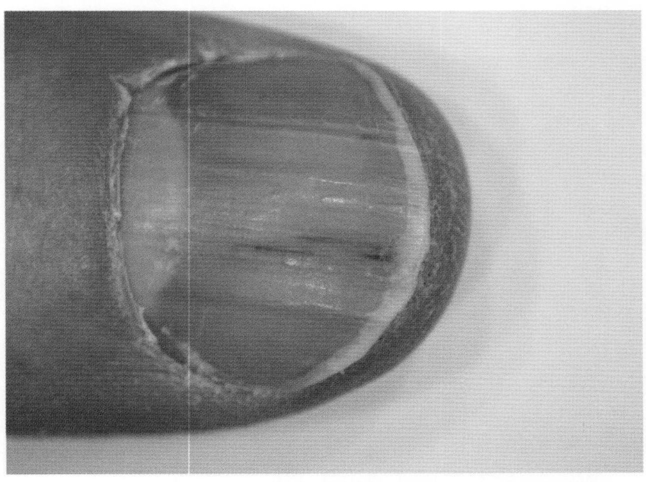

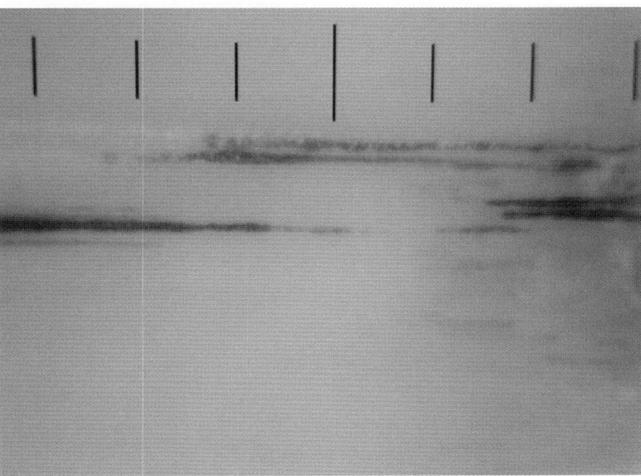

A narrow band or erythronychia originating from the distal lunula with multiple long and short splinter haemorrhages clearly seen on dermoscopy in this case of onychopapilloma.

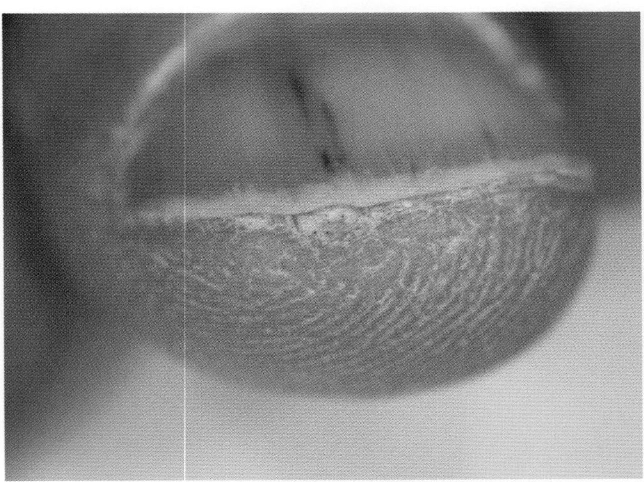

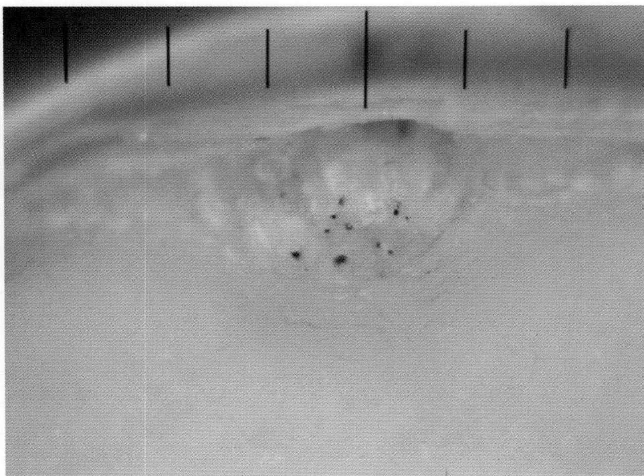

A view of the free edge of the nail plate shows a well-defined subungual keratotic mass: dermoscopy shows focal black haemorrhagic dots without thickening of the overlying nail plate in this onychopapilloma.

Tosti, A. et al. Clinical, dermoscopic, and pathologic features of onychopapilloma: a review of 47 cases. *J Am Acad Dermatol* 2016;74(3):521–526.

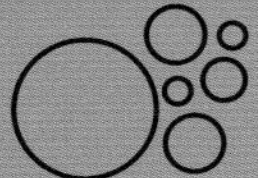

Subungual haematoma

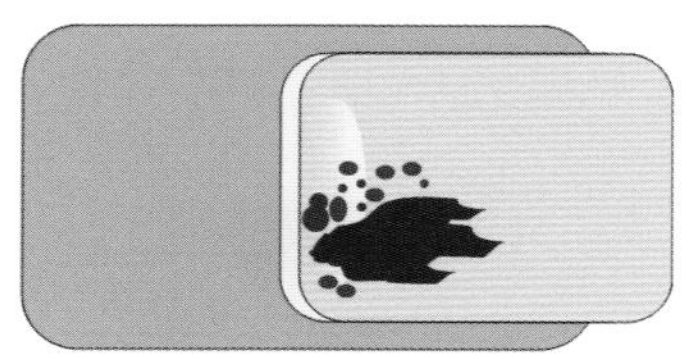

Unlike bruising at other anatomical locations, any bleeding from disrupted nail bed capillaries is slow to resolve as it is trapped beneath the slowly growing nail plate. This presentation typically causes great clinical concern as a history of trauma is often absent and changes may persist for months only clearing as the nail plate advances. As the nail grows, the haemorrhage starts to degrade and resolve, leading to changes in colour from purple to red-brown.

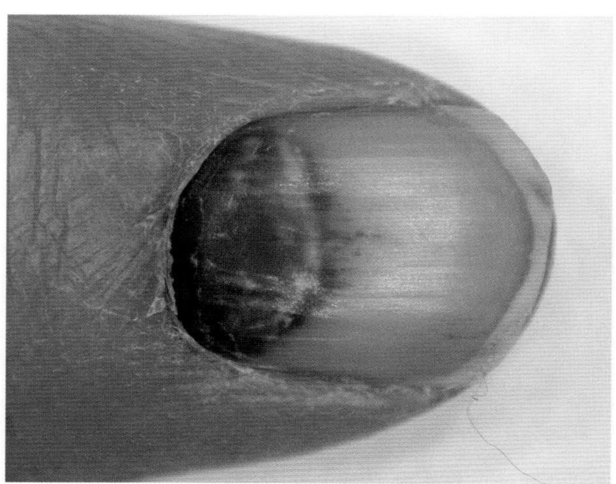

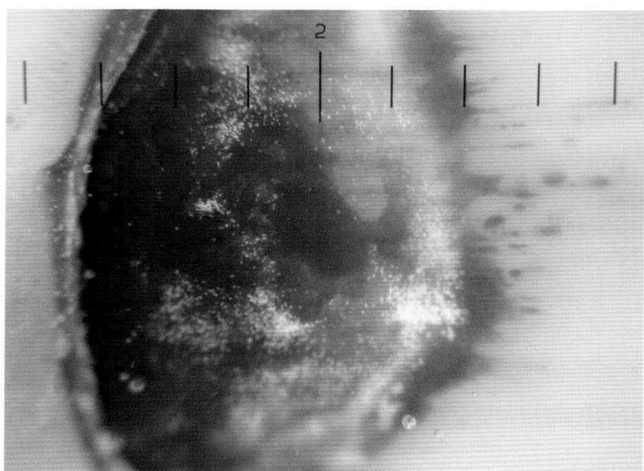

Subungual haematoma of the index finger following trauma: dermoscopy shows a homogeneous purple colour with distal spikes, globules of blood and extensive white granular and globular pigmentation.

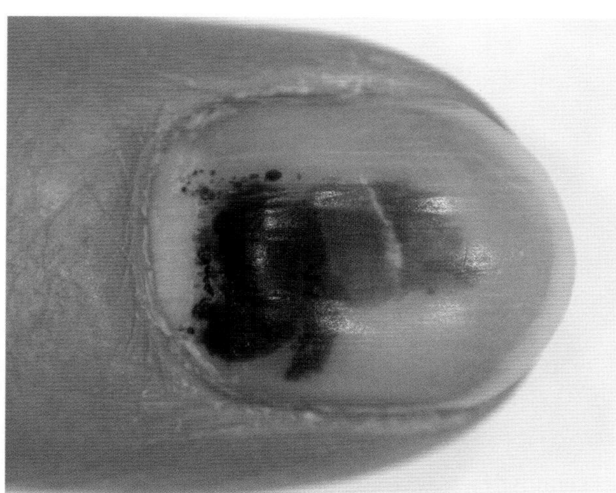

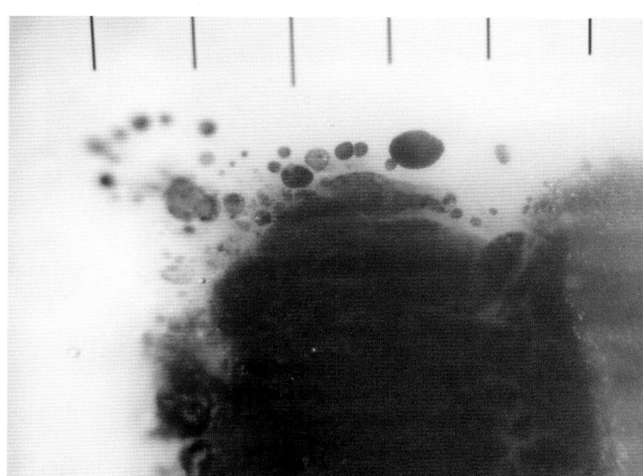

Subungual haematoma of a fingernail with a sizeable purplish blood spill beneath the nail plate: dermoscopy of the proximal margin shows splatter globules with red and purple colour in keeping with haemorrhage.

Braun, R.P. et al. Diagnosis and management of nail pigmentations. *J Am Acad Dermatol*. 2007;156(5):871–874.

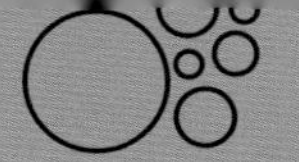

Subungual haematoma cases

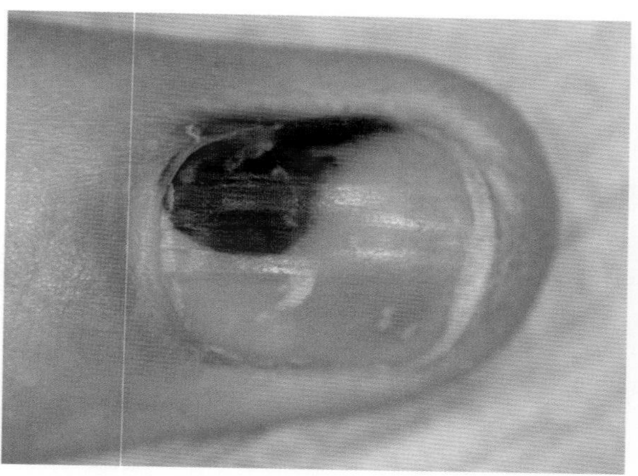

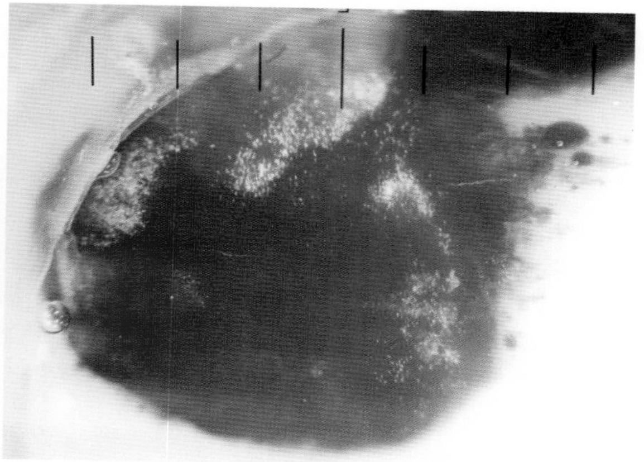

A subungual haemorrhage following trauma to the fingernail: dermoscopy shows homogeneous red and purple pigmentation with granular leukonychia and peripheral globules reflecting a traumatic origin.

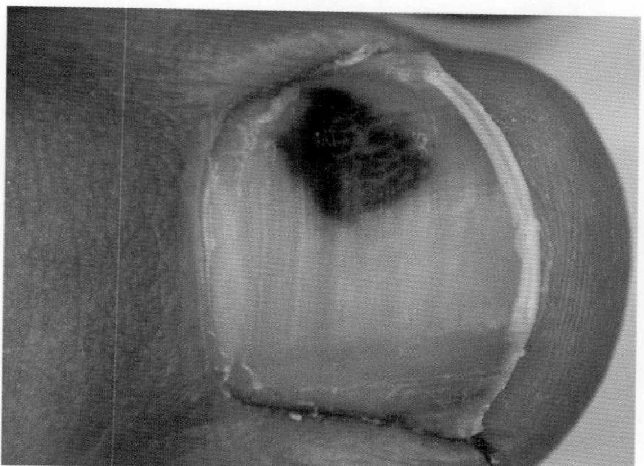

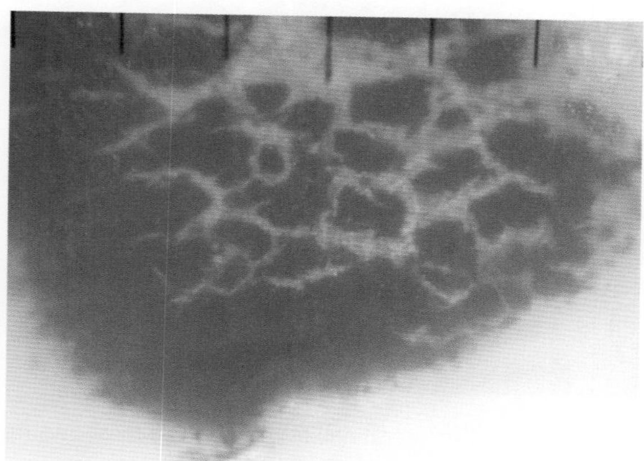

A subungual haemorrhage on the great toe a few weeks post-injury: dermoscopy shows purple homogeneous pigmentation with additional angulated white lines delineating aggregates of the haemorrhage as it starts to break down.

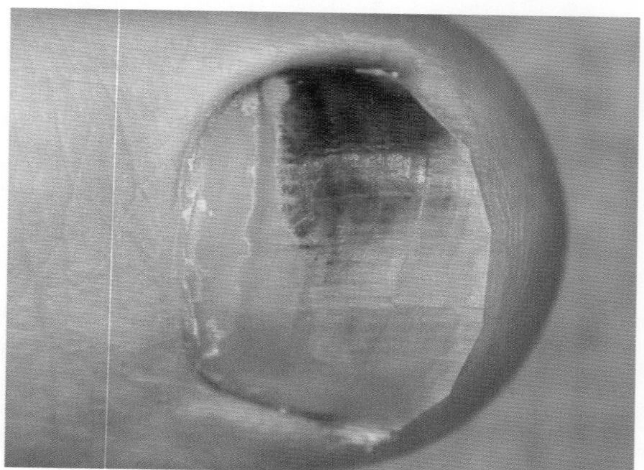

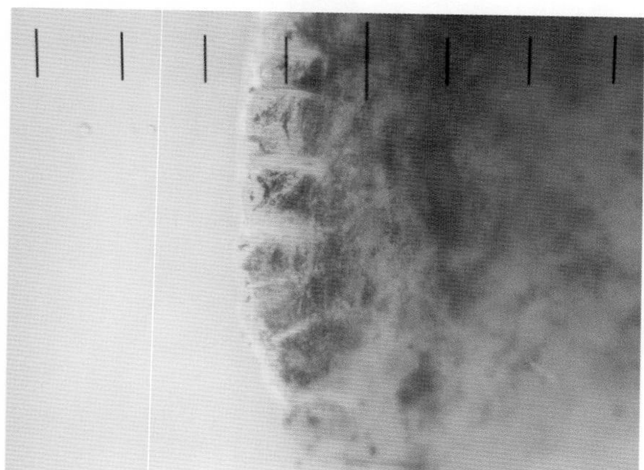

A subungual haemorrharge on the great toe many weeks post-injury: dermoscopy shows clearing of the proximal margin and variable colours as it resolves.

A capillary effect (linear flow of red blood cells along a narrow space) is frequently seen at the distal margin of a subungual haemorrhage. As it resolves, a rounded margin is seen with or without blood spill (globules) at the proximal pole.

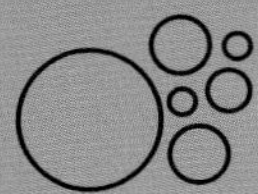

Periungual warts

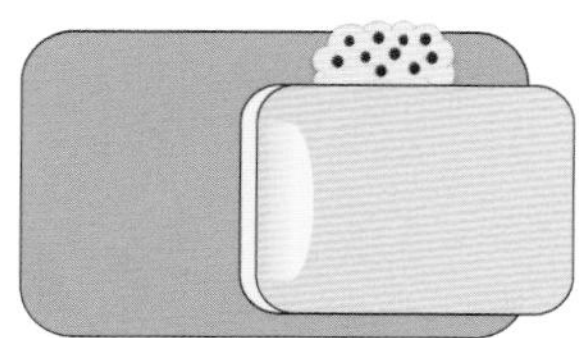

Verrucae or viral warts commonly involve periungual skin. Warts can be easily distinguished from a callus on dermoscopy by the presence of multiple whitish keratotic halos, often with central red/purple dotted vessels. The red dots are often associated with micro-haemorrhages, particularly if the wart has been irritated. When the dots within warts turn black this often implies involution is close. Yellow colouration reflects hyperkeratosis.

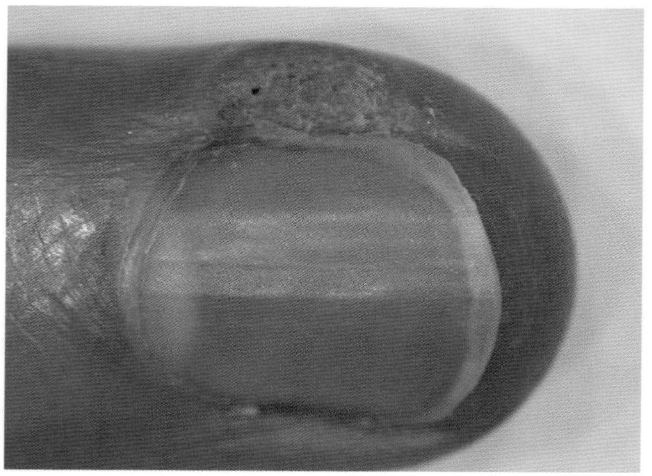

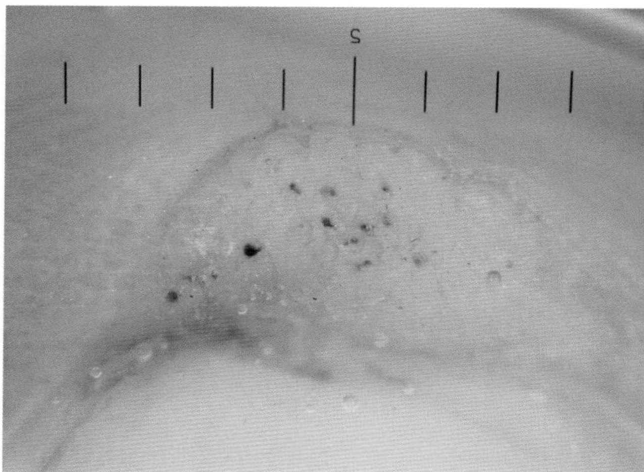

A keratotic plaque on the lateral nail fold: dermoscopy shows multiple purple dots surrounded by keratotic halos, in keeping with a viral wart.

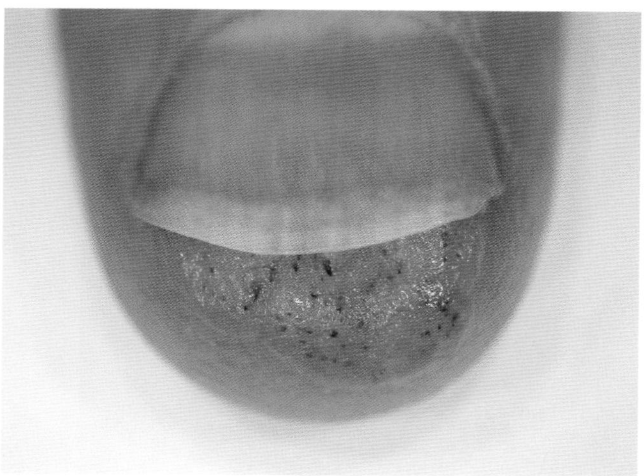

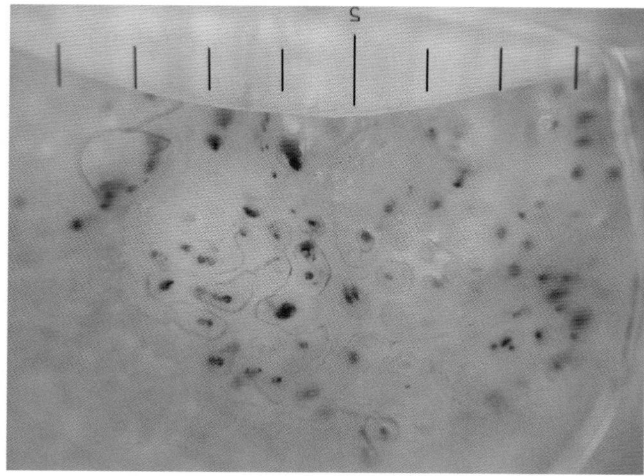

A keratotic plaque on the middle finger hyponychium of a 50-year-old man: dermoscopy shows a mosaic pattern with multiple red purple dots in keratotic halos, in keeping with a viral wart.

Lee, D.Y. et al. The use of dermoscopy for the diagnosis of a plantar wart. Clinical and dermoscopic features of common warts. *J Eur Acad Dermatol Venereol*. 2009;23(6)726–727.

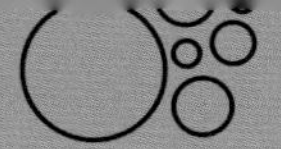

Onychomycosis

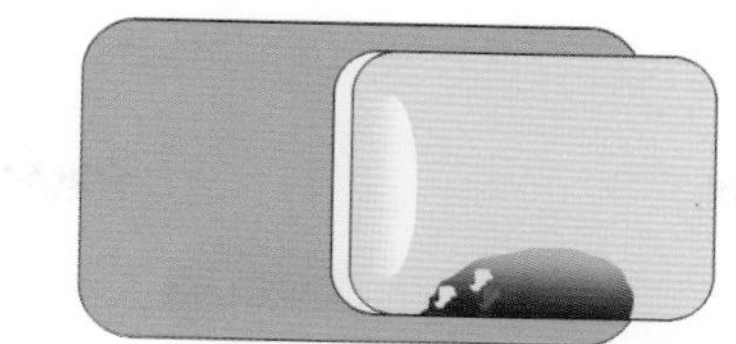

Onychomycosis may present with multifocal changes in the nail plate; however, when it appears as a longitudinal band it may cause diagnostic uncertainty. When pigmentation develops it may broaden distally, providing a helpful clinical feature. The associated onycholysis is often spiky with a jagged proximal border. Nail samples for mycological culture confirm the type of fungus or mould responsible for the infection.

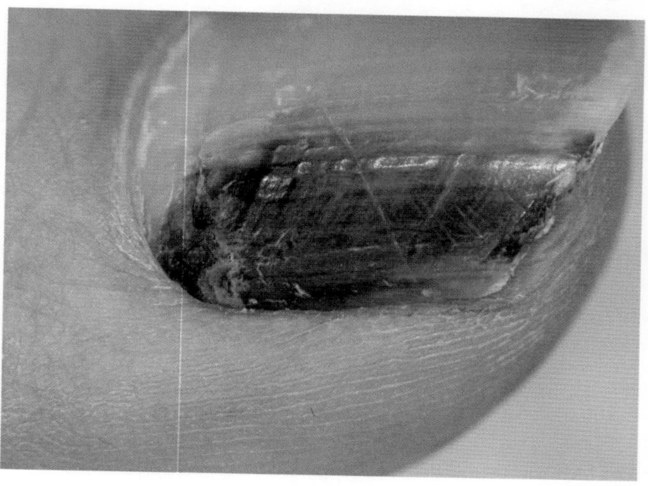

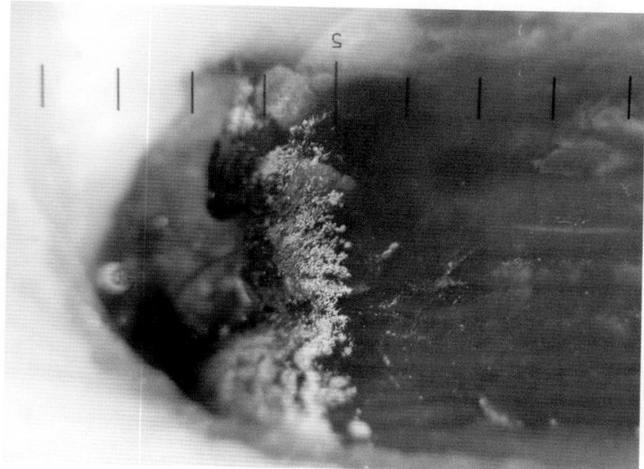

Pigmentation of the lateral nail fold of the great toe: dermoscopy shows variable brown, black and cream-coloured pigmentation broadening distally with dystrophy of the proximal nail plate. *Trichophyton rubrum* was confirmed on culture.

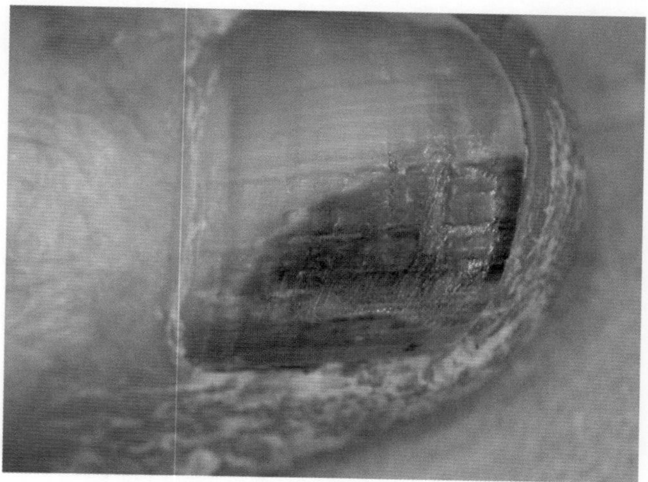

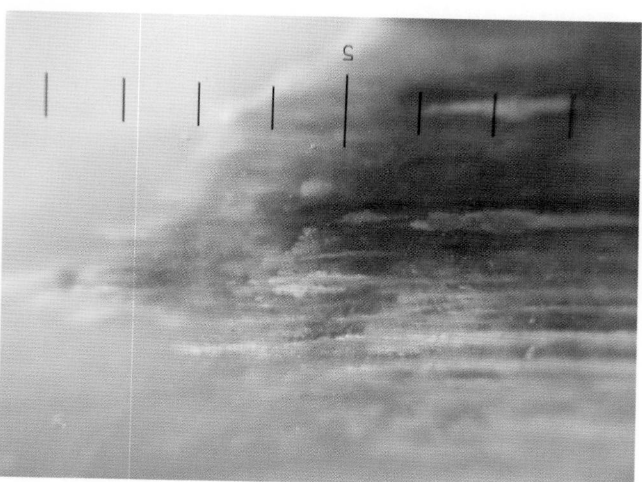

Variable pigmentation of the great toe broadening distally with surrounding hyperkeratosis of the adjacent nail fold: dermoscopy shows multicoloured linear pigmentation broadening distally and proximal yellow-white spikes typical for fungal infection.

Ohn, J. et al. Dermoscopic patterns of fungal melanonychia: a comparative study with other causes of melanonychia. *J Am Acad Dermatol*. 2017;76(3):488–493.

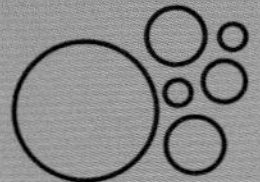

Chloronychia – green nails

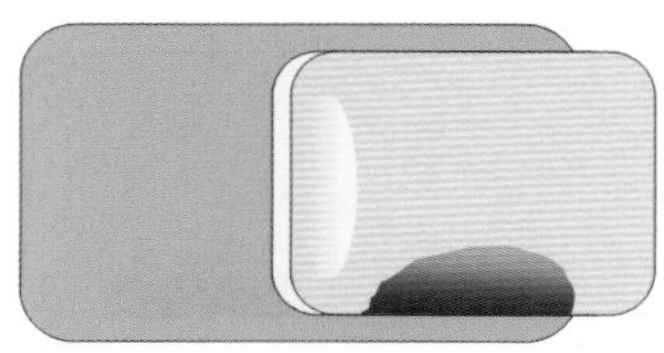

Nail colonisation with *Pseudomonas aeruginosa* creates a vivid bright green colour in addition to the typical offensive odour. It is a common presentation in dystrophic nails with onycholysis.

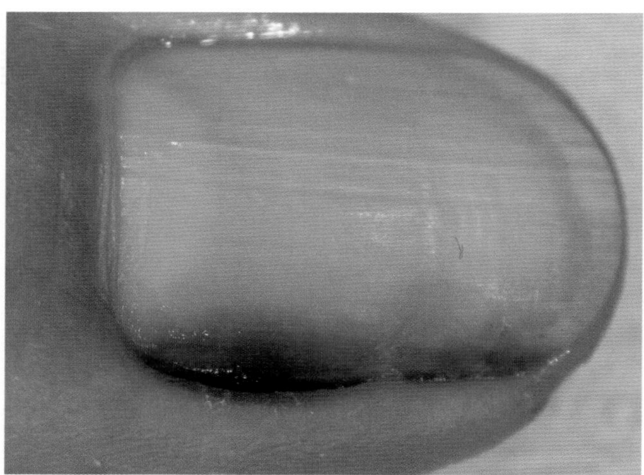

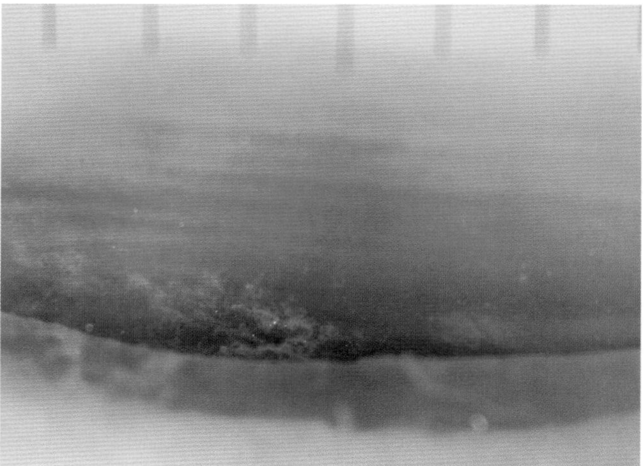

A renal transplant patient with green discoloration of the lateral nail fold of the thumb: dermoscopy shows a homogeneous green colour in keeping with pseudomonas colonisation.

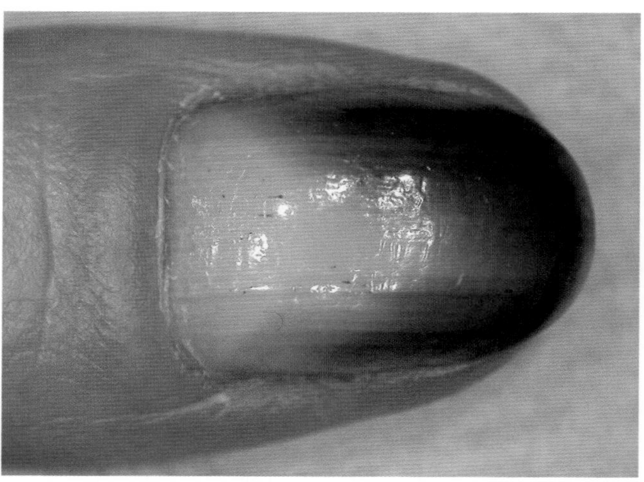

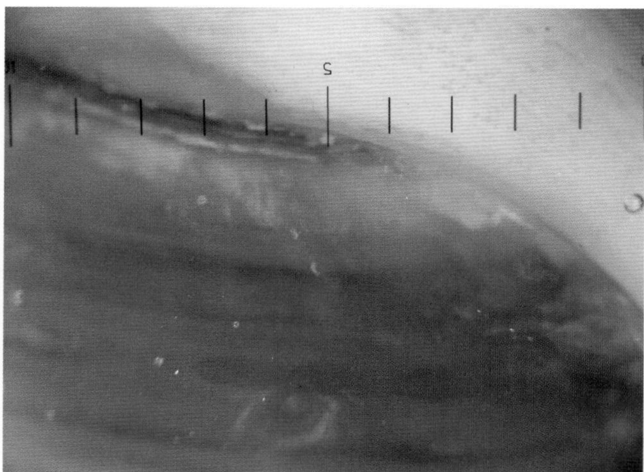

A 50-year-old woman with a solitary bright green discoloration of the index finger nail: dermoscopy shows a bright green homogeneous colour in keeping with pseudomonas colonisation.

The green hue is due to the pigments pyoverdin and pyocyanin produced by the bacteria. Diluted white vinegar soaks may help although the primary cause for the onycholysis must also be addressed.

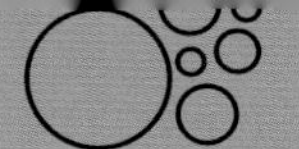

Nail pigmentation – exogenous

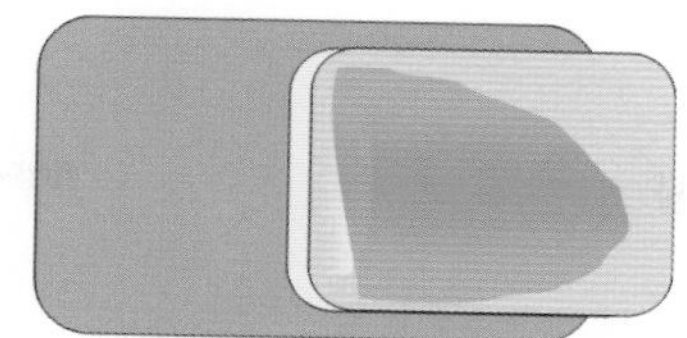

Nail pigmentation is commonly caused by exogenous compounds making contact with the nail plate. A common cause is tar staining from cigarette smoke. If the cause of pigmentation is unknown then it may cause concern to the patient and clinician. Dermoscopy of the nail plate can identify pigment on the surface, confirming an exogenous cause.

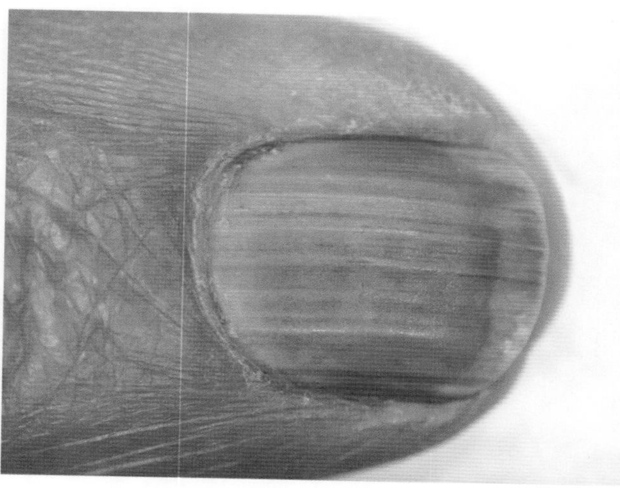

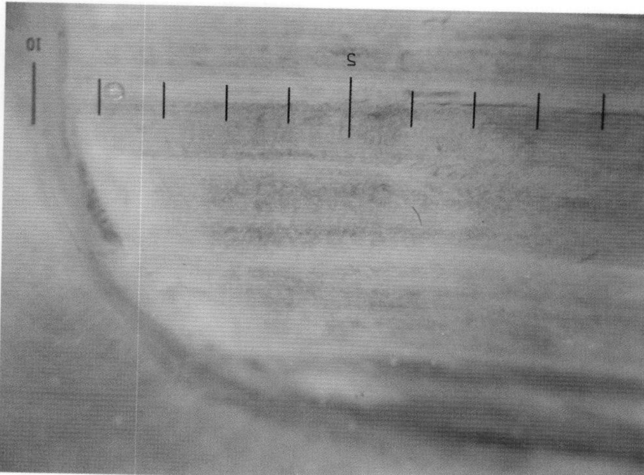

Asymptomatic long-standing tan pigmentation of the nail plate in a smoker: dermoscopy shows light brown/orange pigmentation with clearing before the cuticle, in keeping with tar staining.

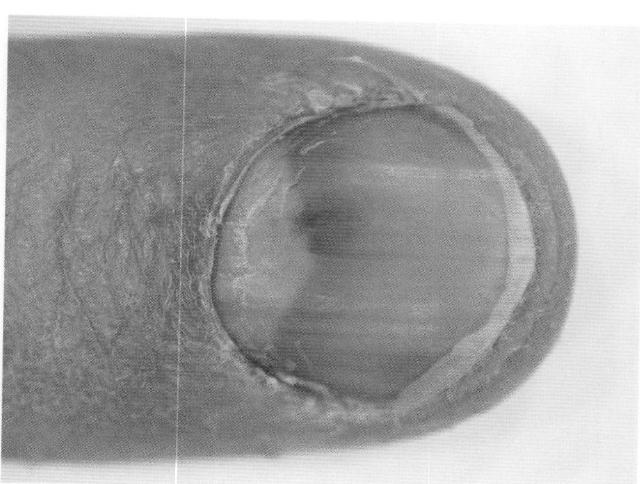

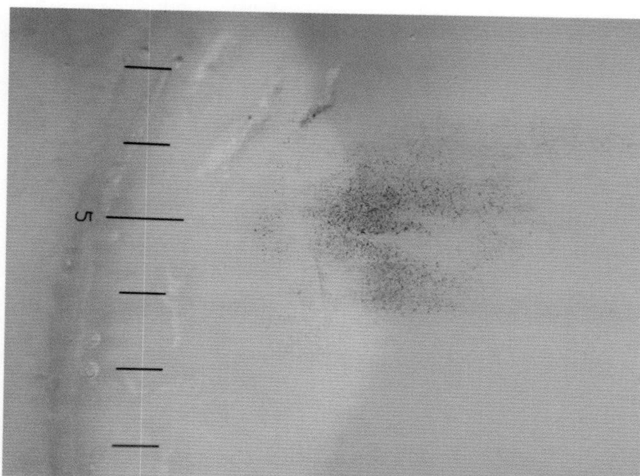

A 50-year-old man with a solitary focus of pigmentation on the index finger nail: dermoscopy shows a focal zone of granular black pigmentation, in keeping with an exogenous cause that was easily removed with paring.

The nail plate can be etched with a file at the proximal margin of pigmentation, which a few months later can be shown to migrate distally. Exogenous pigment should be able to be partially removed with an alcohol wipe.

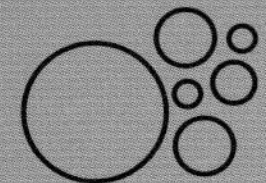

Capillaroscopy

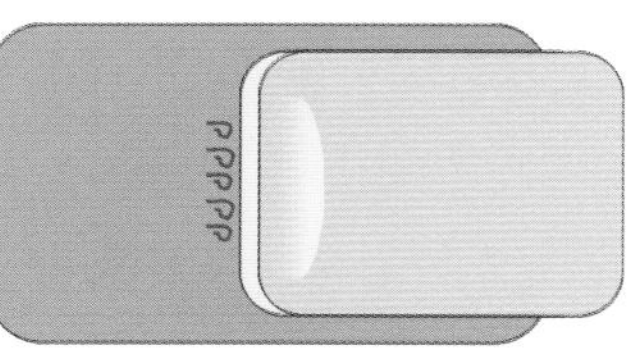

Dilatation of the proximal nail fold capillaries can be seen in connective tissue diseases including dermatomyositis and scleroderma. Visualising these dilated capillaries (capillaroscopy) can be easily achieved with a dermoscope and can provide valuable information for diagnosis.

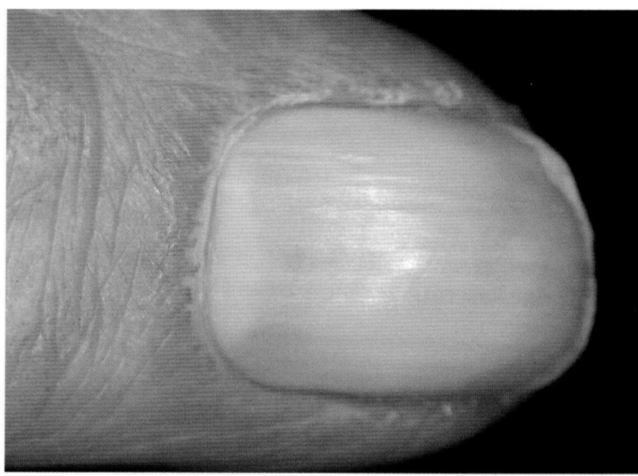

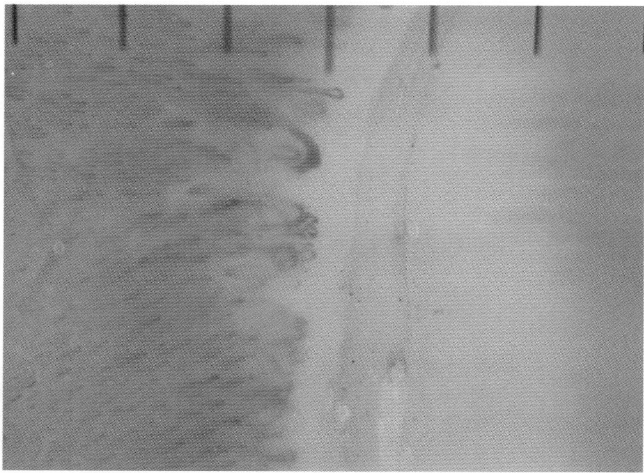

Erythema of the proximal nail folds in a 50-year-old woman with dermatomyositis: on dermoscopy the dilated and looped nail fold capillaries can clearly be seen including some macro-capillaries.

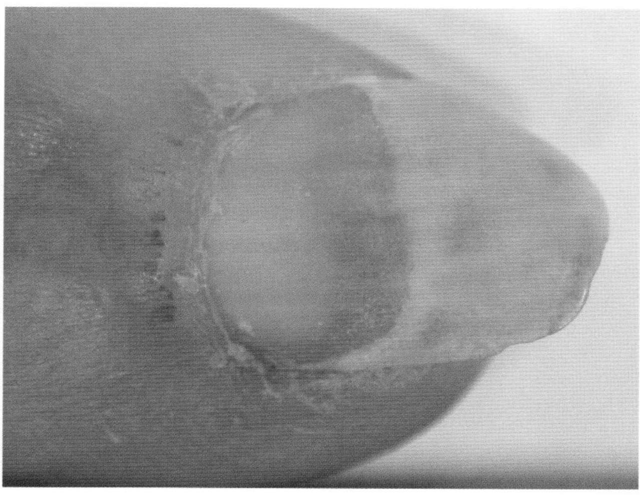

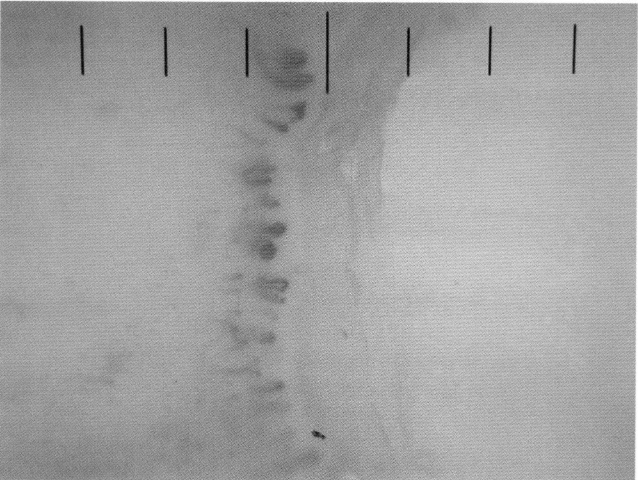

Nail fold changes and tapering of the soft tissues of the terminal phalanges in a 60-year-old woman with scleroderma: dermoscopy shows dilated and looped proximal nail fold capillaries and a ragged cuticle.

Bergman, R. et al. The handheld dermatoscope as a nail-fold capillaroscopic instrument. *Arch Dermatol*. 2003;139(8): 1027–1030.

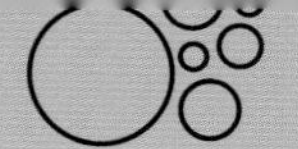

7.3 Facial lesions

Venous lake 200
Mucosal melanosis 201
Milium/keratin cyst 202
Hidrocystoma 203
Epidermoid cysts 204
Pilomatricoma 205
Sebaceous hyperplasia 206
Sebaceous adenoma 207
Sebaceous naevus 208
Malignant adnexal carcinomas 209
Juvenile xanthogranuloma 210
Granulomatous folliculitis 211
Fibrous papule 212
Trichilemmoma 213
Dermal naevus 214
Dermal naevus cases 215
Solar lentigo – fingerprinting 216
Solar lentigo – homogeneous pigmentation 217
Solar lentigo – moth-eaten border 218
Ink spot lentigo 219
Benign lichenoid keratosis 220
Benign lichenoid keratosis – post-inflammation phase 221
Lentigo maligna 222
Lentigo maligna – annular granular pigmentation 223
Lentigo maligna – circles 224
Lentigo maligna – perifollicular pigmentation 225
Lentigo maligna – young adults 226
Lentigo maligna melanoma – I 227
Lentigo maligna melanoma – II 228

Diagnostic Dermoscopy: The Illustrated Guide, Second Edition. Jonathan Bowling.

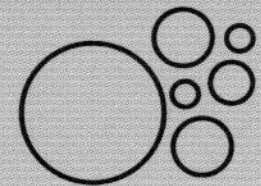

Venous lake

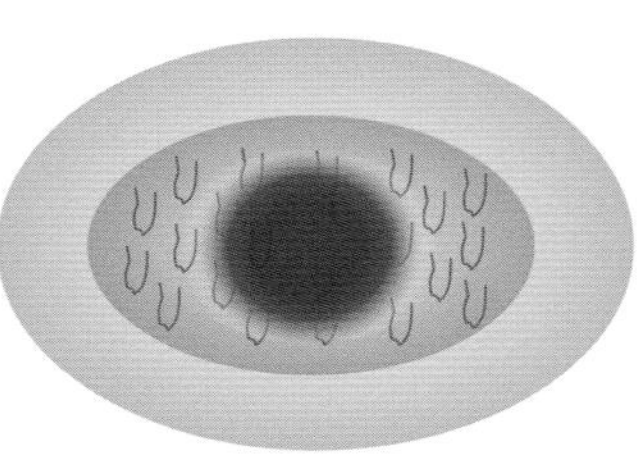

Venous lake is a benign, acquired form of vascular ectasia commonly found on sun-exposed sites of the elderly. The lower lip is the most commonly affected site followed by the helix of the ear, face and neck. They are small, dark blue to purple papules caused by dilatation of post-capillary venules in the upper dermis. Dermoscopy shows a bluish-purple structureless area which is compressible, fading with contact pressure.

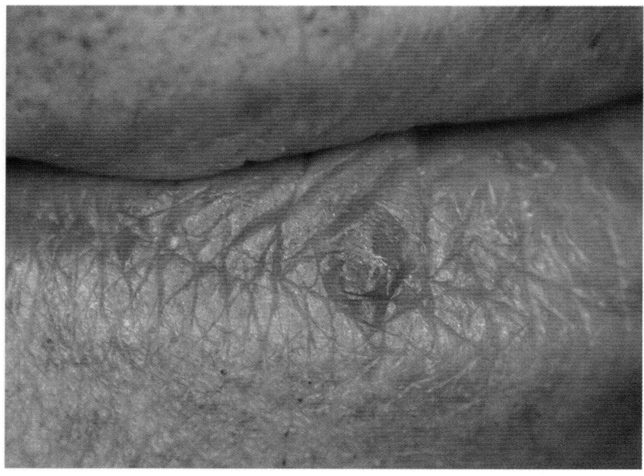

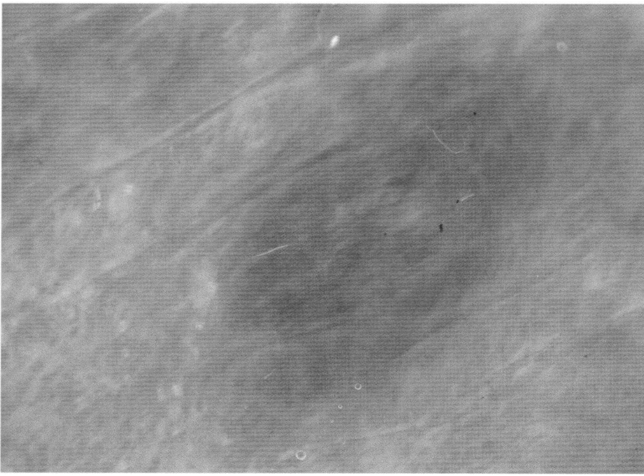

A compressible bluish-purple papule on the lower lip of a 70-year-old woman: dermoscopy shows a bluish-purple structureless area in this venous lake.

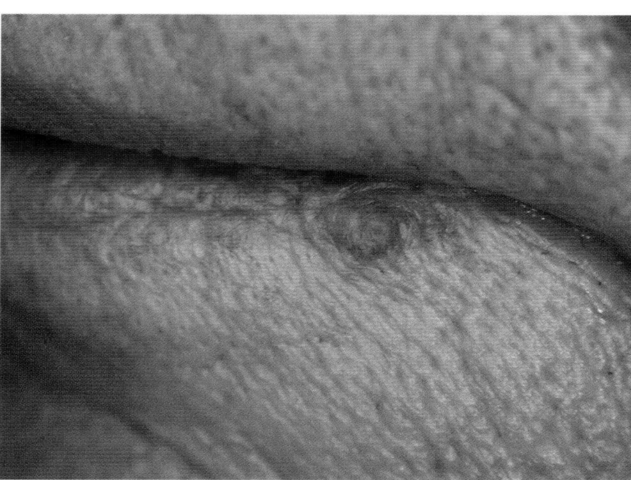

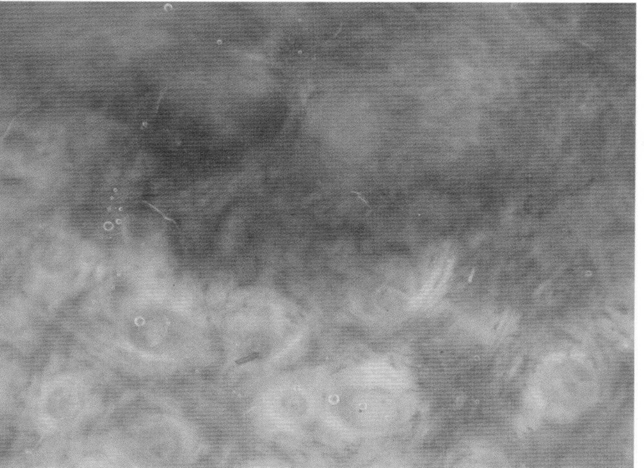

An asymptomatic purple papule on the lower lip of an 80-year-old man: dermoscopy shows a large bluish-purple structureless area with foci of follicular keratin globules in this venous lake.

Lee JS, Mun JH. Dermoscopy of venous lake on the lips: A comparative study with labial melanotic macule. *PLoS One*. 2018;13(10):e0206768.

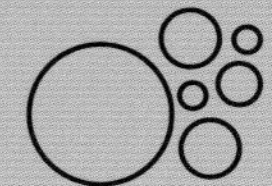

Mucosal melanosis

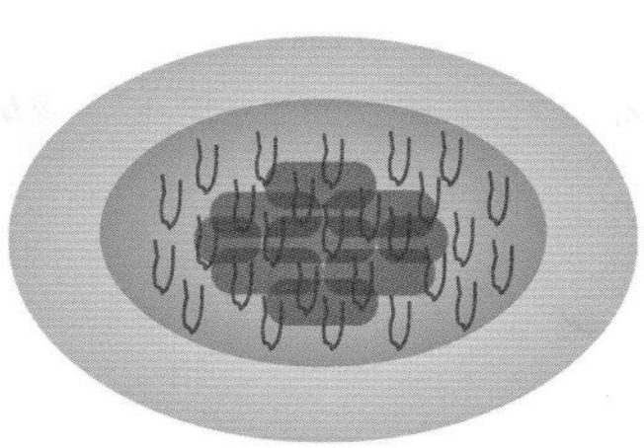

Mucosal melanosis (labial melanotic macule) is a benign pigmented lesion of the mucosae characterised by increased pigmentation of the basal keratinocytes. It most commonly affects the lower lip in patients with a history of high UV exposure. Parallel patterns of pigmentation are the most frequent dermoscopic feature.

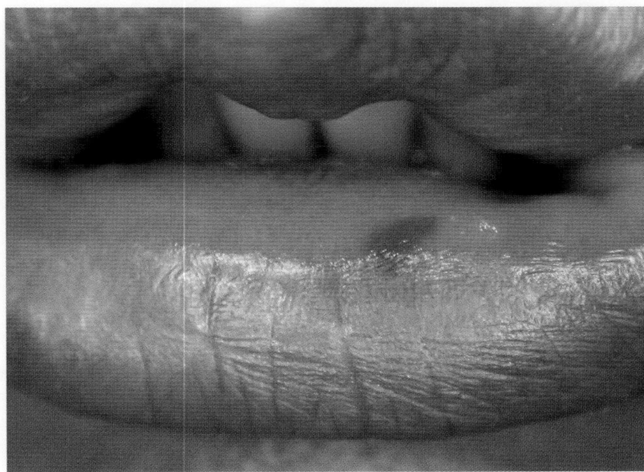

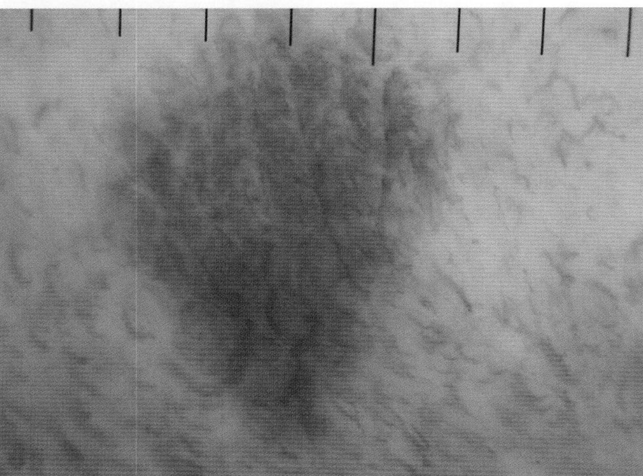

An asymptomatic pigmented macule on the lower lip: dermoscopy shows parallel bands of grey-brown pigmentation and looped vessels in the surrounding mucosa.

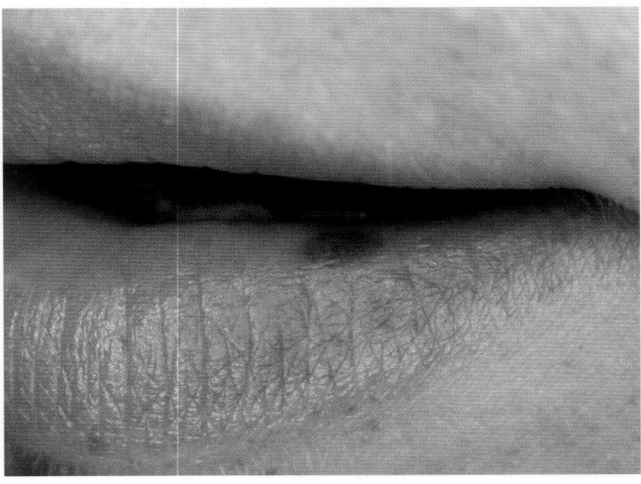

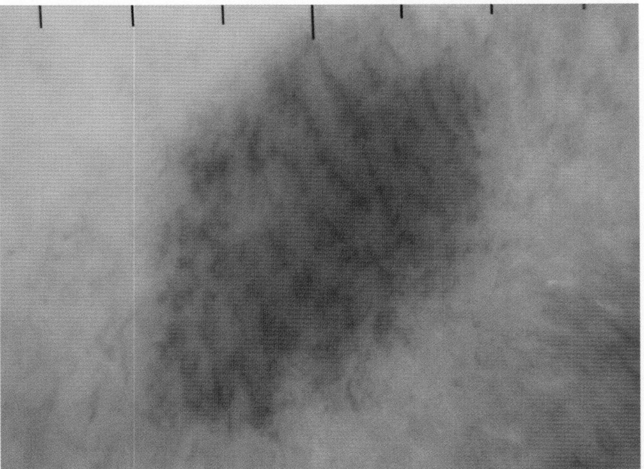

A pigmented macule on the lower lip: dermoscopy shows parallel bands of grey-brown colour and linear vessels in the surrounding mucosa.

Mannone, F. et al. Dermoscopic features of mucosal melanosis. *Dermatol Surg*. 2004;30(8):1118.

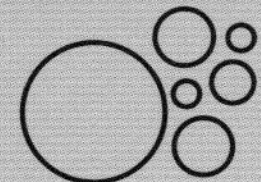

Milium/keratin cyst

Milia or keratin cysts are keratin inclusions within the skin arising from the pilosebaceous apparatus or eccrine sweat duct. They can be solitary or multiple and can be seen in infants, adults and the elderly. They may occur sporadically, following inflammation or injury at the dermoepidermal junction, or following long-term UV exposure.

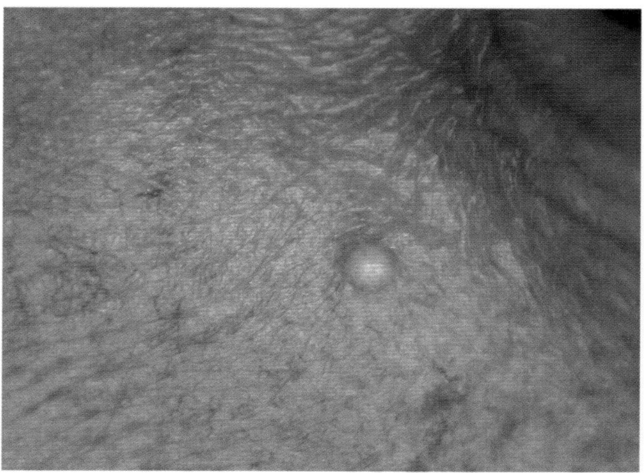

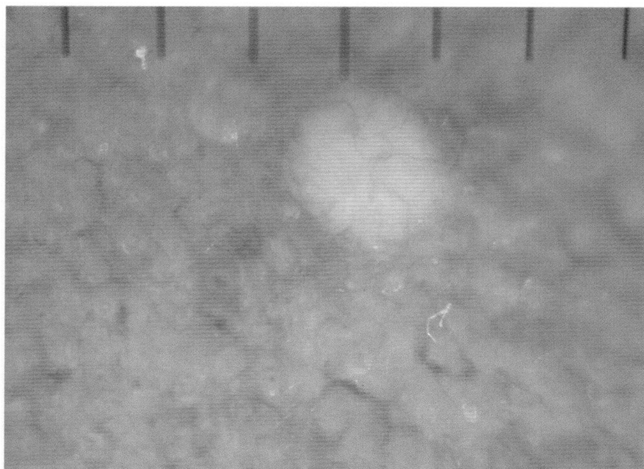

A 2 mm firm yellow papule on the upper cheek of a 60-year-old man: dermoscopy shows a yellow homogeneous area with linear and telangiectatic vessels in a histopathologically confirmed milium.

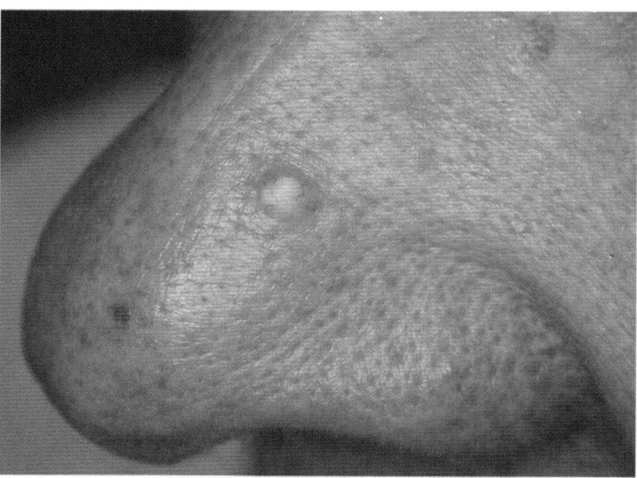

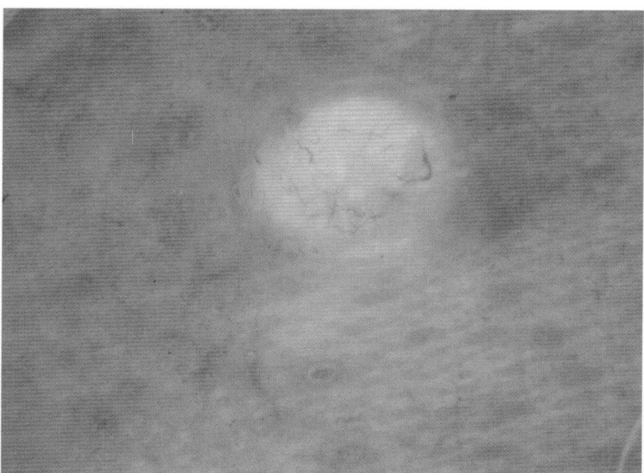

A 3 mm firm yellow papule on the nose of a 60-year-old man: dermoscopy shows a yellow homogeneous area with linear and telangiectatic vessels in a histopathologically confirmed benign milium.

Large milia may share features clinically and dermoscopically with other benign cysts including pilar cysts and epidermoid cysts.

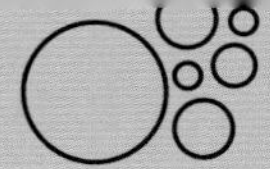

Hidrocystoma

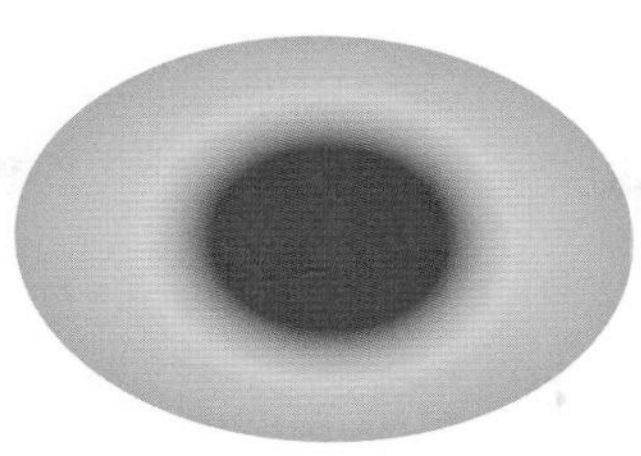

Hidrocystomas are benign tumours of apocrine or eccrine sweat ducts. They can present as either multiple or solitary facial bluish to skin-coloured cystic papules. Dermoscopy can show bluish to opaque homogeneous areas with vessels that are typically arborising. When solitary, they may therefore be difficult to differentiate clinically and dermoscopically from basal cell carcinoma (BCC).

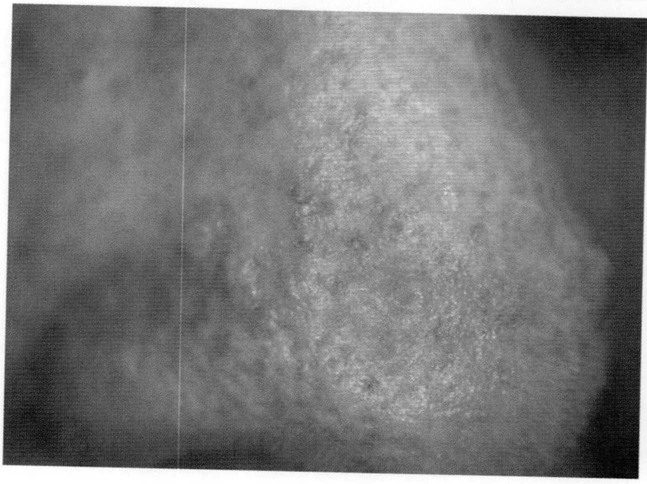

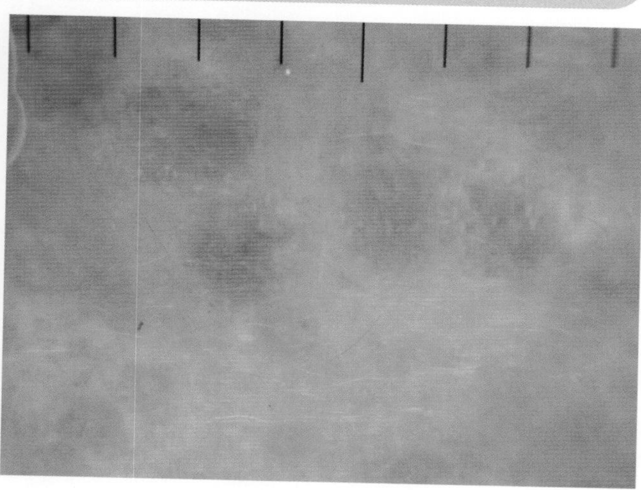

Multiple translucent asymptomatic papules on the nose of a 60-year-old woman: dermoscopy shows multiple monomorphic bluish opaque homogeneous areas, shiny white lines and rosettes confirmed histopathologically as hidrocystomas.

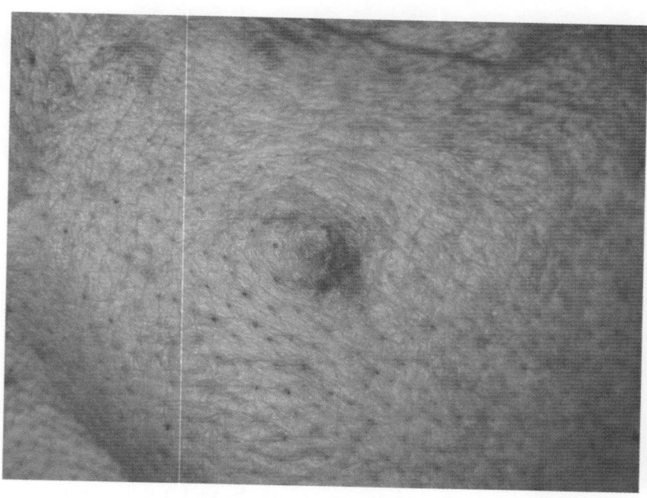

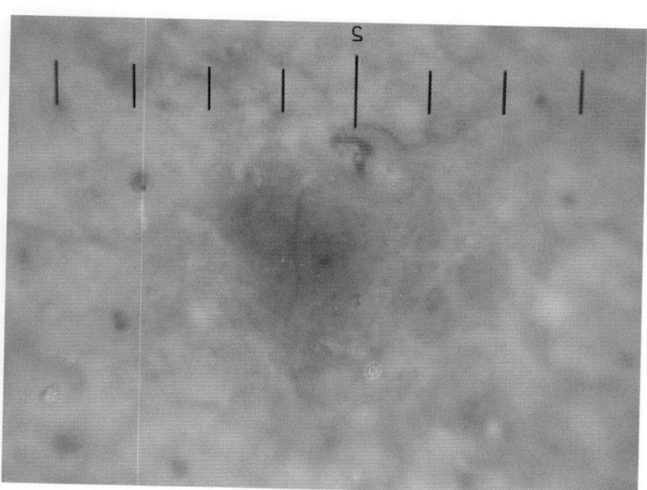

A solitary bluish papule on the cheek of a 70-year-old woman: dermoscopy shows a bluish homogeneous area with linear and telangiectatic vessels in a histopathologically confirmed apocrine hidrocystoma.

Zaballos, P. et al. Dermoscopy of apocrine hidrocystomas: a morphological study. *J Eur Acad Dermatol Venereol.* 2014;28(3):378–381.

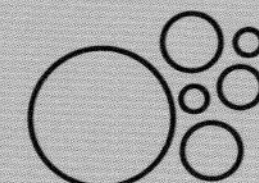

Epidermoid cysts

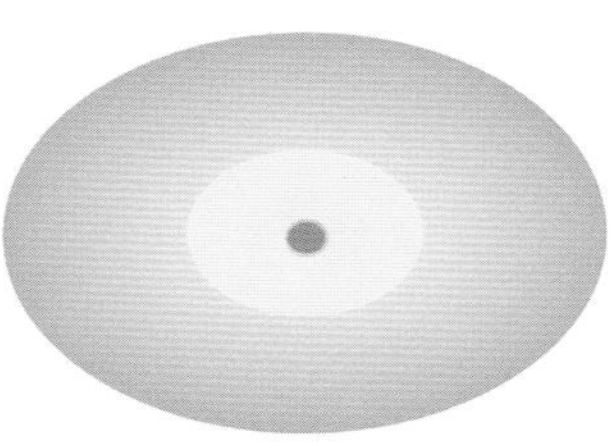

Epidermoid cysts typically appear as an enlarging soft to firm yellow/cream-coloured dermal cyst. A punctum is typically present as a small central keratin focus. Telangiectasia may develop as the cyst enlarges, stretching the overlying epidermis.

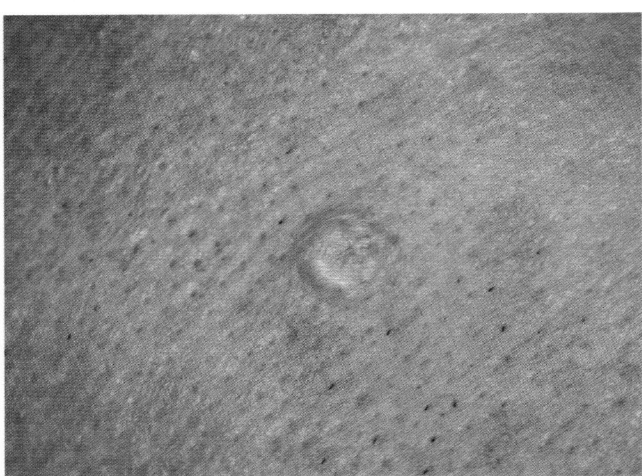

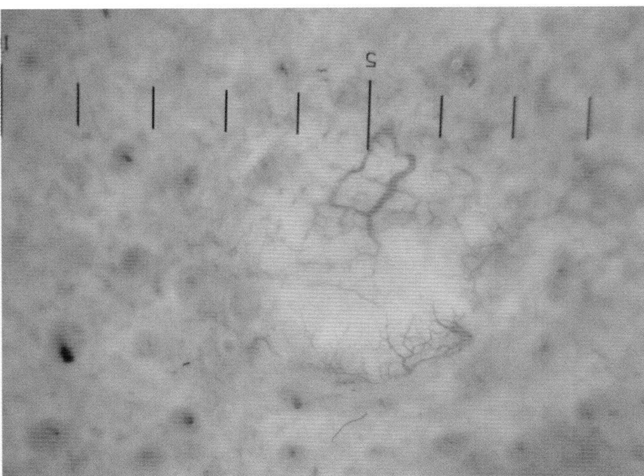

A well-circumscribed 4 mm cream-coloured dermal plaque on the cheek of a 50-year-old man: dermoscopy shows background yellow/cream coloration and linear out-of-focus vessels in this histopathologically confirmed epidermoid cyst.

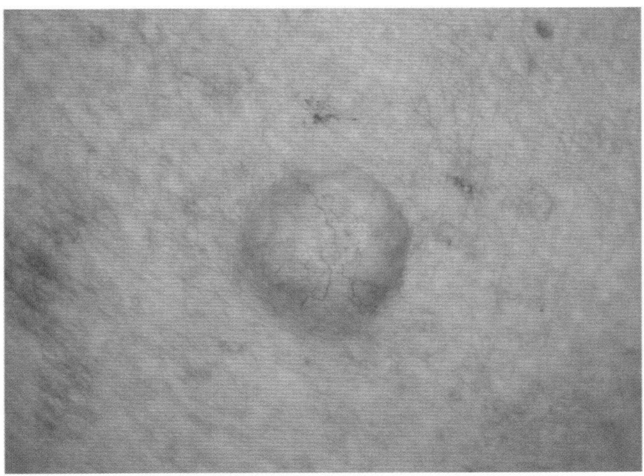

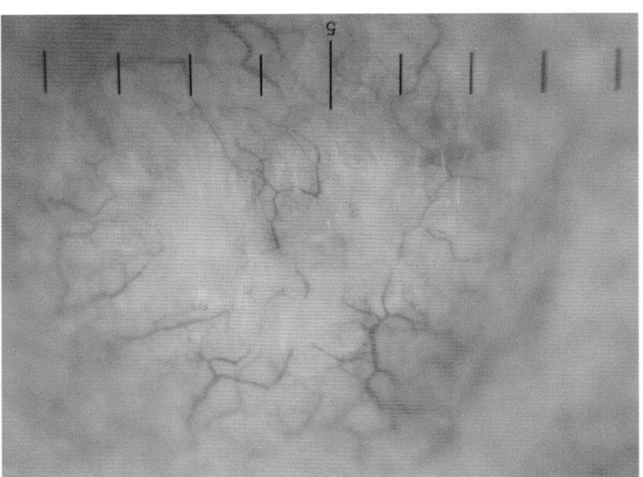

A cream-coloured cyst on the neck of a 70-year-old man: dermoscopy shows a background cream colour, branching linear vessels and shiny white structures in this histopathologically confirmed epidermoid cyst.

Send all excised cysts for histopathology to confirm the diagnosis. Avoid squeezing them as this will cause pain and inflammation on most occasions.

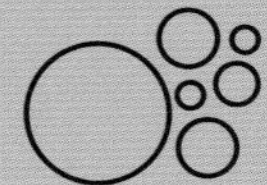

Pilomatricoma

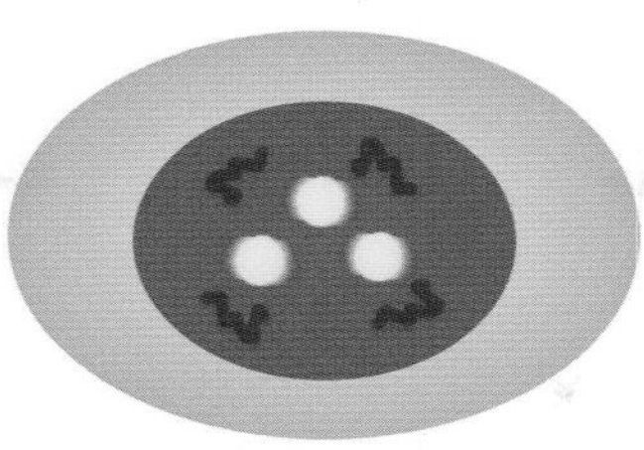

Pilomatricomas may share similar clinical and dermoscopic features with other adnexal skin lesions. Many features are non-specific and hence histopathology should always be considered.

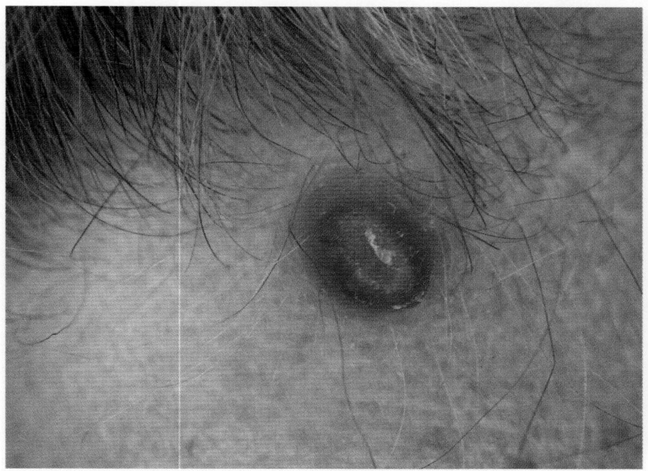

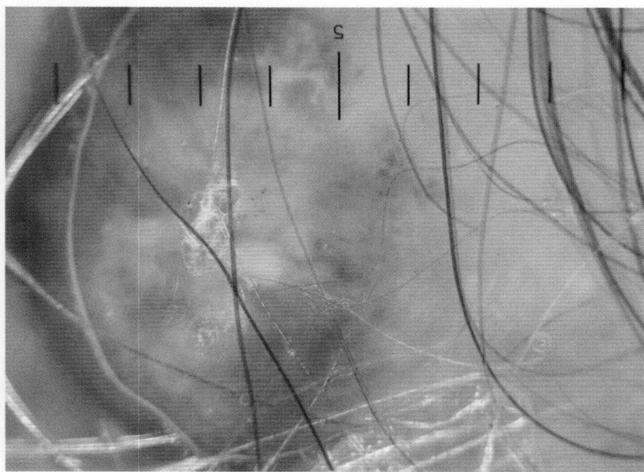

A solitary well-circumscribed erythematous cystic nodule on the forehead of a 70-year-old woman: dermoscopy shows erythema, haemorrhage, whitish structures and irregular vessels in this histopathologically confirmed pilomatricoma.

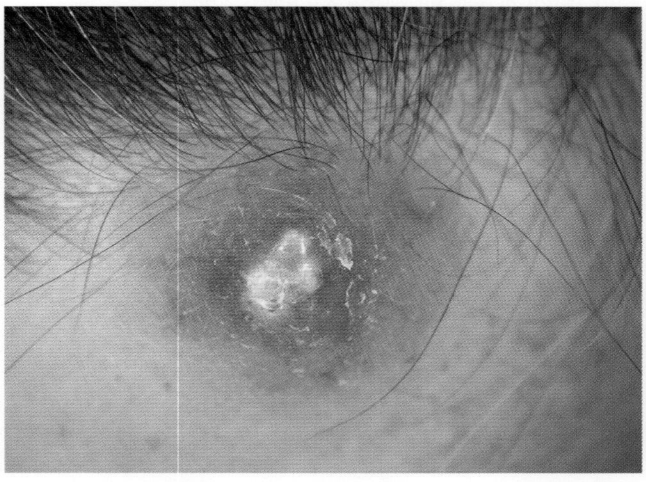

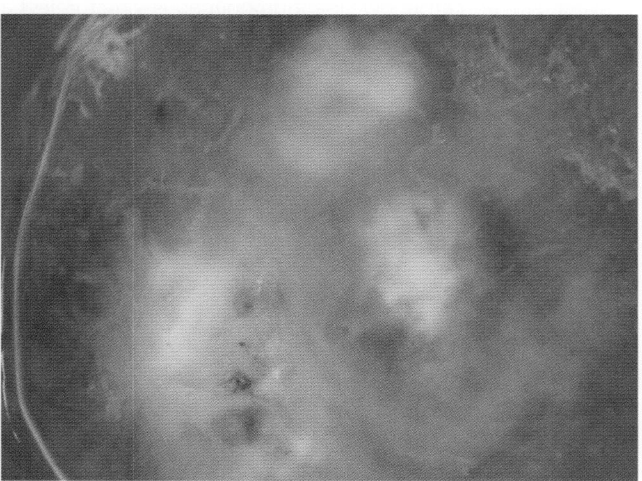

An enlarging erythematous cystic nodule on the forehead of a 60-year-old woman: dermoscopy shows erythema, haemorrhage, whitish structures, ulceration and irregular vessels in this histopathologically confirmed pilomatricoma.

Pilomatricomas are generally very firm.
Zaballos, P. et al. Dermoscopic findings of pilomatricomas. *Dermatology*. 2008;217(3):225–230.

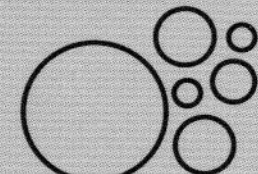

Sebaceous hyperplasia

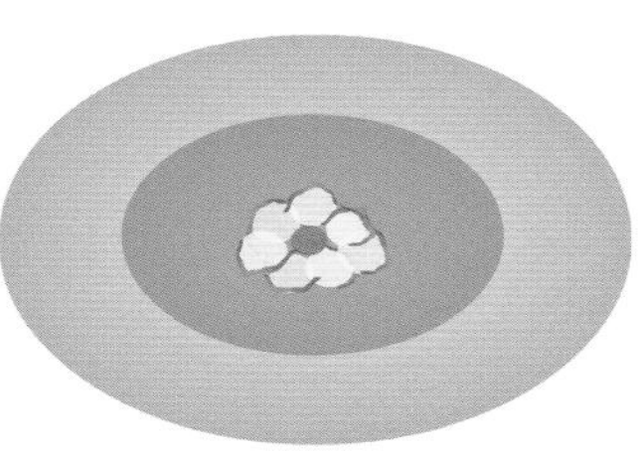

Sebaceous hyperplasia is a common facial lesion that presents as either solitary or, more commonly, multiple skin-coloured/yellow waxy plaques on the face and forehead with linear poorly focused vessels typically marking the periphery of the lesion. These vessels have been described as crown vessels. Sebaceous hyperplasia is often mistaken clinically for BCC.

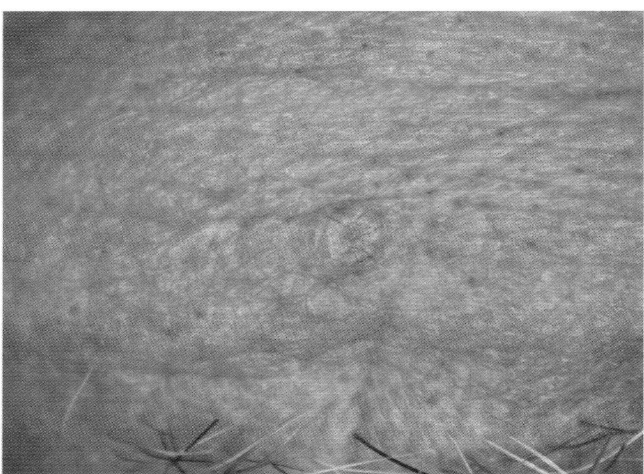

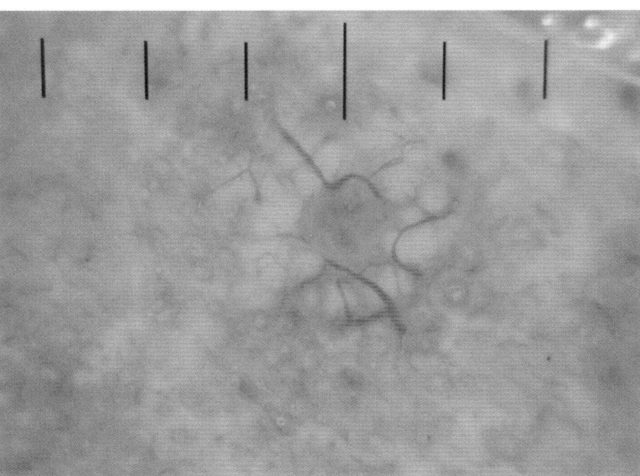

A 2 mm skin-coloured papule on the forehead of a 70-year-old man: dermoscopy shows multiple linear branching crown vessels flowing over and around yellow homogeneous structureless areas with a central pale brown structureless area.

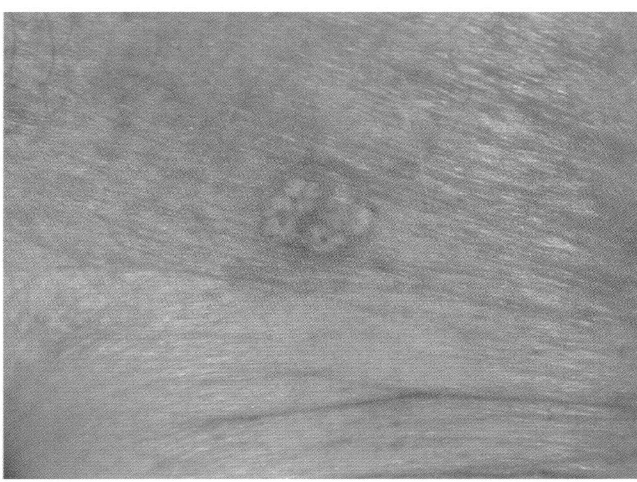

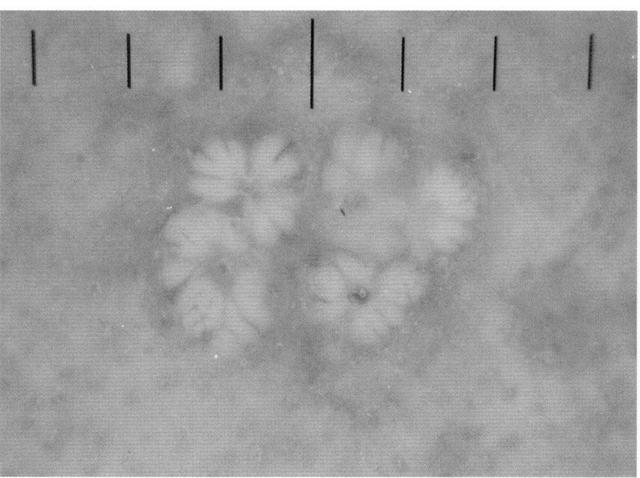

A yellow waxy skin-coloured pre-auricular papule in a 60-year-old woman: dermoscopy shows a cluster of yellow/white sebaceous gland aggregates each with a central comedo-like opening and small peripheral crown vessels.

Take a close look at sebaceous hyperplasia to ensure a BCC is not missed as both may be pearly and facial.

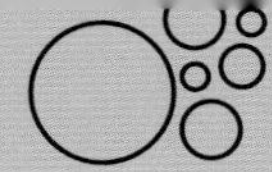

Sebaceous adenoma

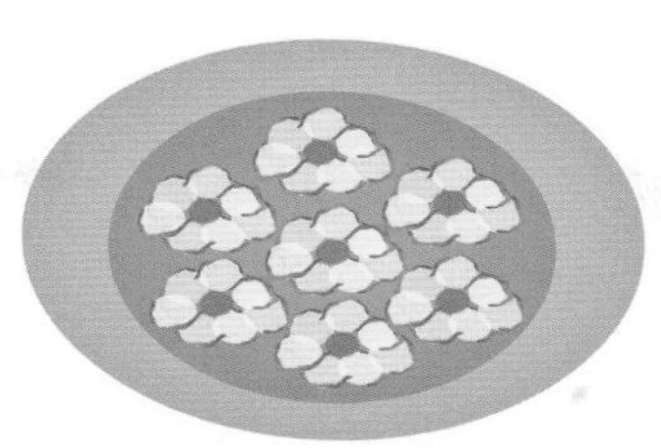

Sebaceous adenomas have the same components dermoscopically as sebaceous gland hyperplasia, namely yellowish sebaceous gland aggregates, comedo-like openings and peripheral curved linear vessels. However, they differ clinically due to the size of the lesion and are linked to Lynch syndrome. Clinically and dermoscopically there is an overlap between a small sebaceous adenoma and a large sebaceous hyperplasia, in which histopathology should be considered.

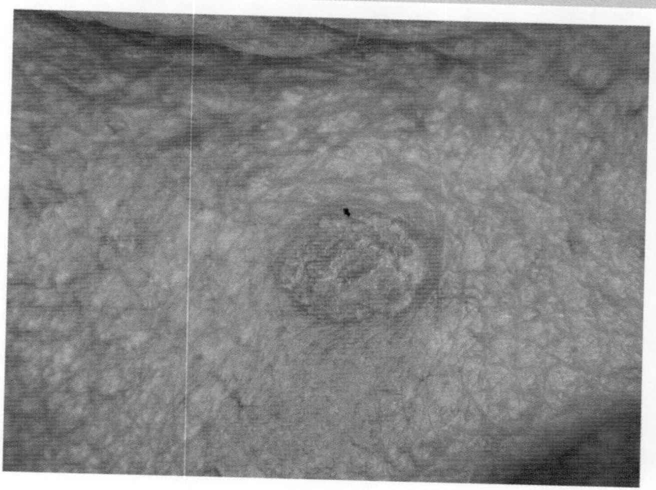

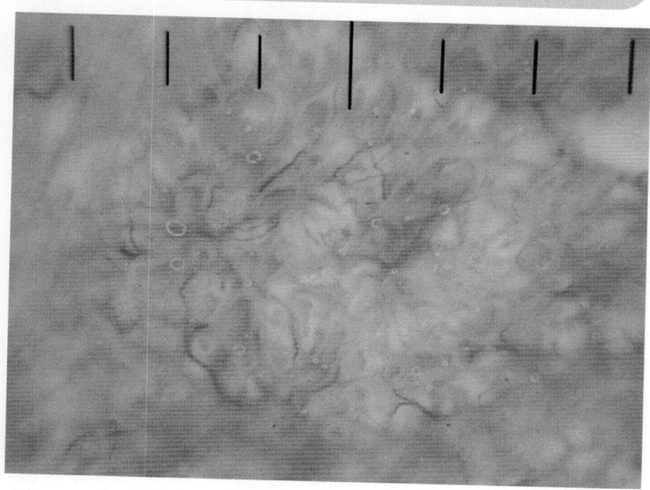

An 8 mm yellow waxy plaque on the cheek of a 70-year-old man: dermoscopy shows sebaceous gland aggregates, comedo-like openings and poorly focused linear branching and curved vessels in this histopathologically confirmed sebaceous adenoma.

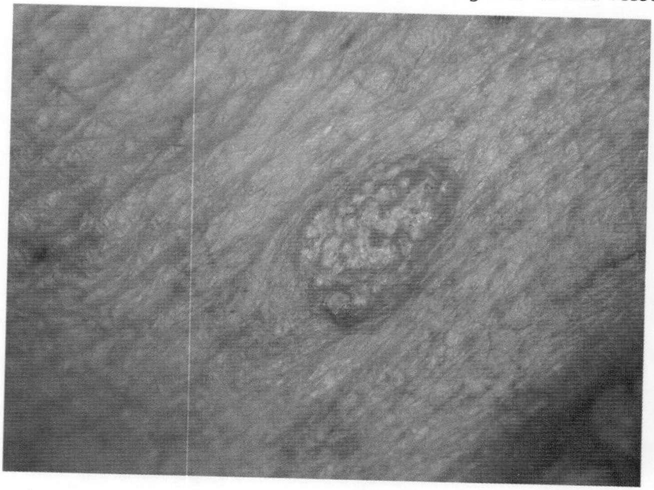

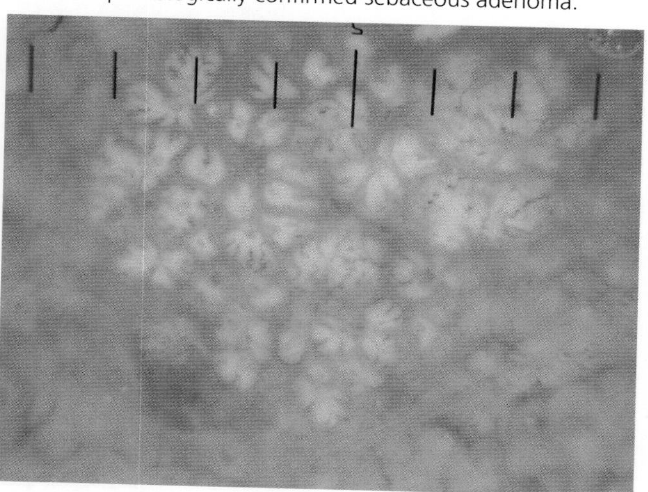

A large waxy yellow plaque on the medial cheek of a 60-year-old man: dermoscopy shows multiple yellow sebaceous gland aggregates and very small localised linear vessels in this histopathologically confirmed sebaceous adenoma.

Consider immunohistochemistry to identify DNA mismatch repair defects in sebaceous adenomas, particularly if there is any family history of colon cancer.

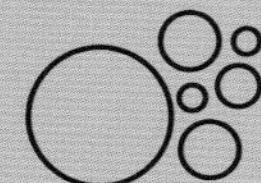

Sebaceous naevus

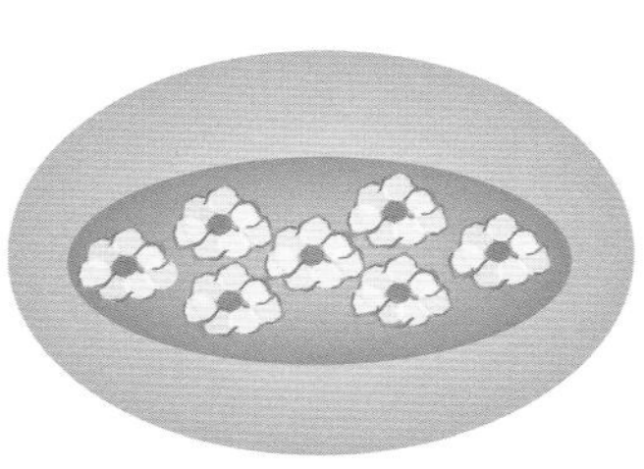

Sebaceous naevus is a congenital lesion that typically presents as a symptomatic yellow waxy plaque on the head or neck. It may increase in size during puberty, leading to cosmetic concern. Additionally, benign neoplasms may develop within them, including trichoepitheliomas and syringocystadenoma papilliferum. Rarely, BCC can arise in a nevus sebaceous.

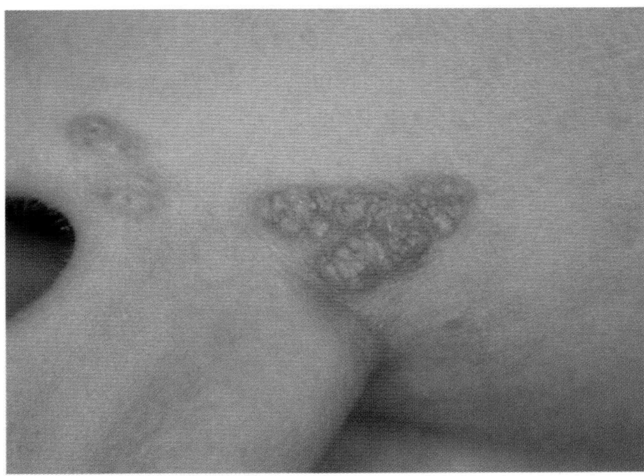

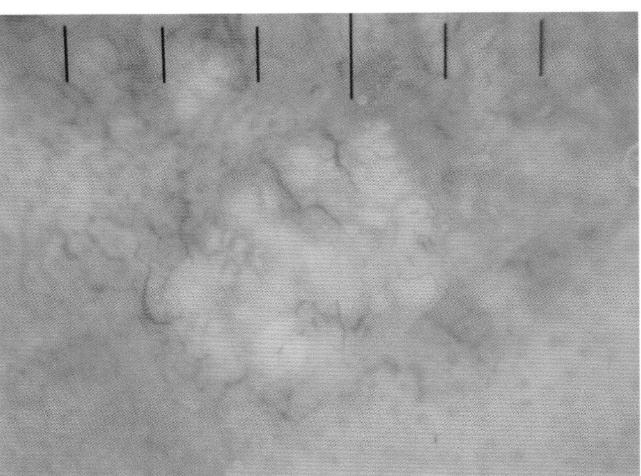

A multifocal waxy yellow pre-auricular plaque in a 14-year-old girl: dermoscopy shows multiple yellow sebaceous gland aggregates with branching poorly focused linear vessels in this histopathologically confirmed sebaceous naevus.

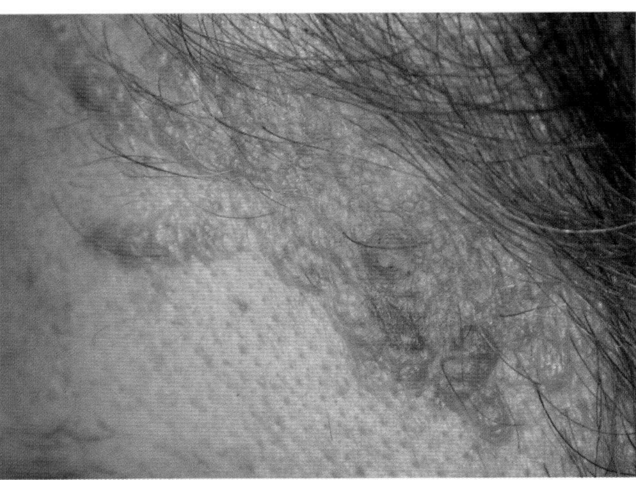

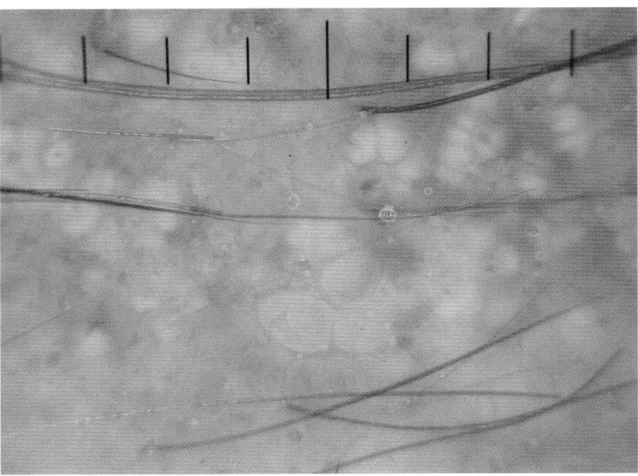

An orange-yellow waxy plaque on the temple of a 40-year-old man: dermoscopy shows discrete yellowish sebaceous gland aggregates outlined by crown vessels and surrounded by erythema in this histopathologically confirmed sebaceous naevus.

Take a close look at sebaceous naevus for signs of additional neoplasms.

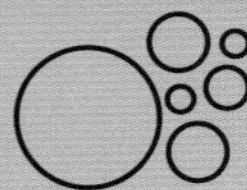

Malignant adnexal carcinomas

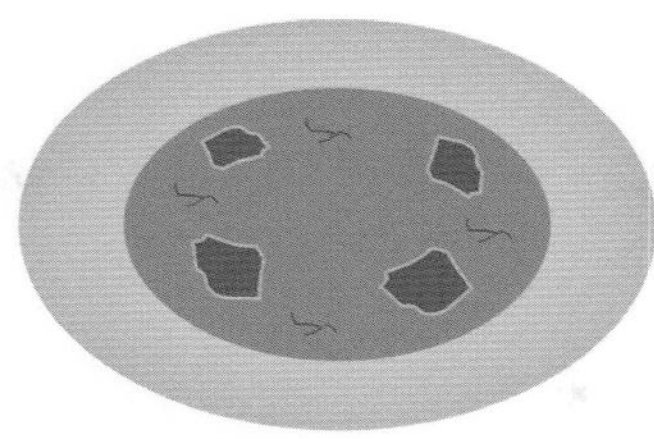

Malignant adnexal carcinomas are a group of rare tumours derived from skin appendages such as hair follicles, sebaceous glands or eccrine and apocrine sweat glands. A few examples are sebaceous carcinoma, commonly developing along the lid margin, or microcystic adnexal carcinoma, a sclerosing sweat duct tumour.

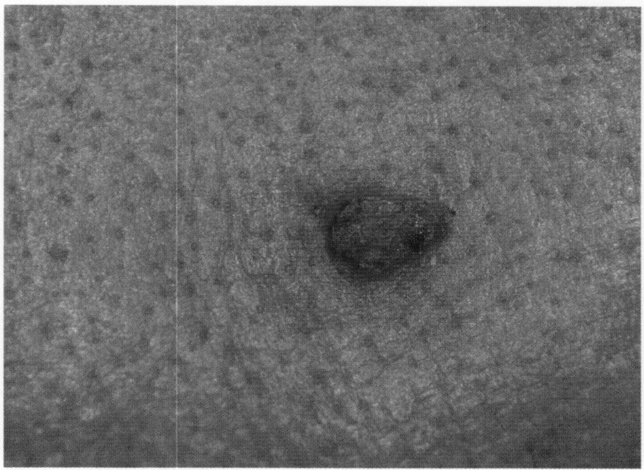

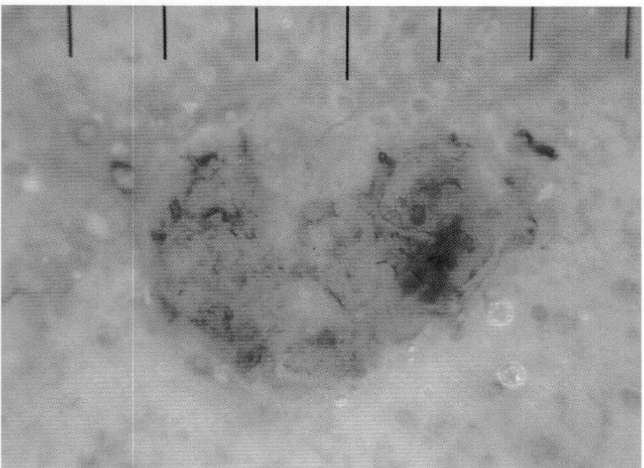

A 4 mm friable orange/yellow plaque on the forehead in a 40-year-old man: dermoscopy shows a background yellow-orange colour with haemorrhage, polymorphous vessels and ulceration in this sebaceous carcinoma.

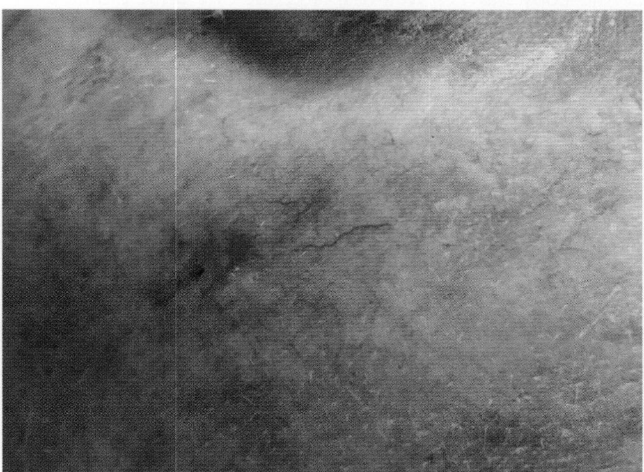

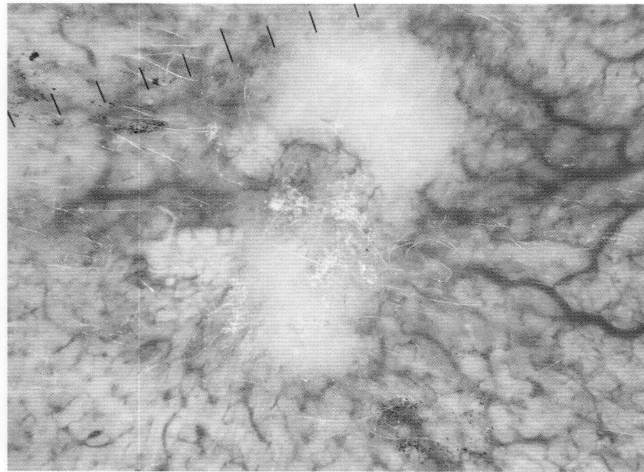

An 8 mm poorly demarcated sclerotic plaque on the cheek of a 55-year old woman: dermoscopy shows white sclerosis and linear branching vessels next to sebaceous gland aggregates surrounded by crown vessels in this microcystic adnexal carcinoma.

Coates, D. et al. Dermoscopic features of extraocular sebaceous carcinoma. *Australas J Dermatol*. 2011;52(3):212–213.

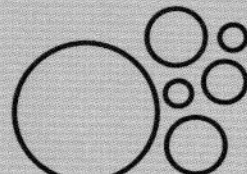

Juvenile xanthogranuloma

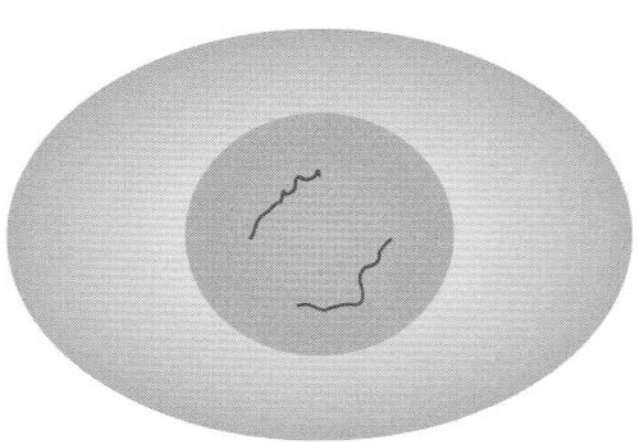

Juvenile xanthogranuloma (JXG) represent non-Langerhans cell proliferations that present typically as a solitary orange papule or nodule on the head and neck. They are rare and typically self-limiting in childhood while spontaneous resolution is less common when they present in adults. JXGs produce a combination of features on dermoscopy with a well-demarcated orange background reflecting granulomatous inflammation, with variable vessels reported.

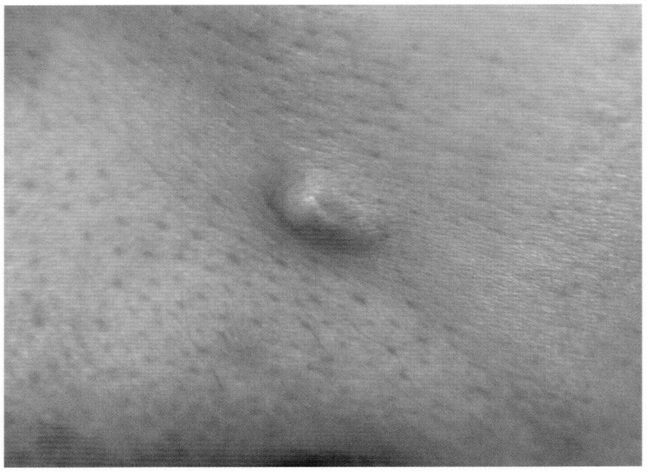

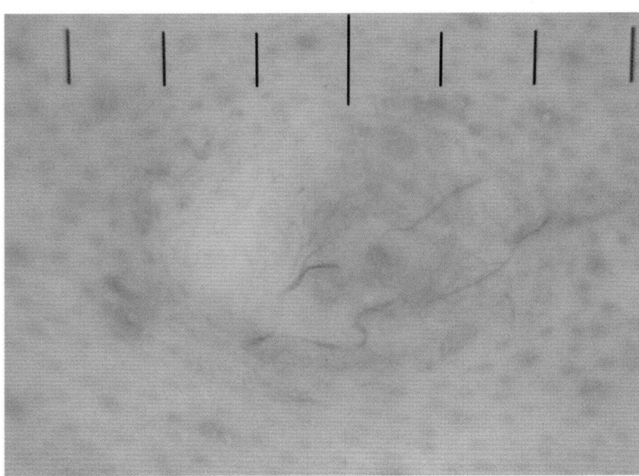

A new enlarging papule on the medial cheek of a 10-year-old girl: dermoscopy shows a well-defined zone of orange pigmentation with multiple fine linear vessels across its surface in this histopathologically confirmed JXG.

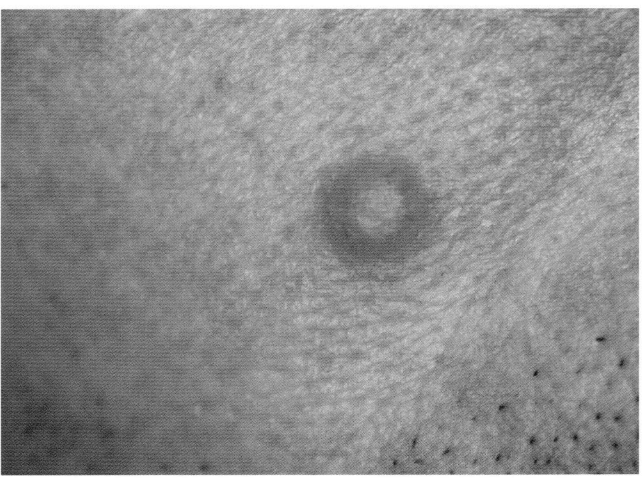

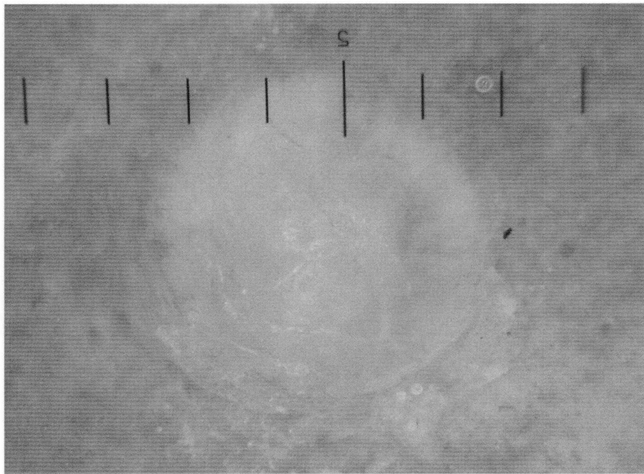

A new enlarging orange papule on the medial cheek of a 30-year-old man: dermoscopy shows a well-demarcated zone of orange pigmentation with multiple fine linear vessels across its surface in this histopathologically confirmed JXG.

Palmer, A. and Bowling, J. Dermoscopic appearance of juvenile xanthogranuloma. *Dermatology*. 2007;215(3):256–259.

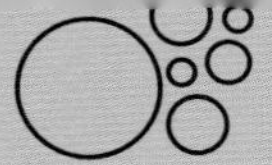

Granulomatous folliculitis

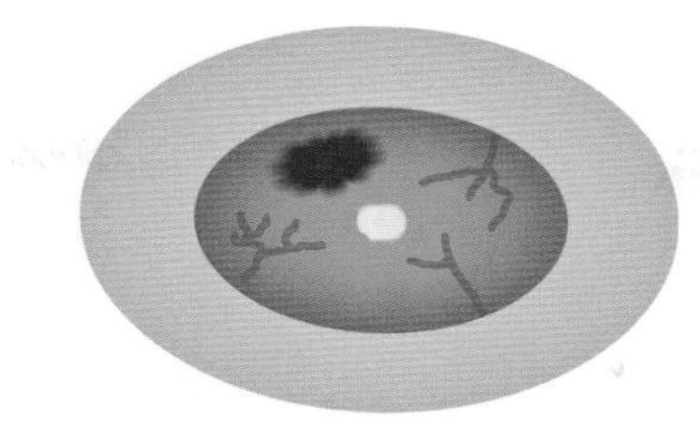

When acneiform lesions rupture within a follicle they cause a focal granulomatous reaction that can last months. Clinically, they can cause diagnostic uncertainty if solitary as the combination of telangiectasia and erythema can mimic BCC, adnexal tumours and other granulomatous conditions. The history in combination with background orange coloration indicate granulomatous inflammation. Sometimes residual yellow/white keratin or haemorrhagic blotches may be seen.

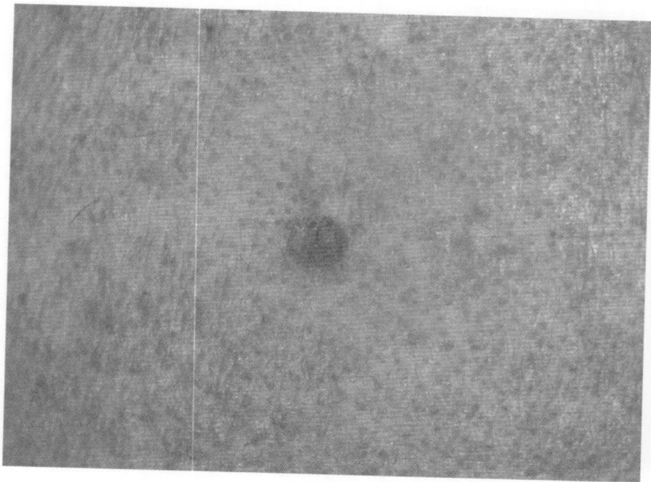

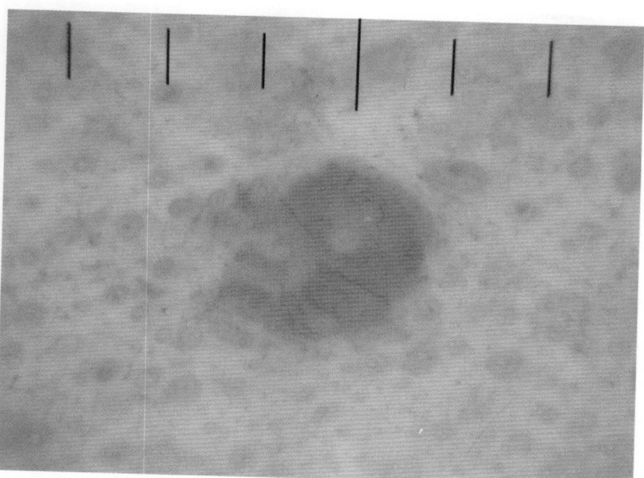

A well-circumscribed 4 mm orange dermal plaque on the forehead of a 35-year-old man mimicking a BCC: dermoscopy shows an orange-pink background and linear branching vessels in this histopathologically confirmed ruptured follicle.

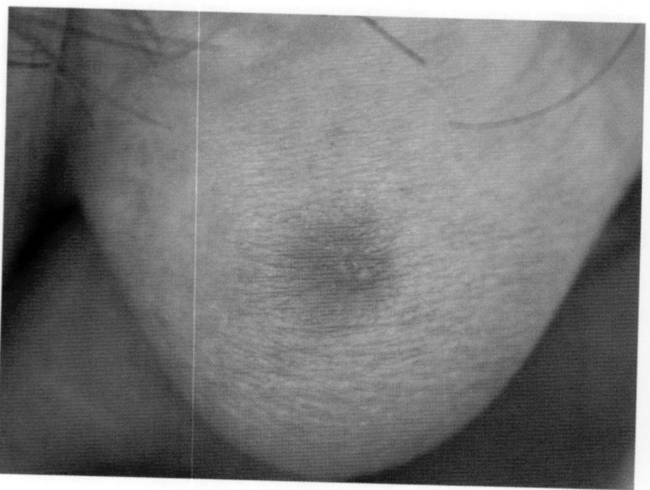

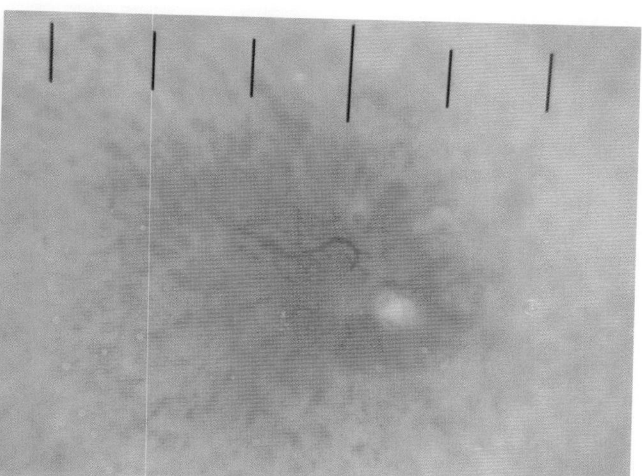

A telangiectatic inflamed plaque on the ear lobe of a 40-year-old woman: dermoscopy shows a background orange colour and multiple branching linear vessels, with a solitary whitish yellow structure (plugged follicle) in this ruptured follicle.

When assessing pink papulonodules on the head and neck, consider diagnostic biopsy if there is clinical uncertainty.

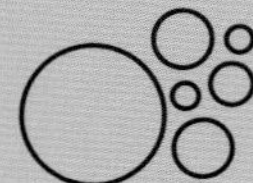

Fibrous papule

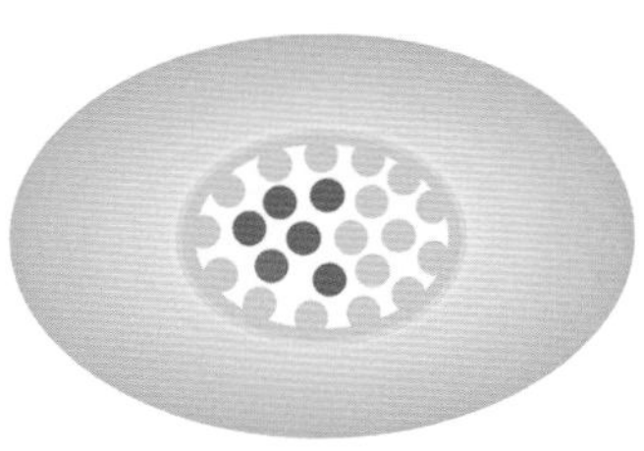

Fibrous papules of the face are a common cause of multiple monomorphic facial papules. They commonly occur on the nose but also across the face. Initially they present as an erythematous papule that tends to progress to form a scarred plaque. Dermoscopy shows dilated vessels during the initial phase, which on compression and blanching may show the evolving perifollicular depigmented fibrotic stroma. The scarring tends to wrap around follicles rather than destroy them.

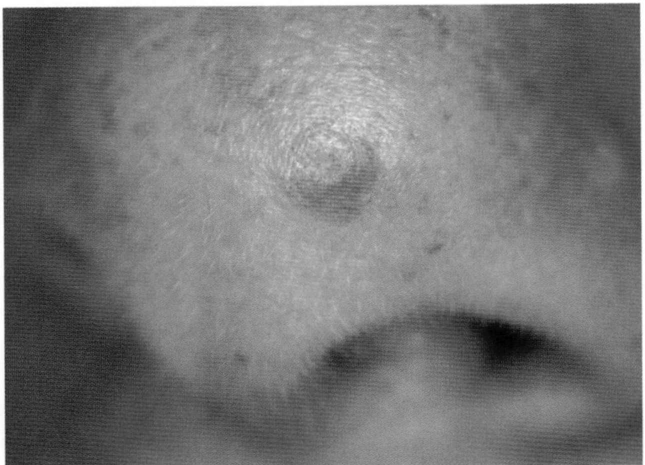

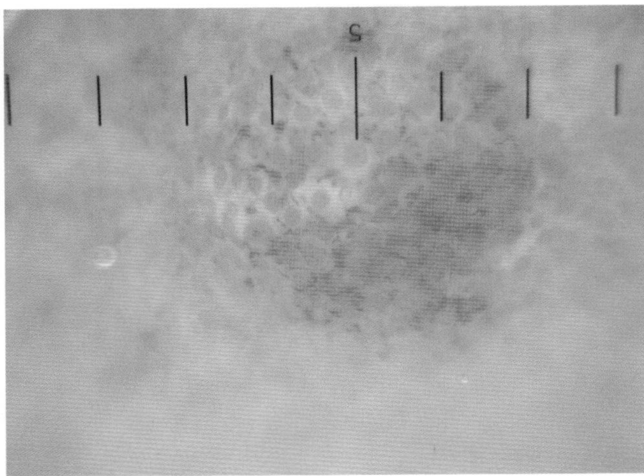

A pink papule on the nasal tip of a 40-year-old woman: dermoscopy shows short curvilinear vessels and perifollicular hypopigmentation indicating scarring in this fibrous papule of the nose.

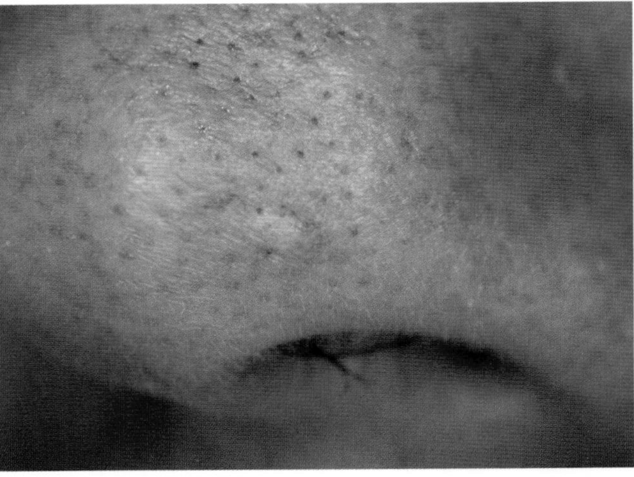

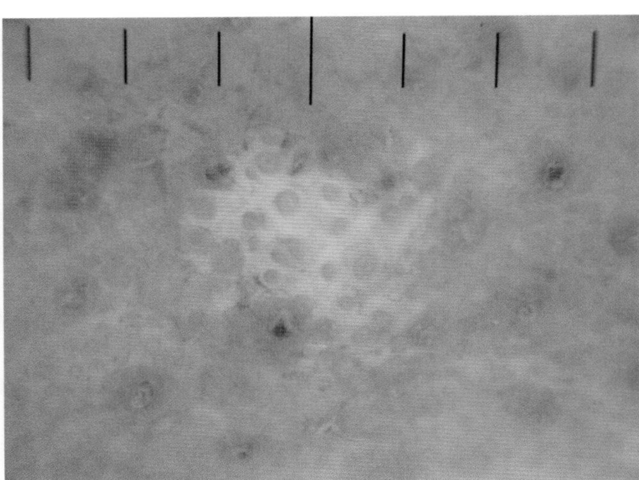

A hypopigmented scarred plaque on the nasal ala of a 60-year-old man: dermoscopy shows a zone of coalescing perifollicular hypopigmentation with no follicular destruction in keeping with fibrous papule of the nose.

If multiple, consider a biopsy to exclude/diagnose multiple fibrofolliculomas, a feature of the Birt–Hogg–Dubé syndrome.

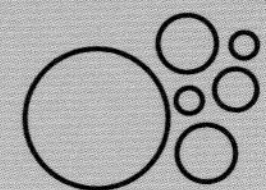

Trichilemmomas

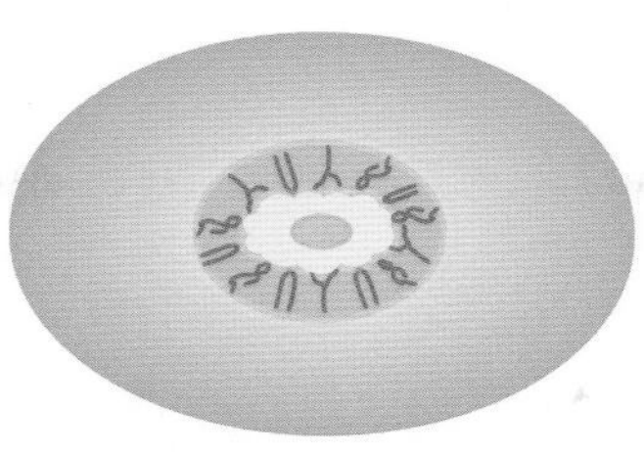

Trichilemmomas or tricholemmomas are rare benign adnexal tumours of the outer root sheath of the hair follicle. They may be sporadic or associated with Cowden syndrome. Dermoscopic features include central keratin, with whitish halos and radial linear vessels. Histopathology is required to confirm the diagnosis as they share clinical and dermoscopic features with other adnexal lesions, BCCs and benign lichenoid keratoses.

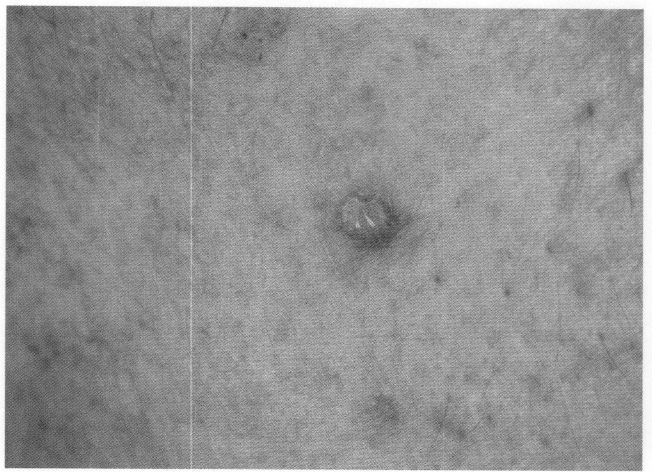

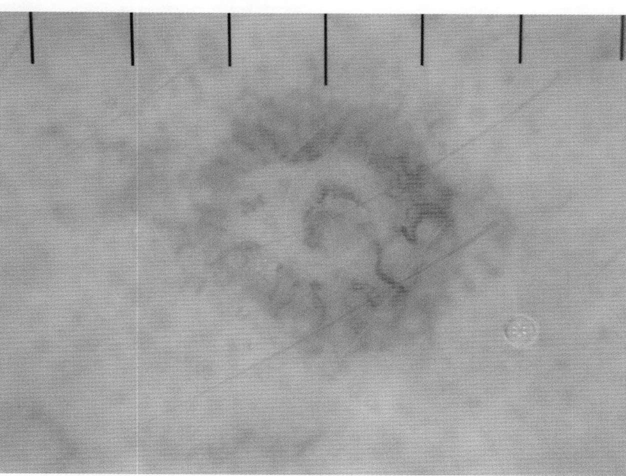

A pink papule on the cheek of a 60-year-old woman: dermoscopy shows a central scale surrounded by a whitish homogeneous area and peripheral radial linear blood vessels and erythema in this histopathologically confirmed trichilemmoma.

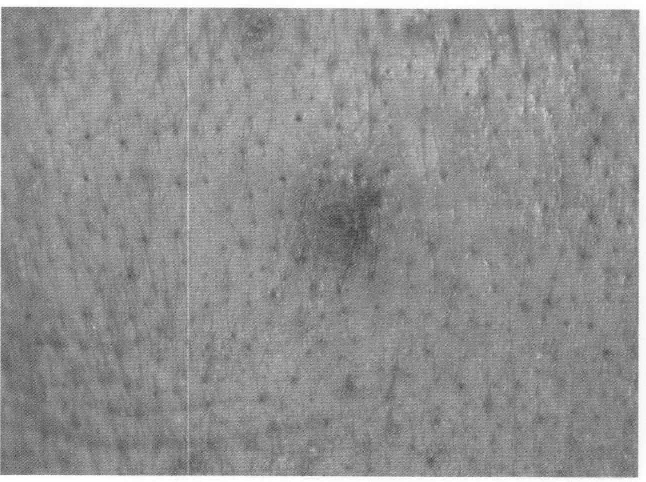

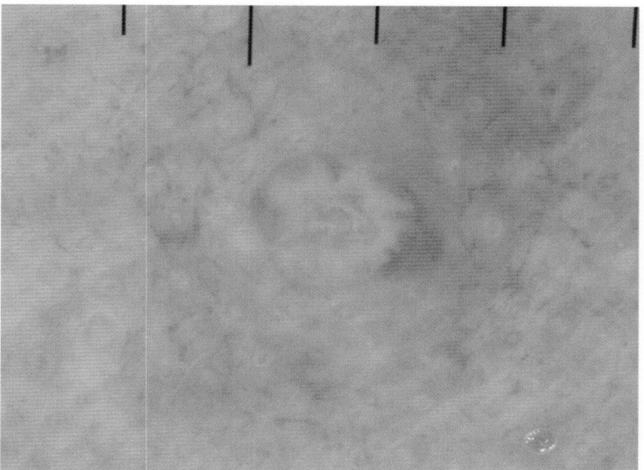

A pink papule on the forehead of a 55-year-old woman: dermoscopy shows central keratin with a surrounding whitish homogeneous area with peripheral erythema in this histopathologically confirmed trichilemmoma.

Horcajada-Reales, C. et al. Dermoscopic pattern in facial trichilemmomas: red iris-like structure. *J Am Acad Dermatol.* 2015;72(1 Suppl.):S30–32.

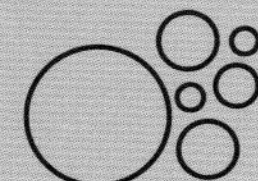

Dermal naevus

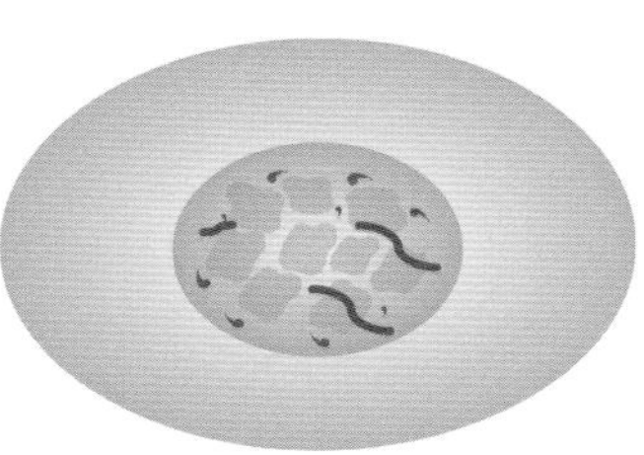

Facial dermal naevi are frequently skin-coloured with few dermoscopic features. Typically the vascular pattern comprises linear vessels, which are curved and flow in and out of focus. These short curved vessels have been described as comma-shaped. Pigmented structures of junctional naevi are absent, but pigment remnants of cobblestone morphology may be seen.

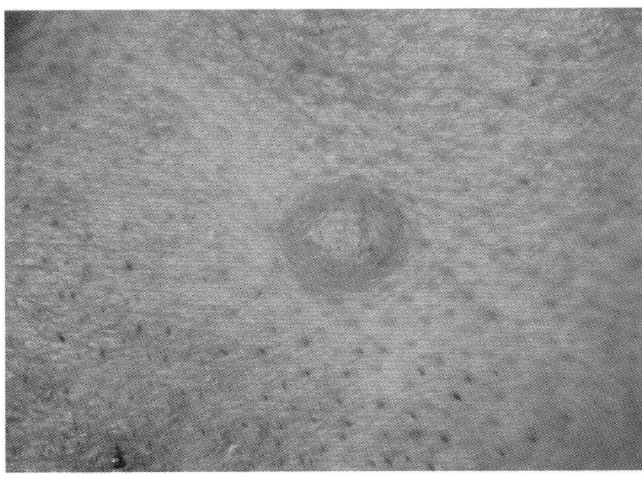

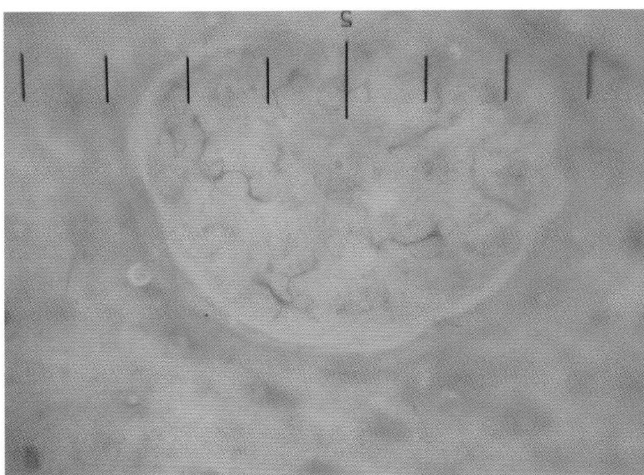

A skin-coloured papule on the melolabial sulcus of a 40-year-old man: dermoscopy shows multiple linear curved blood vessels flowing in and out of focus in this histopathologically confirmed dermal naevus.

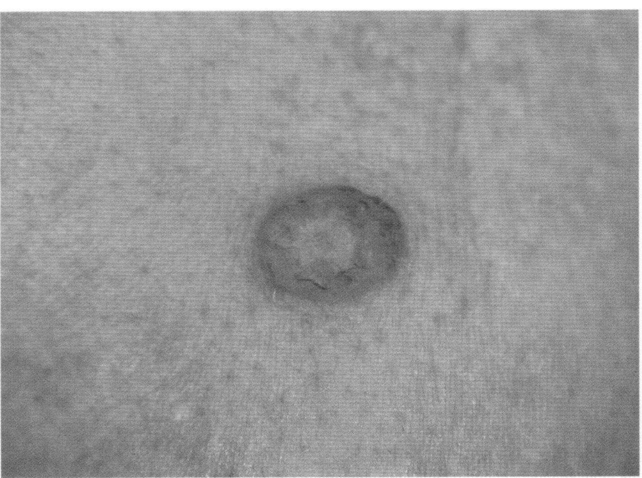

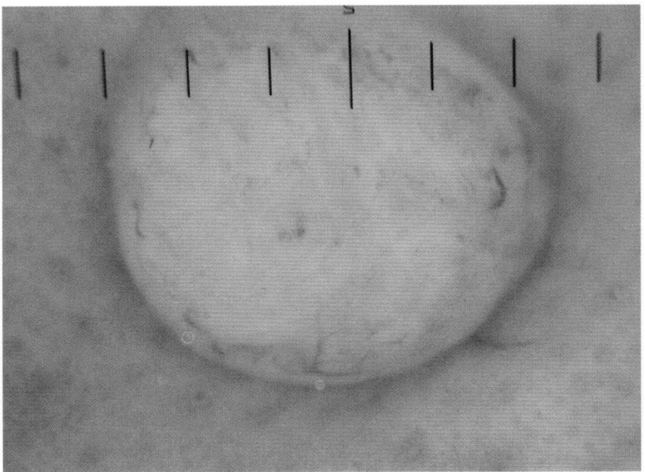

A skin-coloured papule on the forehead of a 50-year-old woman: dermoscopy shows few peripheral short curvilinear vessels (the central vessels are compressed) and minimal pigment remnants in this histopathologically confirmed dermal naevus.

Take a close look at any dermal naevi on the nose to ensure a BCC is not missed.

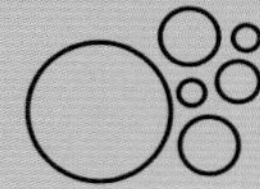

Dermal naevus cases

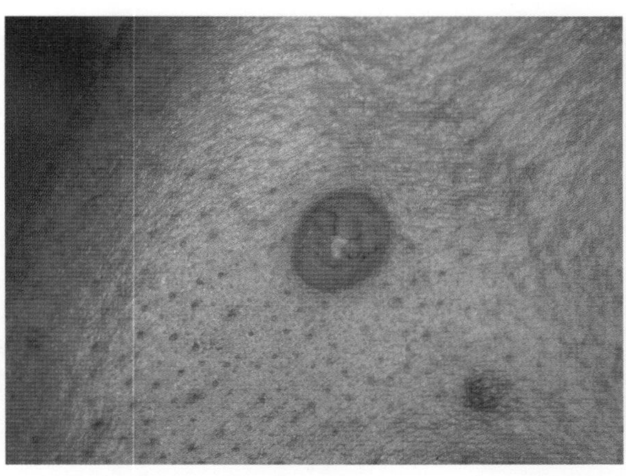

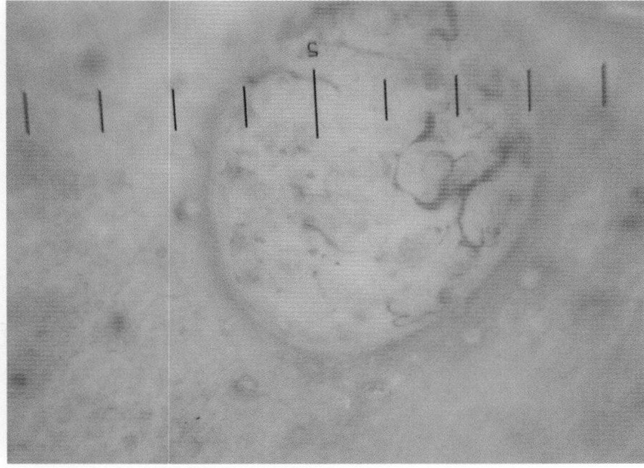

A skin-coloured papule with prominent vessels on the nasal sidewall of a 50-year-old man: dermoscopy shows poorly focused branching comma vessels and pigment remnants in this histopathologically confirmed dermal naevus.

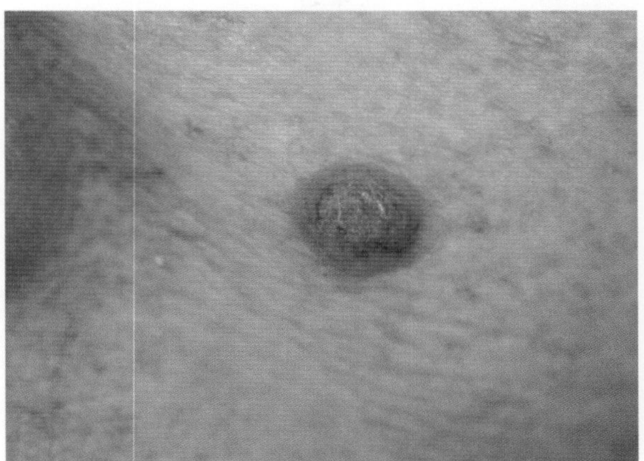

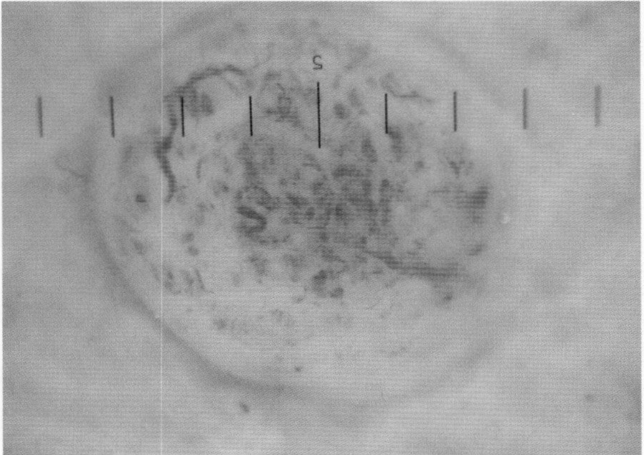

A lightly pigmented papule with prominent vessels on the melolabial sulcus of a 40-year-old woman: dermoscopy shows central cobblestone pigmented structures and peripheral branching comma vessels in this dermal naevus.

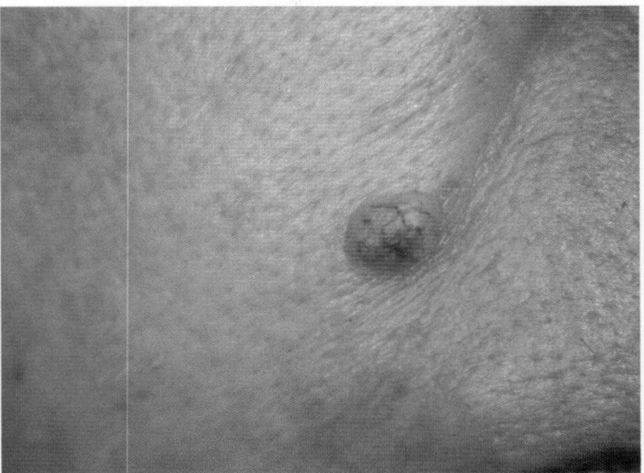

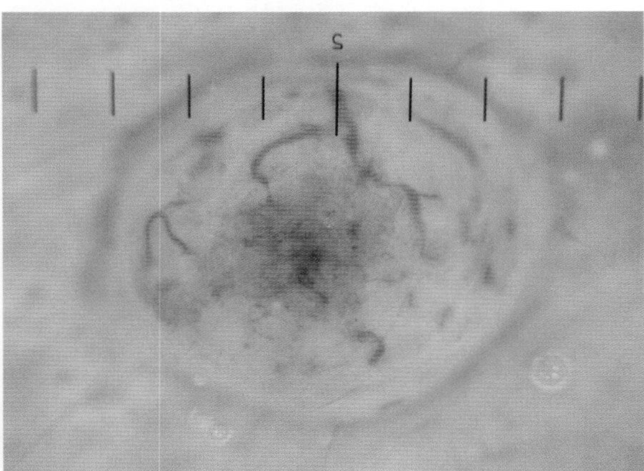

A lightly pigmented papule with prominent vessels on the melolabial sulcus of a 50-year-old woman: dermoscopy shows central brown pigment remnants and peripheral comma vessels in this dermal naevus.

Dermal naevi may show minimal pigmentation; applying pressure to occlude the vascular component may help to illustrate any background pigmented structures to aid diagnosis.

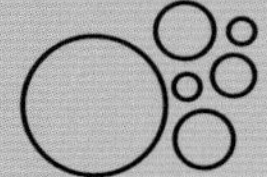

Solar lentigo – fingerprinting

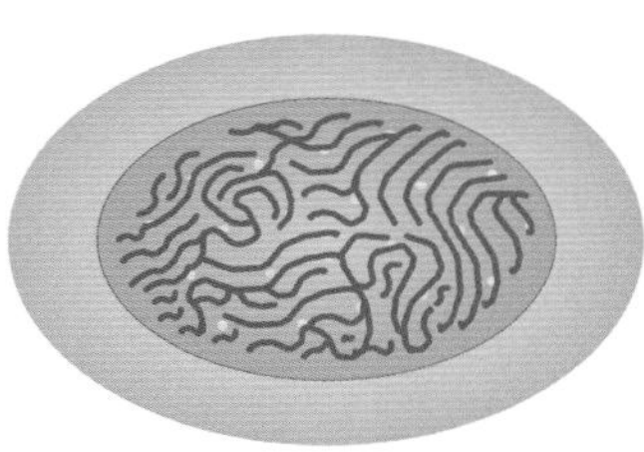

Facial solar lentigines may develop a pigmented pattern composed predominantly of short lines and circles, giving the appearance of fingerprinting. The short lines tend to run parallel to each other and curve around or radiate towards the brown circles of follicular apertures. In contrast to lentigo maligna, solar lentigines typically have a clear-cut peripheral margin with moth-eaten borders, uniform brown colour and symmetry of pigmentation around follicles.

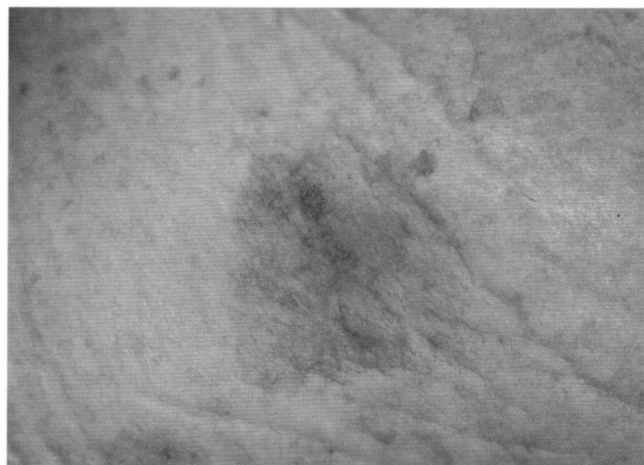

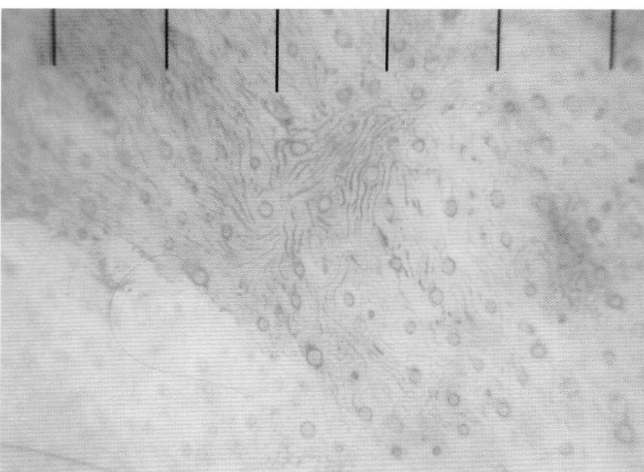

A large pigmented macule on the jawline of an 80-year-old woman: dermoscopy shows brown short parallel lines and brown circles, creating a fingerprint pattern in addition to a well-defined peripheral moth-eaten border in this solar lentigo.

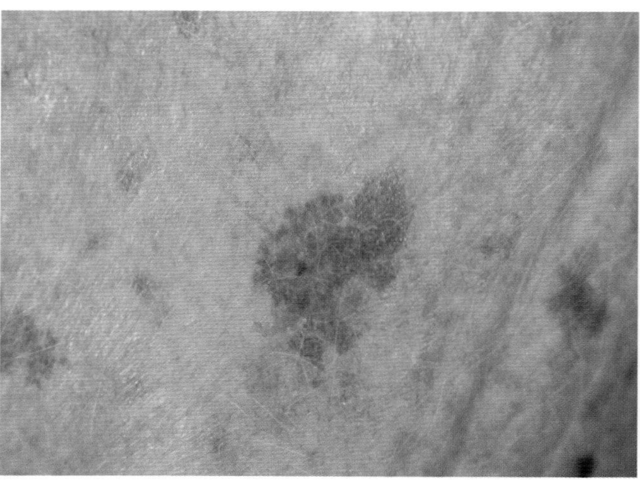

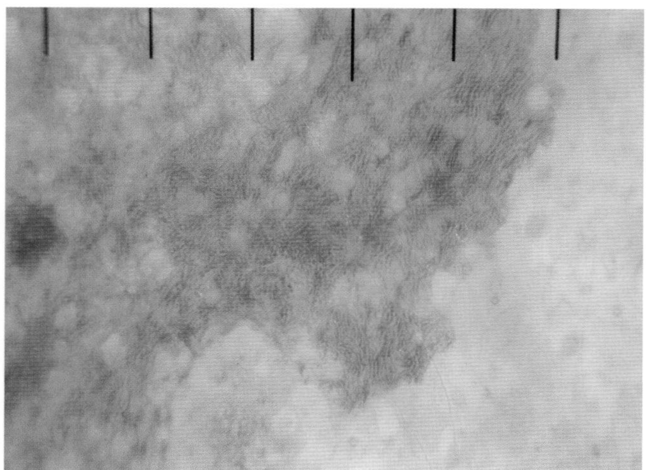

A large pigmented macule on the cheek of another 80-year-old woman: dermoscopy shows parallel and branching brown lines radiating towards and delineating the follicular apertures and a well-defined peripheral moth-eaten border.

Solar lentigines may show combinations of patterns of pigmentation composed of short brown lines and circles, including reticular and fingerprinting.

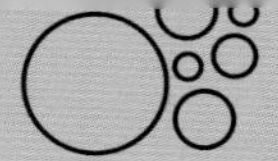

Solar lentigo – homogeneous pigmentation

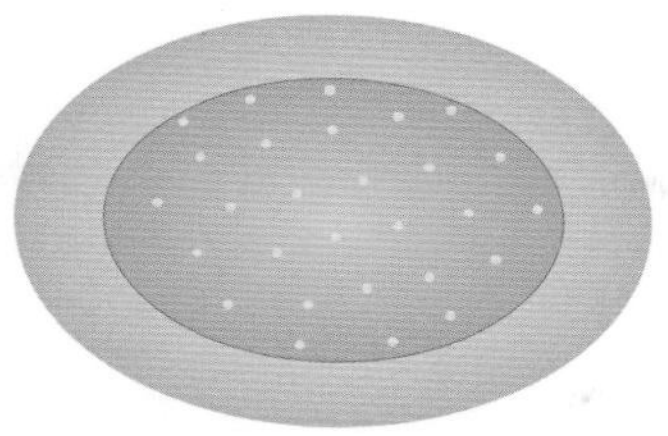

Closer inspection of solar lentigines on dermoscopy can show uniform tan pigmentation with multiple foci of perifollicular hypopigmentation and fragmentation of pigmentation at the peripheral border. In contrast, lentigo maligna typically has more variable colouration and asymmetrical perifollicular pigmentation.

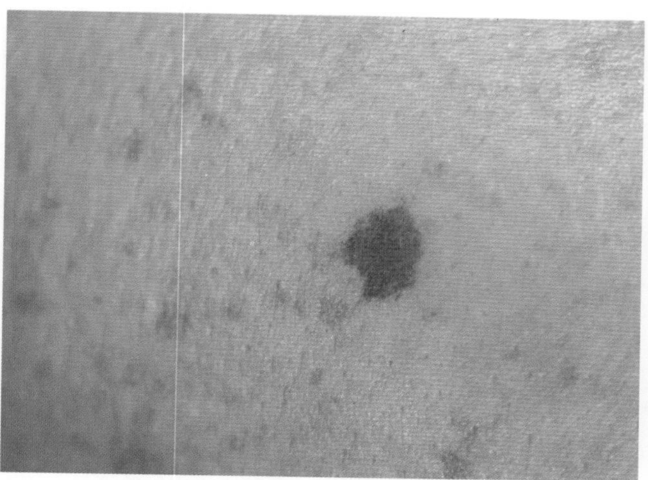

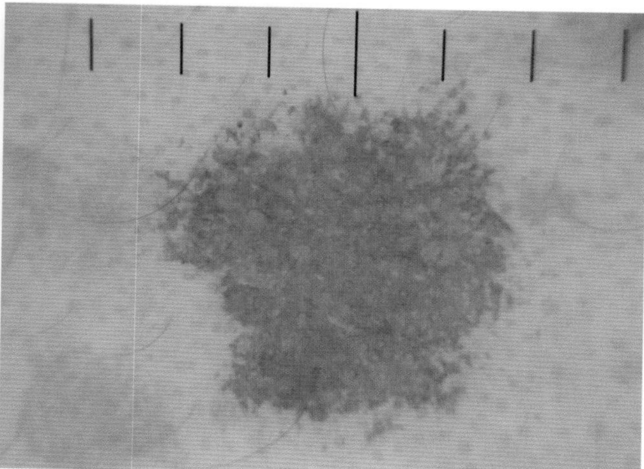

A pigmented macule on the zygoma of a 70-year-old woman: dermoscopy shows homogeneous tan pigmentation with regular reduced pigmentation at the follicular aperture and peripheral fragmentation of pigmentation in this solar lentigo.

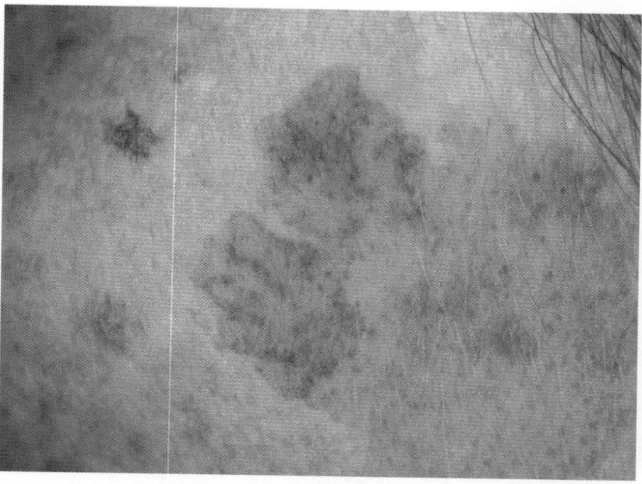

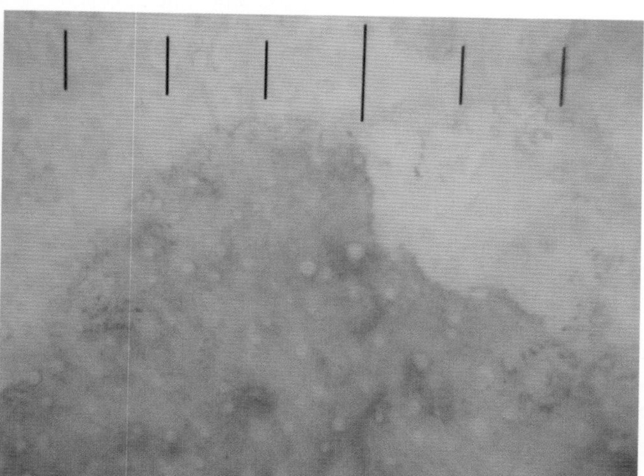

A large pigmented patch on the lateral cheek of an 80-year-old woman: dermoscopy shows homogeneous tan coloration with multiple foci of hypopigmentation around adnexal openings, in addition to a well-defined peripheral border.

The peripheral margin of solar lentigines may show 'fragmented' islands of pigmentation corresponding to the evolving clinical nature of these lesions.

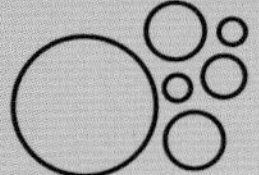

Solar lentigo – moth-eaten border

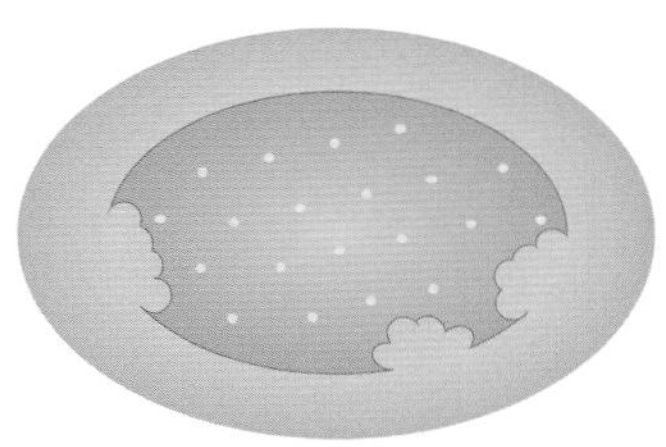

Closer inspection of solar lentigines on dermoscopy can show uniform tan pigmentation with multiple foci of perifollicular hypopigmentation with or without hairs and a well-defined 'moth-eaten' peripheral border. Lentigo maligna, on the other hand, typically presents with an ill-defined peripheral margin.

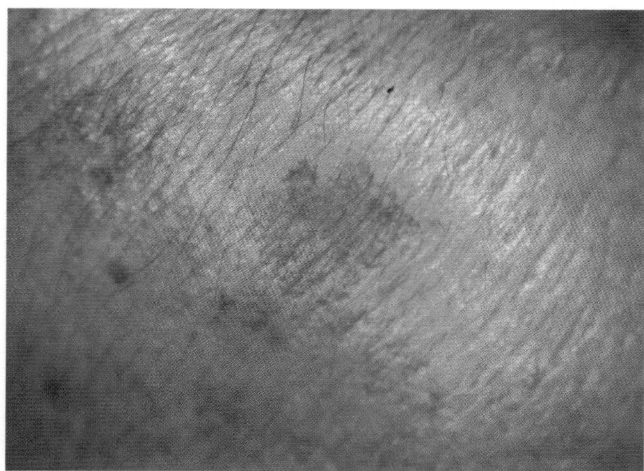

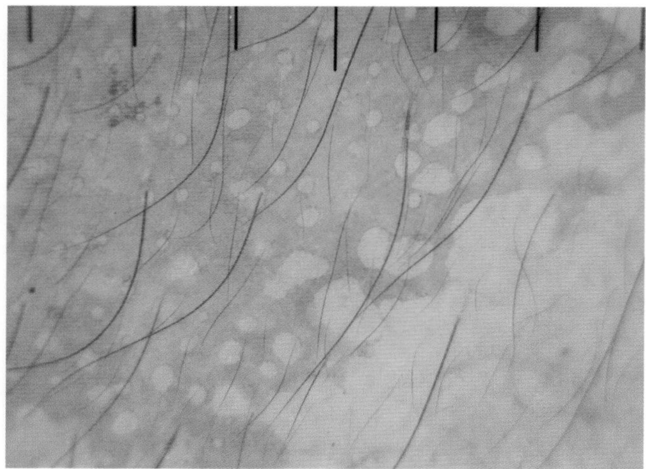

A pigmented macule on the zygoma of a 65-year-old woman: dermoscopy shows homogeneous tan pigmentation with uniform pigmentation around the follicles and a peripheral well-defined moth-eaten border in this solar lentigo.

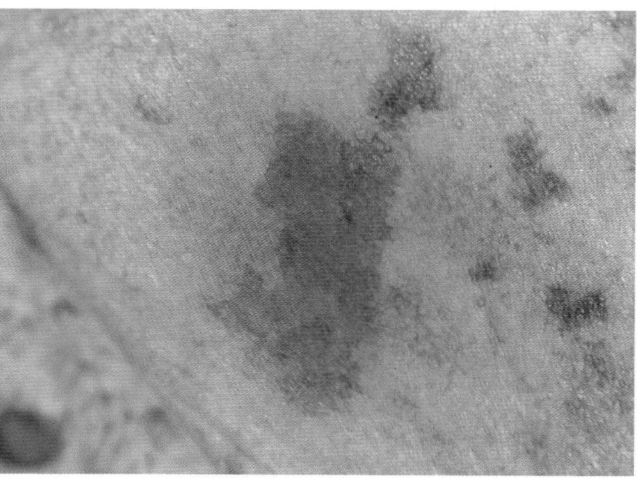

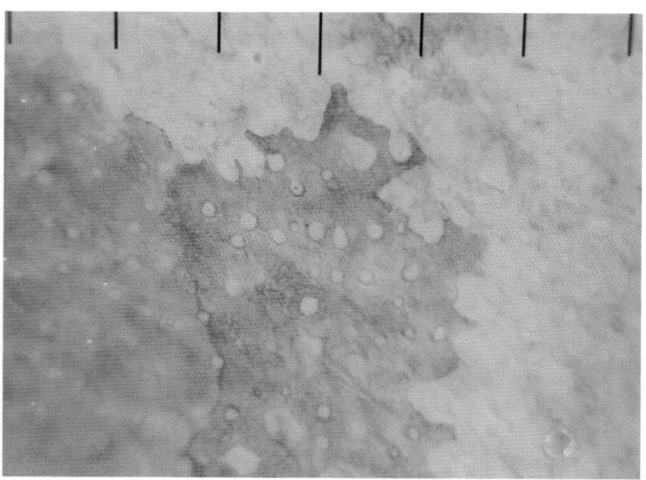

A large pigmented macule on the medial cheek of a 70-year-old woman: dermoscopy shows homogeneous tan coloration, early fingerprinting and a scalloped moth-eaten peripheral border in this solar lentigo.

Lallas, A. et al. Diagnosis and management of facial pigmented macules. *Clin Dermatol*. 2014;32(1):94–100.

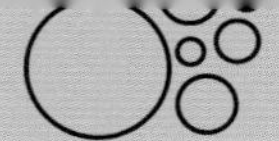

Ink spot lentigo

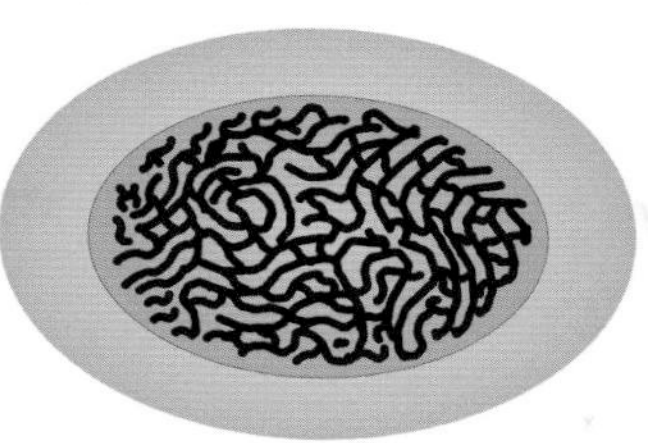

Ink spot lentigines on the face share similar dermoscopic features with solar lentigines though they may cause diagnostic uncertainty due to hyperpigmentation. The peripheral margin may show discohesion or fragmentation of pigmentation. In the Carney complex, multiple ink spot lentigines may be seen involving the conjunctiva and mucosae.

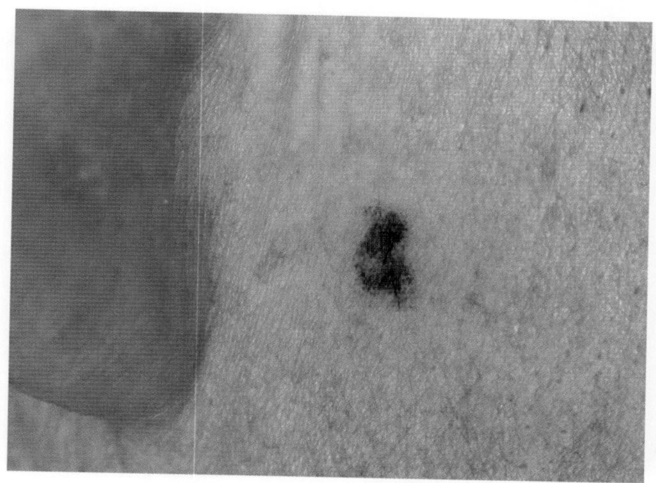

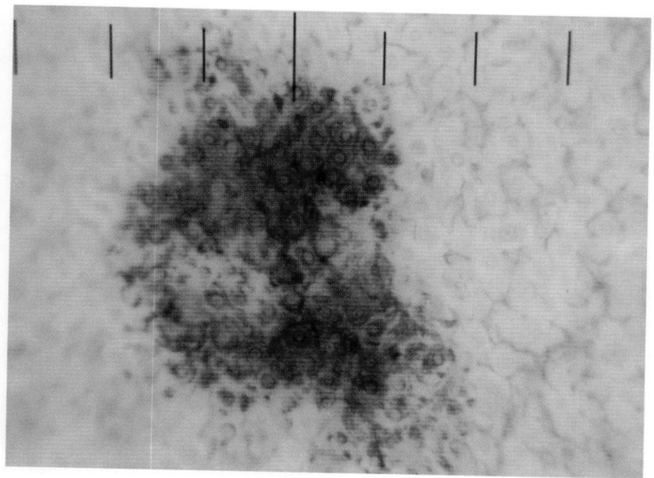

A hyperpigmented macule on the cheek of a 60-year-old woman: dermoscopy shows hyperpigmented concentric perifollicular circles and a peripheral clear-cut margin with multiple fragmented foci of pigmentation in this histopathologically confirmed ink spot lentigo.

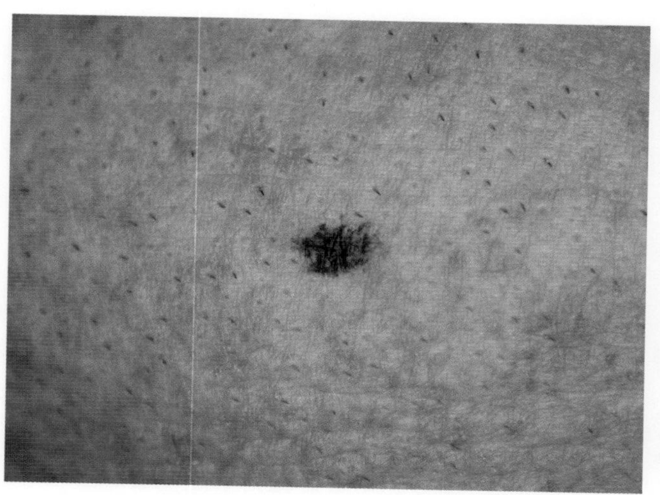

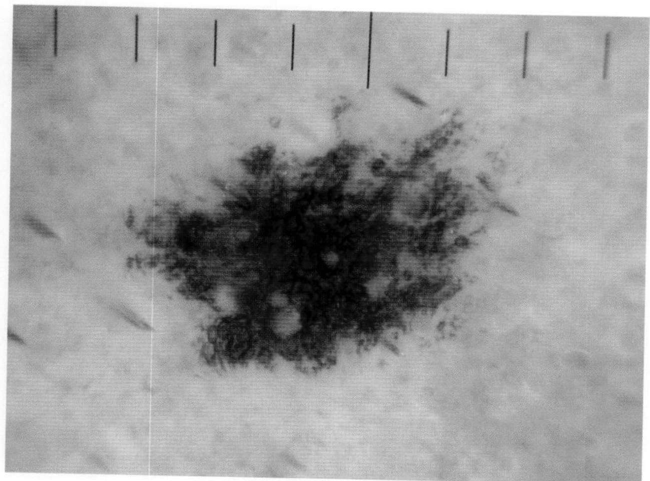

A well-defined hyperpigmented macule on the cheek of a 60-year-old man: dermoscopy shows perifollicular hyperpigmentation, pigmented circles and a clear-cut fragmented peripheral margin in this histopathologically confirmed ink spot lentigo.

Consider a diagnostic biopsy if there is any concern.

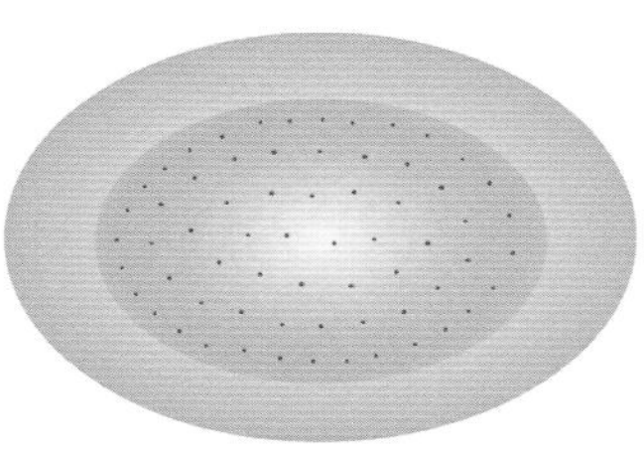

A benign lichenoid keratosis (lichen-planus like keratosis) commonly presents as a changing skin lesion with inflammation/ regression developing in a seborrhoeic keratosis or solar lentigo. This focal change can cause diagnostic uncertainty as the mixture of pigmentation and inflammation can make diagnosis at an early phase difficult. Importantly, during the inflammatory phase the area of inflammation is located at the footprint of the pre-existing skin lesion.

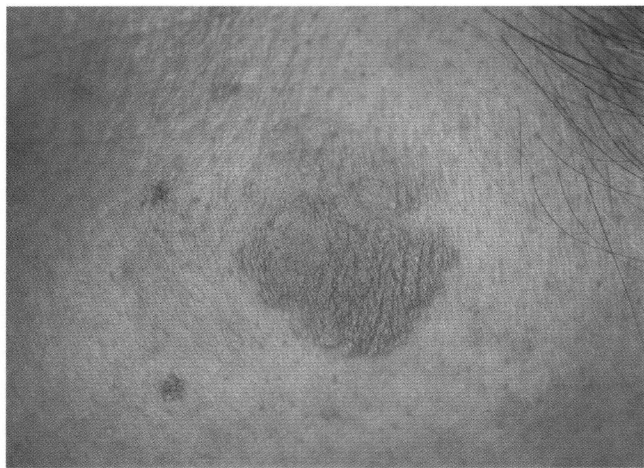

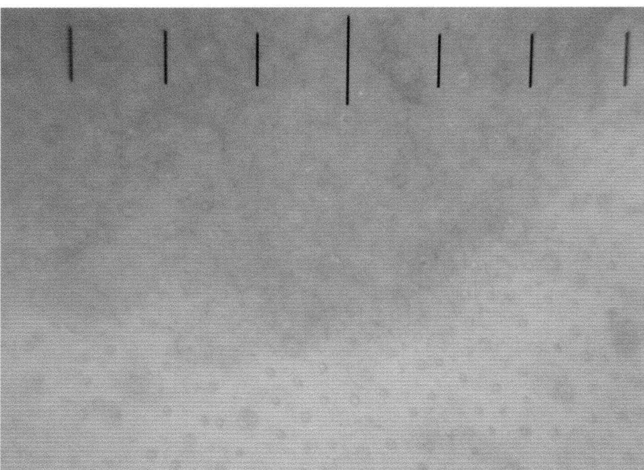

A large flat seborrhoeic keratosis on the zygoma of a 60-year-old woman with a recent onset of inflammation: dermoscopy shows homogeneous tan and pink colouration with clear demarcation in the inflammatory phase of benign lichenoid keratosis.

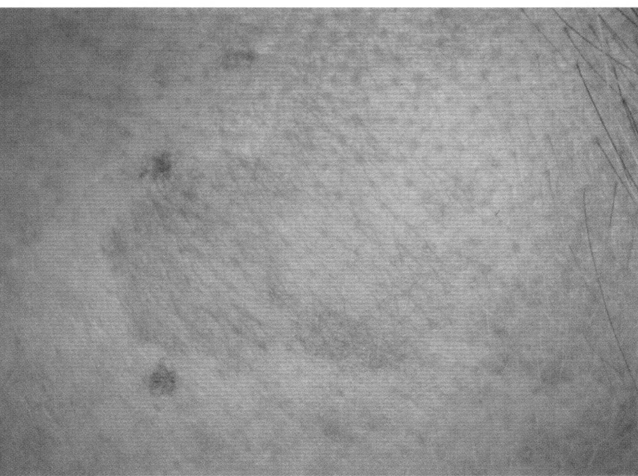

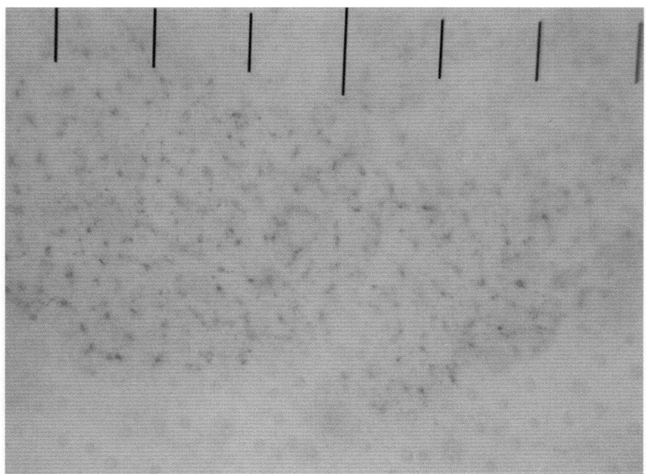

The same lesion two months later following topical steroid application shows resolution of the inflammatory component: dermoscopy shows granular grey pigmentation in keeping with post-lichenoid inflammation pigmentation.

Consider a diagnostic biopsy if the diagnosis is in doubt.

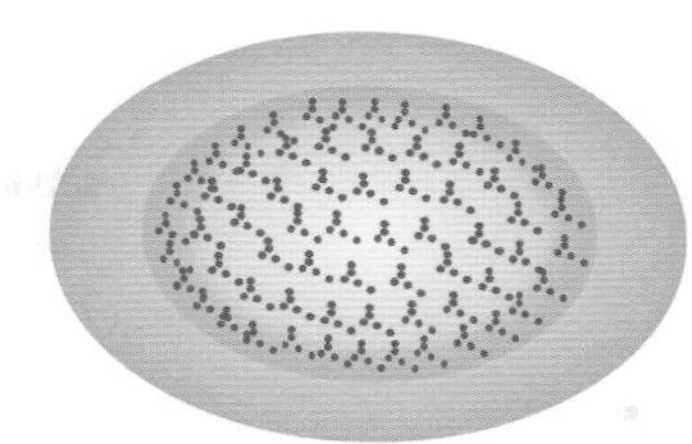

Once the inflammatory phase has passed the post-inflammatory pigmentation of a benign lichenoid keratosis can be clearly seen. The pigmentation is uniform in density and evenly scattered across the lesion. In addition to the history and clinical examination, three dermoscopic features help to differentiate between a benign lichenoid keratosis from lentigo maligna: uniform grey granular pigmentation, symmetry of pigmentation around the follicles and a well-defined peripheral margin.

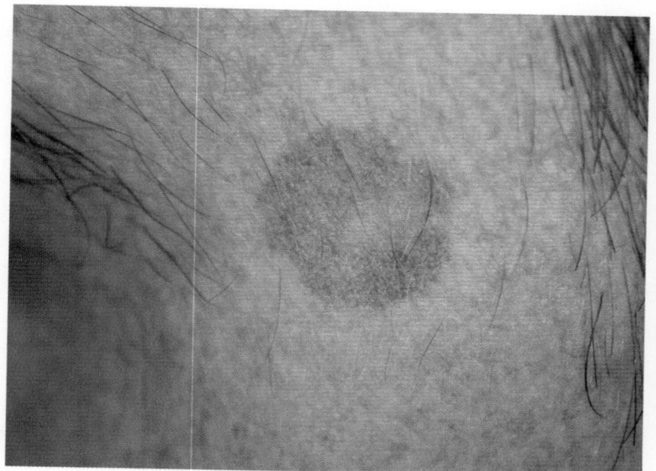

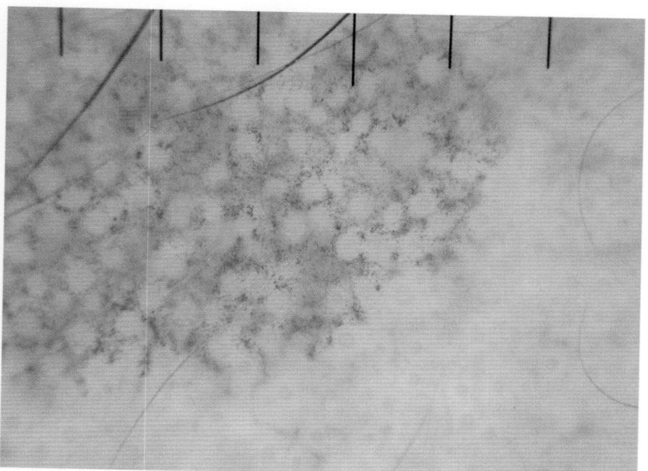

A grey pigmented macule on the temple of a 45-year-old man: dermoscopy shows uniform grey granular perifollicular pigmentation, a well-defined peripheral margin and poorly focused dilated background vessels.

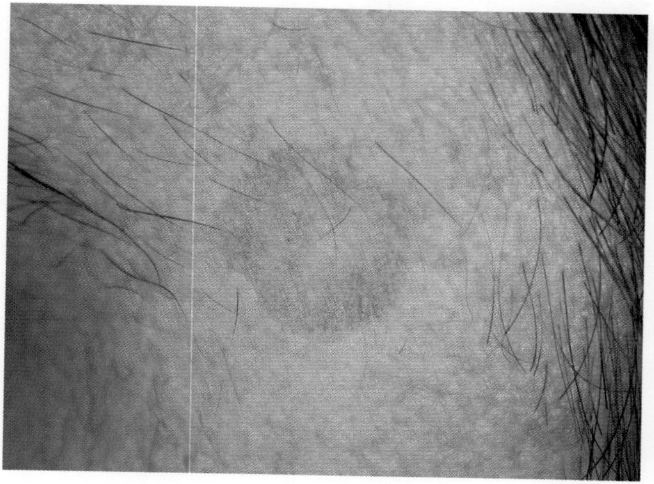

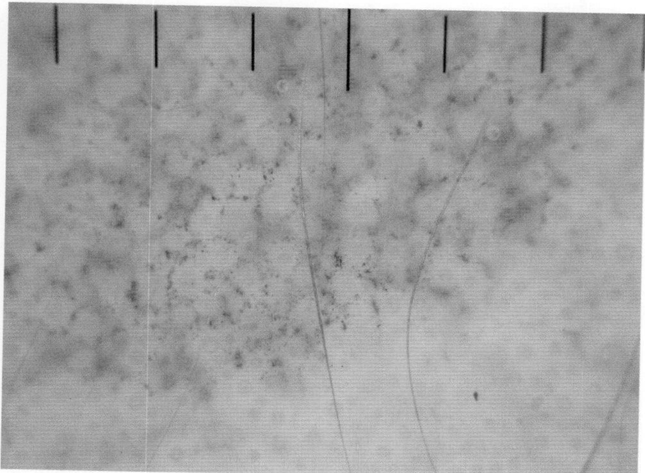

The same lesion two months later following no active treatment: dermoscopy shows a reduction in intensity of the granular grey pigmentation and ongoing mild background vascular dilatation.

The grey granular pigmentation will typically clear over many months.

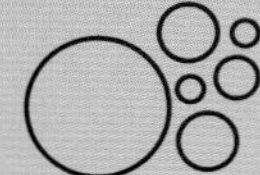

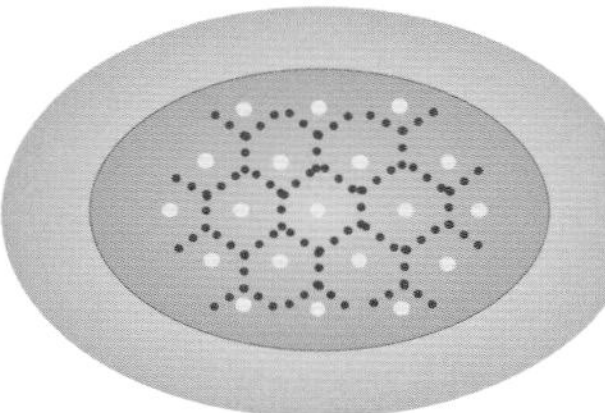
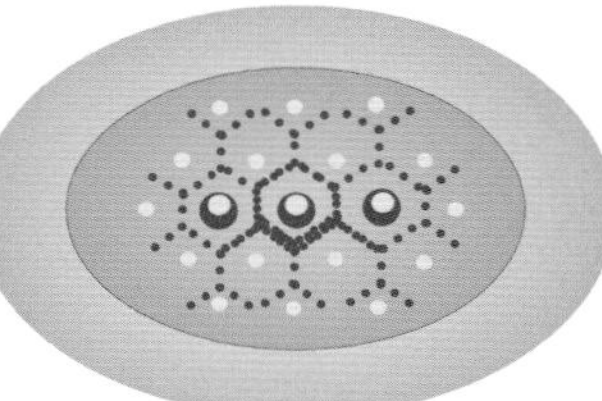
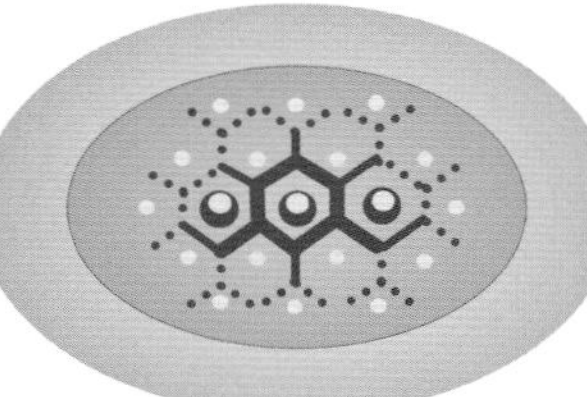
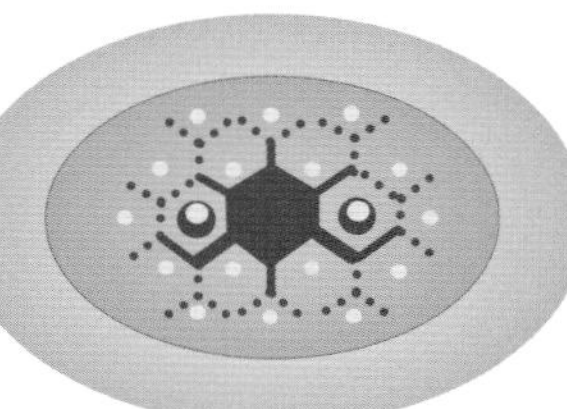

Stolz proposed a dermoscopic model of progression of lentigo maligna. As the lentiginous proliferation develops, dermoscopic features progress from annular granular pigmentation to asymmetry of perifollicular pigmentation, rhomboidal structures and, finally, follicular destruction as the tumour becomes invasive. Three dermoscopic clues to look for are: irregular brown/grey granular pigmentation, irregular perifollicular pigmentation, ill-defined peripheral margins.

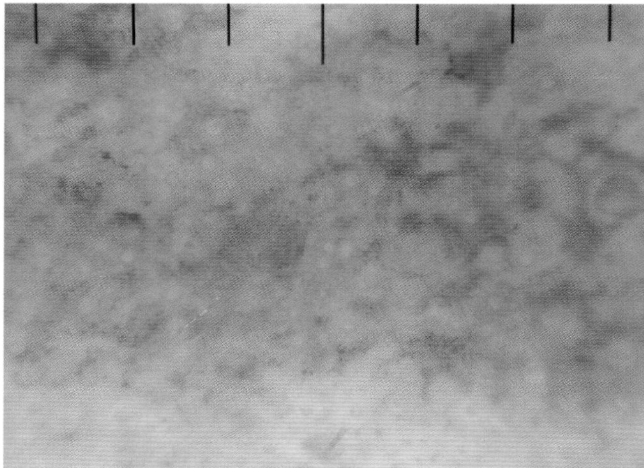

Annular granular pigmentation.

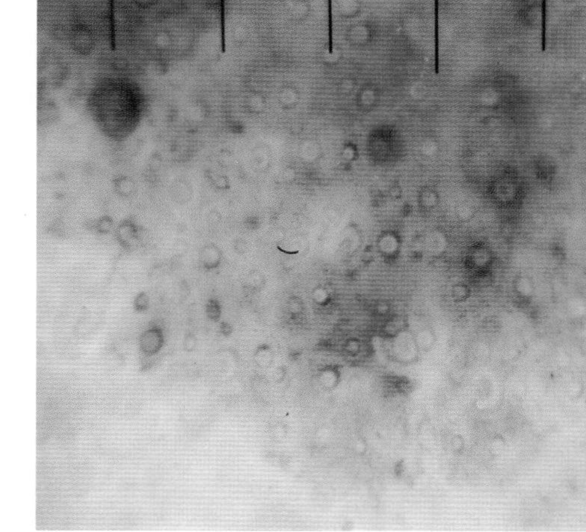

Asymmetrical perifollicular pigmentation.

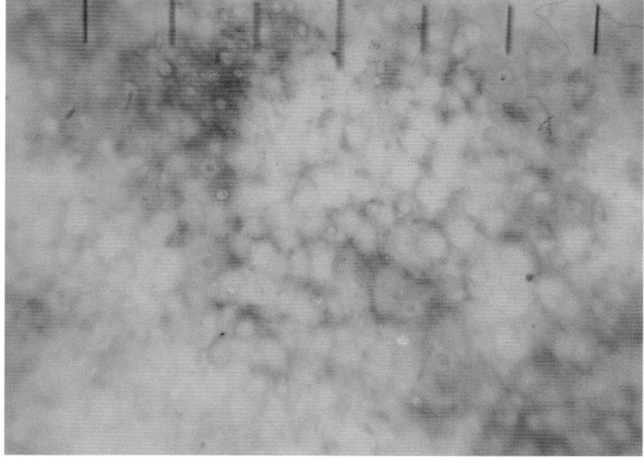

Rhomboidal structures, angulated/zig-zag lines or polygons.

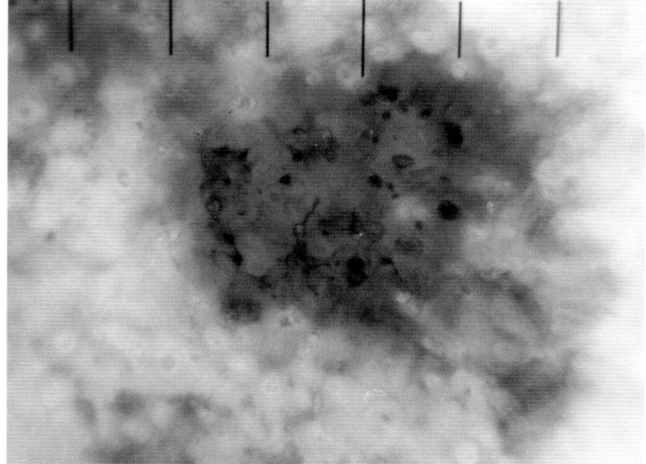

Follicular destruction.

Schiffner, R. et al. Improvement of early recognition of lentigo maligna using dermatoscopy. *J Am Acad Dermatol*. 2000;24(1):25–32.

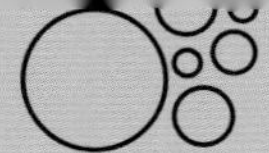

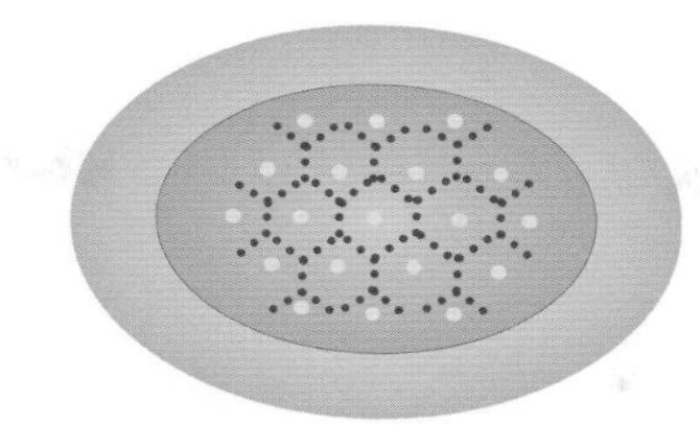

Lentigo maligna is usually the dominant facial pigmented lesion, whereas solar lentigines are multiple and more similar in colour. Common features distinguishing a lentigo maligna from solar lentigo include the following: an ill-defined peripheral margin, brown granular pigmentation and asymmetry of pigmentation around follicles.

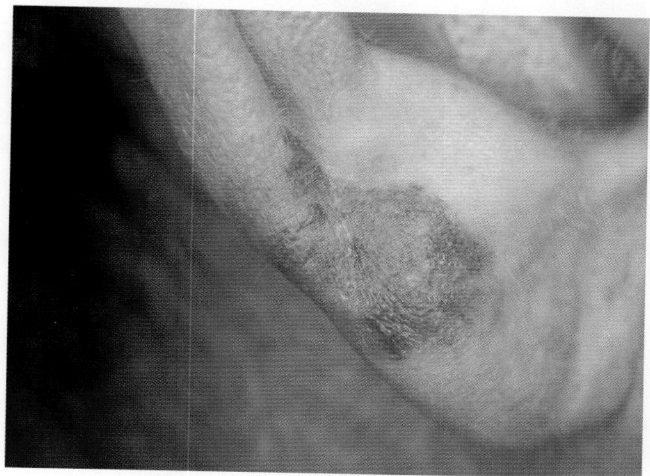

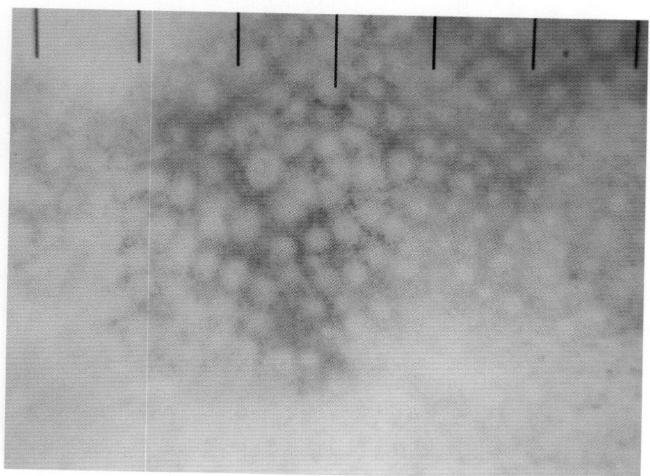

An irregular pigmented macule on the earlobe of a 50-year-old man: dermoscopy shows brown annular granular pigmentation with rhomboidal structures and an ill-defined peripheral margin in this lentigo maligna.

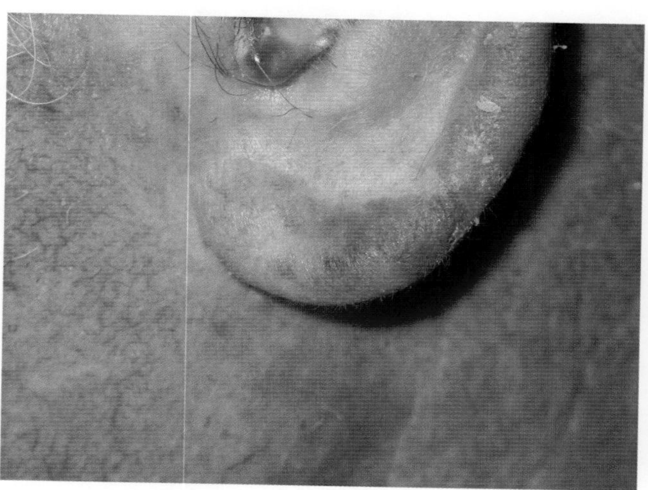

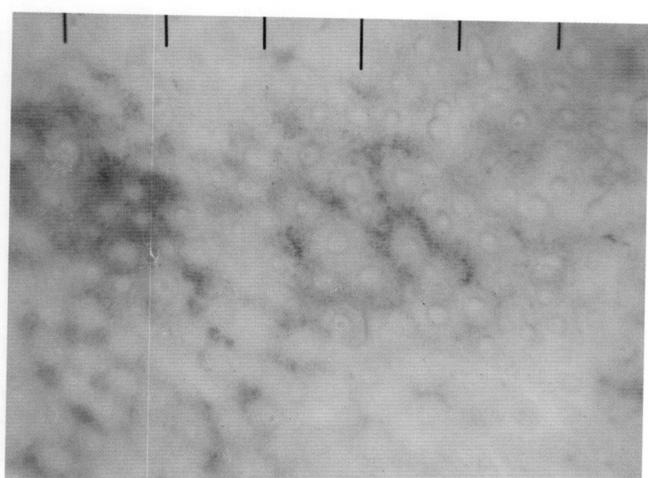

An irregular pigmented macule on the earlobe of a 75-year-old man: dermoscopy shows annular granular pigmentation, irregular perifollicular pigmentation, angulated lines and an ill-defined peripheral margin in this lentigo maligna.

Tanaka, M. et al. Key points in dermoscopic differentiation between lentigo maligna and solar lentigo. *J Dermatol*. 2011;38(1):53–58.

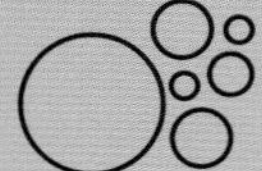

Lentigo maligna – circles

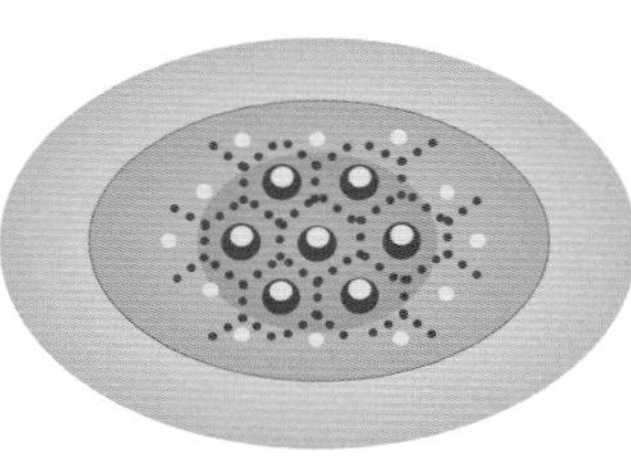

Lentigo maligna in areas with high follicular density may show increased pigmentation around these follicles, giving an appearance of pigmented circles.

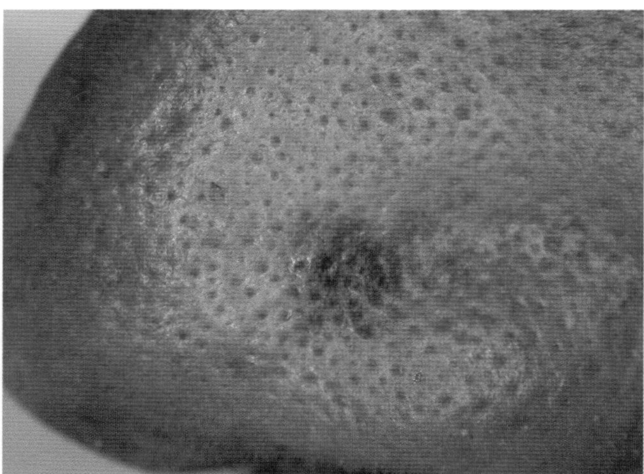

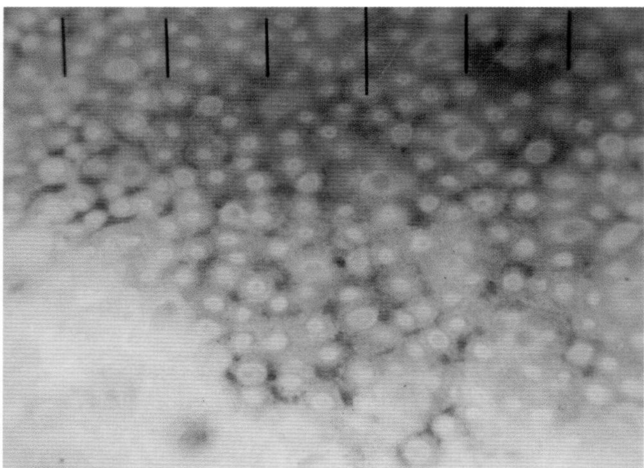

An irregular pigmented macule on the nose of a 60-year-old man: dermoscopy shows irregular perifollicular pigmentation and circles within circles in this lentigo maligna.

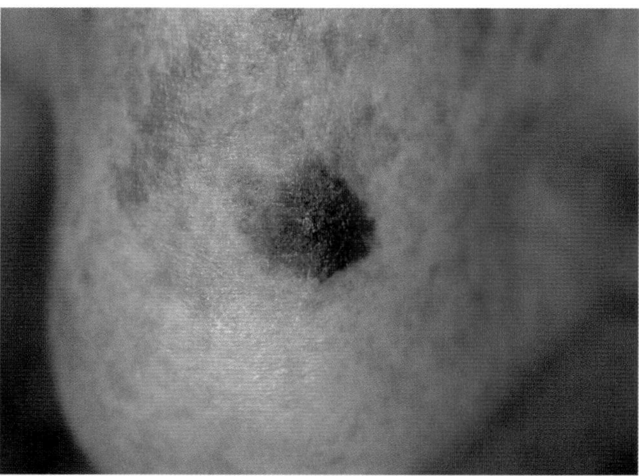

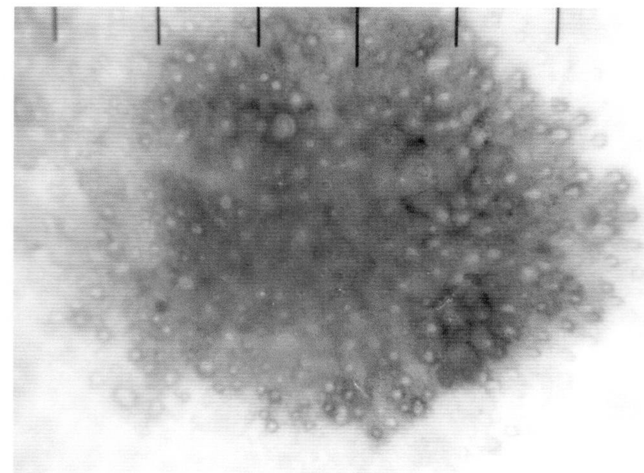

An irregular hyperpigmented macule on the nose of a 75-year-old woman: dermoscopy shows irregular granular brown perifollicular pigmentation and circles around follicular openings in this lentigo maligna.

Lallas, A. et al. The dermoscopic inverse approach significantly improves the accuracy of human readers for lentigo maligna diagnosis. *J Am Acad Dermatol*. 2021;84(2):381–389.

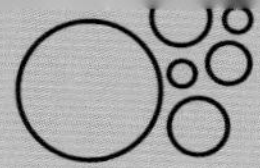

Lentigo maligna – perifollicular pigmentation

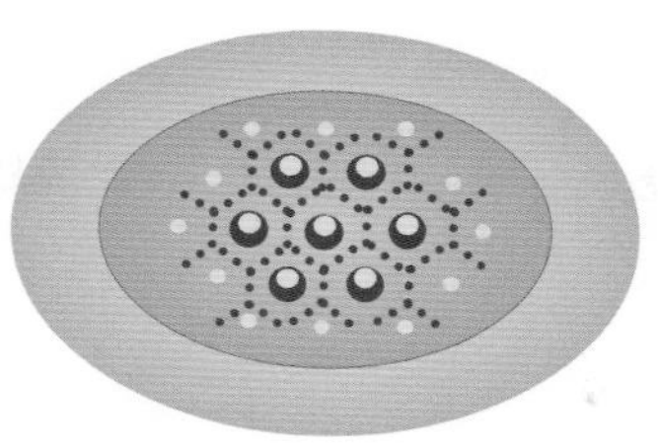

Lentigo maligna may present with a predominant folliculocentric pattern with follicular pigmentation. Dermoscopy shows irregular pigmented circles or semicircles of brown and grey pigmentation. Early invasive disease can be difficult to predict on clinical and dermoscopic examination.

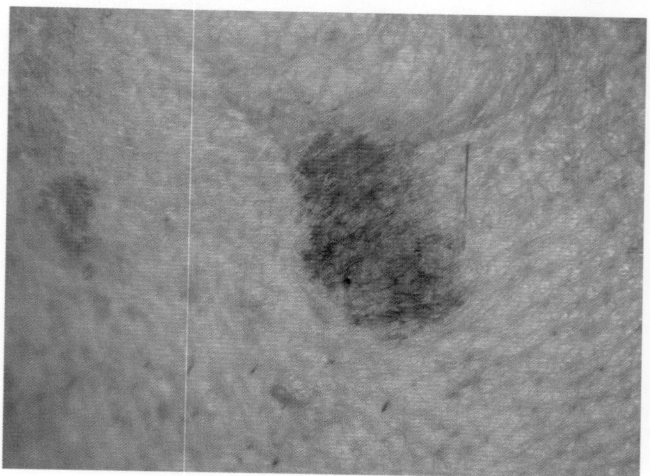

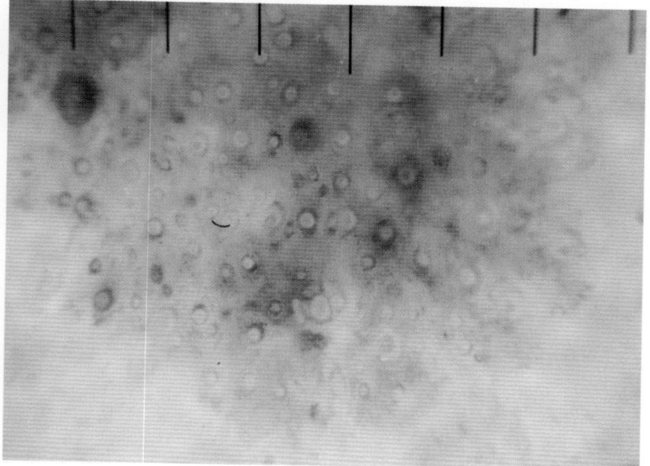

An irregular pigmented macule on the cheek of a 70-year-old man: dermoscopy shows multiple irregular pigmented brown and grey circles on a pink background in this 0.3 mm thick lentigo maligna melanoma.

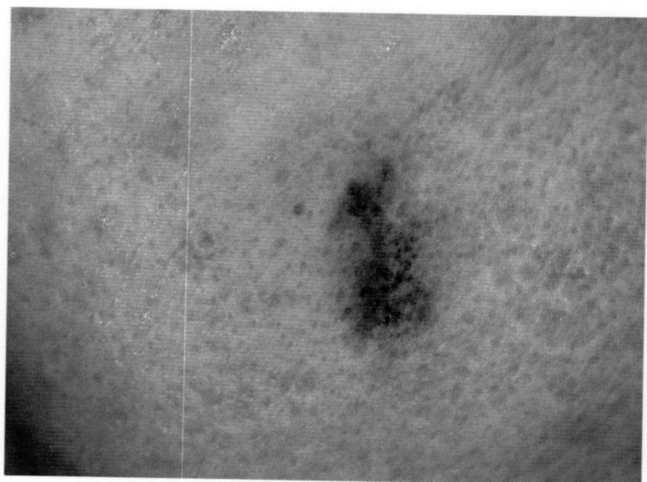

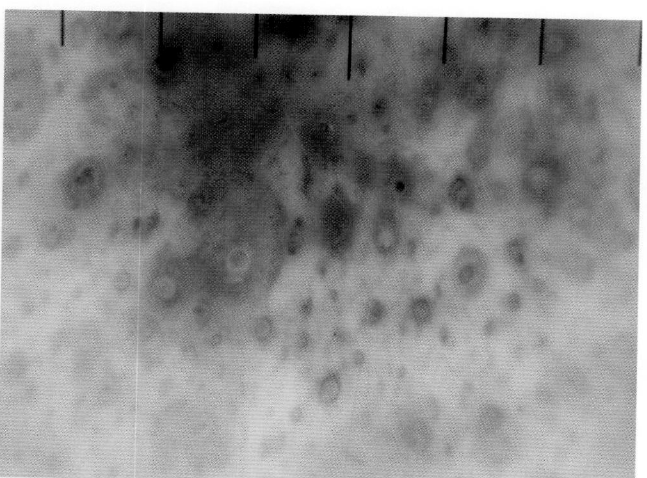

An irregular hyperpigmented macule on the cheek of a 65-year-old man: dermoscopy shows irregular hyperpigmented circles and granular grey pigmentation in this 1.7 mm thick lentigo maligna melanoma.

Tschandl, P. et al. Dermatoscopy of flat pigmented facial lesions. *J Eur Acad Dermatol Venereol*. 2015;29(1):120–127.

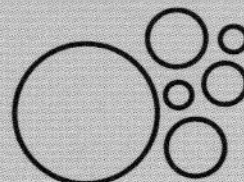

Lentigo maligna – young adults

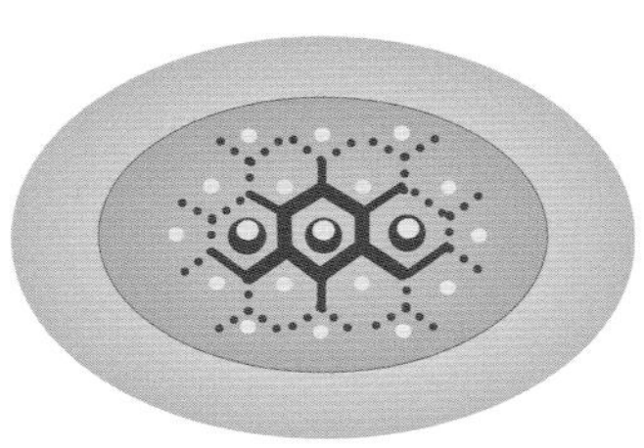

Lentigo maligna should be considered in adults, not just the elderly, with irregular pigmented macules and risk factors for melanoma. Signs to look for include irregular granular pigmentation, ill-defined peripheral margins and irregular perifollicular pigmentation.

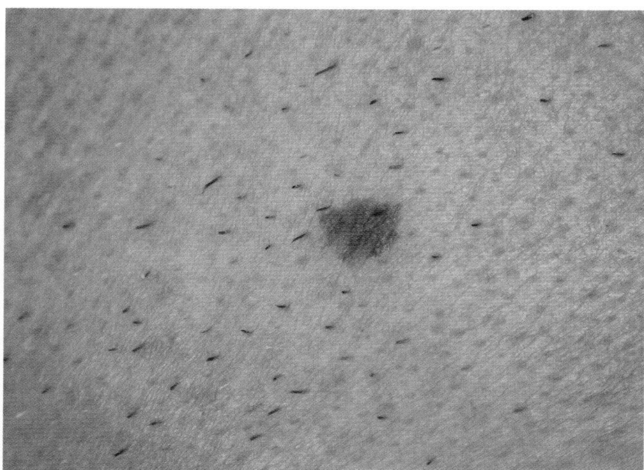

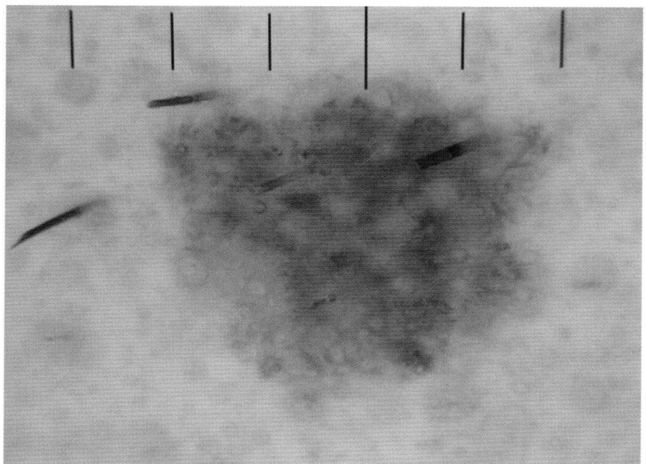

A well-defined 4 mm pigmented macule on the cheek of a 30-year-old man: dermoscopy shows irregular brown and blue-grey granular pigmentation in this lentigo maligna.

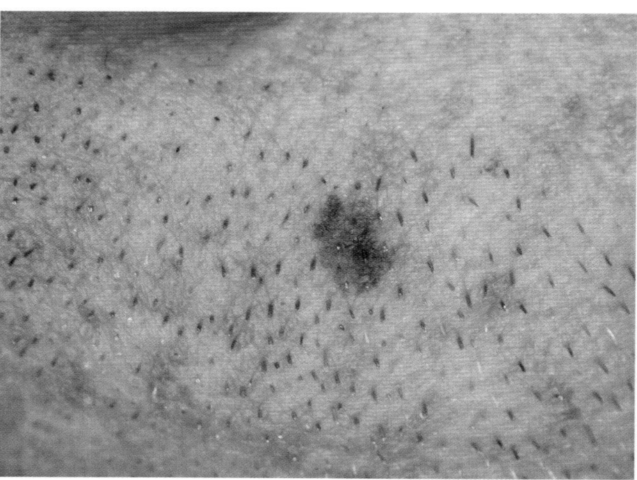

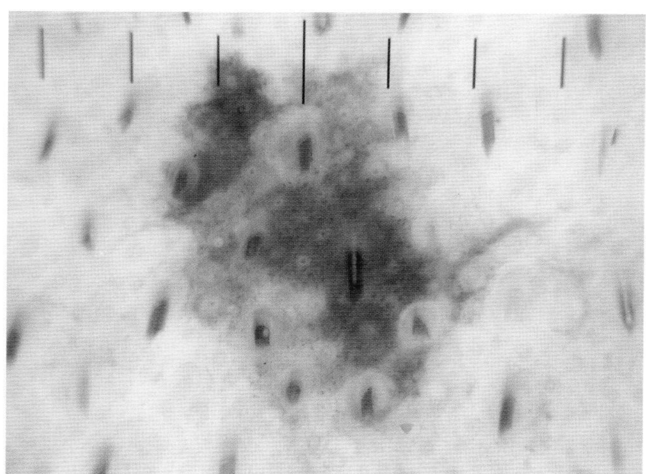

A well-defined 4 mm hyperpigmented macule on the upper lip of a 25-year-old man: dermoscopy shows irregular brown and blue-grey granular pigmentation as well as irregular perifollicular pigmentation in this lentigo maligna.

Ferrara, G. et al. Lentigo maligna in a young adult. *Dermatology*. 2008;217(1):66–68.

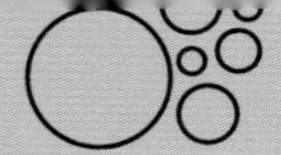

Lentigo maligna melanoma – I

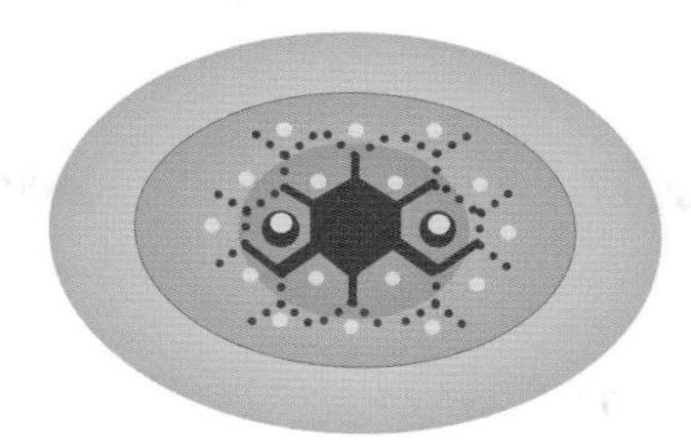

Lentigo maligna with hyperpigmented blotches giving rise to follicular destruction is a good indicator of invasive disease.

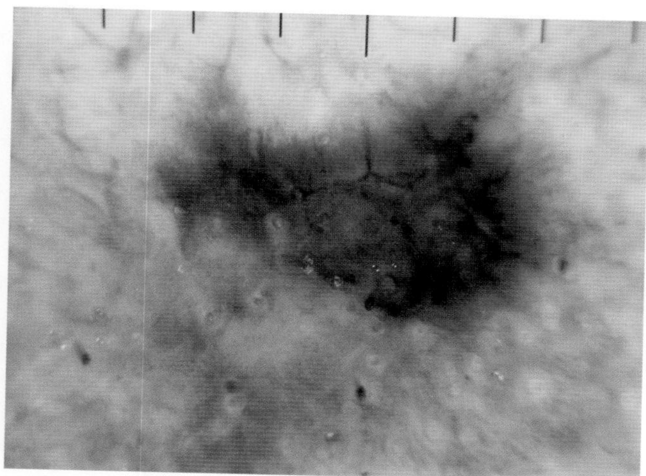

A solitary hyperpigmented macule on the cheek of a 75-year-old man: dermoscopy shows a hyperpigmented blotch, angulated lines, loss of follicular detail and background irregular pigmentation in this 0.7 mm thick lentigo maligna melanoma.

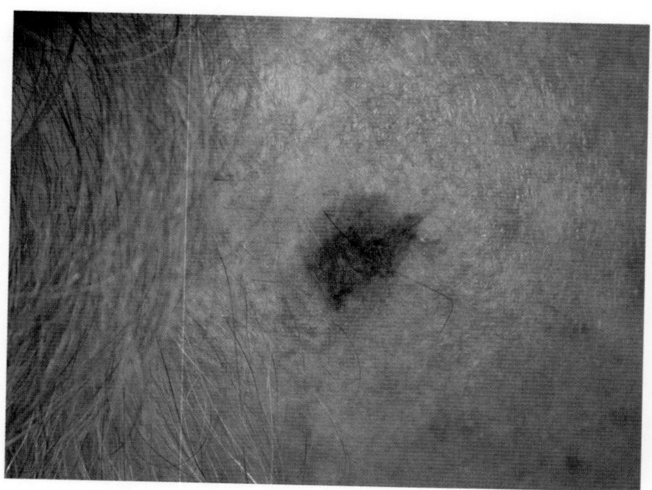

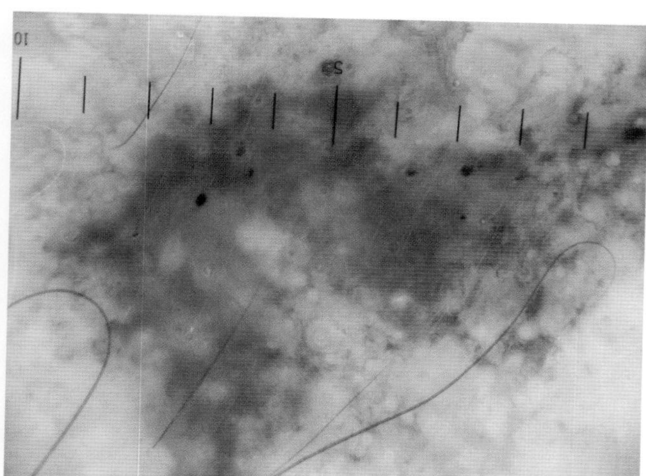

An irregularly pigmented macule on the temple of a 65-year-old man: dermoscopy shows irregular hyperpigmentation with loss of follicular structures in this 1.1 mm thick lentigo maligna melanoma.

It may be difficult to predict invasion or Breslow thickness in a hyperpigmented lentigo maligna melanoma.

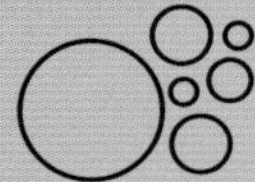

Lentigo maligna melanoma – II

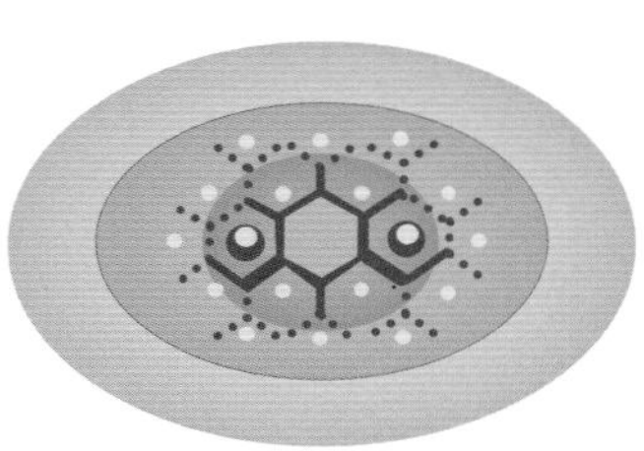

Pink structureless areas with follicular destruction is a good indicator of invasive disease within a lentigo maligna.

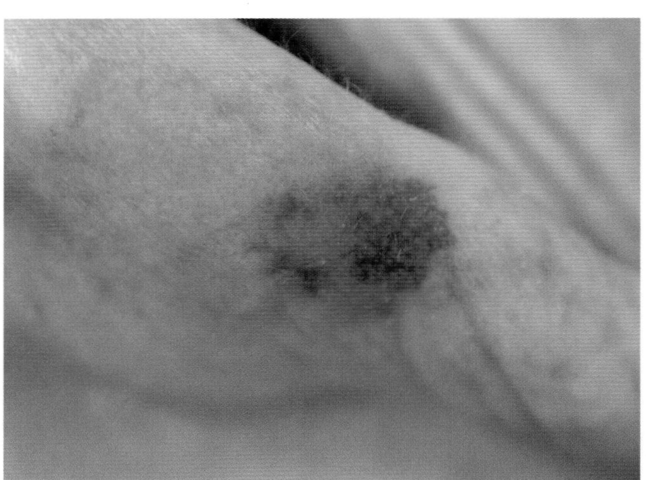

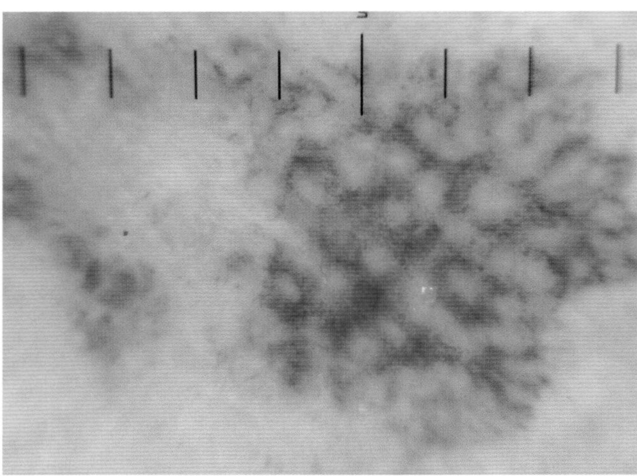

A pink and pigmented macule on the ear of an 80-year-old man: dermoscopy shows annular granular pigmentation with rhomboidal structures and a pink structureless area corresponding to a focus of invasion in this 0.3 mm thick lentigo maligna melanoma.

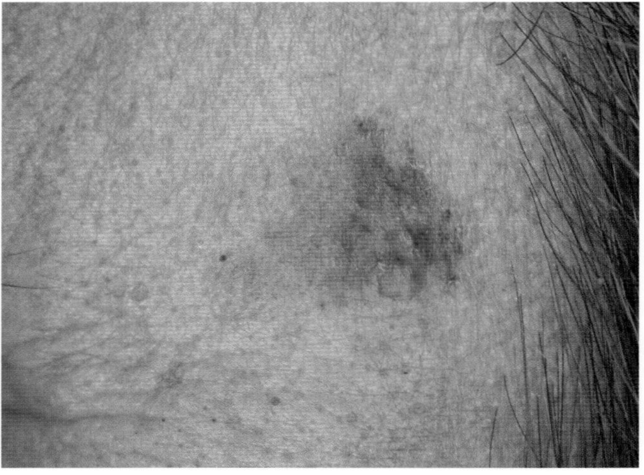

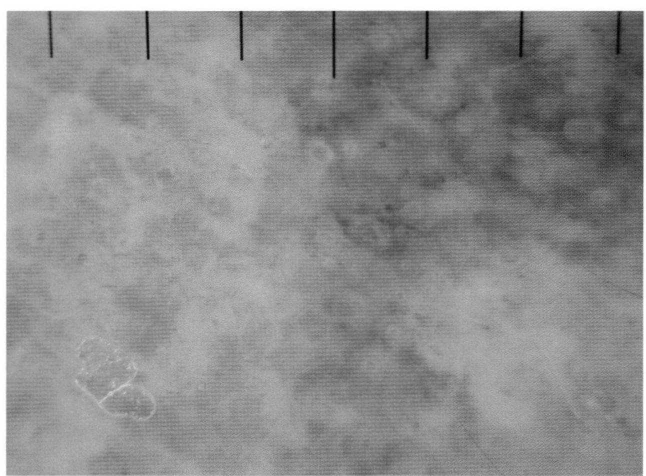

A hypomelanotic macule on the temple of a 60-year-old man: dermoscopy shows a pink structureless area with loss of follicular detail and irregular granular perifollicular pigmentation in this 0.5 mm thick lentigo maligna melanoma.

Pralong, P. et al. Dermoscopy of lentigo maligna melanoma: report of 125 cases. *Br J Dermatol*. 2012;167(2):280–287.

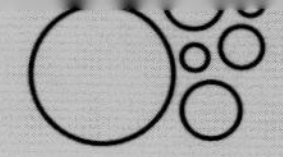

7.4 Scalp lesions

Scalp naevus – dermal 230
Scalp naevus – junctional 231
Scalp naevus – blue 232
Scalp naevus – reticular homogeneous 233
Scalp seborrhoeic keratosis 234
Scalp seborrhoeic keratosis cases 235
Scalp melanoma – thin 236
Scalp melanoma – thin cases 237
Scalp melanoma – thick 238
Scalp metastases 239
Scalp basal cell carcinoma 240
Scalp basal cell carcinoma cases 241
Scalp B-cell lymphoma 242
Scalp cylindromas/spiradenomas 243
Scalp sarcoidosis 244

Diagnostic Dermoscopy: The Illustrated Guide, Second Edition. Jonathan Bowling.

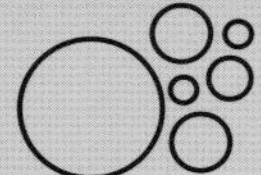

Scalp naevus – dermal

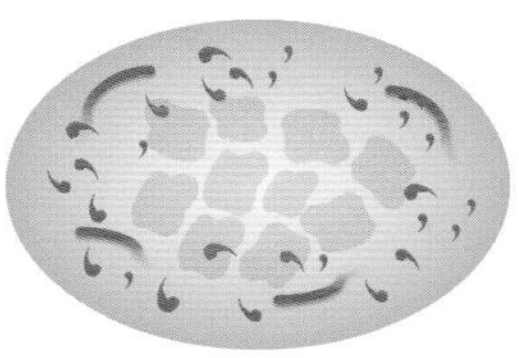

A common presentation of a scalp naevus is a skin-coloured soft exophytic lobulated papule. They may present with focal bleeding following trauma. Dermoscopy can show large cobblestone aggregates with or without pigmentation as well as curvilinear (comma-shaped) and looped (hairpin) vessels.

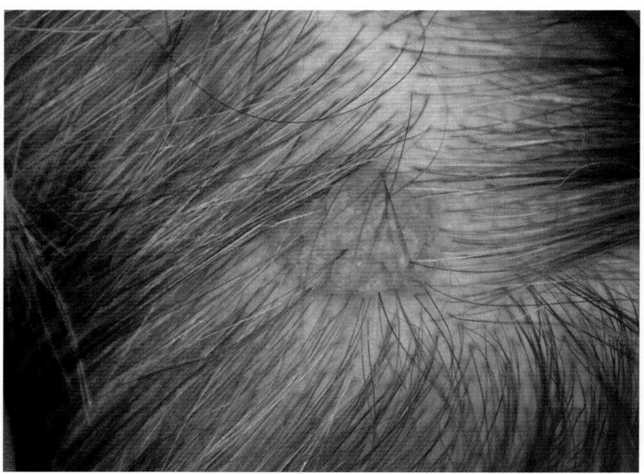

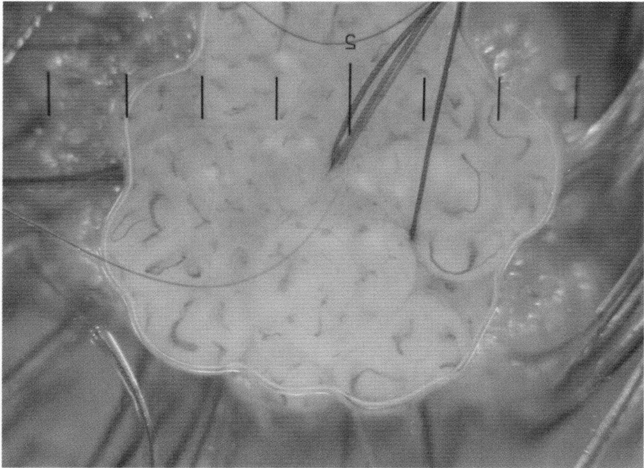

A skin-coloured exophytic lobulated papule on the scalp of a 50-year-old woman: dermoscopy shows multiple monomorphic pink lobules with curvilinear and looped vessels in this dermal naevus.

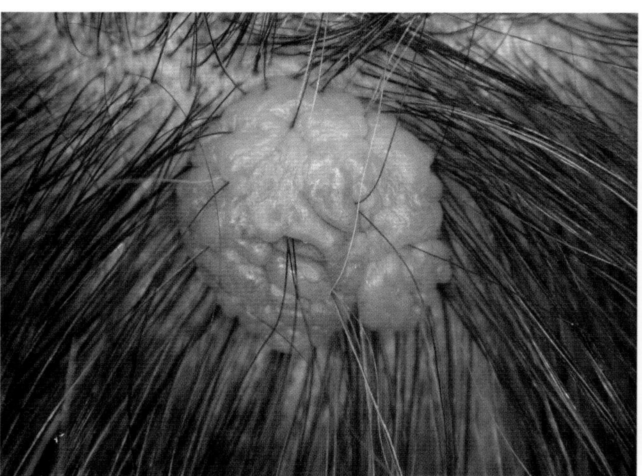

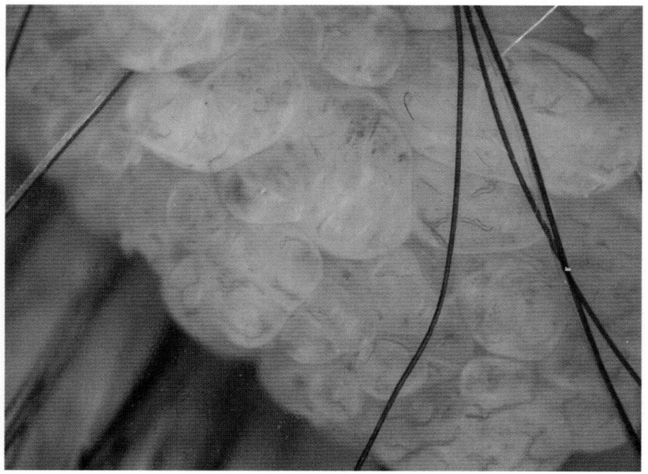

A solitary soft lobulated exophytic nodule on the scalp of a 60-year-old woman: dermoscopy shows cobblestone morphology with pigment remnants as well as curvilinear and looped vessels in this dermal naevus.

Zalaudek, I. et al. Proposal for clinical-dermoscopic classification of scalp naevi. *Br. J. Dermatol*. May 2014;170(5):1065–1072.

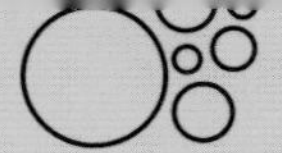

Scalp naevus – junctional

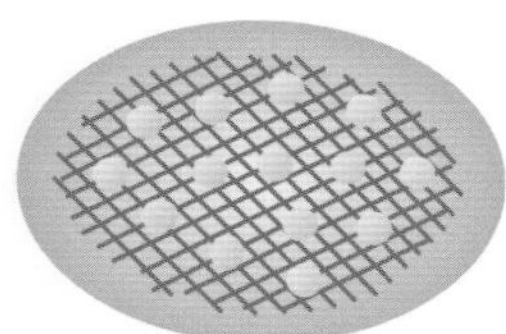

Junctional naevi of the scalp are often observed as an incidental finding. They do not have a raised profile and thus do not tend to present as a traumatised lesion. The high density of follicles impact the dermoscopy pattern seen with either a uniform homogeneous or reticular pattern with perifollicular hypopigmentation.

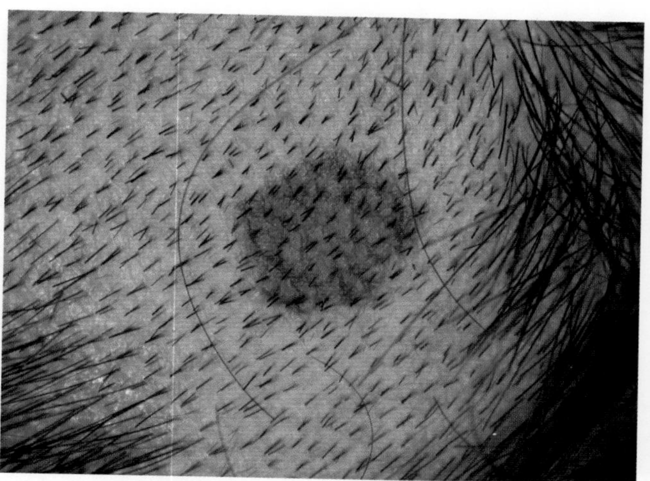

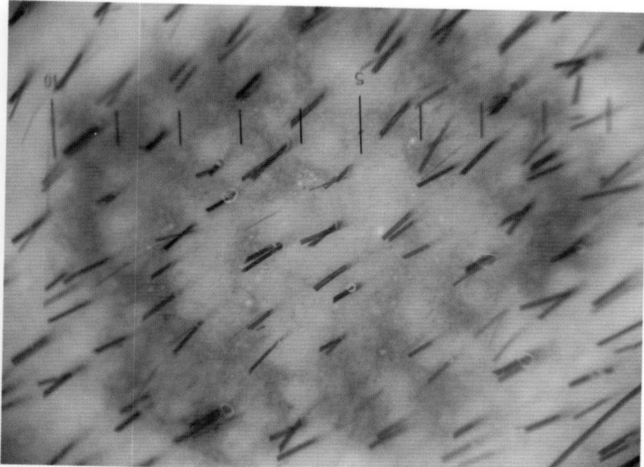

An incidental pigmented scalp macule on a 30-year-old man following a haircut: dermoscopy shows a clearly defined symmetrical brown homogeneous pattern of pigmentation with perifollicular hypopigmentation in this junctional naevus.

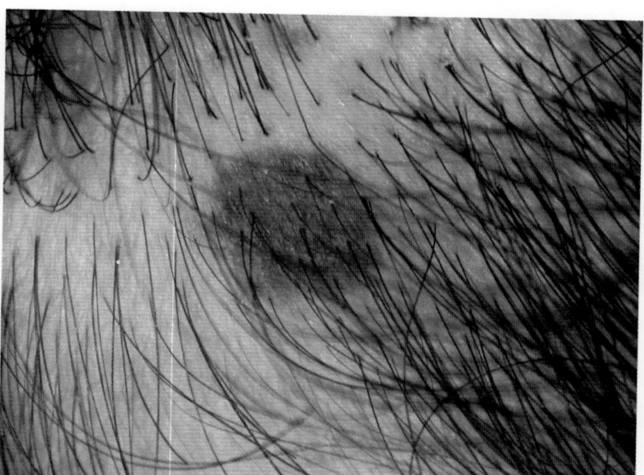

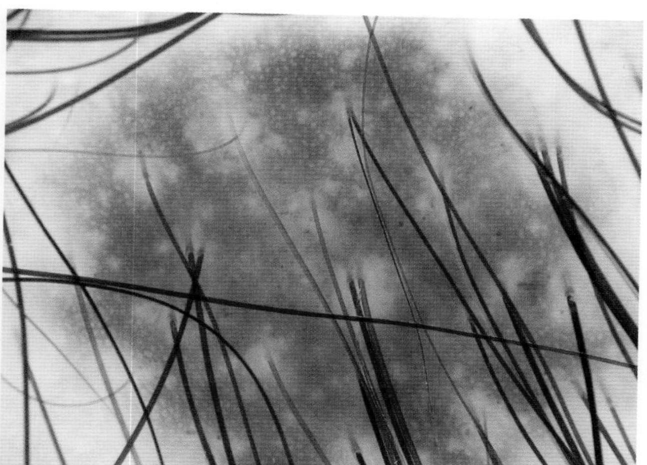

A hyperpigmented macule on the parietal scalp of a 30-year-old man with a history of melanoma: dermoscopy shows a symmetrical pattern of homogeneous and reticular pattern with perifollicular hypopigmentation in this junctional naevus.

A scalp melanocytic lesion with asymmetry, irregularity of pigmentation and/or an atypical pigment network should be treated with the utmost suspicion.

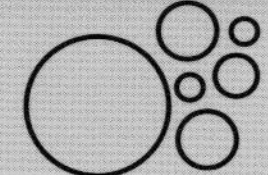

Scalp naevus – blue

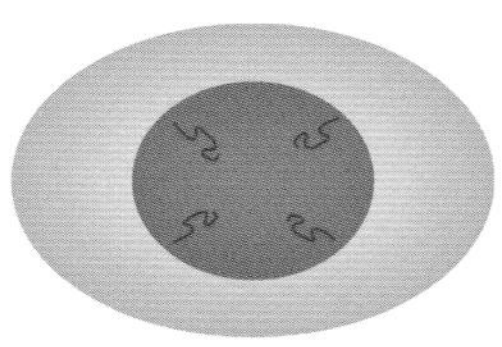

Scalp blue naevi often present a diagnostic challenge. Firstly, by definition they present as a hyperpigmented dermal melanocytic lesion. Secondly, a documented history of stability over many years may be lacking. Thirdly, they may present with additional vascular features giving increased diagnostic uncertainty. Therefore, careful examination of blue naevi-like scalp lesions should be undertaken and excision should be considered.

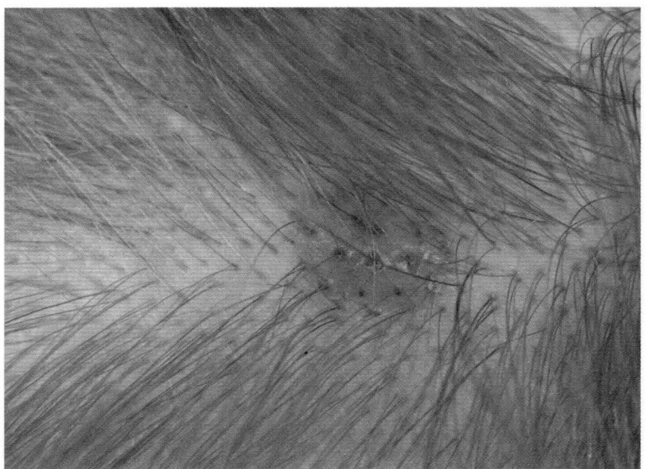

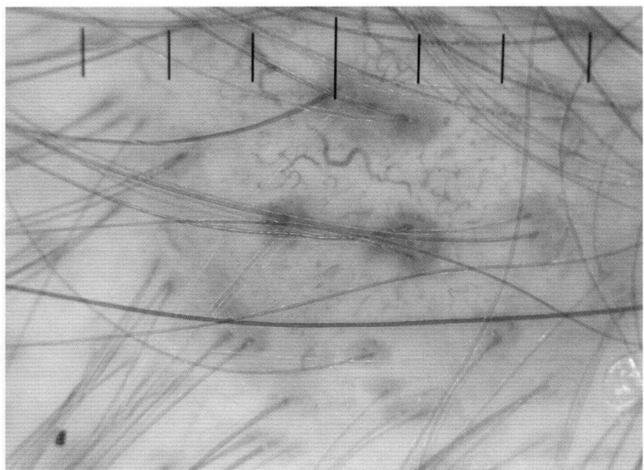

A pale blue dermal papule on the vertex of the scalp in a 20-year-old man: dermoscopy shows a pale lesion with perifollicular hyperpigmentation and poorly focused linear branching vessels in this histopathologically confirmed blue naevus.

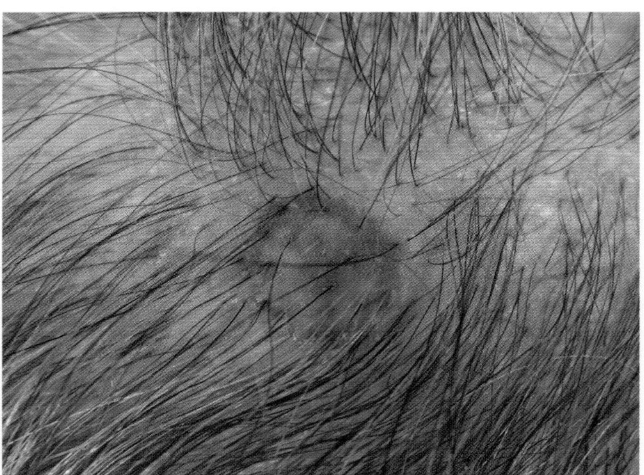

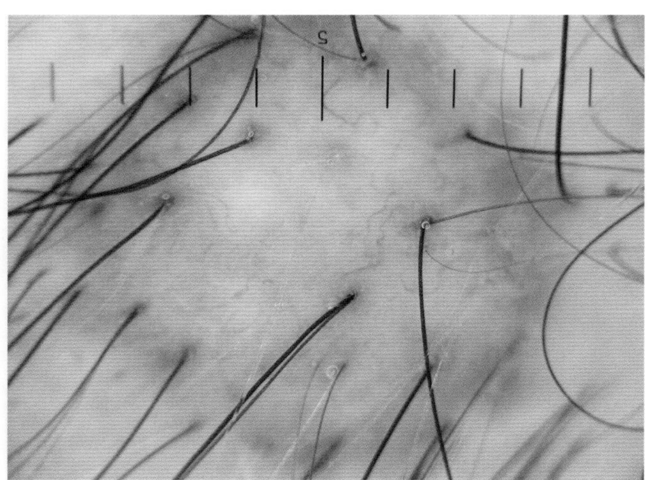

A hyperpigmented slate blue plaque on the parietal scalp of a 70-year-old man: dermoscopy shows slate blue and white colouration with perifollicular hyperpigmentation and multiple atypical vessels in this histopathologically confirmed blue naevus.

Up to 13% of blue naevi have a vascular pattern whilst 4% show ill-defined peripheral streaks, which may raise concern for melanoma.

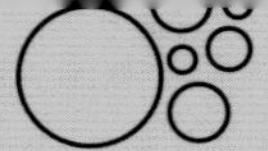

Scalp naevus – reticular homogeneous

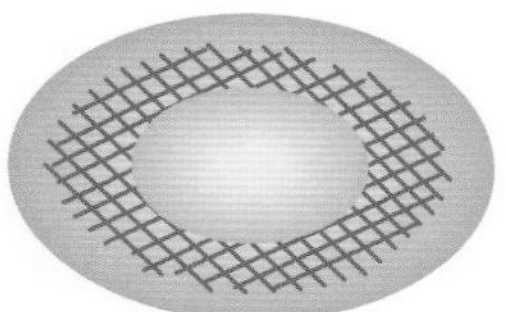

A common presentation of scalp naevi in children and adults with light skin is a symmetrical tan/brown annular macule surrounding a raised and hypopigmented central dermal component. These are compound naevi which are frequently located on the parietal or temporal area. Dermoscopy shows a typical reticular and homogeneous pattern with peripheral hyperpigmentation and central hypopigmentation. This type of nevus is sometimes referred to as an 'eclipse nevus'.

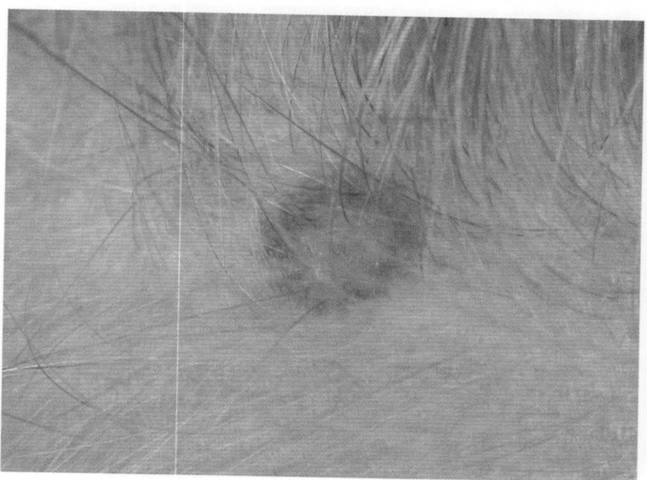

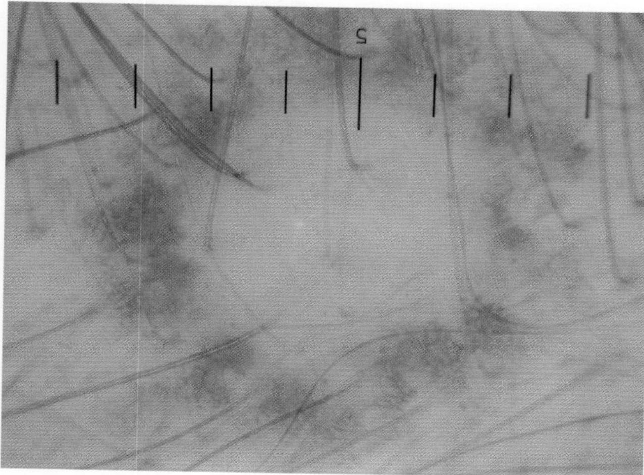

An annular pigmented macule on the temporal scalp of a light-skinned 15-year-old girl: dermoscopy shows a central structureless area with uniform peripheral tan reticular pigmentation in this 'eclipse naevus'.

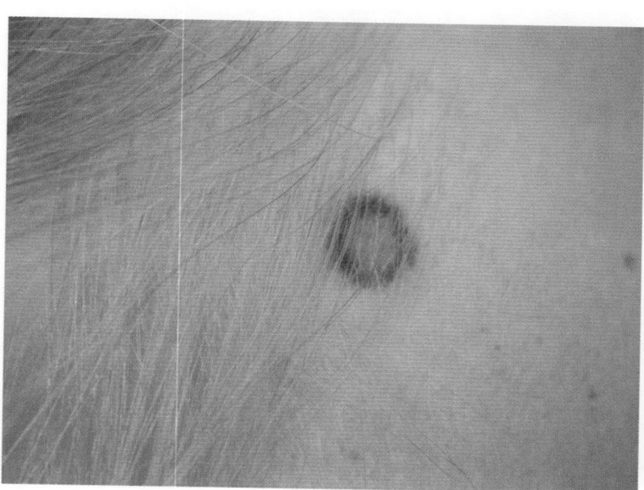

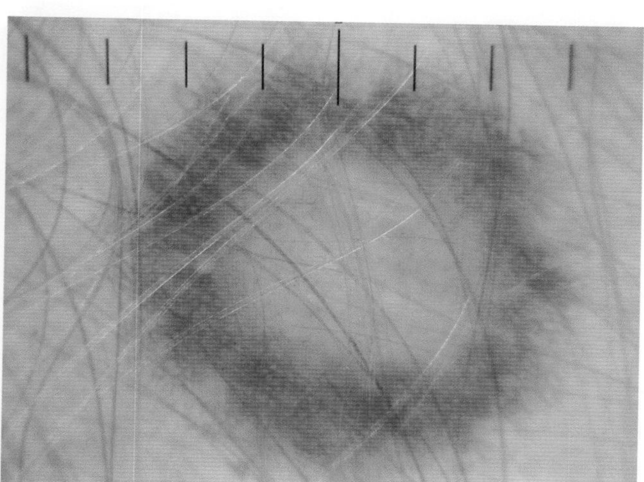

An annular pigmented macule on the scalp of a fair-skinned 10-year-old girl: dermoscopy shows uniform reticular peripheral tan/brown pigmentation in this 'eclipse naevus'.

Suh, K. and Bolognia, J. Signature naevi. *J Am Acad Dermatol*. 2009;(60(3):508–514.

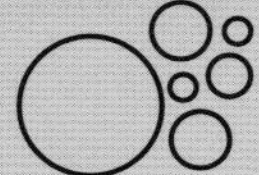

Scalp seborrhoeic keratosis

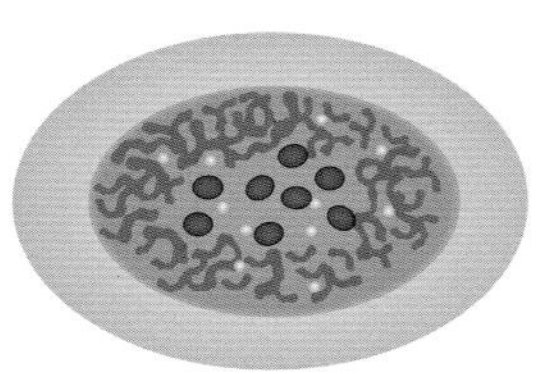

Scalp seborrhoeic keratoses share the same clinical and dermoscopic features as seborrhoeic keratoses elsewhere on the body, with the additional feature of increased density of hair follicles. Clinically they may cause diagnostic concern and, when hyperpigmented, may mimic melanocytic lesions.

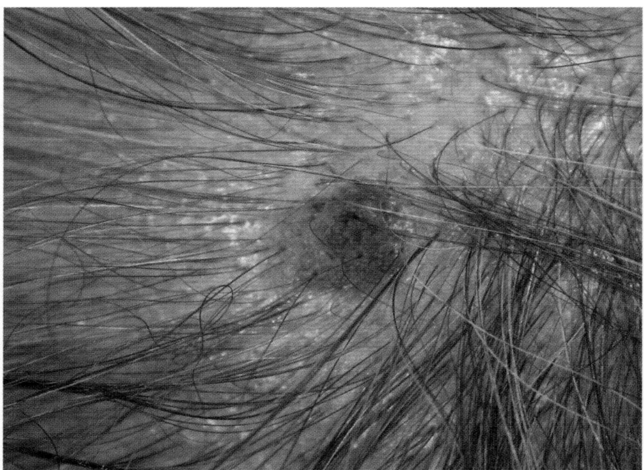

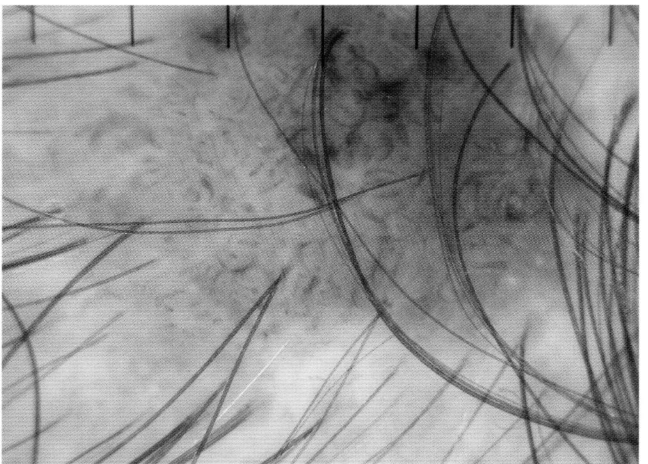

A warty pigmented plaque on the scalp of a 60-year-old man: dermoscopy shows a cerebriform pattern with hairpin vessels in this scalp seborrhoeic keratosis.

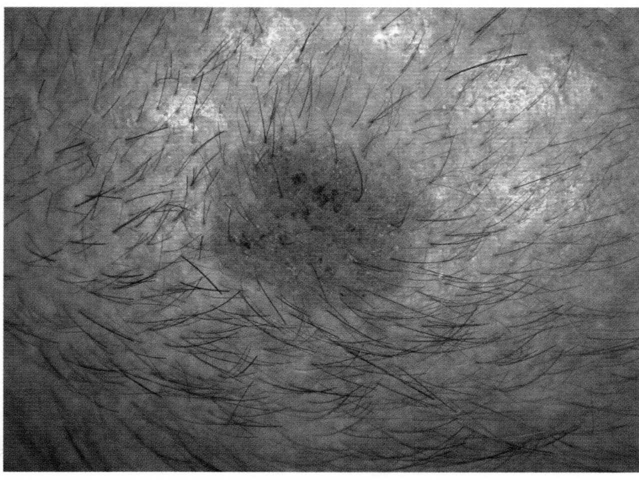

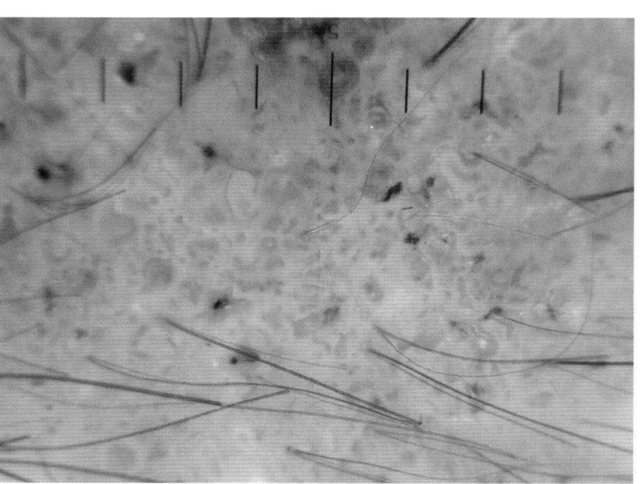

A pink and brown keratotic plaque on the scalp of a 60-year-old man: dermoscopy shows hairpin vessels and comedo-like openings in this seborrhoeic keratosis.

Braun, R.P. et al. Dermoscopy of pigmented seborrheic keratosis: a morphological study. *Arch Dermatol*. 2002;138(12): 1556–1560.

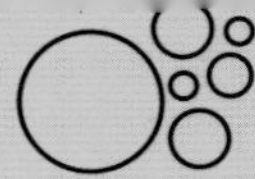

Scalp seborrhoeic keratosis cases

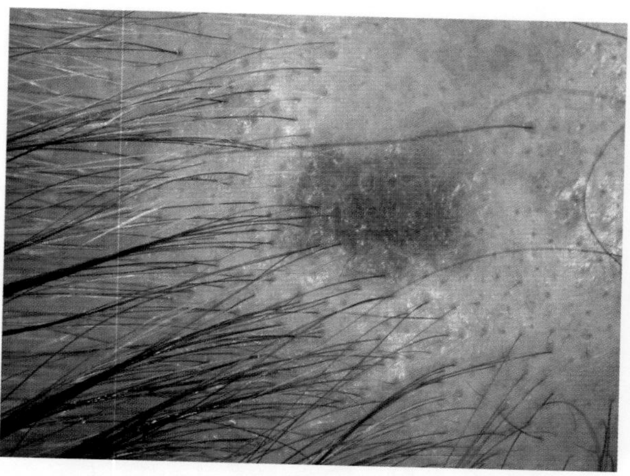

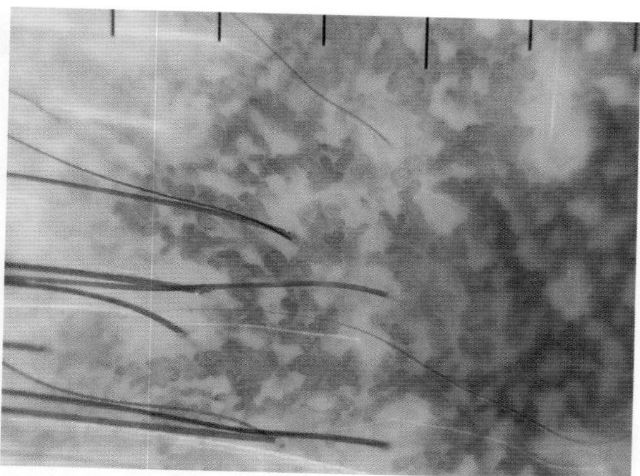

A tan macule on the parietal scalp of a 70-year-old man: dermoscopy shows cerebriform (or brain-like) pigmentation in this early evolving seborrhoeic keratosis.

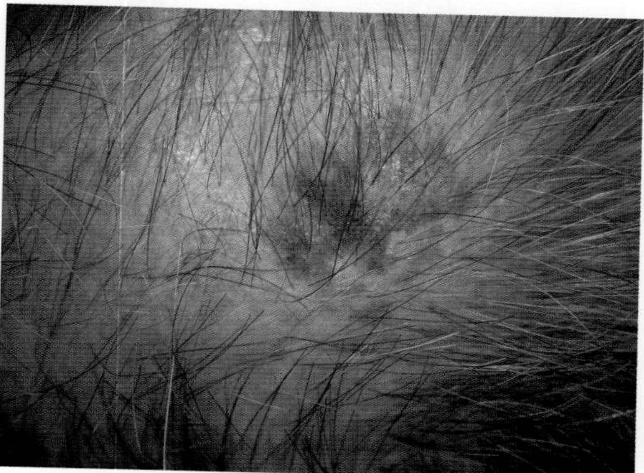

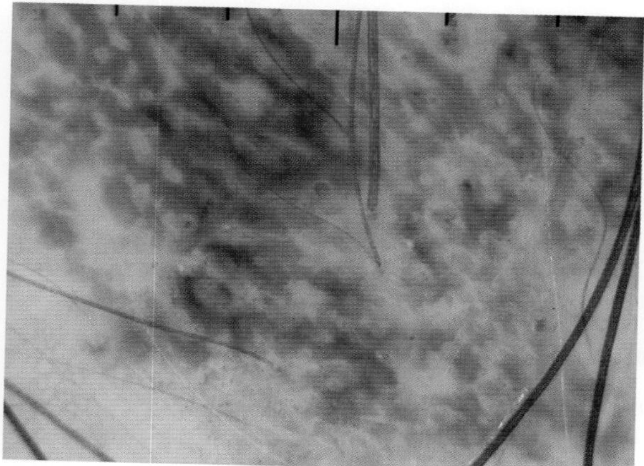

An irregularly shaped brown macule on the vertex of a 60-year-old man: dermoscopy shows preserved terminal hairs, a uniform brown cerebriform pattern and comedo-like openings in this seborrhoeic keratosis.

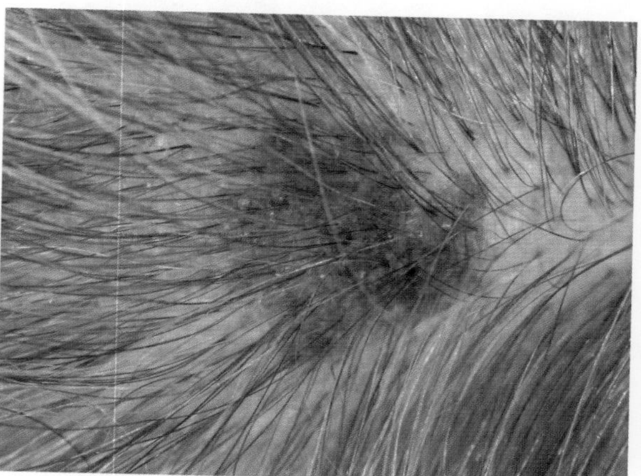

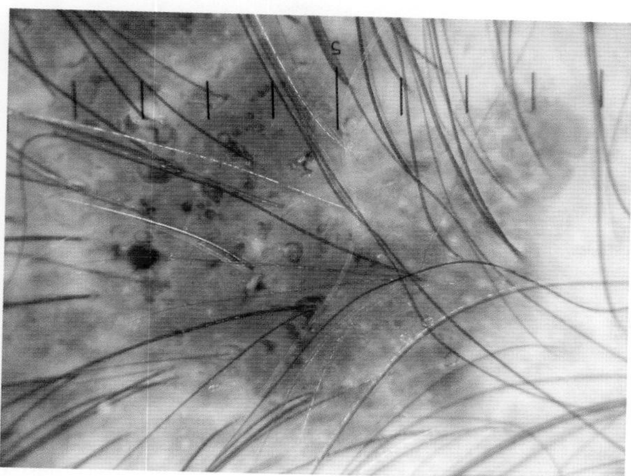

A hyperpigmented and hyper keratotic plaque on the vertex of the scalp of a 50-year-old man: dermoscopy shows comedo-like openings, milia-like cysts and peripheral cerebriform features in this seborrhoeic keratosis.

Take a close look at scalp seborrhoeic keratoses to ensure no suspicious or malignant features are present. Patients will rarely be able to give a clear history as these are typically concealed.

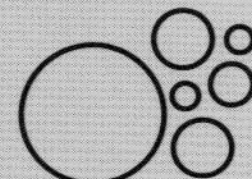

Scalp melanoma – thin

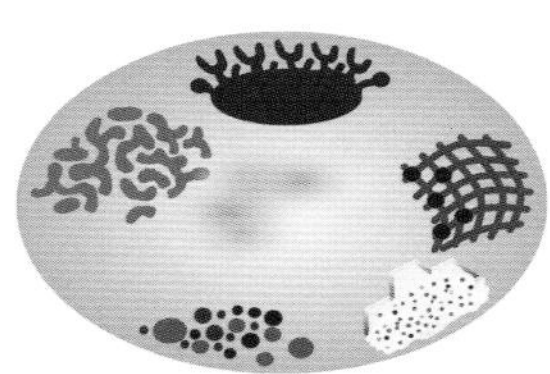

Scalp melanoma can mimic seborrhoeic keratoses or solar lentigines. Diagnostic features may be subtle and biopsy should be considered for equivocal lesions.

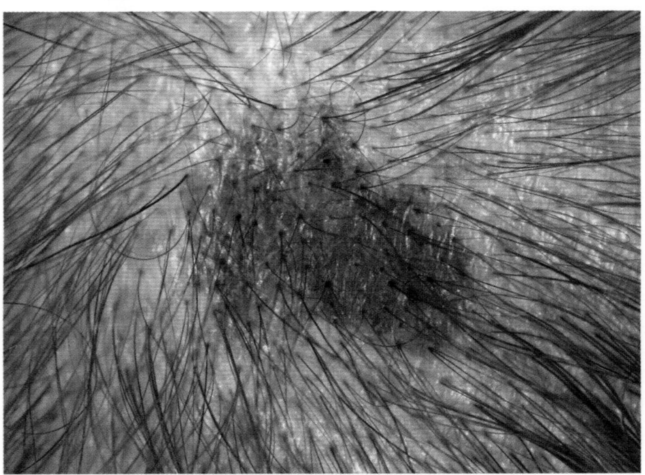

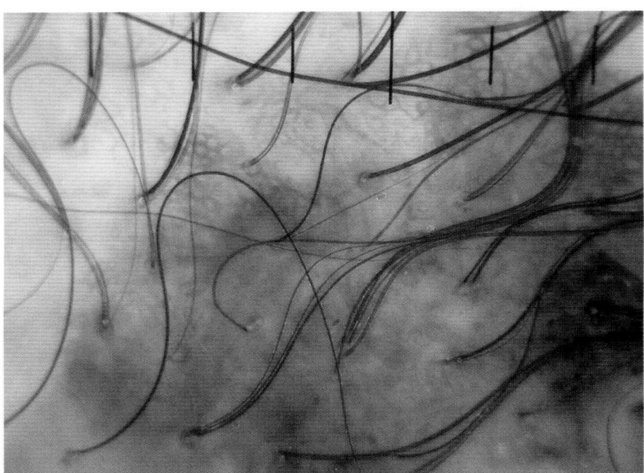

A hyperpigmented macule on the scalp of a 30-year-old man: dermoscopy shows atypical pigment network, irregular pigmented dots, isolated asymmetric pigmented follicular openings and blue-grey granules in this melanoma in situ.

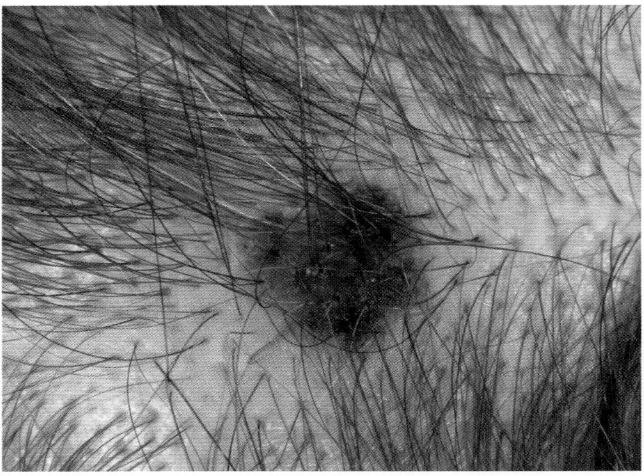

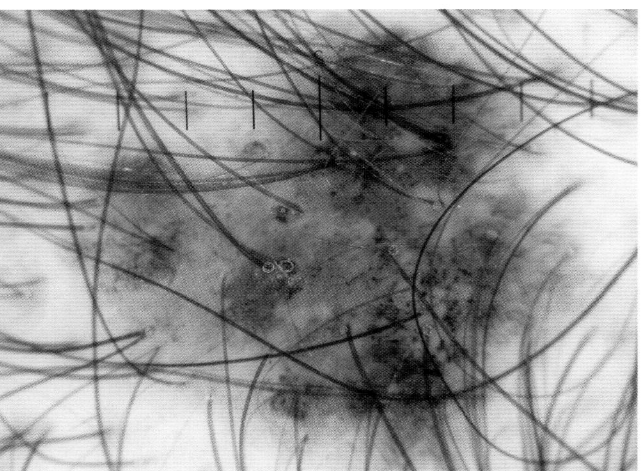

A hyperpigmented macule on the scalp of a 40-year-old man: dermoscopy shows a disordered multicoloured lesion with atypical pigment network, irregular pigmented dots and blue-grey granular pigmentation in this melanoma in situ.

Stanganelli, I. et al. Dermoscopy of scalp tumours: a multi-centre study conducted by the International Dermoscopy Society. *J Eur Acad Dermatol Venereol*. 2012;26(8):953-63.

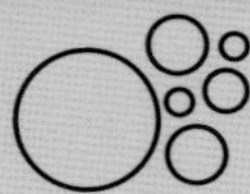

Scalp melanoma – thin cases

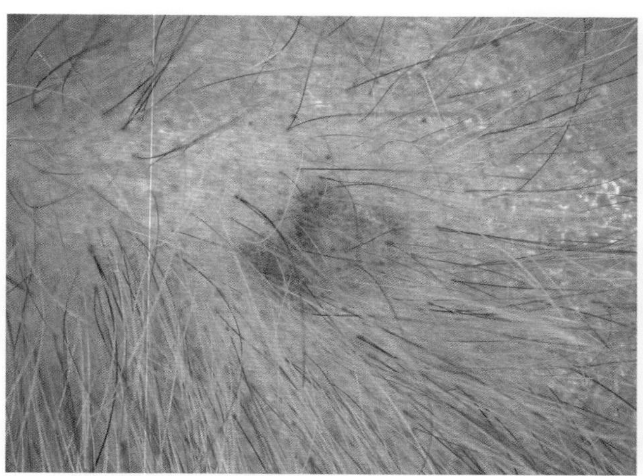

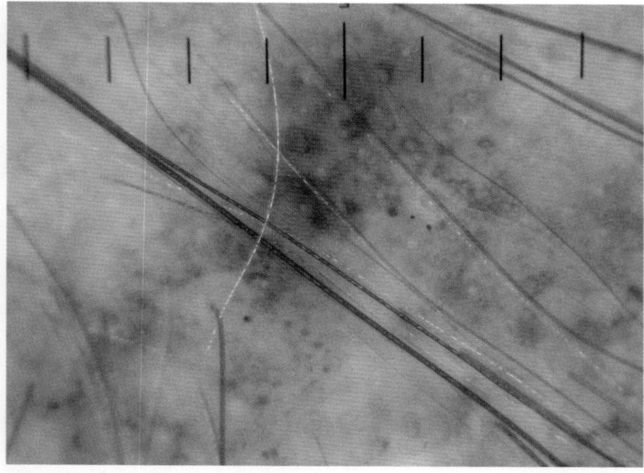

A subtle lightly pigmented macule on the parietal scalp of an 80-year-old man: dermoscopy shows irregular brown-grey granular pigmentation with pigment globules and irregular follicular pigmentation in this lentigo maligna.

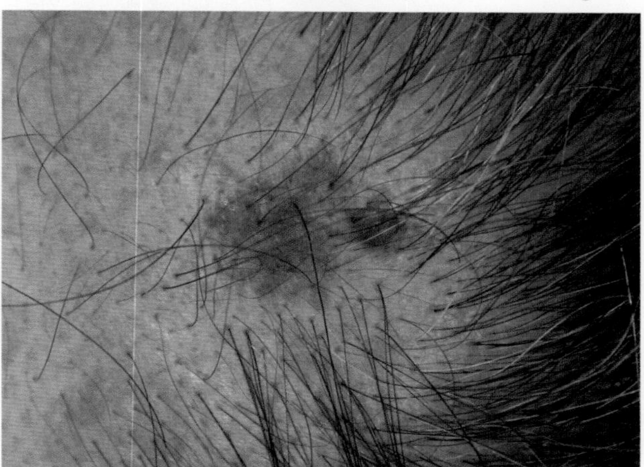

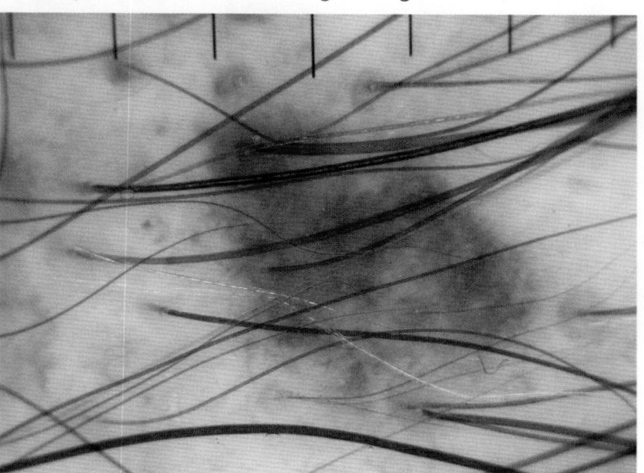

An irregular pigmented macule on the scalp of an 80-year-old man: dermoscopy shows irregular brown-grey granular pigmentation and irregular follicular pigmentation in this 0.6 mm thick lentigo maligna melanoma.

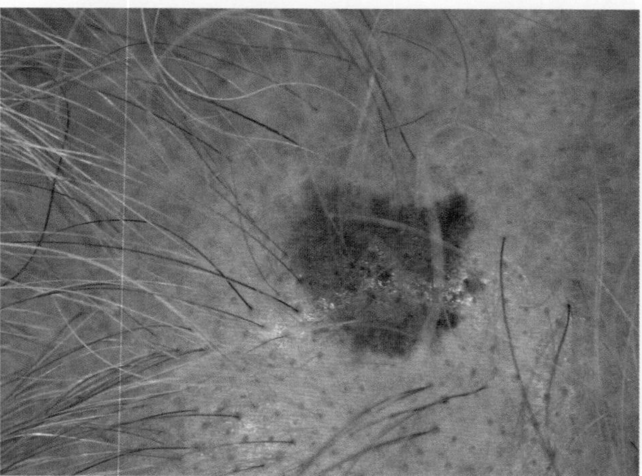

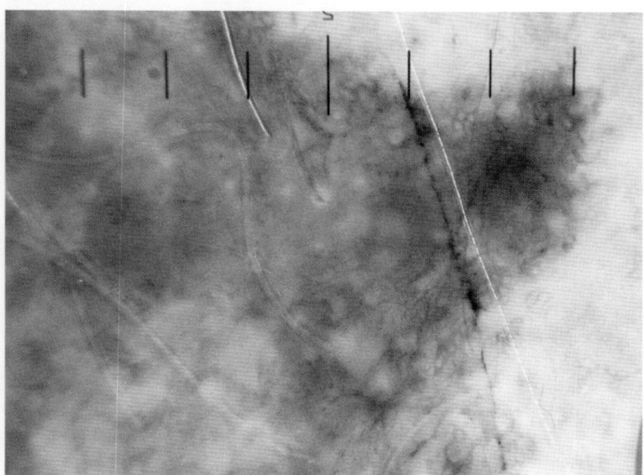

A pigmented macule on the scalp in a 70-year-old man: dermoscopy shows irregular brown-grey granular pigmentation, irregular follicular pigmentation and angulated lines in this 0.2 mm thick lentigo maligna melanoma.

Don't forget to examine the scalp when performing a total body skin examination.

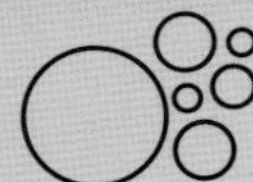

Scalp melanoma – thick

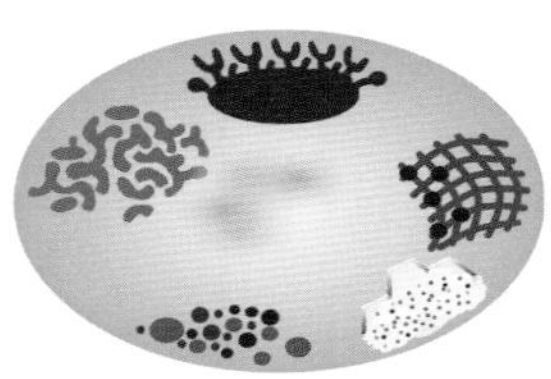

Thick melanomas on the scalp may mimic other thick skin tumours including seborrhoeic keratoses and blue naevi. Diagnostic features may be subtle and close examination should be considered for all scalp pigmented skin lesions.

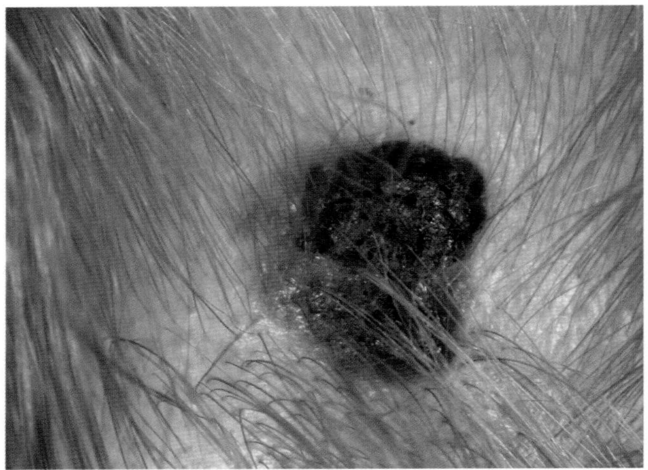

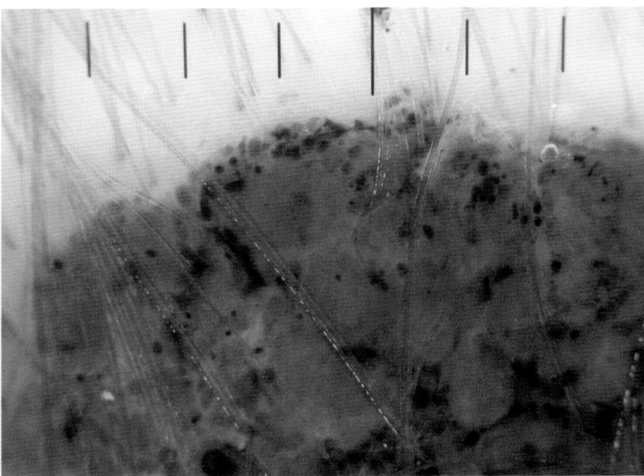

A hyperpigmented warty plaque on the scalp mimicking a seborrhoeic keratosis in a 35-year-old man: dermoscopy shows irregular pigmented globules, black dots and a blue-whitish veil in this 2.3 mm thick superficial spreading melanoma.

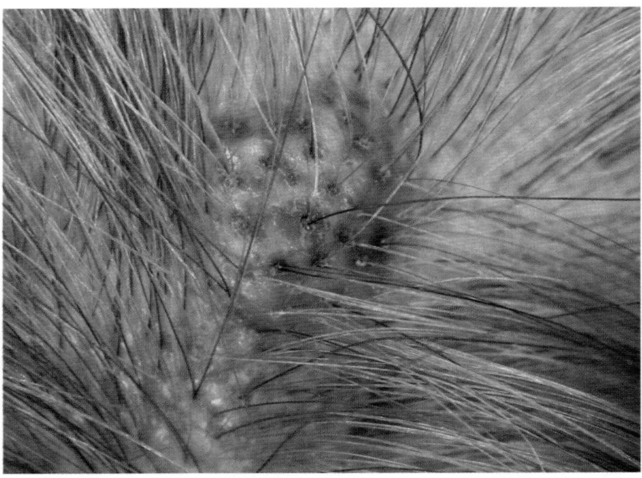

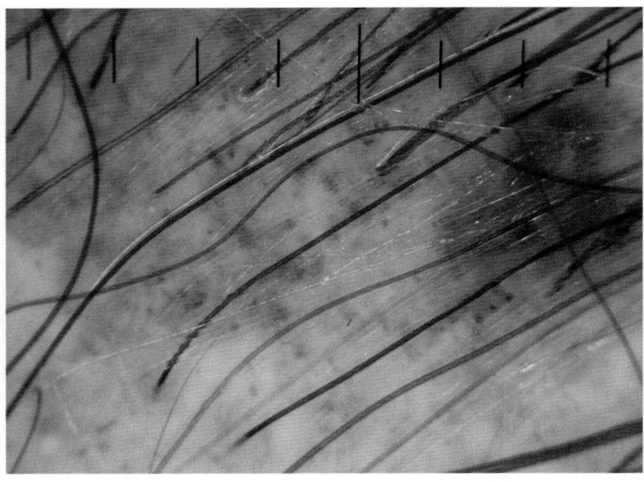

A blue-grey pigmented nodule of the scalp with an ill-defined inferior border in a 45-year-old man: dermoscopy of the border shows irregular grey-brown granules and globules in this 4.3 mm thick lentigo maligna melanoma.

Examine the whole peripheral margin of thick scalp lesions.

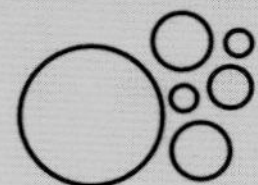

Scalp metastases

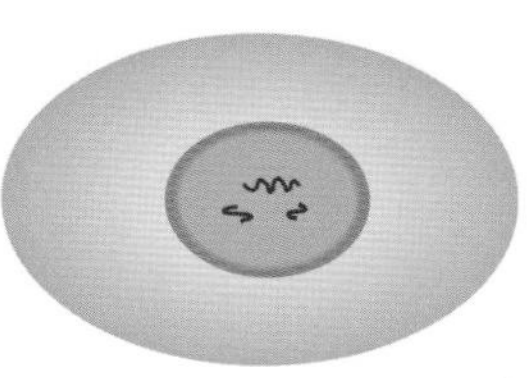

The scalp is a common site for metastases. Dermoscopic features include structureless areas, irregular vessels and haemorrhagic blotches as well as milky red areas.

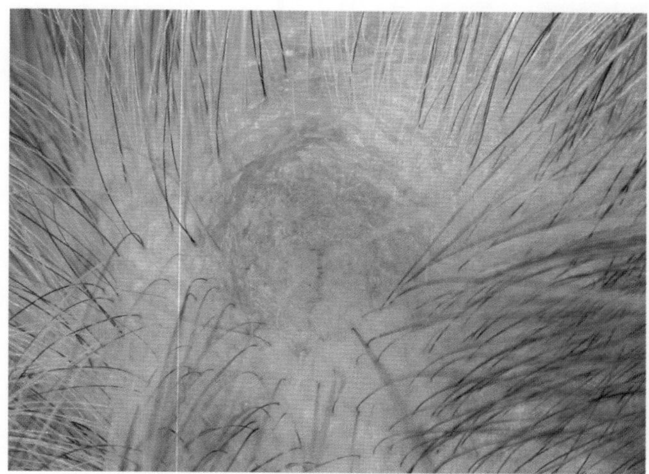

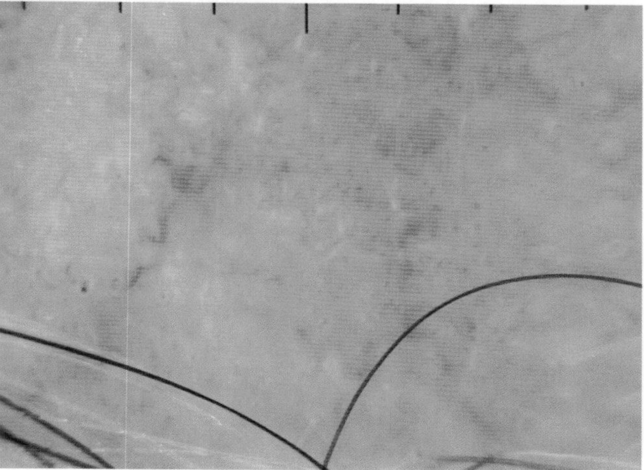

One of several pink plaques on the scalp in an 80-year-old woman with adenocarcinoma of the breast: dermoscopy shows structureless areas and poorly focused irregular vessels and shiny white structures in this cutaneous metastasis.

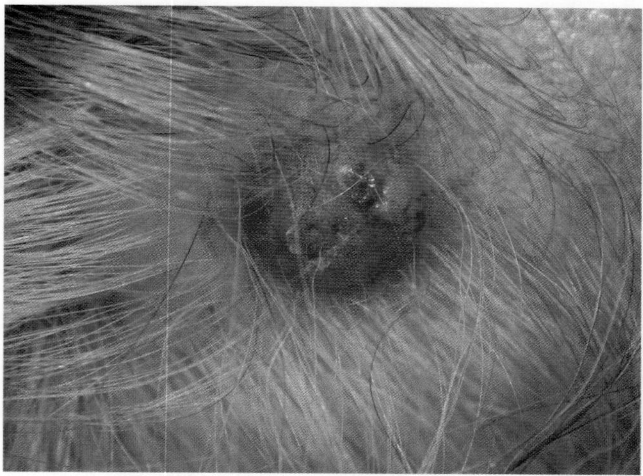

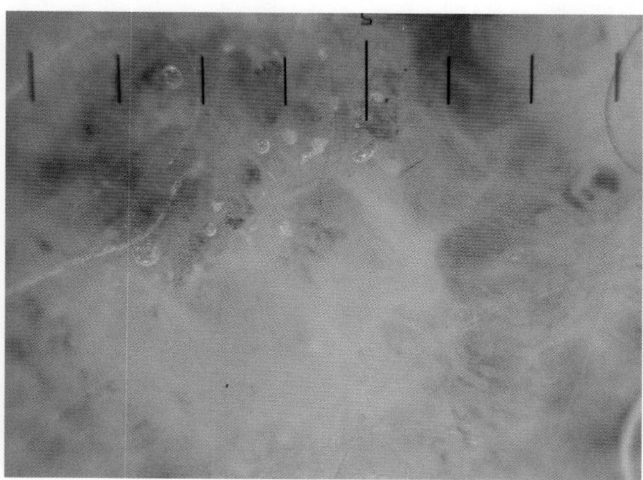

A pink nodule on the scalp of a 75-year-old man with a history of colorectal adenocarcinoma: dermoscopy shows a purple blotch, ill-defined vessels, erosions and structureless areas in this metastatic deposit from colorectal adenocarcinoma.

Lung, breast, colorectal and liver cancers may metastasise to the scalp. Consider biopsy of unusual scalp lesions in patients with history of these malignancies. Search for scalp plaques and nodules in patients with a known history of systemic malignancy.

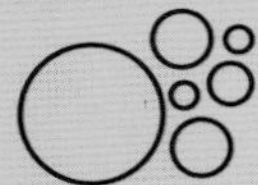

Scalp basal cell carcinoma

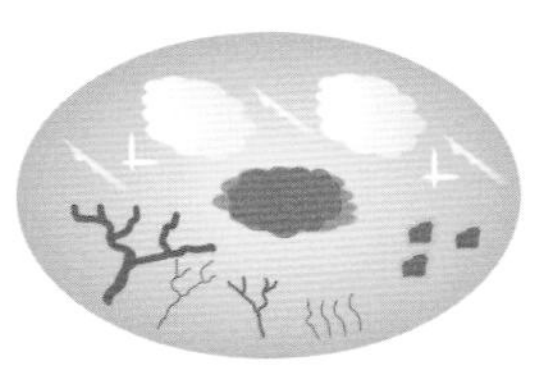

Basal cell carcinoma (BCC) may be found on the scalp. They are found more commonly along the part-line and crown in those with a full head of hair. Patients at risk of skin cancer should have their scalp examined as part of the skin cancer examination.

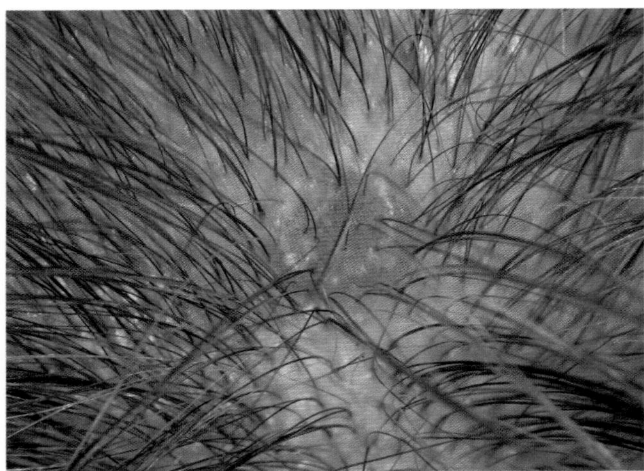

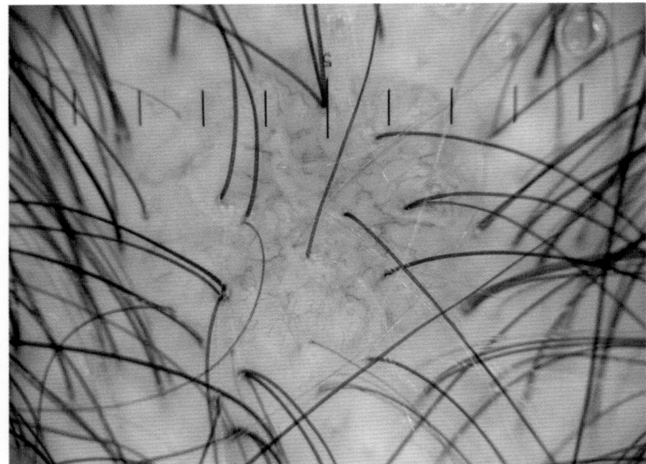

A 70-year-old woman with a history of high UV exposure and previous BCC with a new scalp lesion: dermoscopy shows sharply defined arborising vessels in this histopathologically confirmed nodular BCC.

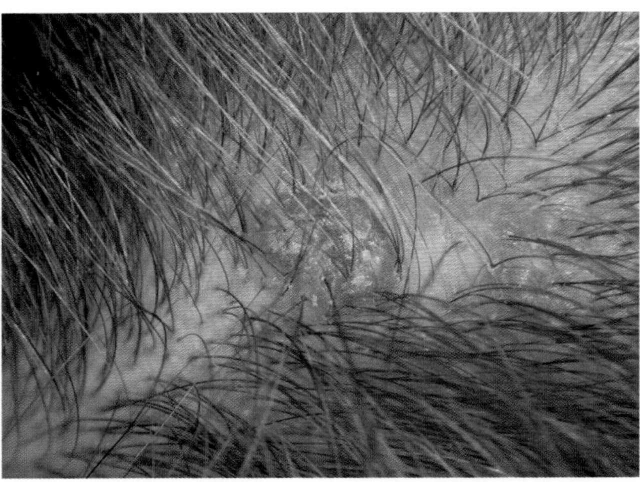

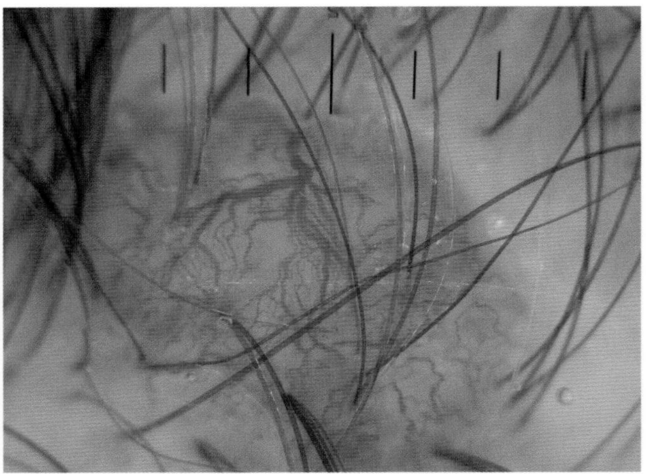

A new scalp papule in a 50-year-old woman: dermoscopy shows arborising vessels within a pink matrix in this histopathologically confirmed nodular BCC.

Scalp BCCs share similar dermoscopic features with other pink scalp tumours such as poorly differentiated squamous cell carcinoma and amelanotic nodular melanoma. Await histopathology before confirming a diagnosis.

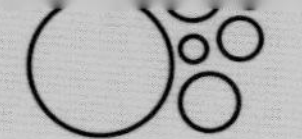

Scalp basal cell carcinoma cases

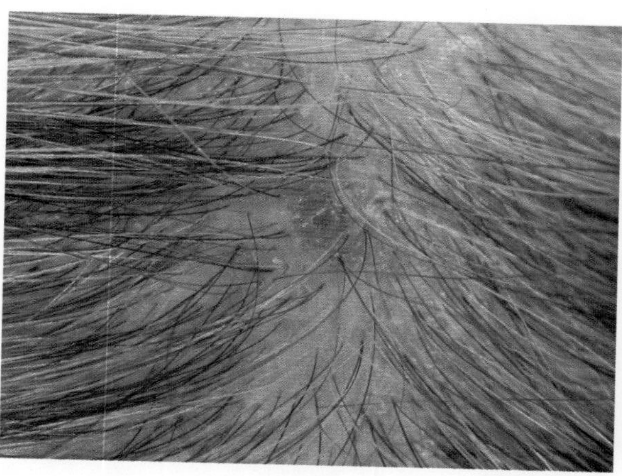

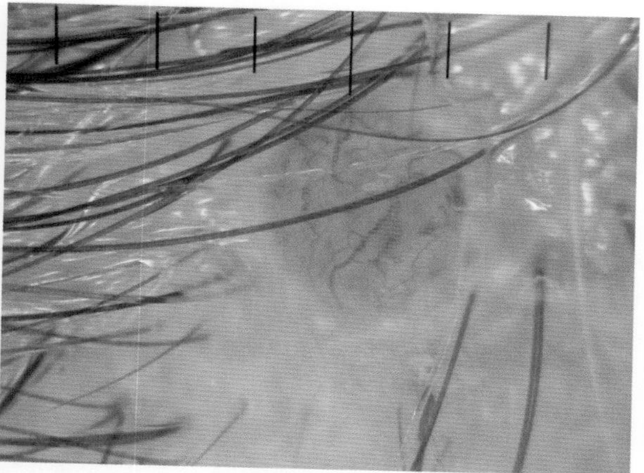

A small 2 mm pink papule on the part-line of a 70-year-old woman: dermoscopy shows a pink background colour with sharply focused linear branching vessels in this nodular BCC.

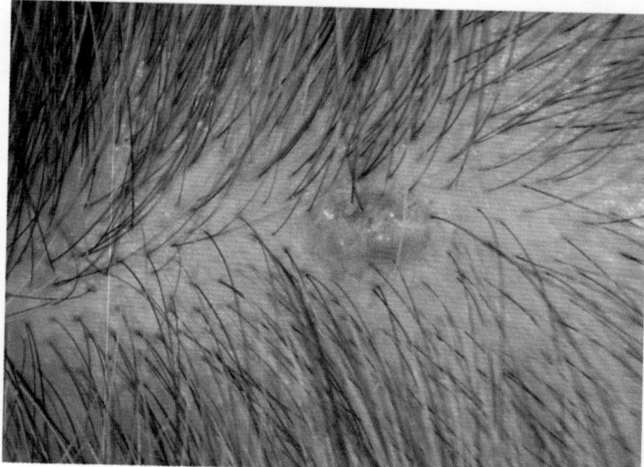

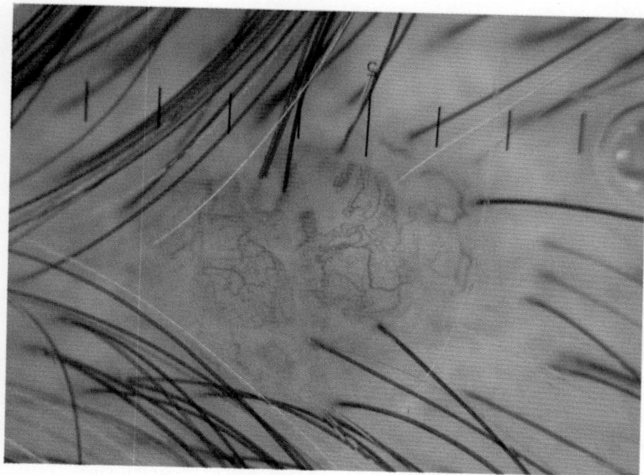

A 5 mm plaque on the vertex of the scalp in a 70-year-old woman: dermoscopy shows sharply focused linear branching vessels in this nodular BCC.

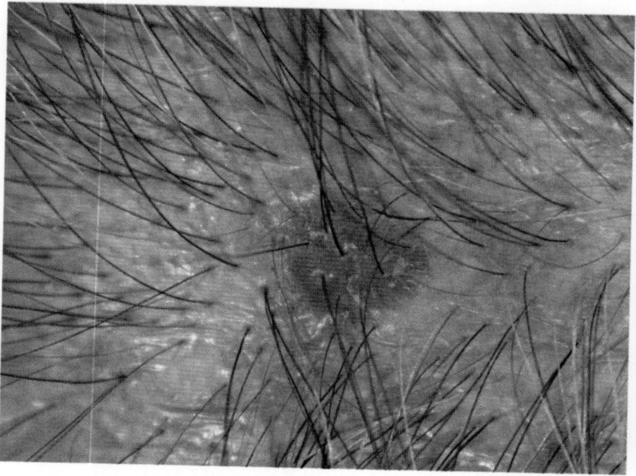

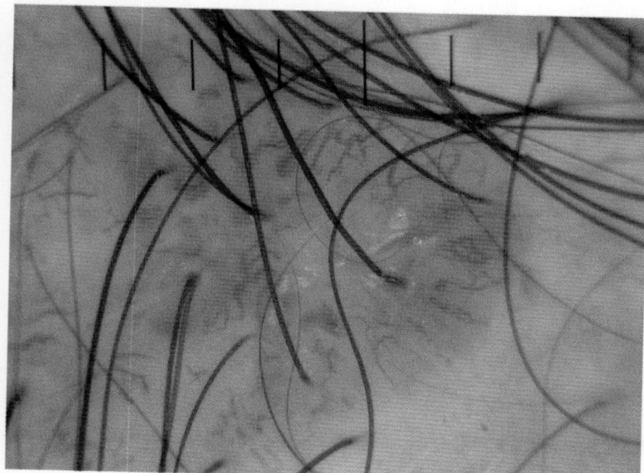

A pink telangiectatic plaque on the vertex of the scalp in a 70-year-old man: dermoscopy shows sharply focused linear branching and irregular vessels in this nodular BCC.

Consider close examination of the vertex and parting line to look for scalp BCC.

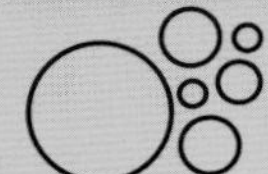

Scalp B-cell lymphoma

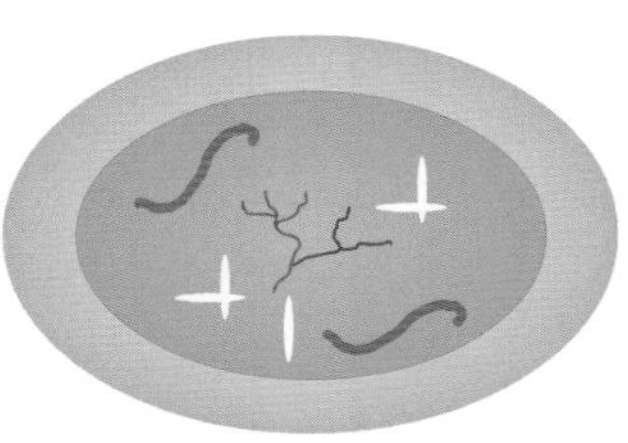

One type of uncommon pink scalp tumour are B-cell lymphomas, most typically primary cutaneous follicle centre lymphoma (PCFCL). They may present clinically as multiple pink plaques that don't tend to ulcerate. Common dermoscopic features include serpentine (linear) vessels and salmon-pink background colouration. Dermoscopy is not specific and diagnosis should be confirmed by combining the clinical features with histopathology and immunohistochemistry.

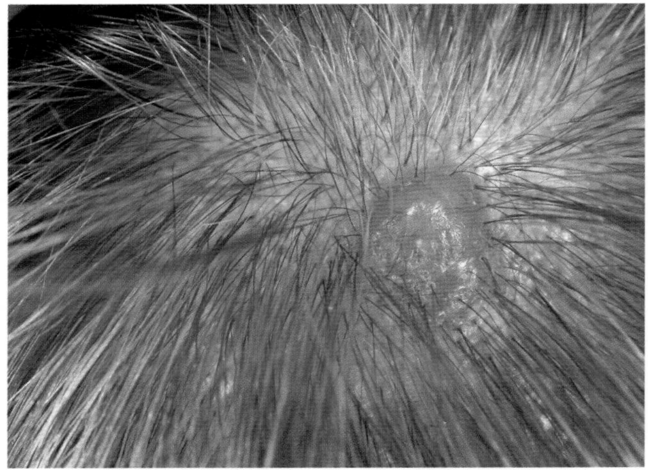

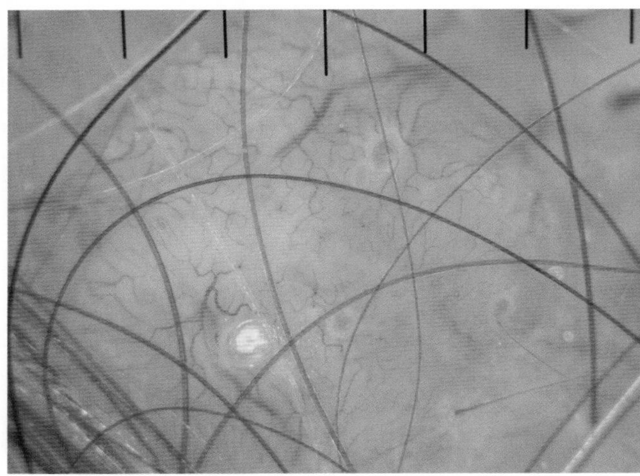

A 60-year-old man with multiple asymptomatic enlarging scalp plaques: dermoscopy shows a pink structureless area with sharply focused linear branching vessels and perifollicular hyperkeratosis in this histopathologically confirmed PCFCL.

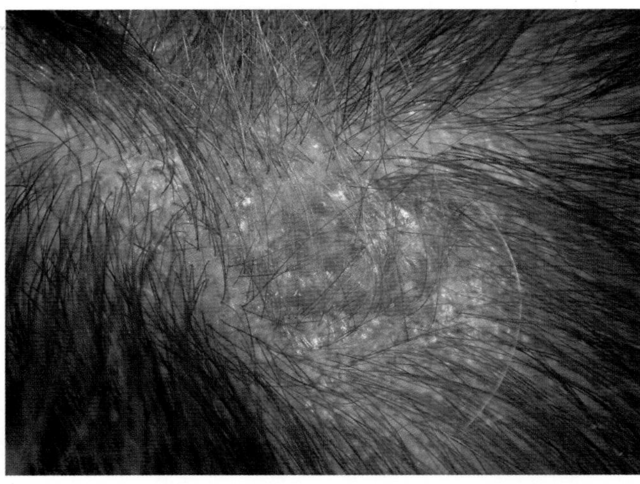

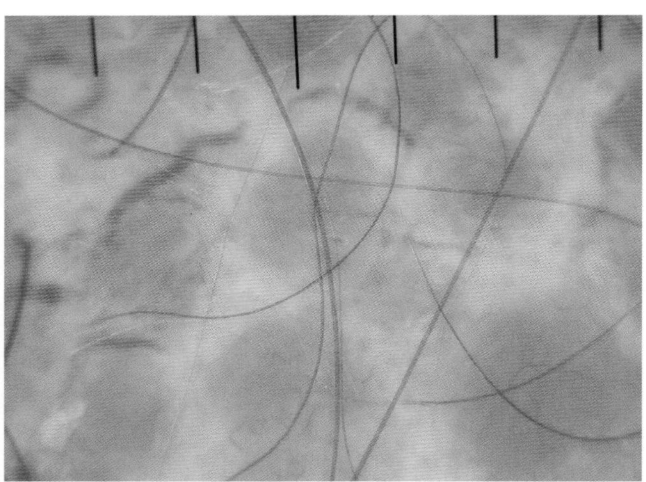

A second firm pink plaque on the scalp of the same 60-year-old man: dermoscopy shows poorly focused serpentine linear vessels with salmon-pink structureless aggregates in this histopathologically confirmed PCFCL.

Geller, S. et al. Dermoscopy and the diagnosis of primary cutaneous B-cell lymphoma. *J Eur Acad Dermatol Venereol*. 2018;32(1):53–56.

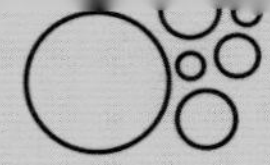

Scalp cylindromas/spiradenomas

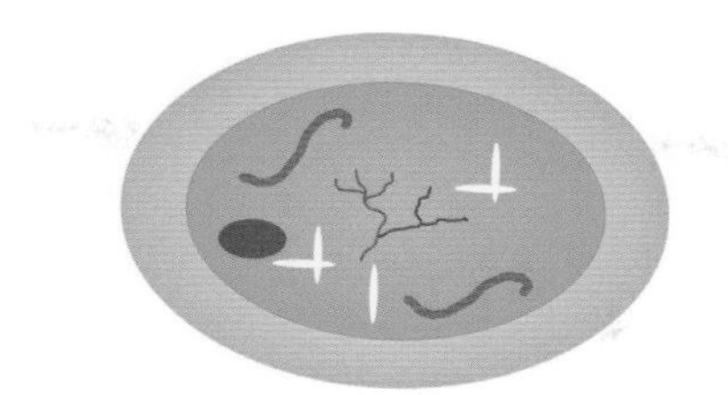

Uncommon pink scalp tumours include cylindromas and spiradenomas. They tend not to show ulceration or erosions unless traumatised. They may be sporadic and solitary or multiple and associated with Brooke–Spiegler syndrome caused by mutations in the CYLD gene. When solitary they mimic many skin tumours and histopathology is required to confirm the diagnosis.

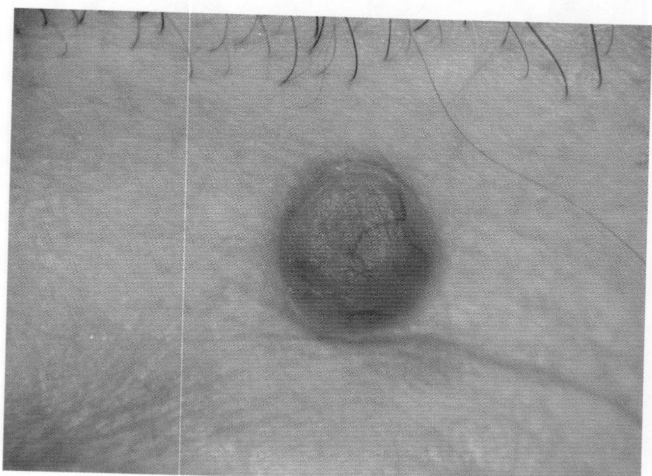

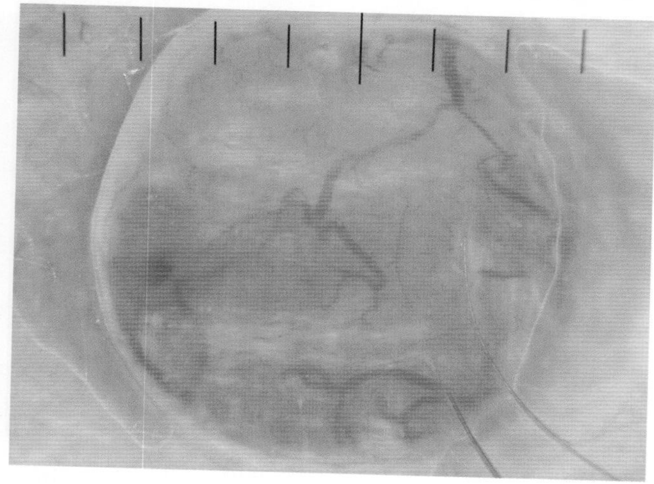

A pink exophytic pre-auricular nodule in a 60-year-old woman: dermoscopy shows a pink structureless area with poorly focused linear branching vessels and shiny white structures in this histopathologically confirmed cylindroma.

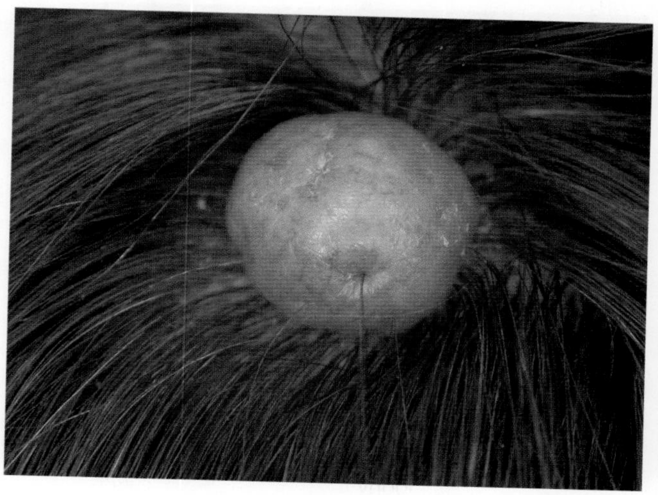

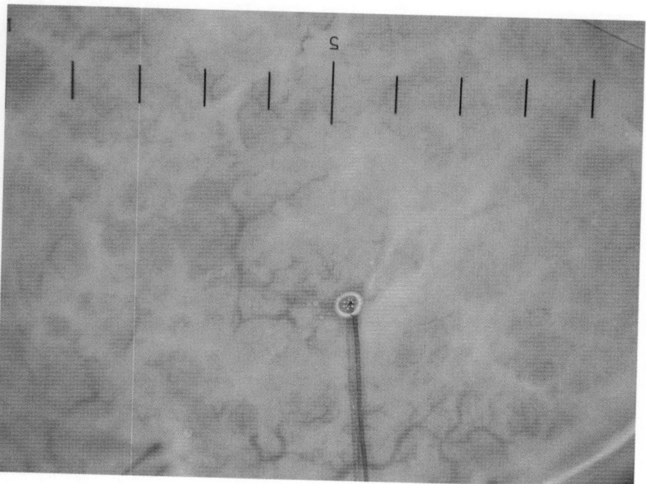

A firm exophytic nodule on the scalp of a 50-year-old woman: dermoscopy shows poorly focused linear branching vessels and pink structureless areas in this histopathologically confirmed cylindroma.

Lallas, A. et al. Dermoscopy of solitary cylindroma. *Eur J Dermatol*. 2011;21(4):645–646.

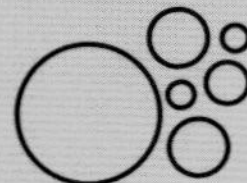

Scalp sarcoidosis

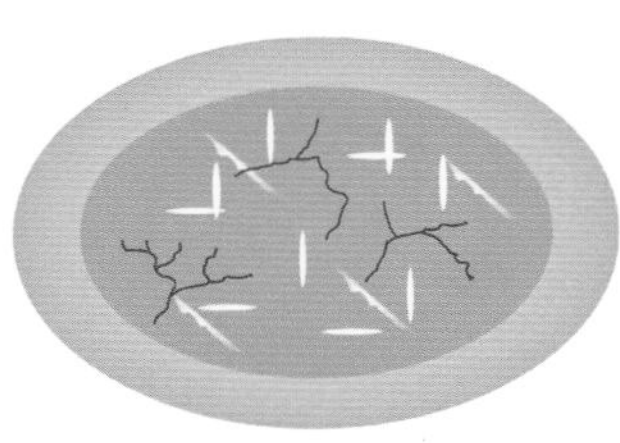

The scalp is an uncommon site for sarcoidosis. It may present as an orange granulomatous plaque or papules on the scalp with reduced density of follicles and telangiectasia on dermoscopy.

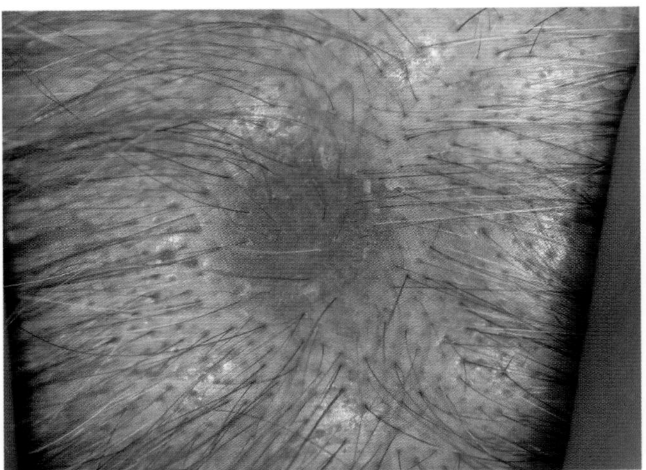

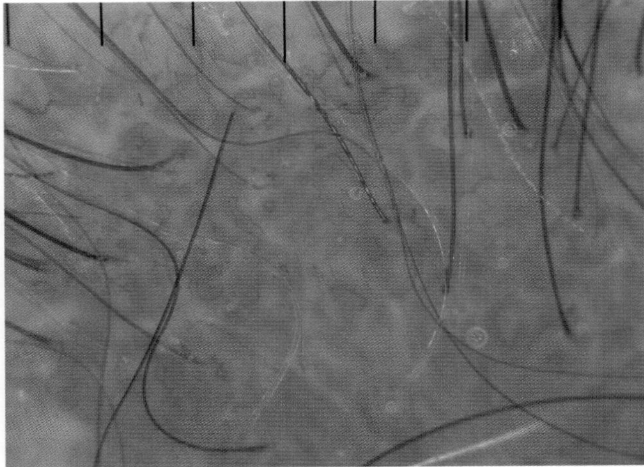

An orange plaque on the scalp in a 70-year-old man: dermoscopy shows linear irregular vessels with orange colouration and reduced follicular density confirmed as scalp sarcoidosis on histopathology.

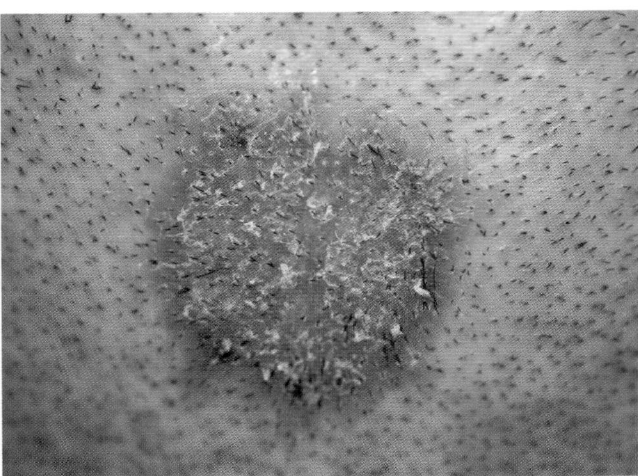

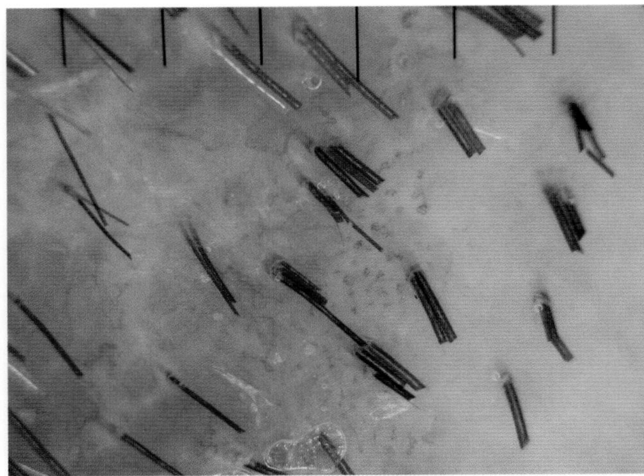

A scaly orange telangiectatic plaque on the scalp of a 45-year-old man: dermoscopy shows orange background colour with linear irregular and branching vessels confirmed as scalp sarcoidosis on histopathology.

Torres, F. et al. Trichoscopy as a clue to the diagnosis of scalp sarcoidosis. *Int J Dermatol*. 2011;50(3):358–361.

7.5 Trichoscopy

Alopecia areata 246
Androgenetic alopecia 247
Frontal fibrosing alopecia 248
Lichen planopilaris 249
Discoid lupus erythematosus 250
Tufted folliculitis 251
Steroid-induced telangiectasia 252
Pseudopelade 253
Circle hairs 254
Trichostasis spinulosa 255
Picker's nodule 256
Traction/frictional alopecia 257
Pseudonits 258

Diagnostic Dermoscopy: The Illustrated Guide, Second Edition. Jonathan Bowling.

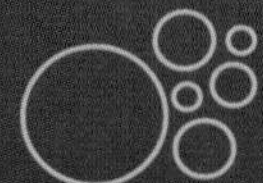

Alopecia areata

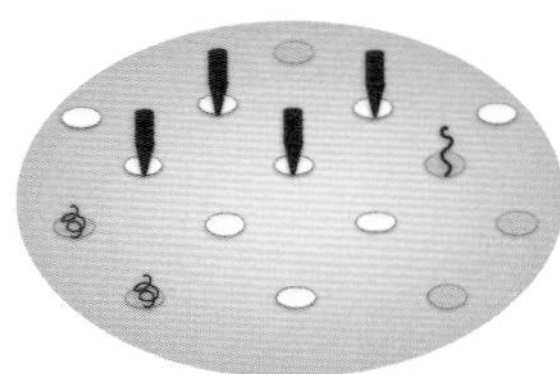

Alopecia areata is a common form of inflammatory non-scarring hair loss characterised by well-circumscribed patches of hair loss with preservation of the follicular ostia. On dermoscopy, typical features of exclamation/tapered hairs, yellow and/or black dots as well as dystrophic and coiled hairs may be seen.

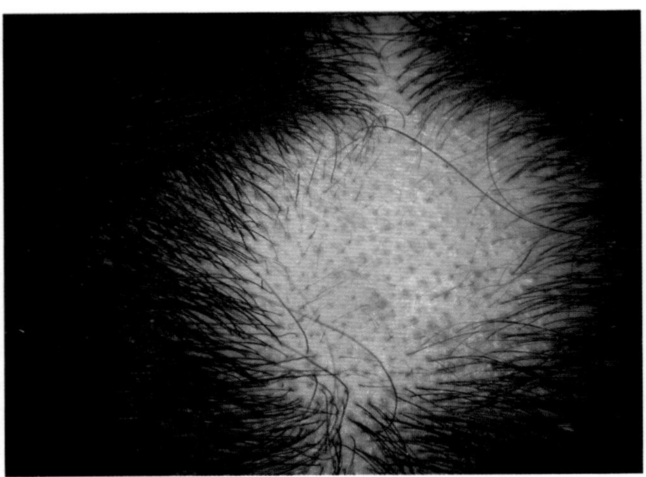

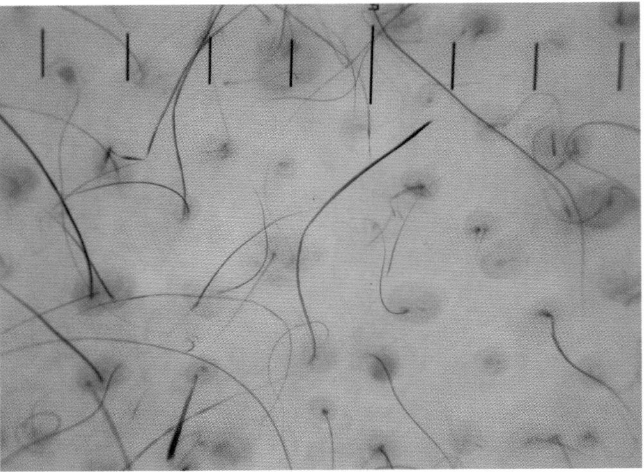

A solitary well-circumscribed patch of non-scarring hair loss on the posterior vertex of a 20-year-old woman: dermoscopy shows yellow dots, exclamation hairs and dystrophic hairs, with preservation of the follicular ostia in this case of alopecia areata.

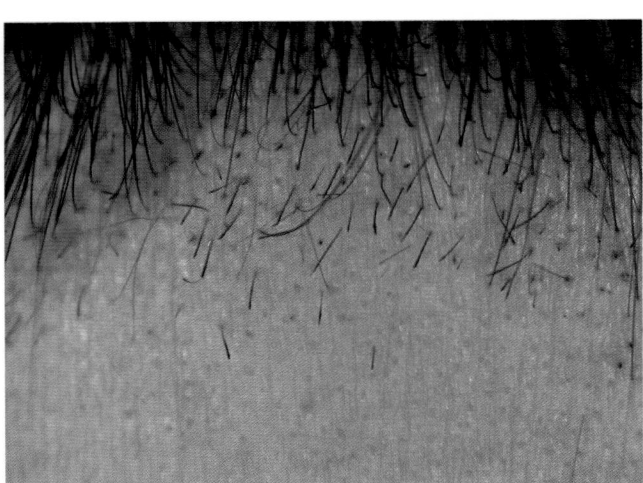

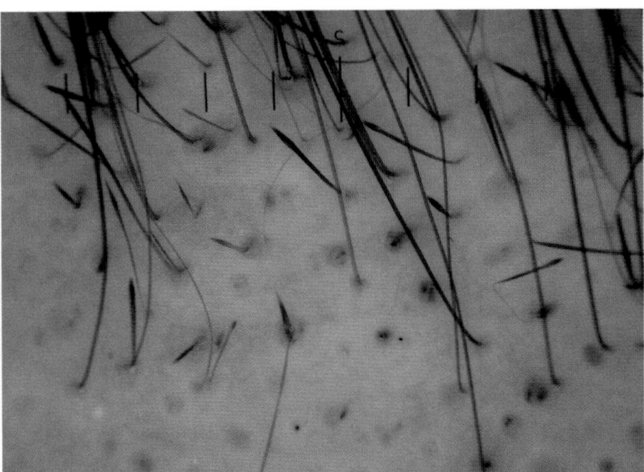

A well-defined patch of alopecia on the occiput of a 30-year-old woman: dermoscopy shows multiple exclamation/tapered hairs plus yellow and black dots in this case of alopecia areata.

Miteva, M. and Tosti, A. Hair and scalp dermatoscopy. *J Am Acad Dermatol.* 2012;67(5):1040–1048.
Waśkiel, A. et al. Trichoscopy of alopecia areata: an update. *J Dermatol.* 2018;45(6):692–700.

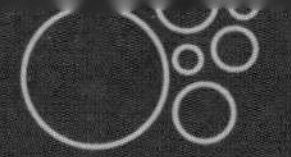

Androgenetic alopecia

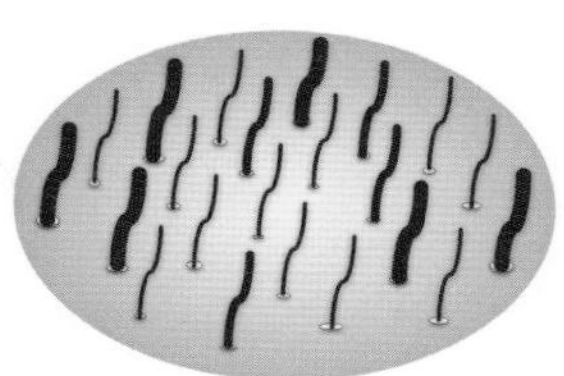

Androgenetic alopecia is a diffuse non-scarring type of hair loss with a patterned distribution. Dermoscopy of hair follicles and hair shaft (trichoscopy) within affected areas shows an increase in the number of vellus (miniaturised) hairs compared with non-affected sites. Repeat trichoscopic imaging at these sites can be useful in monitoring treatment response.

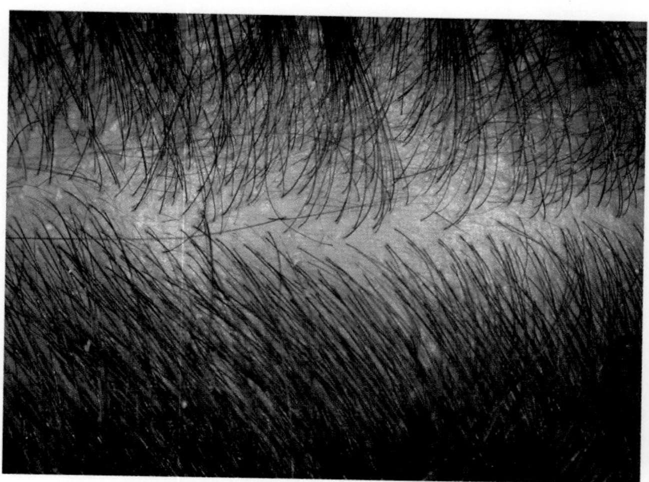

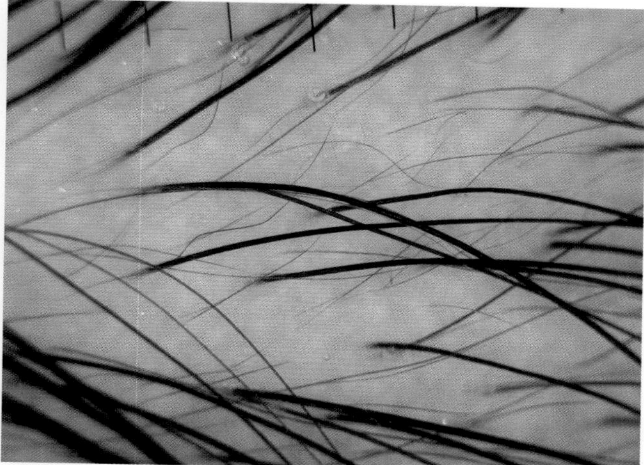

An area of patterned diffuse hair loss with reduced hair density at the vertex of a 50-year-old Indian woman: trichoscopy shows an increase in vellus hairs in keeping with androgenetic alopecia.

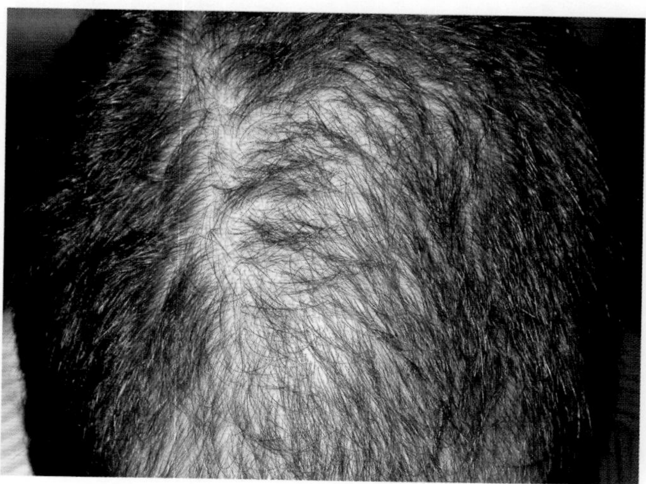

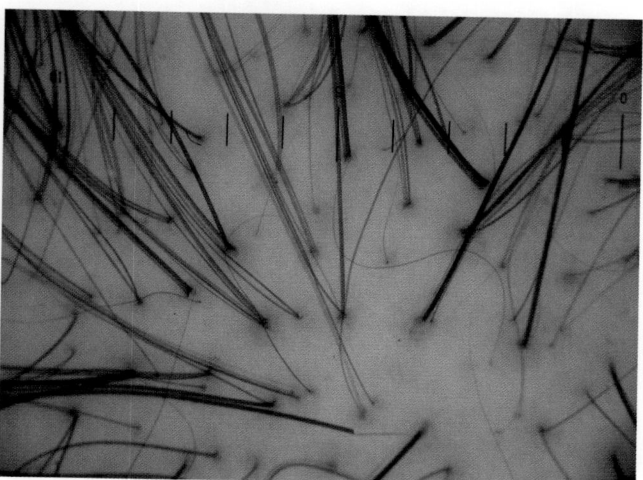

An area of patterned diffuse hair loss at the vertex of a 30-year-old man: trichoscopy shows an increase in vellus hairs consistent with androgenetic alopecia.

Hair diameter diversity greater than 20% is diagnostic of androgenetic alopecia.

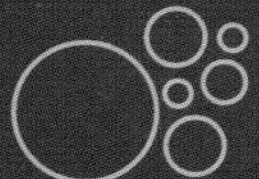

Frontal fibrosing alopecia

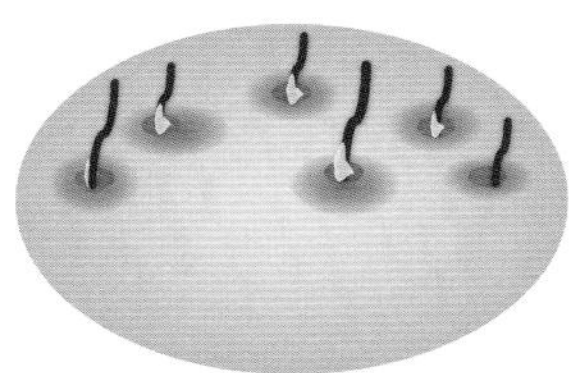

Frontal fibrosing alopecia is a type of lymphocytic scarring alopecia with a band-like distribution involving the frontal hair margin. An early feature is the loss of marginal hairs, the shorter fine hairs at the boundary between mature hairs of the scalp and the vellus hairs of the forehead. Trichoscopy shows peripilar casts, more visible in dry dermoscopy, and peripilar erythema, both indicators of active inflammation. Isolated hair follicles and loss of follicular ostia indicate a scarring process.

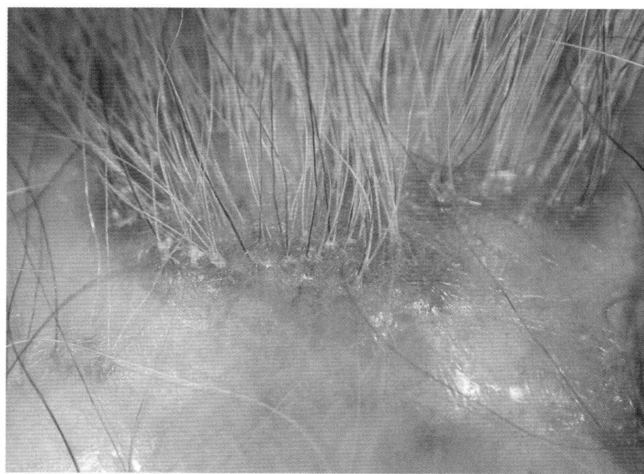

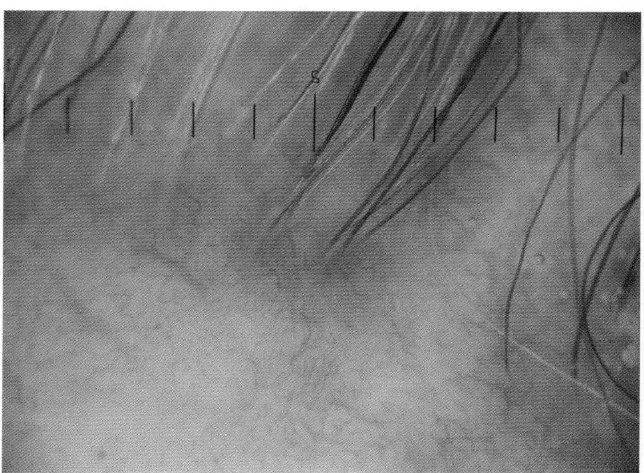

Visible inflammation and hair loss at the anterior hair margin with peripilar casts and scarring in a 70-year-old woman: gel immersion dermoscopy illustrates peripilar erythema but not peripilar casts in keeping with frontal fibrosing alopecia.

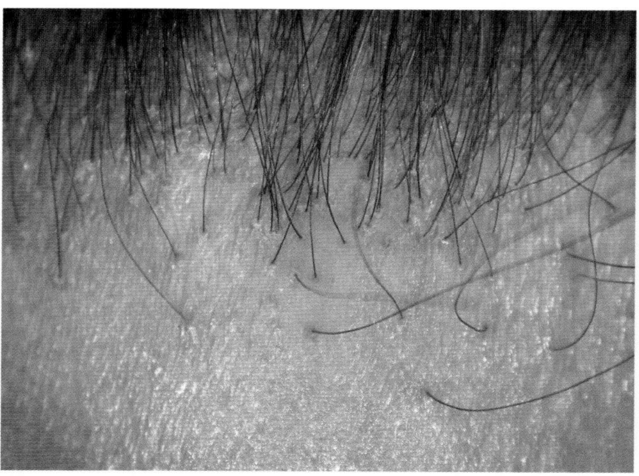

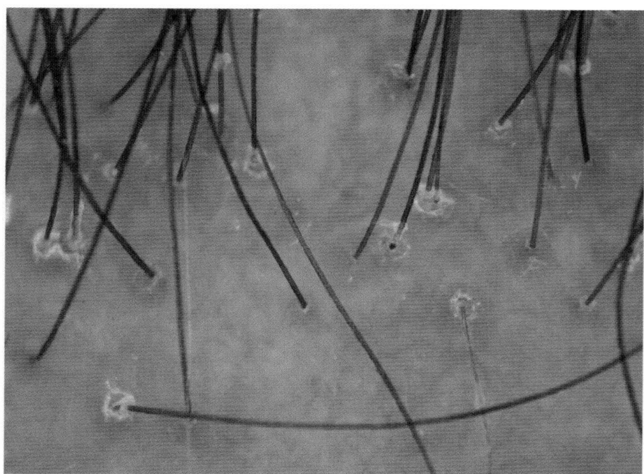

Scarring alopecia affecting the anterior hairline in a 65-year-old woman: dry dermoscopy shows peripilar casts, loss of follicular ostia and widespread background erythema in keeping with frontal fibrosing alopecia.

Martínez-Velasco, M.A. et al. Frontal Fibrosing Alopecia Severity Index: A trichoscopic visual scale that correlates thickness of peripilar casts with severity of inflammatory changes at pathology. *Skin Appendage Discord*. 2018;4(4):277–280.

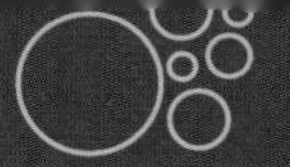

Lichen planopliaris

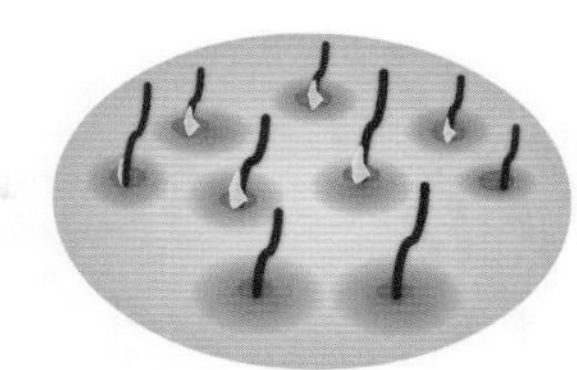

Lichen planopilaris is a type of lymphocytic scarring alopecia characterised by diffuse or focal patches of hair loss often in a more generalised scalp distribution. There is clinical, dermoscopic and histopathological overlap with frontal fibrosing alopecia. Trichoscopy shows peripilar casts and erythema, both indicators of active inflammation. Elongated linear vessels, and loss of follicular ostia are also observed.

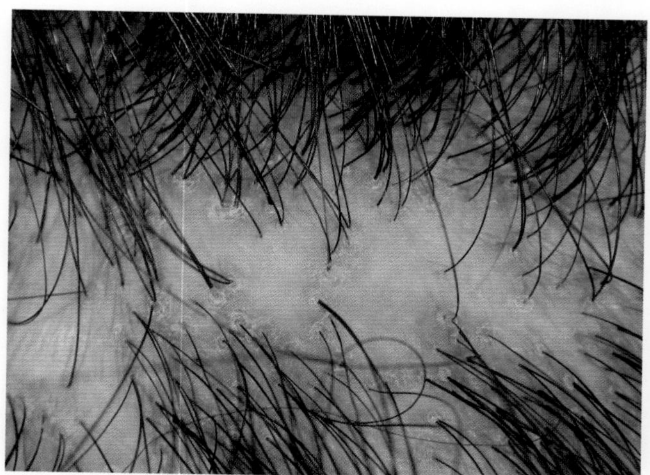

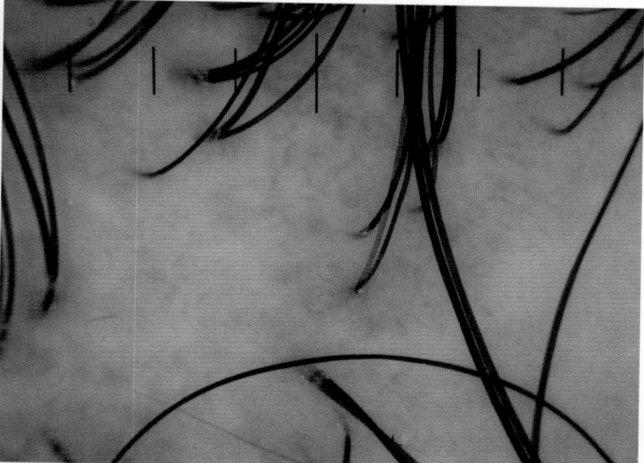

Patches of scarring alopecia across the vertex of the scalp with perifollicular scales and erythema in this 70-year-old woman: gel immersion dermoscopy shows peripilar erythema, loss of follicular ostia and linear vessels in keeping with lichen planopilaris.

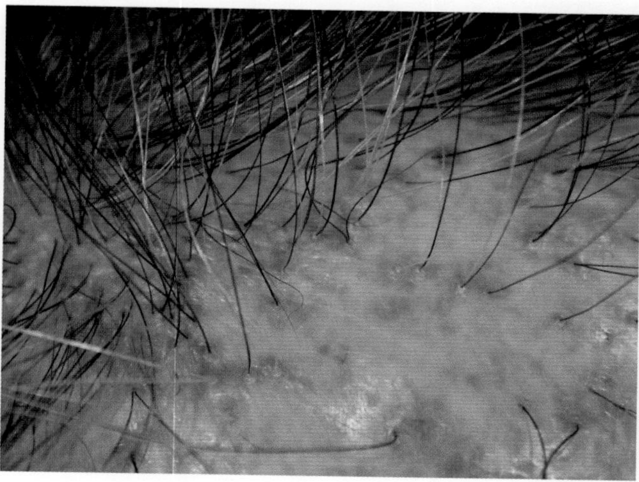

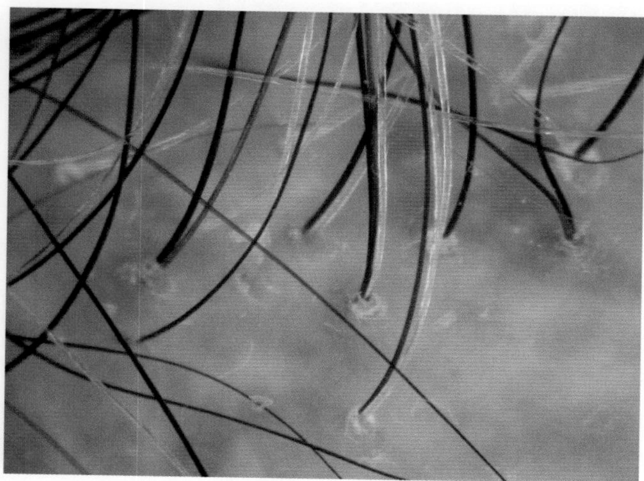

Multifocal patches of scarring alopecia across the scalp with erythema and scales in this 70-year-old woman: dry dermoscopy shows peripilar casts, peripilar erythema and loss of follicular ostia in keeping with lichen planopilaris

Rakowska, A. et al. Trichoscopy of cicatricial alopecia. *J Drugs Dermatol*. 2012;11(6):753–758.

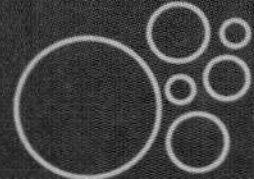

Discoid lupus erythematosus

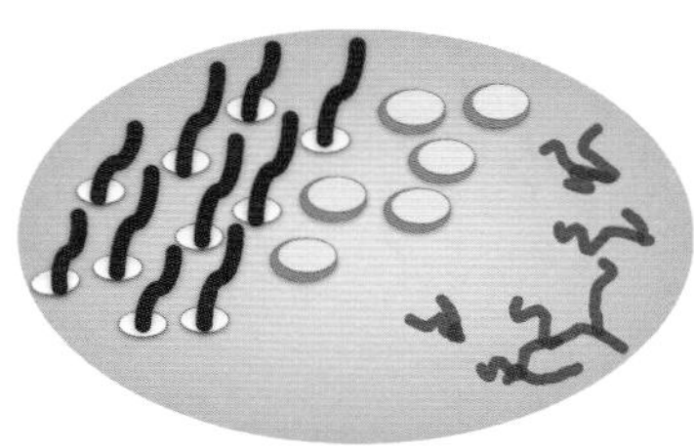

Discoid lupus erythematosus of the scalp is a lymphocytic scarring alopecia that typically presents as localised patches of scarring alopecia. It shares clinical features with many of the lymphocytic scarring alopecias. Dermoscopy may show a variety of features including follicular plugging, scarring alopecia and variable vessel types.

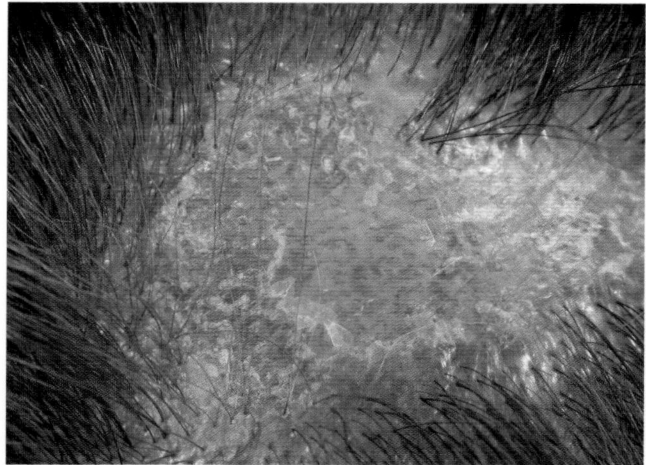

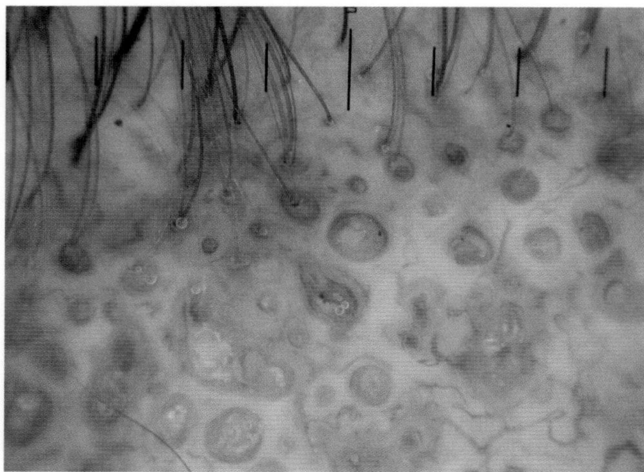

A 70-year-old woman with multiple plaques of scarring alopecia: dermoscopy shows scarring alopecia, keratotic follicular plugging and ectatic linear and irregular vessels confirmed as discoid lupus erythematosus on histopathology.

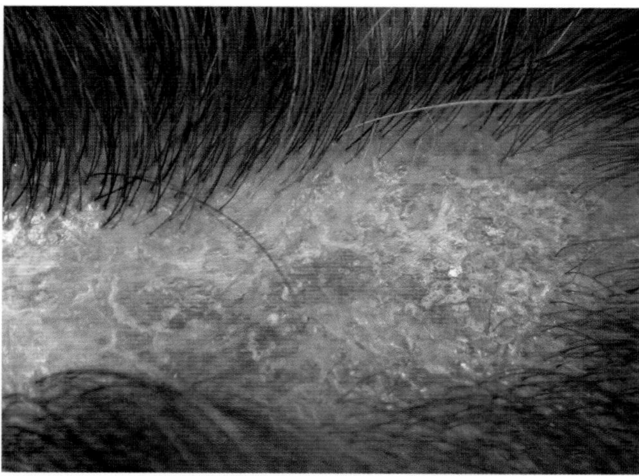

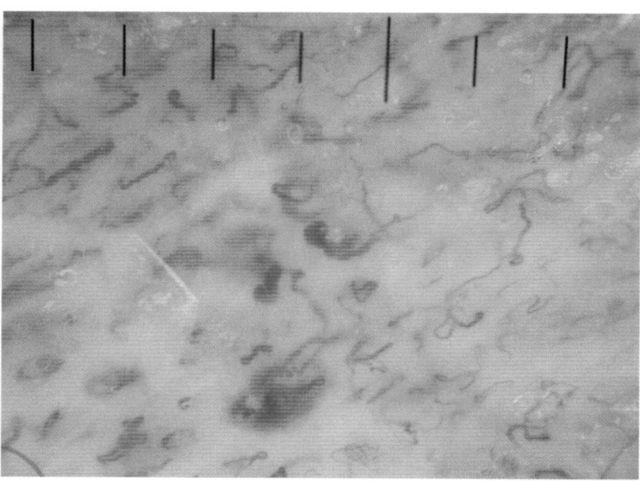

A further telangiectatic plaque on the scalp of the same 70-year-old woman: dermoscopy shows broad, ectatic and tortuous linear vessels.

Duque-Estrada, B. et al. Dermoscopy patterns of cicatricial alopecia resulting from discoid lupus erythematosus and lichen planopilaris. *An Bras Dermatol*. 2010;85(2):179–183.

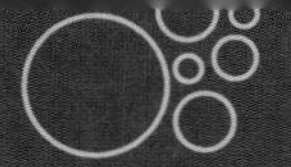

Tufted folliculitis

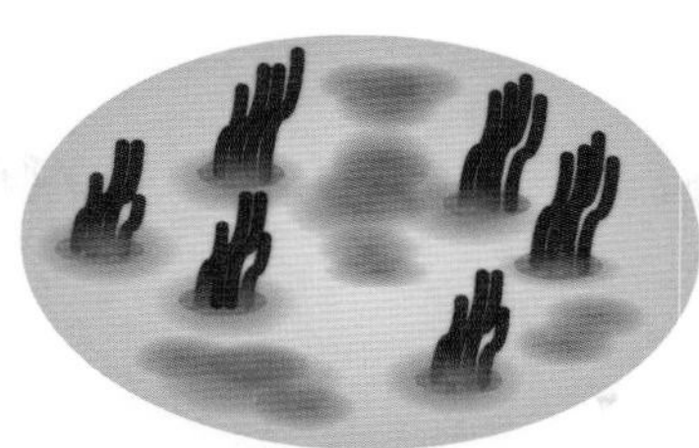

Tufting is a clinical feature seen across the spectrum of neutrophilic scarring alopecias, which include tufted folliculitis, folliculitis decalvans and dissecting cellulitis. Common clinical features include intense inflammation, scarring, crusting and tufting, where multiple hairs twist and emerge through a common follicular ostium. Trichoscopy can help illustrate tufting, scarring, interfollicular or perifollicular erythema and dilated vessels.

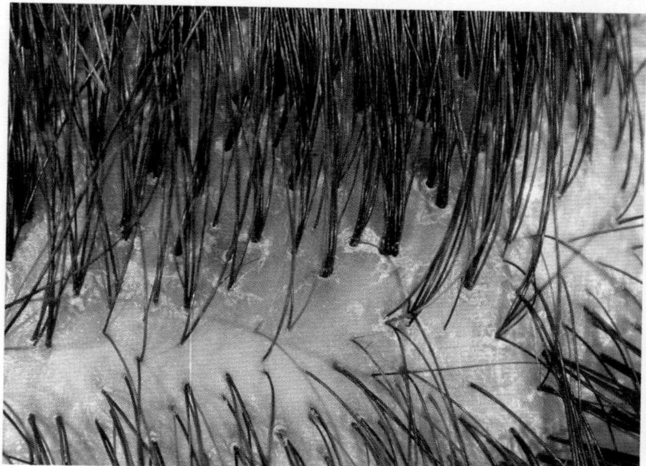

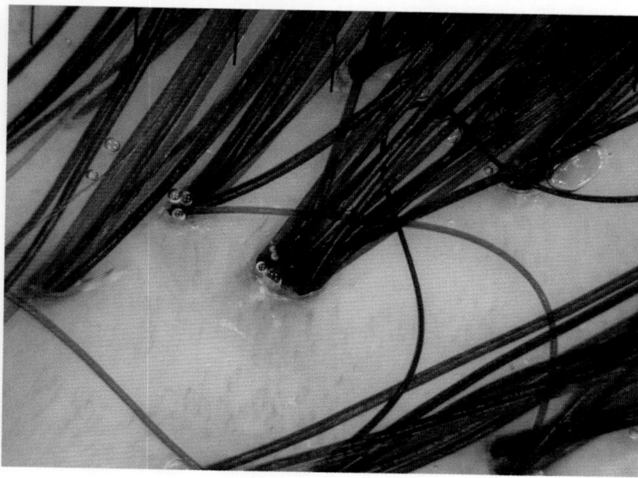

A patch of localized inflammation and scarring alopecia on the parietal scalp of a 30-year-old man: dermoscopy shows tufting and dilated perifollicular and interfollicular linear vessels in this case of tufted folliculitis.

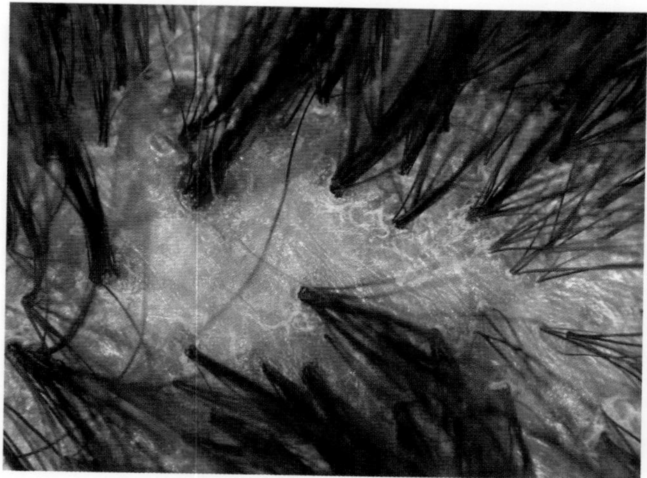

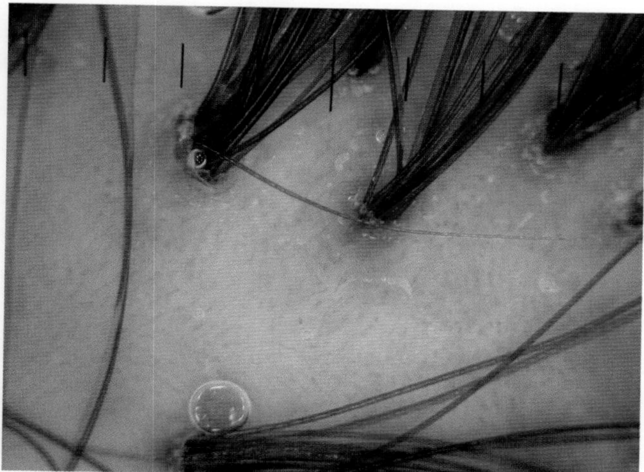

Widespread scalp scarring and inflammation in a 50-year–old man: dermoscopy shows tufting and marked dilated perifollicular and interfollicular linear vessels in this case of folliculitis decalvans.

Uchiyama, M. et al. Histopathologic and dermoscopic features of 42 cases of folliculitis decalvans: a case series. *J Am Acad Dermatol.* 2020;S0190–9622(20):30515–30516.

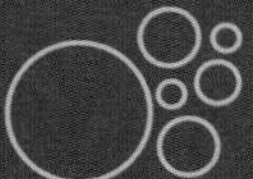

Steroid-induced telangiectasia

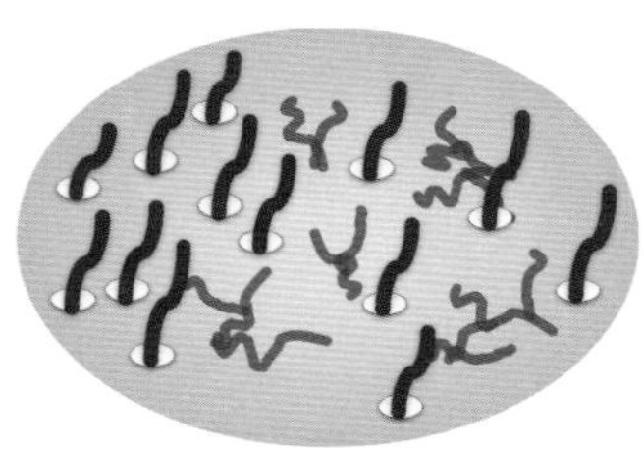

Following prolonged topical steroid use, vessels in the dermal vascular plexus may be seen through a combined process of skin atrophy and vascular dilatation and proliferation. Clinically this erythema may be thought to be active inflammation. Trichoscopy can show the erythema is caused by steroid-induced telangiectasia and not perifollicular erythema.

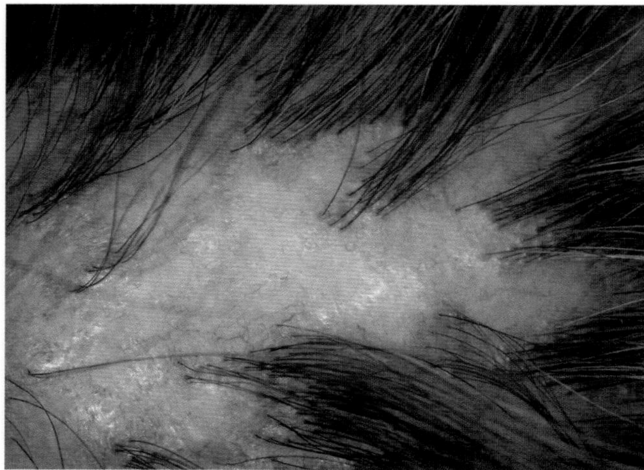

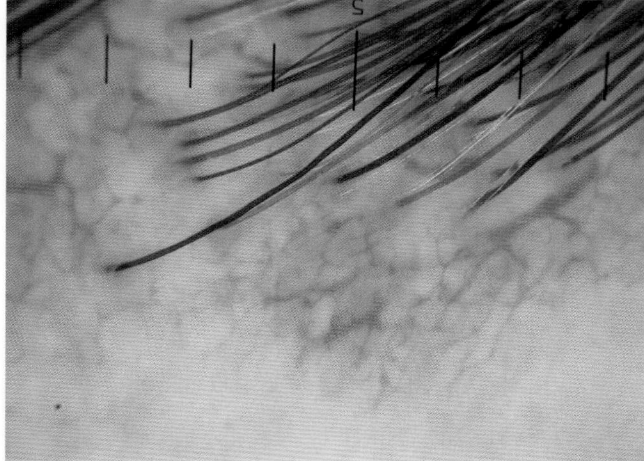

Lichen planopilaris of the scalp treated with prolonged topical steroids in a 50-year-old woman: dermoscopy shows atrophy with broad linear vessels of the dermal plexus in keeping with steroid-induced telangiectasia.

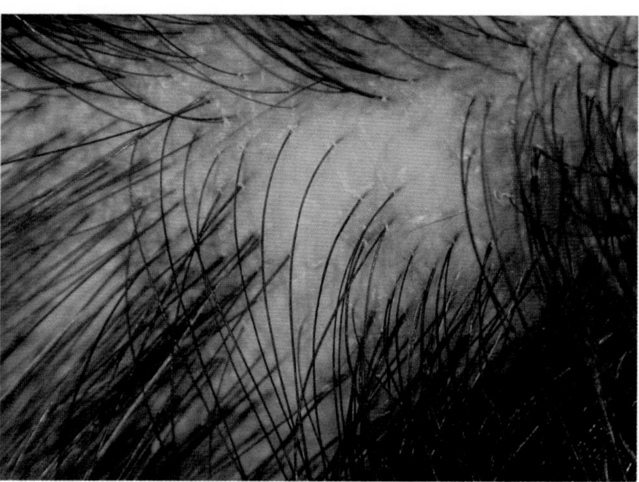

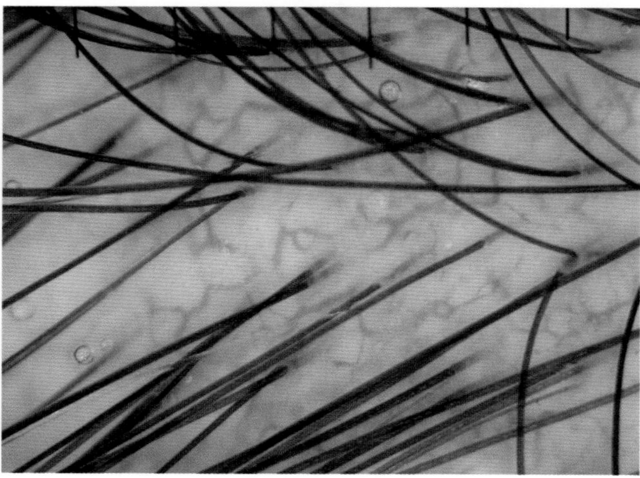

Lichen planopilaris of the scalp treated with prolonged topical steroids in another 50-year-old woman: dermoscopy shows a vascular network of poorly focused ectatic linear vessels in keeping with steroid-induced telangiectasia.

Pirmez, R. Trichoscopy of steroid-induced atrophy. *Skin Appendage Disord*. 2017;3(4):171–174.

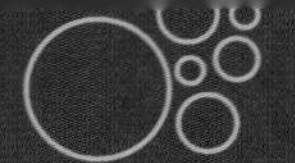

Pseudopelade

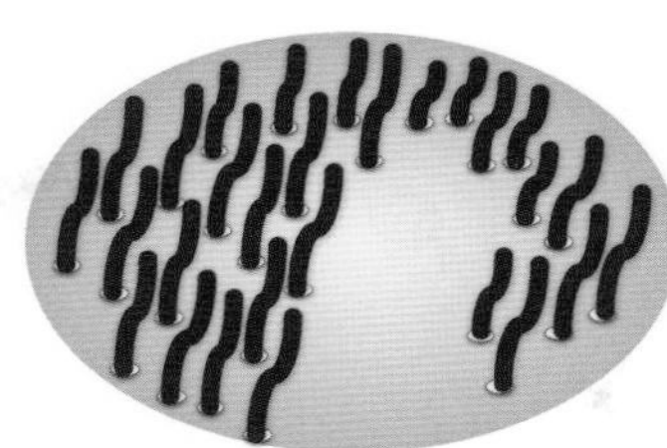

Pseudopelade is a non-specific scarring end-stage of scalp diseases resulting in alopecia. It may present as an idiopathic form of scarring, but it is most likely associated with the lymphocytic scarring alopecias, with clinically smooth, skin-coloured patches of alopecia over the parietal and vertex areas. Trichoscopy shows loss of follicle ostia and absence of inflammation.

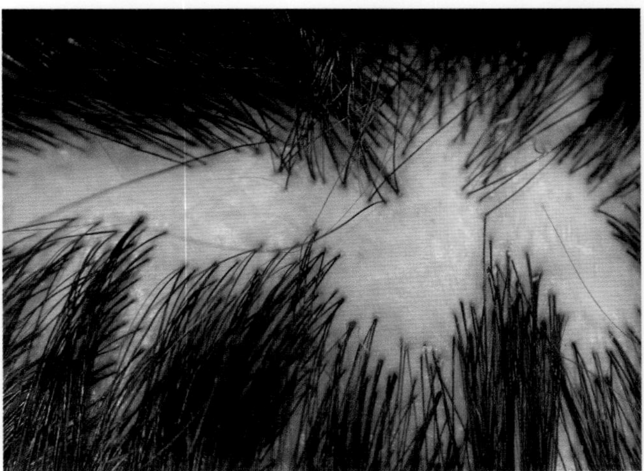

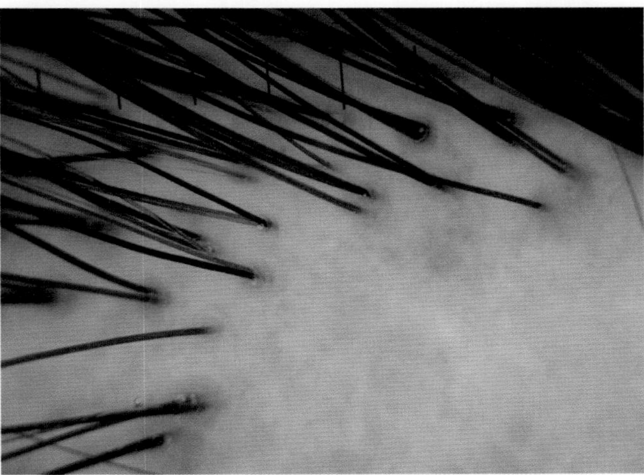

An irregular patch of scarring alopecia on the parietal scalp of a 25-year-old man: dermoscopy shows loss of follicular ostia and no signs of inflammation (perifollicular erythema or dilated vessels) in this case of idiopathic pseudopelade.

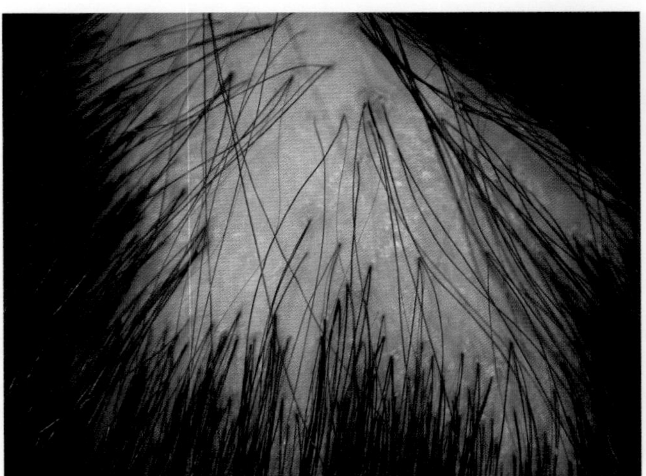

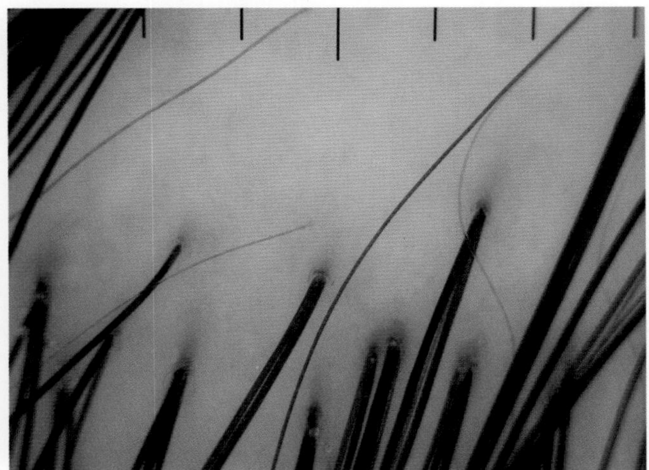

A large patch of scarring alopecia on the posterior vertex of a 40-year-old man: dermoscopy shows loss of follicular ostia without signs of inflammation in this case of pseudopelade.

Consider a biopsy to determine the diagnosis and disease activity following a clinical and trichoscopic examination.

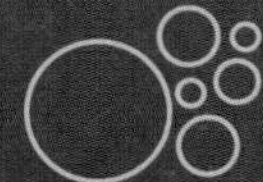

Circle hairs

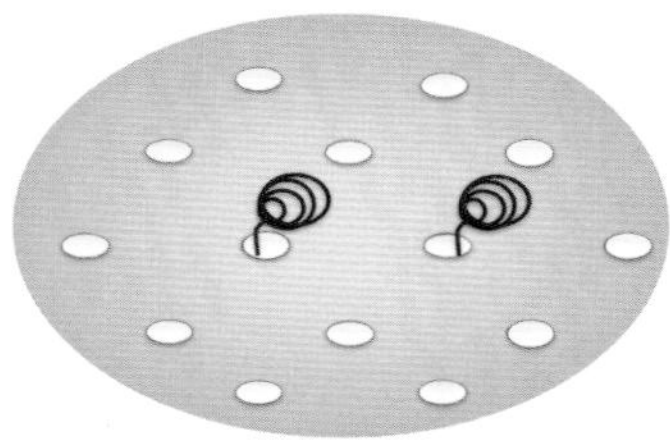

Solitary ingrown or circle hairs rarely cause diagnostic concern, but they may be associated with secondary skin changes such as inflammation and scarring. When extensive and multiple they may cause diagnostic concern and mimic follicular keratinising conditions. They can clearly be seen on dermoscopy/trichoscopy as dark subcorneal coiled hairs.

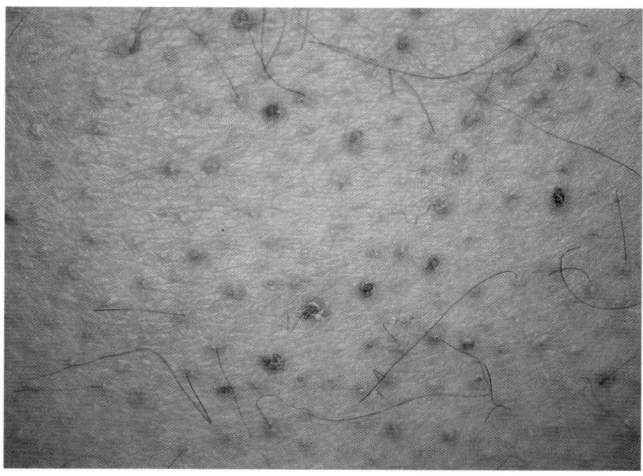

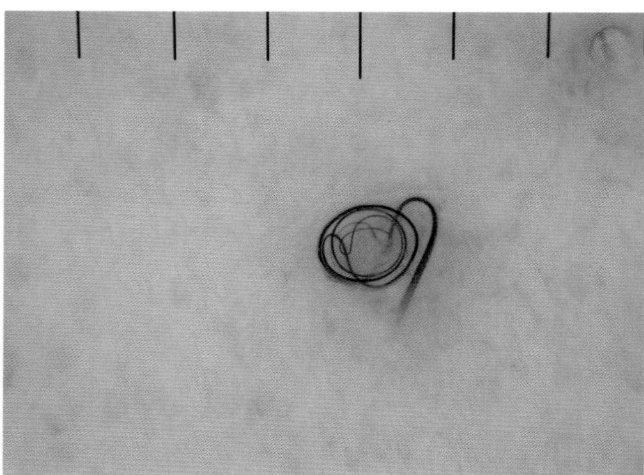

Multiple follicular papules on the posterior thighs of a 50-year-old man: dermoscopy shows coiled or circle hairs.

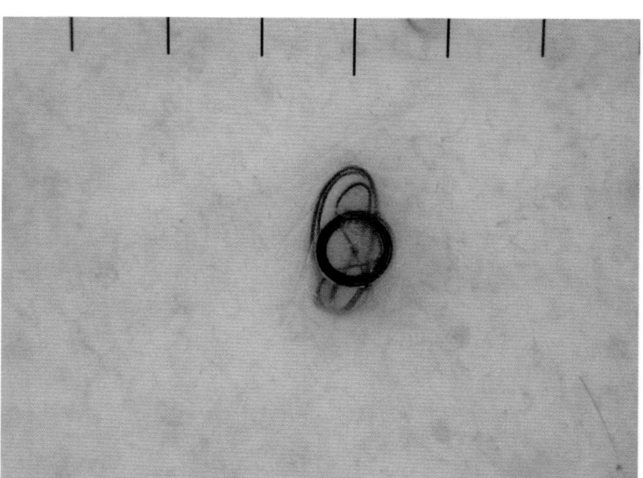

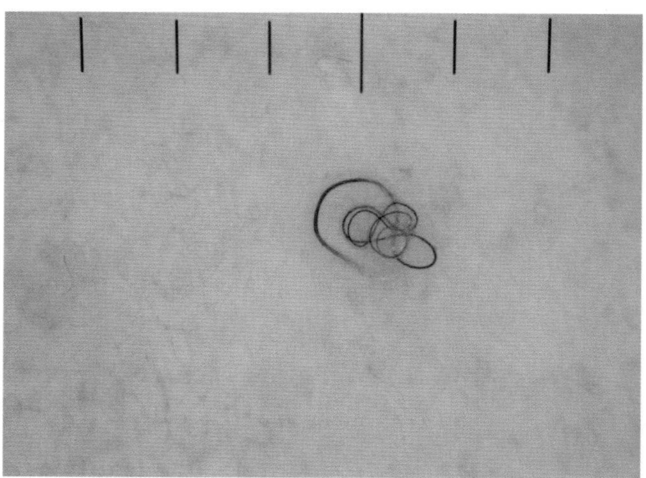

Further images of coiled circle hairs.

Follicular keratinisation is a feature of many different dermatologic conditions. Consider a diagnostic biopsy if any diagnostic doubt remains following clinical history, examination and dermoscopy.

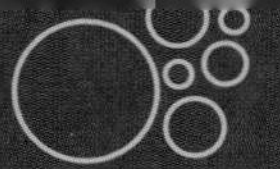

Trichostasis spinulosa

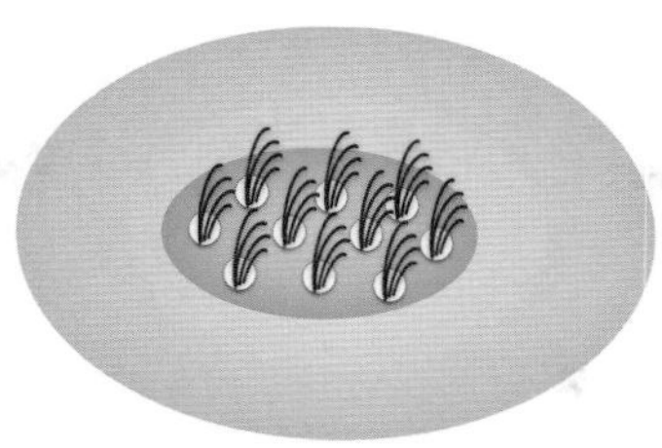

Trichostasis spinulosa can be a localised feature within skin lesions such as dermal naevi or an incidental finding. Multiple vellus hairs erupt through a follicle ostium, which are clearly seen on trichoscopy.

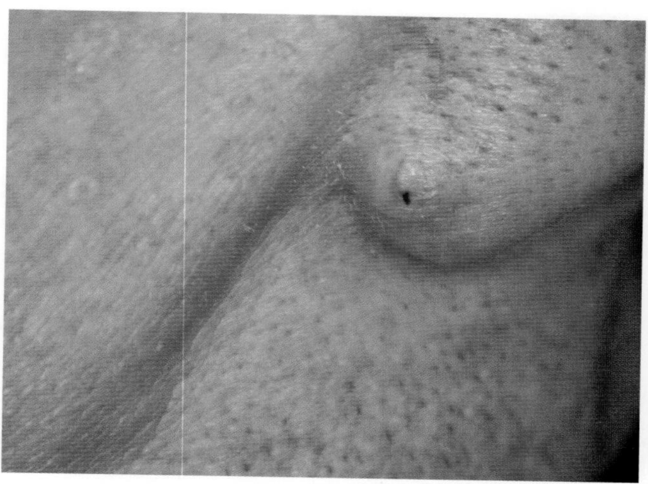

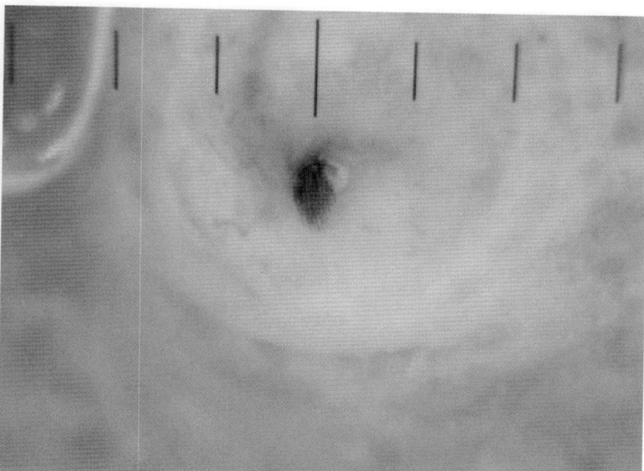

A dermal naevus on the nasal ala of a 60-year-old man: trichoscopy shows multiple vellus hairs protruding through a follicle ostium.

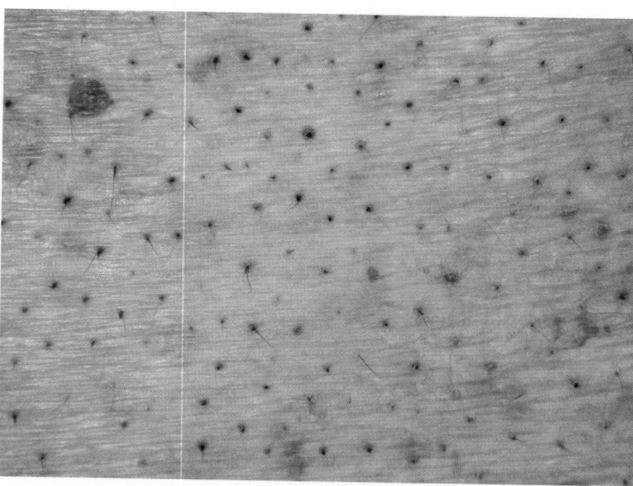

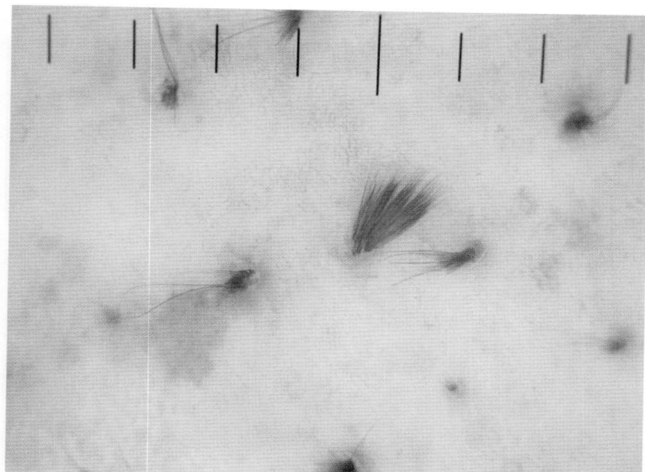

Multiple follicle papules on the flanks of a 30-year-old man: dermoscopy shows multiple vellus hairs protruding through various follicle ostia in keeping with trichostasis spinulosa.

Pozo, L. et al. Dermoscopy of trichostasis spinulosa. *Arch Dermatol*. 2008;144(8):1088.

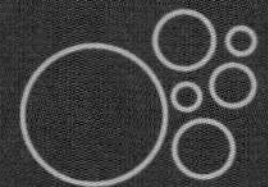

Picker's nodule

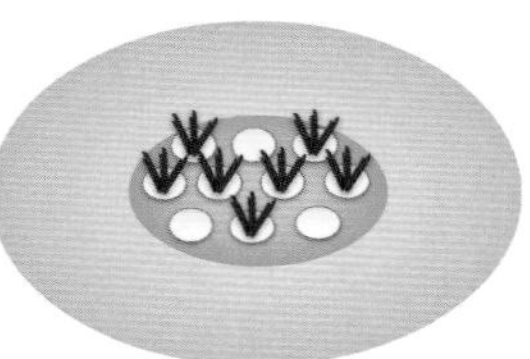

A picker's nodule (lichen simplex chronicus) represents thickening of the skin caused by repetitive trauma, often habitual. When on the scalp, the increase in hair density creates a scar-like plaque or nodule with multiple broken hairs and split hairs (trichoptilosis). Trichoscopy can illustrate the focal traumatic change in hair shafts, thus aiding diagnosis.

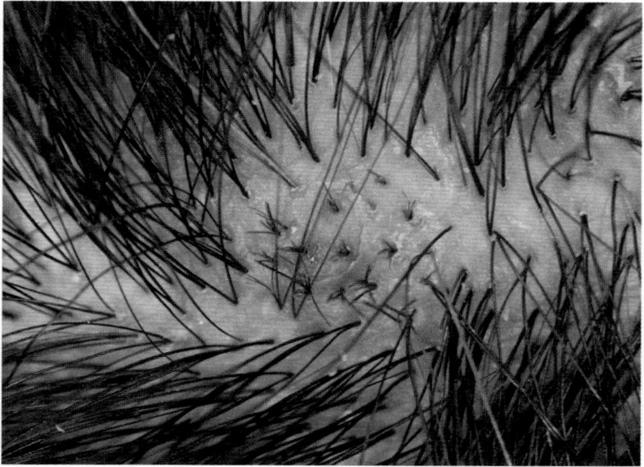

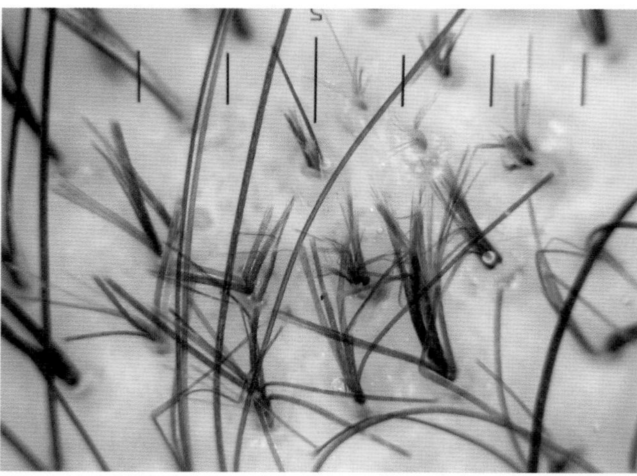

A solitary plaque on the parietal scalp of a 50-year-old man: trichoscopy shows multiple broken hairs and trichoptilosis in keeping with a picker's nodule.

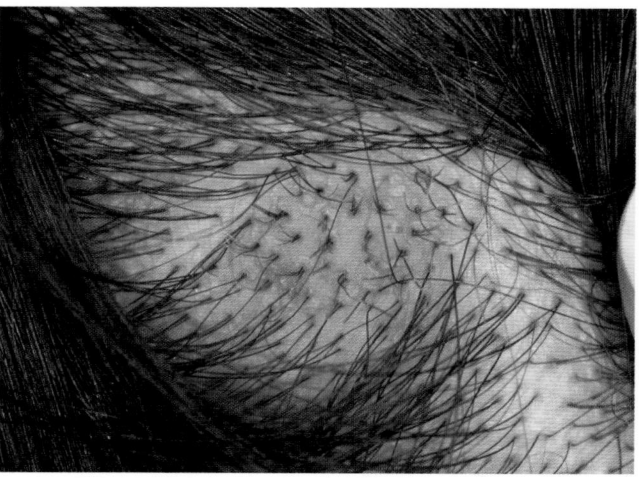

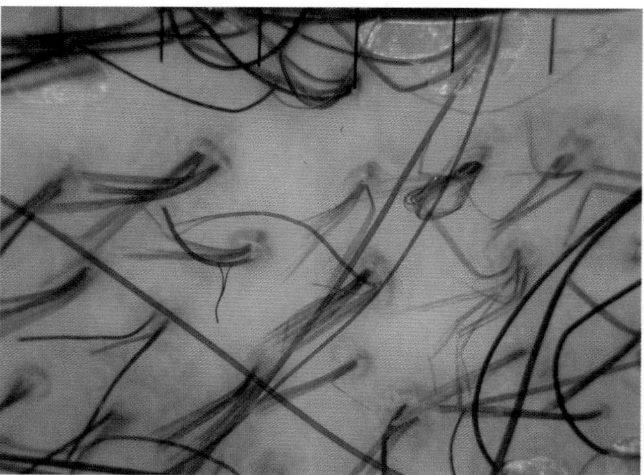

A solitary plaque on the occipital scalp of a 40-year-old man: trichoscopy shows multiple broken hairs and trichoptilosis in keeping with a picker's nodule.

Consider a biopsy if concerns regarding diagnosis and disease activity remain following a clinical and trichoscopic examination.

Traction/frictional alopecia

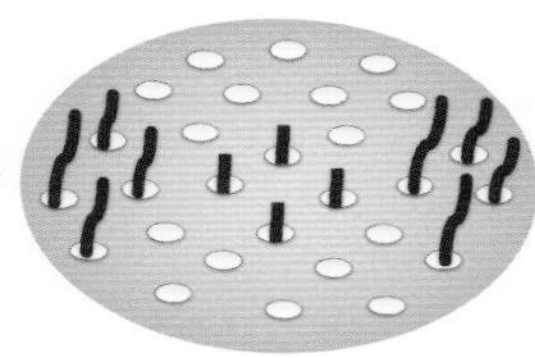

Traction alopecia is a type of hair loss caused by constant pulling of the hair over a long period of time. Common causes are braids and tight ponytails. Trichotillomania (trichotillosis) is a form of traction alopecia resulting from repetitive trauma (rubbing, pulling, or plucking) to the scalp. Trichoscopy shows hairs of differing lengths, broken hairs and an absence of yellow dots or exclamation/tapered hairs that are seen in alopecia areata.

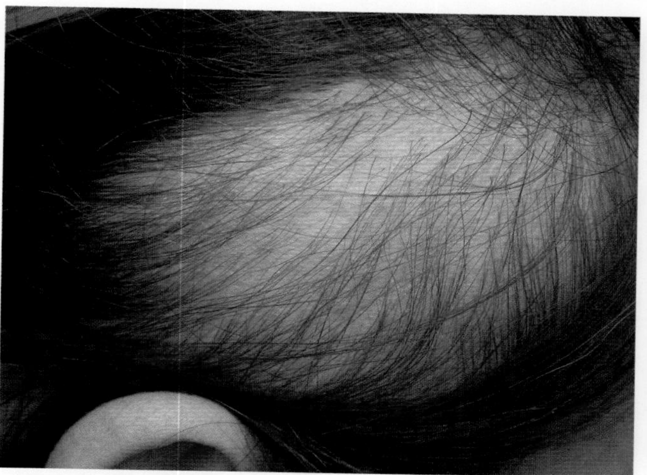

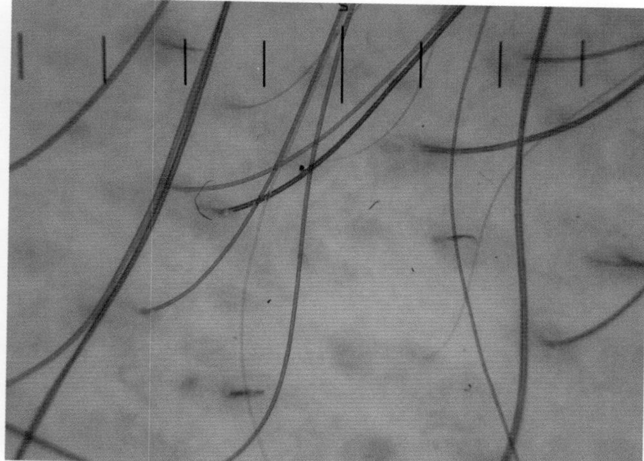

Biparietal hair loss in a 20-year-old woman with a history of traction alopecia from tight ponytails: dermoscopy shows hair loss and broken hairs.

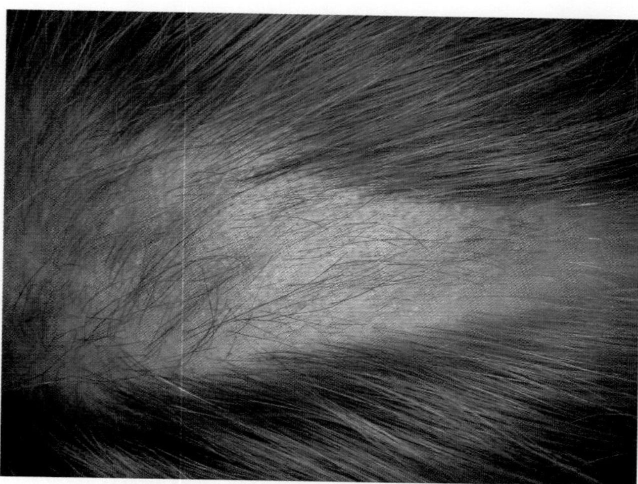

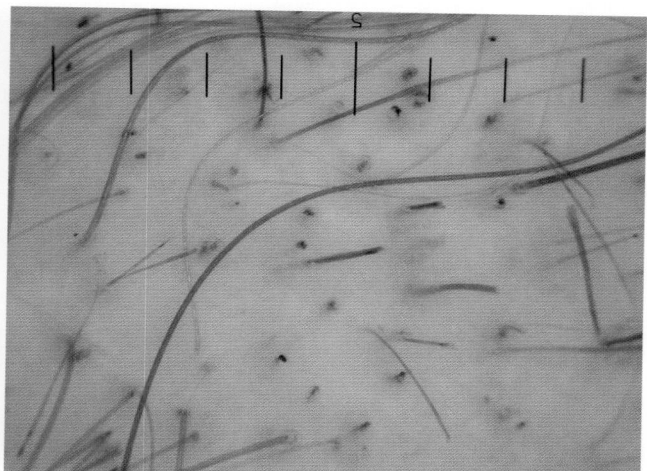

A triangular patch of reduced hair density on the vertex scalp of a 12-year-old boy: trichoscopy shows multiple broken hairs, black dots and hairs of different lengths.

Abraham, L.S. et al. Dermoscopic clues to distinguish trichotillomania from patchy alopecia areata. *An Bras Dermatol.* 2010;85(5):723–726.

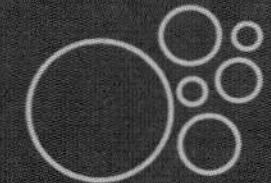

Pseudonits

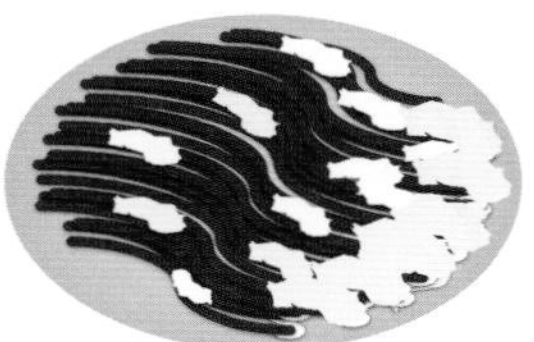

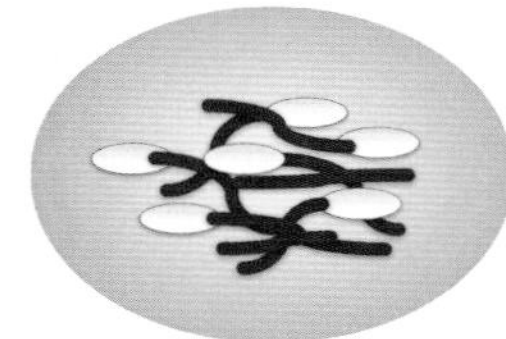

Pseudonits are white structures found along hair shafts of the scalp that mimic the nits of head lice. Inflammatory scaling conditions such as psoriasis, seborrhoeic dermatitis or pityiasis amiantacea are common causes. Dreadlocks can also generate pseudonits when the bulbs of telogen hairs are retained and entangled in neighbouring hair. Dermoscopy can help differentiate keratin structures, hair casts and telogen bulbs from true nits.

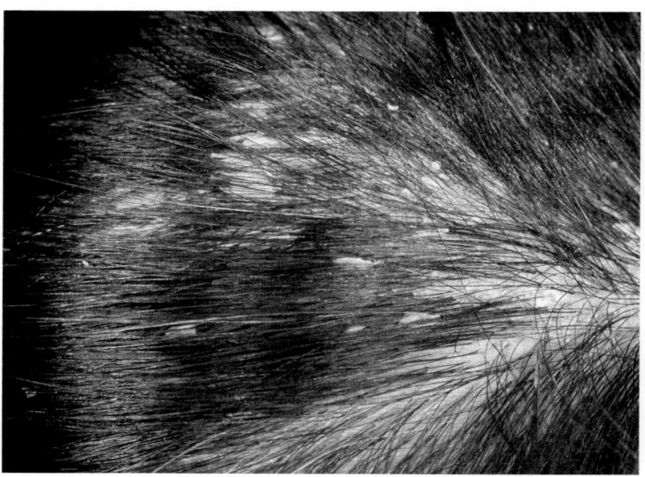

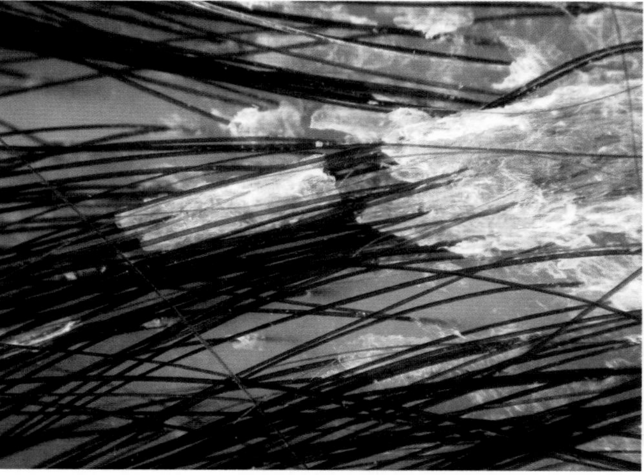

Pityriasis amiantacea with adherent scale on the scalp of a 50-year-old woman: dermoscopy clearly shows multiple keratin aggregates of scale on hair follicles.

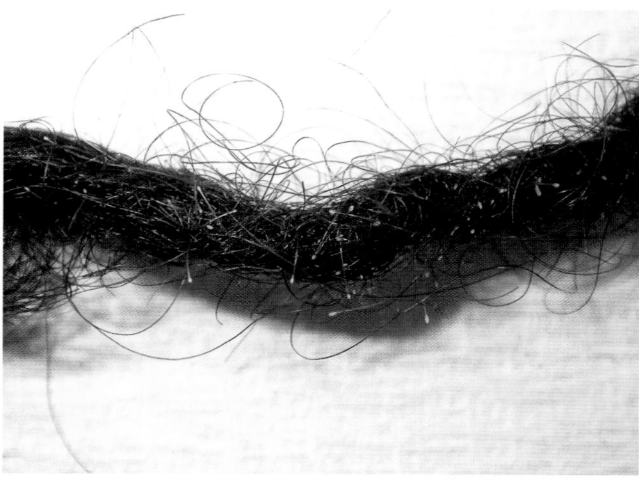

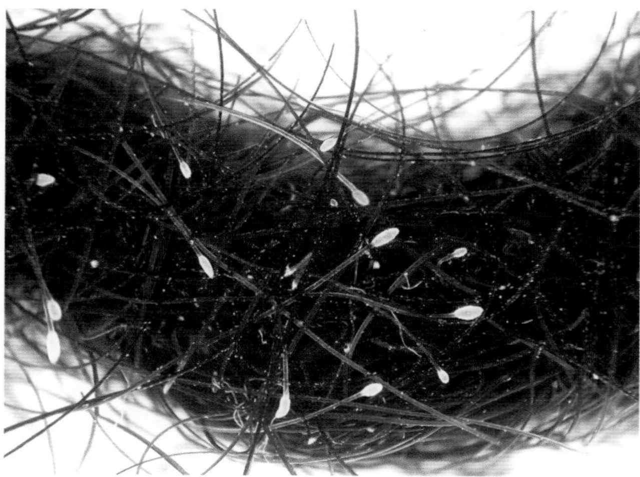

A sample of a dreadlock in a 20-year-old man: dermoscopy clearly shows retained hair with bright white telogen bulbs.

Salih, S. and Bowling, J.C. Pseudonits in dreadlocked hair: a lousey case of nits. *Dermatology*. 2006;213(3):245.

8 Vascular lesions

Telangiectasia 260
Spider telangiectasia 261
Subcorneal haematoma – parallel pattern 262
Subcorneal haematoma – parallel pattern cases 263
Subcorneal haematoma – homogeneous pattern 264
Subcorneal haematoma – homogeneous pattern cases 265
Haemangiomas – red 266
Haemangiomas – purple 267
Angiokeratomas 268
Lymphangiomas 269
Pyogenic granulomas 270
Pyogenic granulomas – acral cases 271
Vascular tumours 272
Purpura – traumatic 273

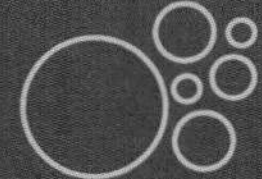

Telangiectasia

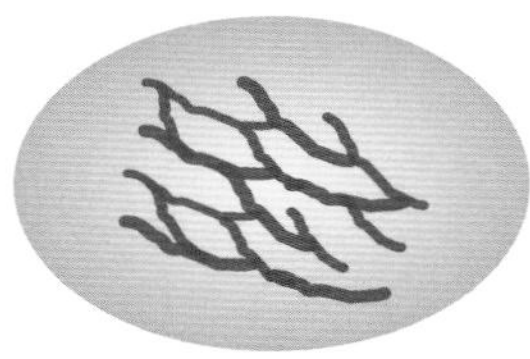

Telangiectatic macules may be seen as part of photodamaged skin or as a benign feature on normal skin. Typically, the vessels are of a similar size and run a horizontal course parallel to the skin surface in a deeper dermal plane, creating vessels that are poorly focused.

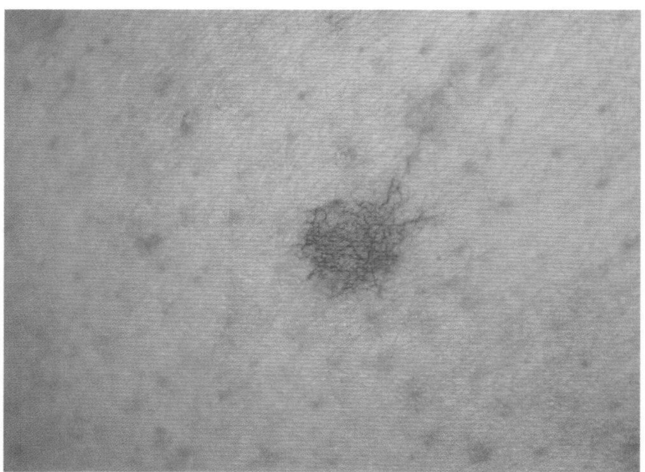

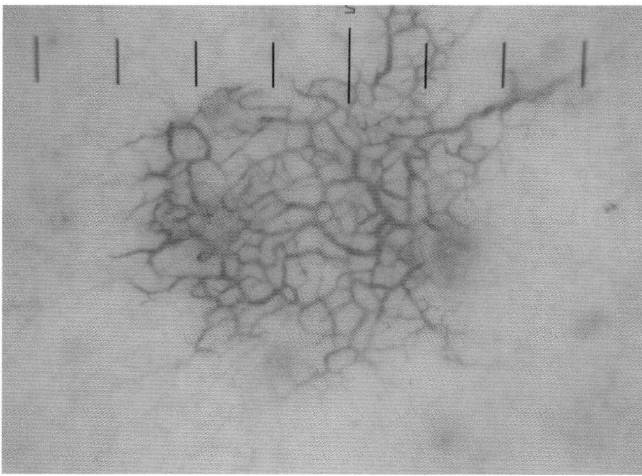

An asymptomatic long-standing pink macule on the upper arm of a 60-year-old woman: dermoscopy shows a well-circumscribed reticular zone of regular anastomosing and poorly focused linear vessels.

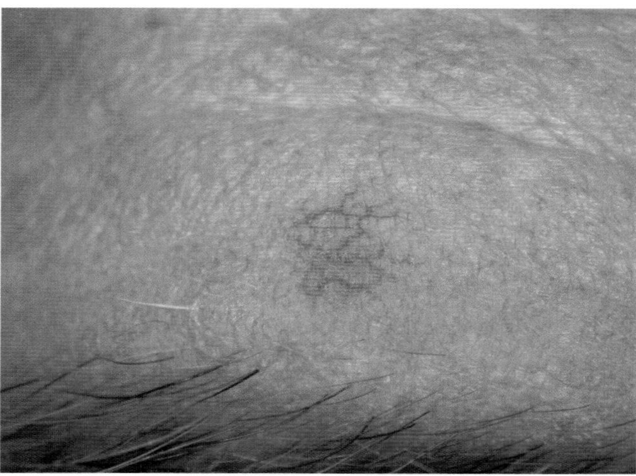

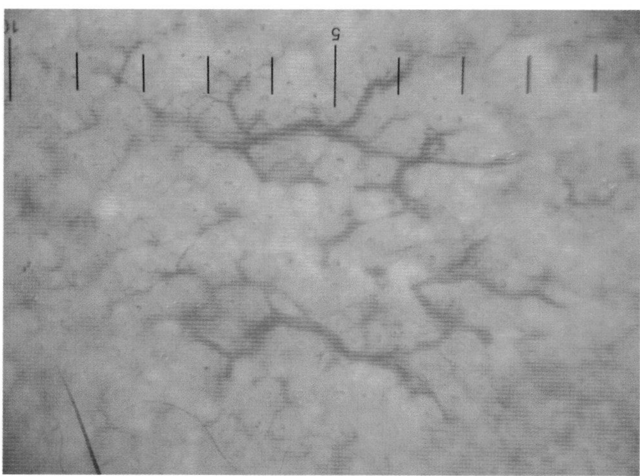

A 70-year-old man with a solitary telangiectatic macule on the forehead: dermoscopy shows a focal zone of poorly focused broad telangiectatic branching linear vessels.

If solitary and urticate on rubbing consider a diagnostic biopsy to exclude mastocytosis.

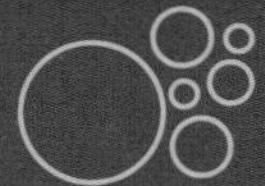

Spider telangiectasia

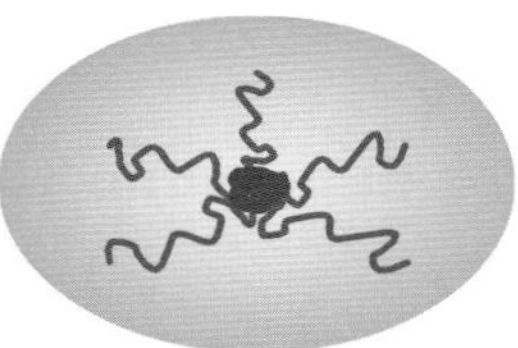

Spider telangiectasia (formerly known as spider naevi) are focal telangiectatic macules with a characteristic central feeding arteriole running perpendicular to the skin surface, from which the dilated vessels radiate. The radiating vessels are poorly focused and run a horizontal course through the skin blanching with pressure. They are a normal feature of skin and are common in children, especially on the cheeks below the lower eyelids.

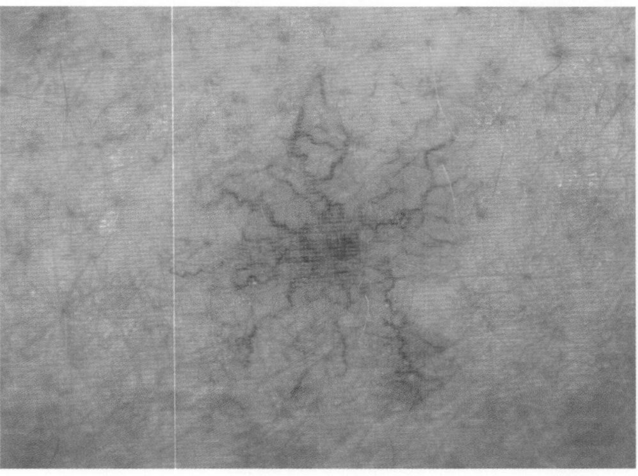

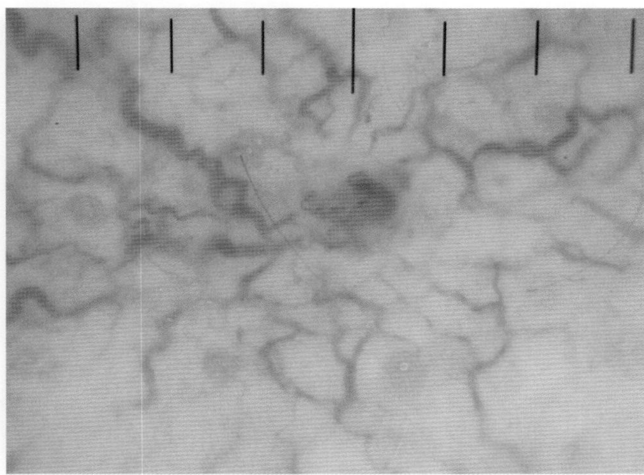

A typical spider telangiectasia with a central dilated vessel: dermoscopy clearly shows a central dilated vessel with radiating linear poorly focused vessels.

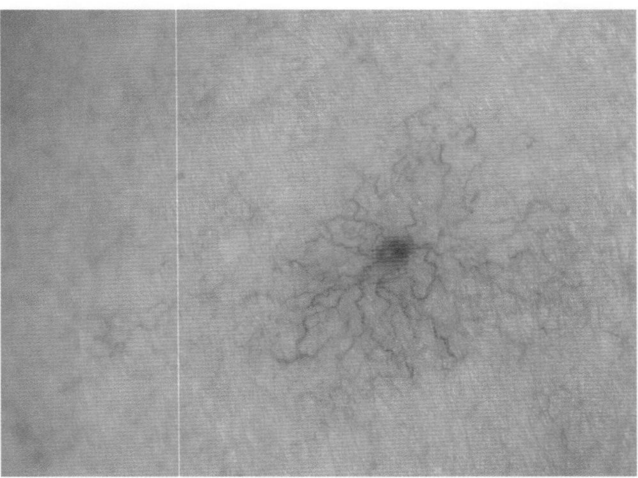

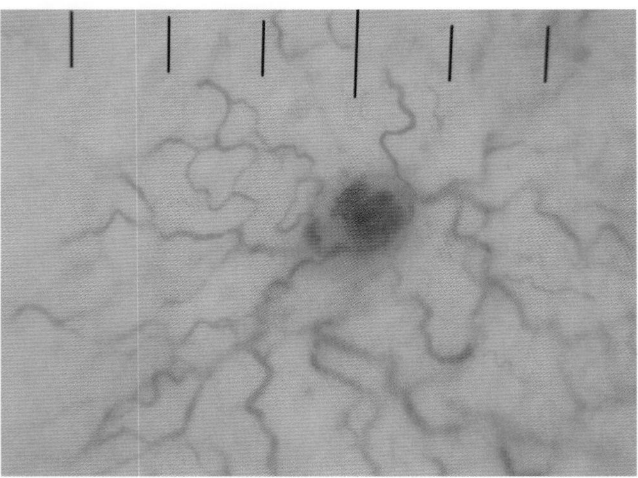

A similar spider telangiectasia: dermoscopy shows a central tortuous dilated vessel with multiple radial linear vessels that are poorly focused.

To demonstrate these to a patient, face a mirror then use a glass slide to compress the lesion then relax to watch the central vessel re-fill. In adults with multiple spider telangiectasia consider screening for signs of chronic hepatic disease.

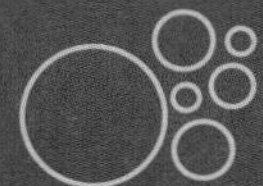

Subcorneal haematoma – parallel pattern

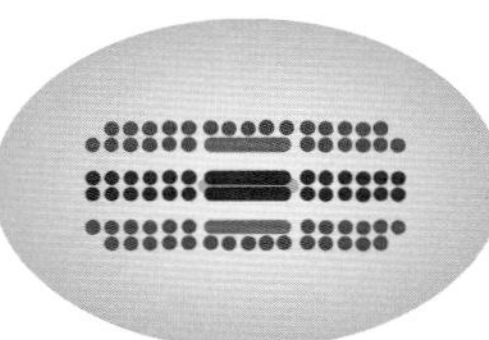

Bleeding into acral skin can give rise to either a parallel pattern of purpura, a homogeneous or variable pigmented red-purple/black blotch. The colours seen depend upon the volume of blood and the age of the lesion. Older lesions may show variable colours due to degradation of the haematoma.

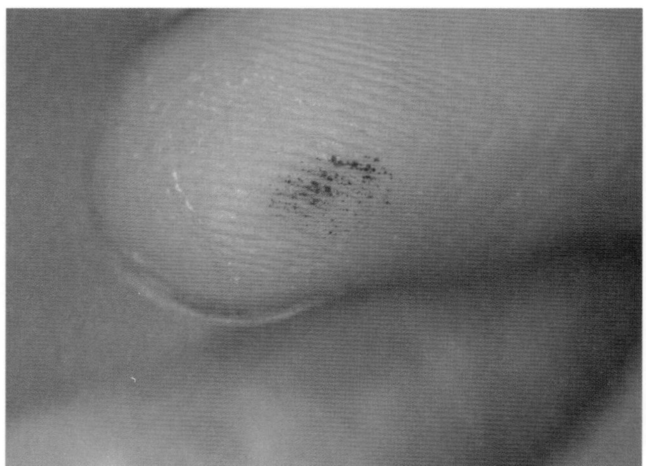

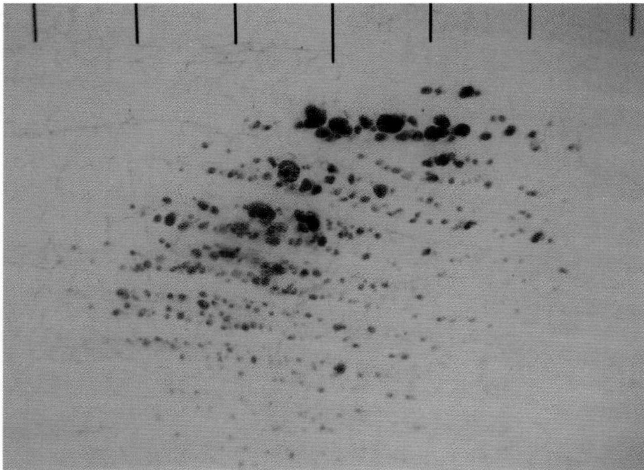

Pinch trauma to the finger causing an obvious haematoma: dermoscopy shows a parallel arrangement of purple and red globules of blood.

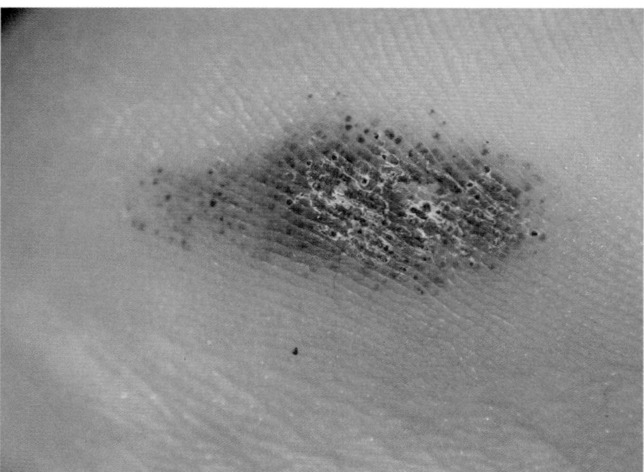

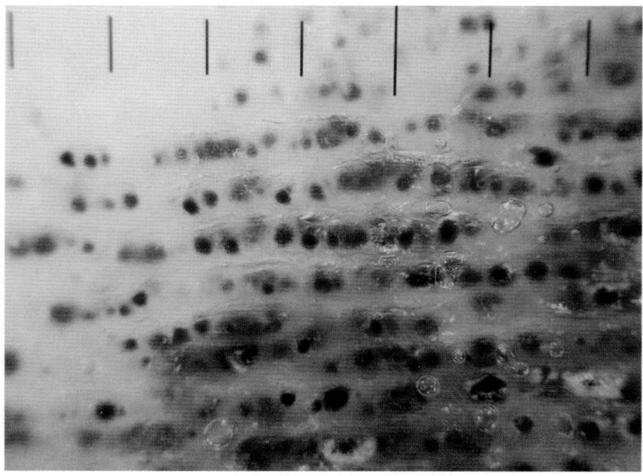

Asymptomatic trauma to the heel in a sportsman causing pigmentation: dermoscopy shows multiple parallel lines of red and purple globules along the lines of the acral ridges. This pattern has been previously described as "pebbles on the ridges".

Saida, T. et al. Dermoscopy for acral pigmented skin lesions. *Clin Dermatol*. 2002;20(3):279–285.

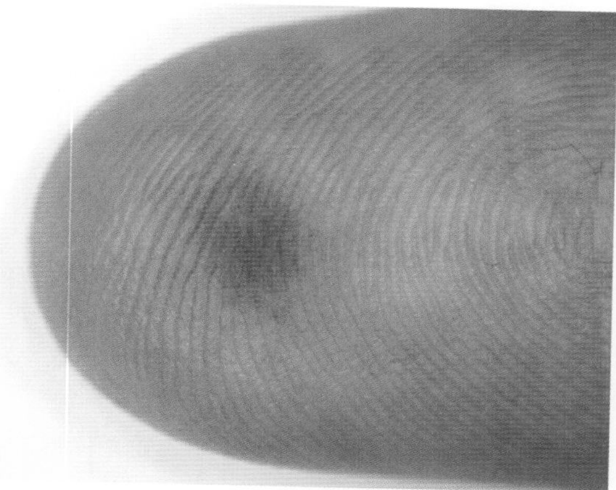
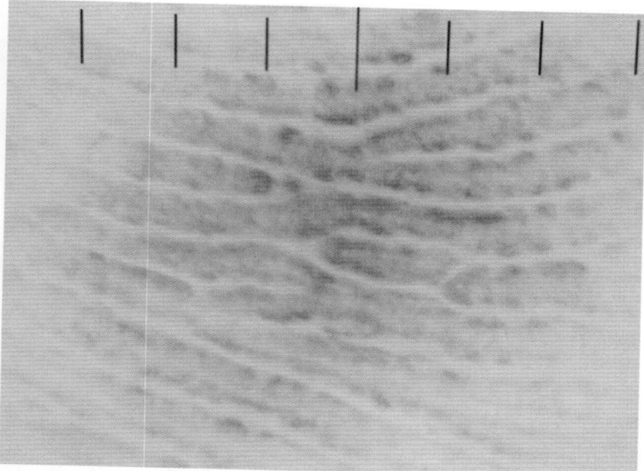

A tan macule on the pulp of the finger in keeping with a resolving subcorneal haematoma: dermoscopy shows the parallel ridge pattern where the blood occupies the ridge of the dermatoglyphics.

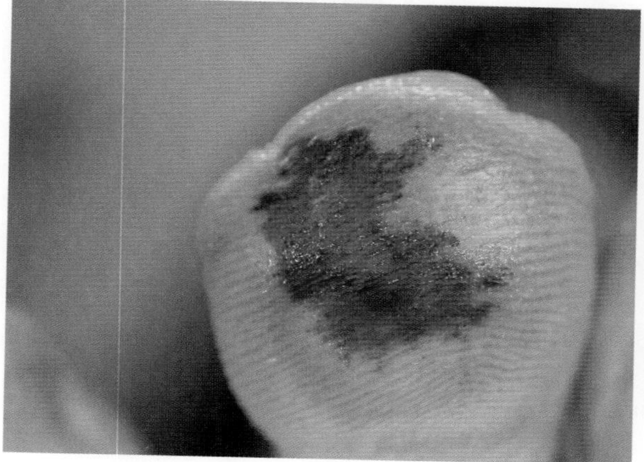
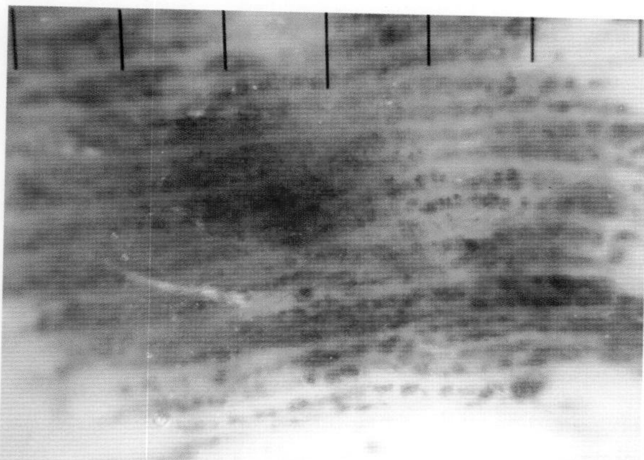

A haemorrhagic macule on the toe of a diabetic man with peripheral neuropathy: dermoscopy confirms the parallel ridge pattern of blood within the dermatoglyphics.

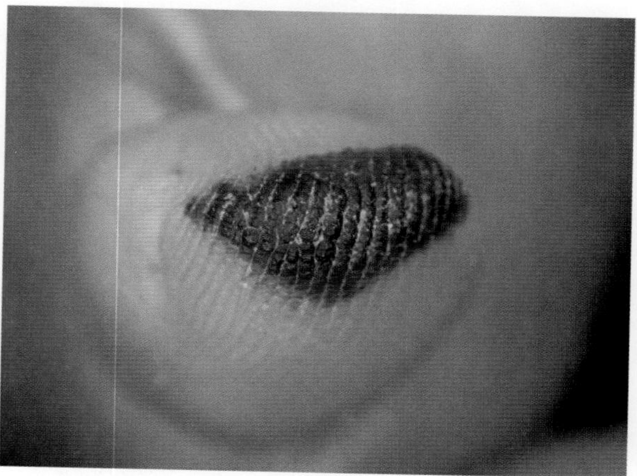
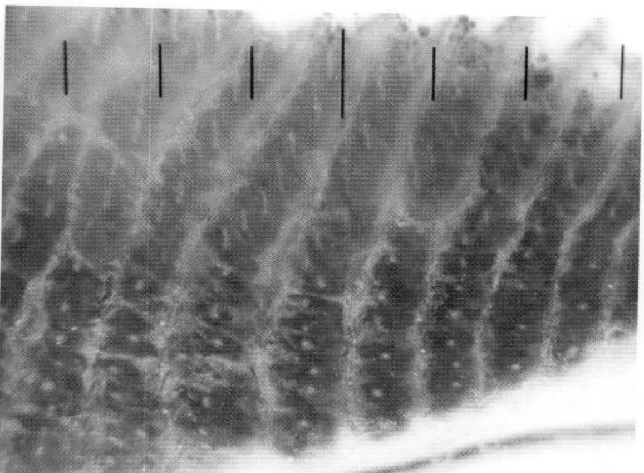

A sporting injury producing a well-defined purple plaque on the toe: dermoscopy shows filling of the ridge of the acral dermatoglyphics with homogeneous purple blood and white dots (prominent eccrine duct openings).

Fake tan, blue naevus, congenital naevus or ethnic pigment may also show a parallel ridge pattern.

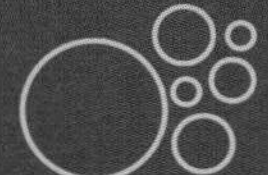

Subcorneal haematoma – homogeneous pattern

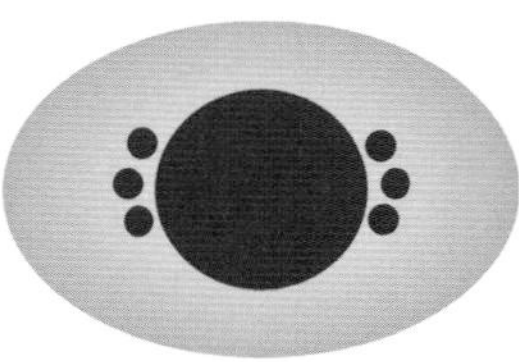

Trauma to the skin, and particularly to acral skin, may give rise to bleeding and the development of a subcorneal haematoma. Dermoscopically the parallel ridge pattern may be seen or alternatively a homogeneous deeply pigmented lesion. Where there is no clear history of trauma, these purple-black macules on acral skin can be mistaken for melanoma.

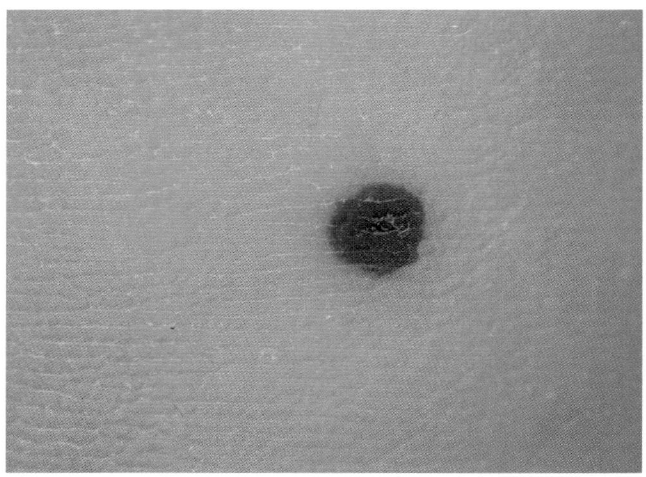

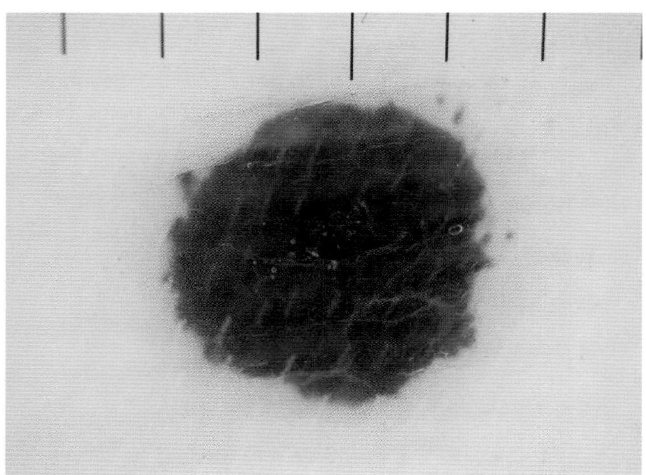

A new hyperpigmented macule on the sole following hiking: dermoscopy clearly shows purple homogeneous pigmentation with peripheral purple globules.

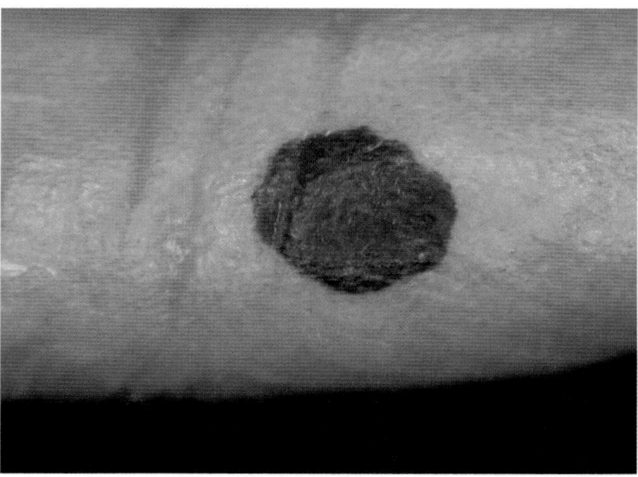

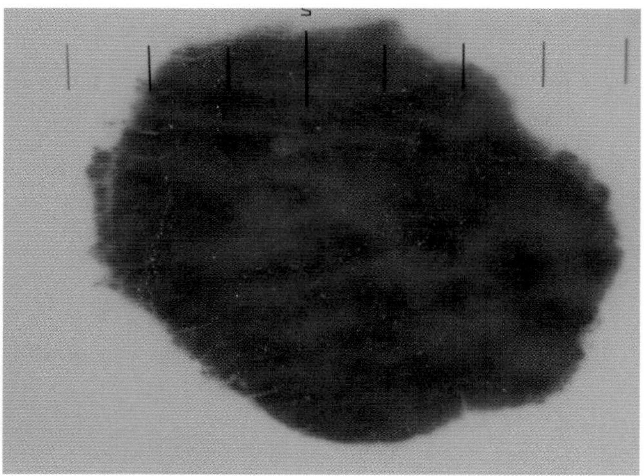

Trauma to the finger causing a large purple haemorrhagic macule: dermoscopy shows homogeneous dark purple colour centrally and discrete brighter purple globules at the margin

In hyperpigmented subcorneal haematomas, diagnostic features may be subtle. Therefore, look for the diagnostic clues of purple globules at the peripheral margin. These globules are akin to the splatter or splash of spilling any liquid.

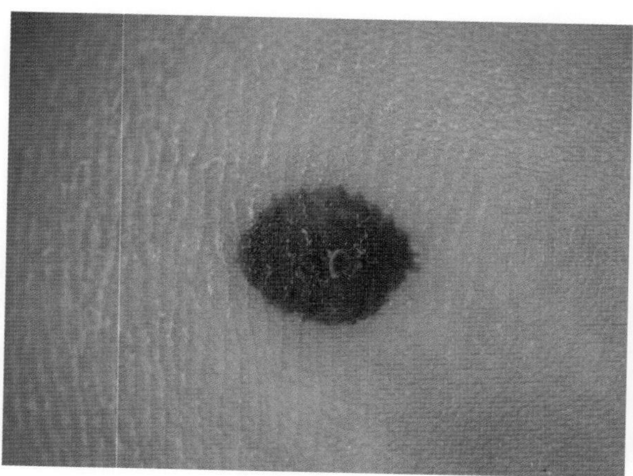

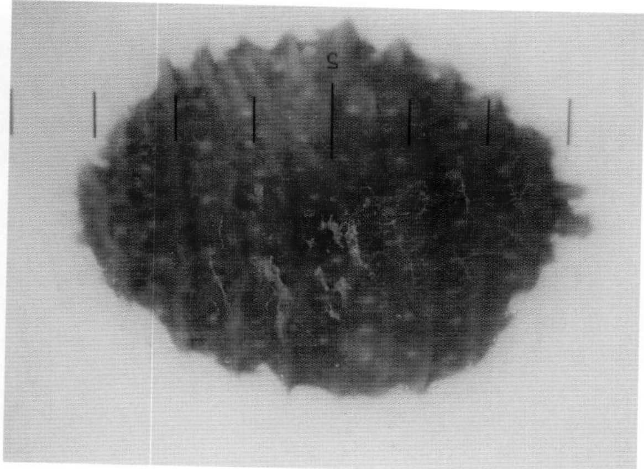

A blood red homogeneous macule on the finger following trauma: dermoscopy show homogeneous red pigmentation corresponding to blood outlining the dermatoglyphics.

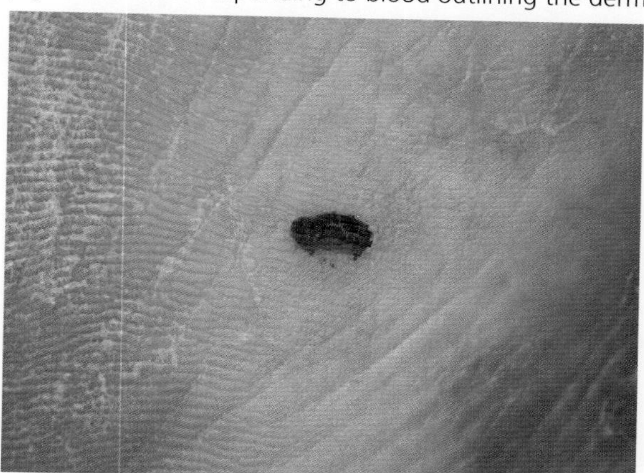

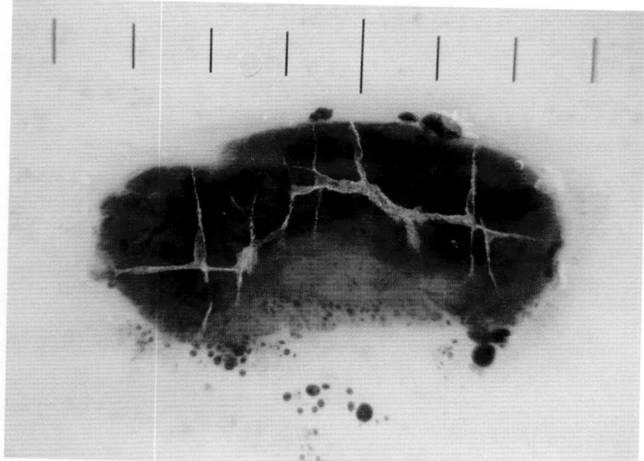

A haemorrhagic macule on the sole starting to resolve: dermoscopy shows breakdown of the blood with fragmentation and peripheral red globules.

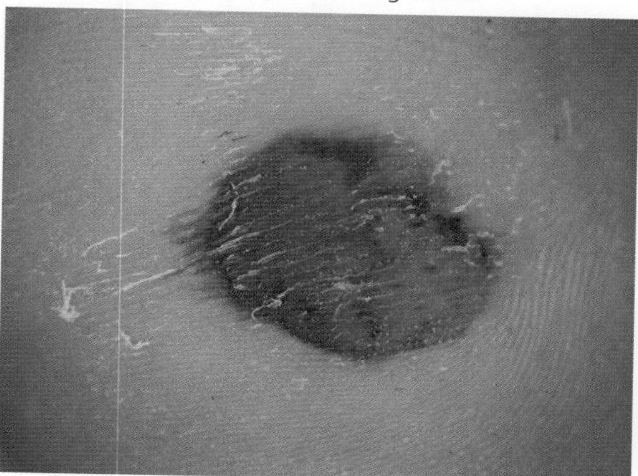

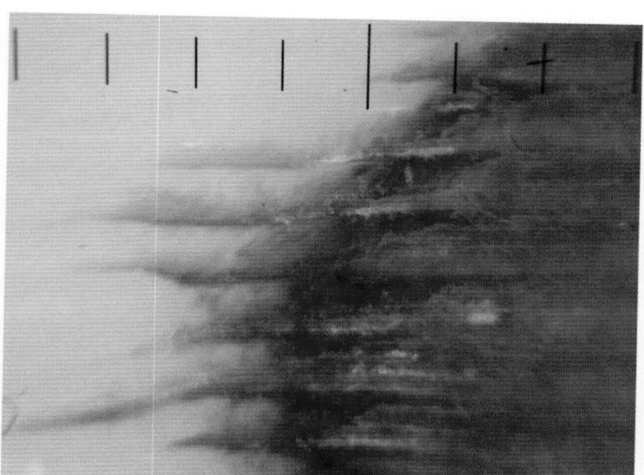

A sporting injury to the heel: dermoscopy shows large red/purple homogeneous pigmentation extending laterally into the acral furrows.

When dermoscopy confirms a subcorneal haematoma superficial paring or curettage can be used to identify and remove the dried blood which is reached easily and without discomfort.

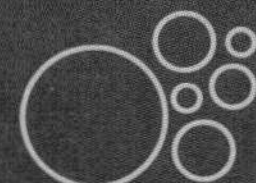

Haemangiomas – red

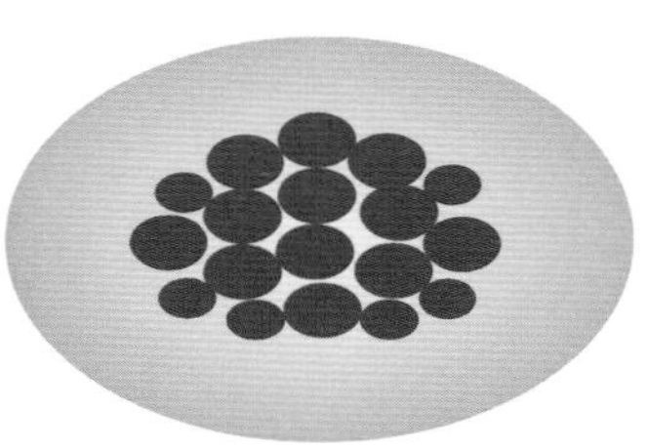

Haemangiomas are common benign vascular tumours. They may present as solitary or multiple red or purple macules, plaques, papules or nodules. Histopathologically, haemangiomas consist of dilated subepidermal blood vessels, which may form large vascular spaces that, following trauma, may thrombose. They are also known as 'cherry' angiomas or Campbell de Morgan spots. Dermoscopy shows multiple, uniform red globules or lacunae.

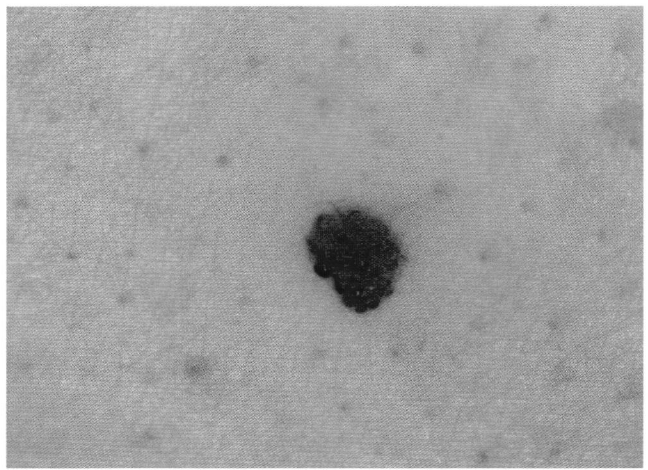

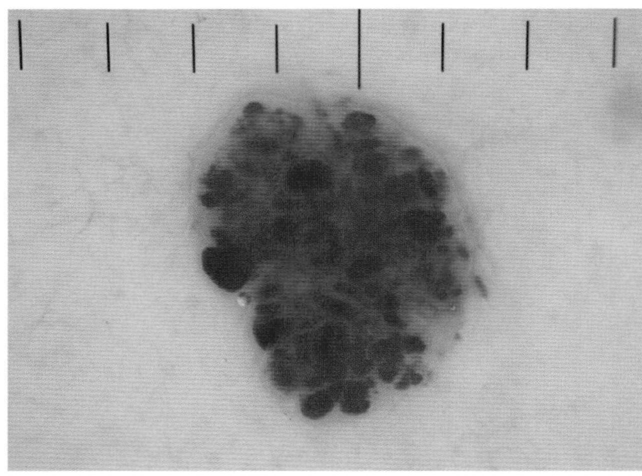

Multiple 'cherry red' vascular macules, plaques and papules across the trunk and proximal limbs in a 40-year-old woman: dermoscopy shows uniform bright red globules/lacunae resembling a bunch of grapes.

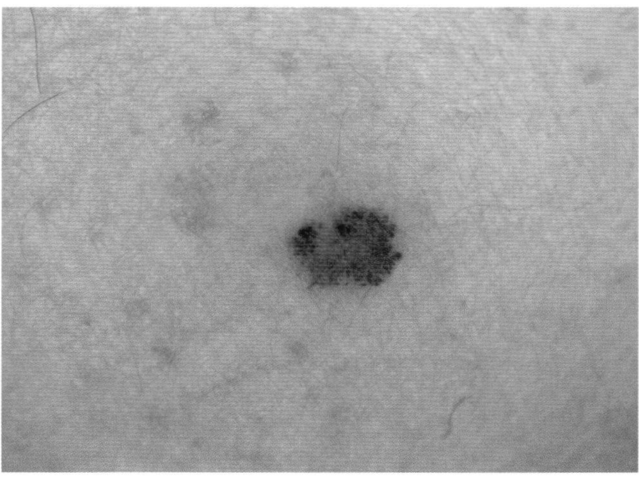

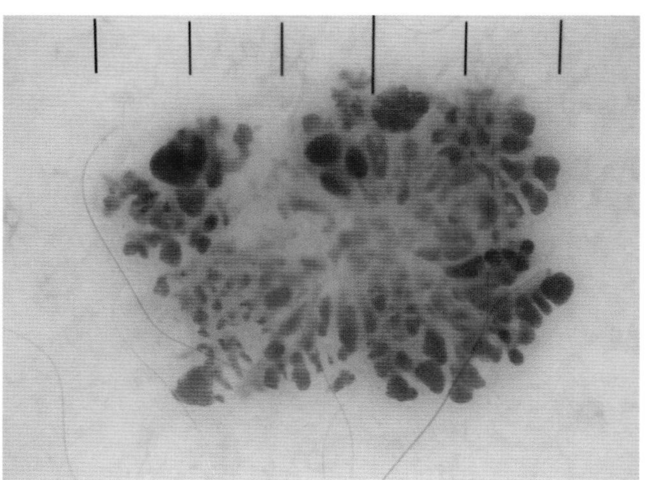

A solitary erythematous macule on the outer thigh of a 50-year-old woman: dermoscopy shows multiple homogeneous red globules/lacunae in keeping with a benign haemangioma.

Piccolo, V. et al. Dermatoscopy of Vascular Lesions. *Dermatol Clin.* 2018;36(4):389–395.

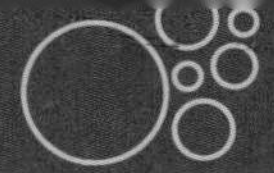

Haemangiomas – purple

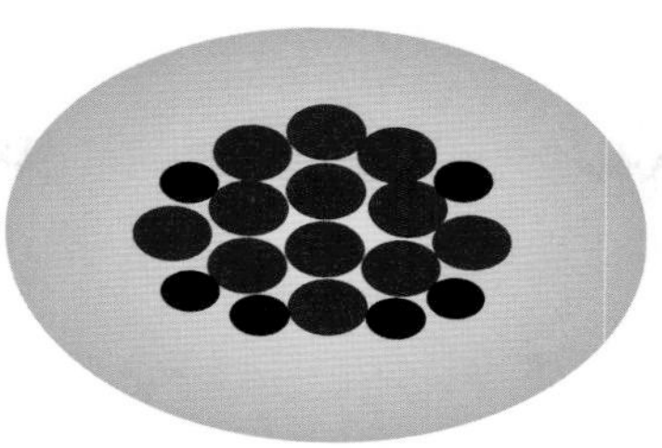

Haemangiomas lying deeper in the dermis are typically well-demarcated with whitish lines/septae dividing the lesion and delineating the peripheral margin of the lacunae seen dermoscopically. Importantly, each lacune is composed of a single homogeneous purple colour.

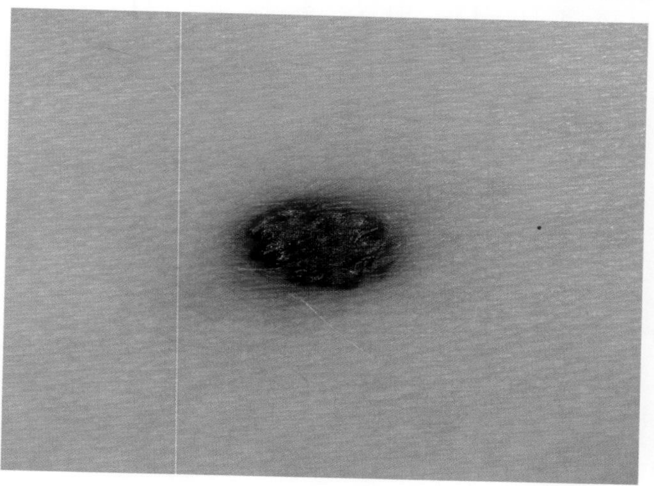

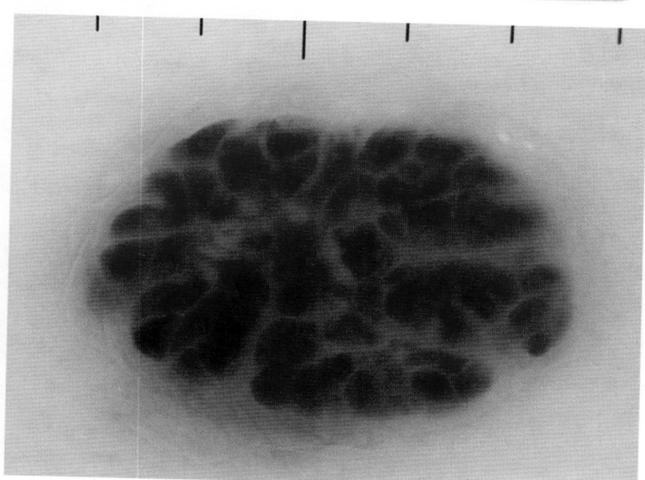

A purple plaque on the lower back of a 30-year-old woman: dermoscopy shows homogeneous purple lacunae forming a cobblestone pattern.

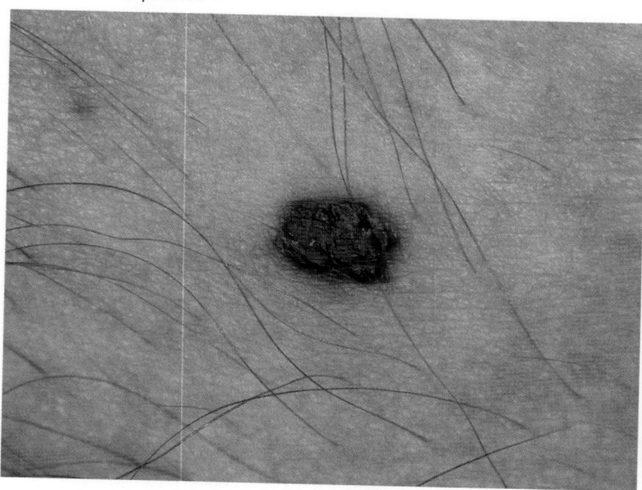

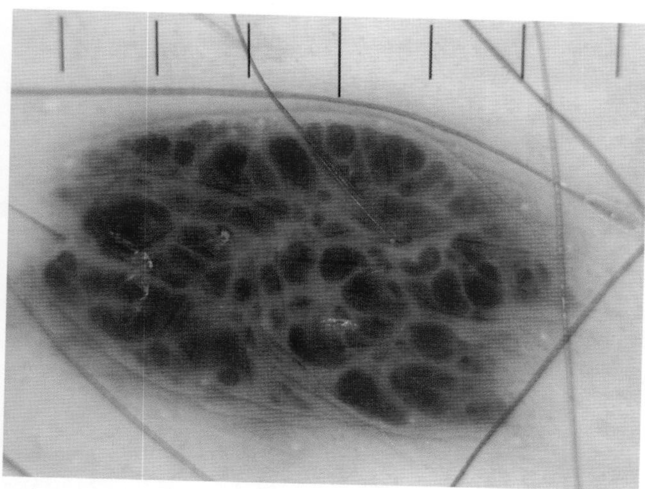

A purple plaque on the posterior thigh of a 25-year-old man: dermoscopy shows uniformly pigmented purple lacunae in a cobblestone pattern.

The colour of the lacunae seen on dermoscopy depends on the degree of oxygenation and presence or otherwise of thrombosis. Consider excisional biopsy if there is any diagnostic doubt, variability of pigmentation, or atypical vessels within the lacune.

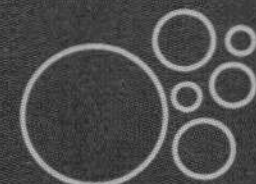

Angiokeratomas

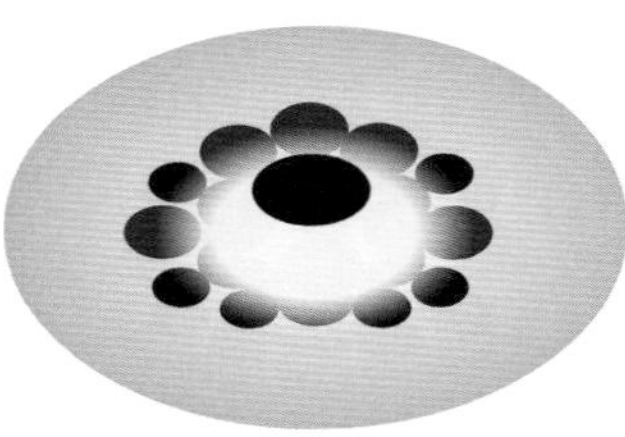

In angiokeratomas dark lacunae are frequently seen reflecting thrombosis within the vascular spaces. The whitish veil seen in angiokeratomas is due to hyperkeratosis and acanthosis overlying the vascular spaces. Inflammation and red blood cell extravasation may present as peripheral erythema.

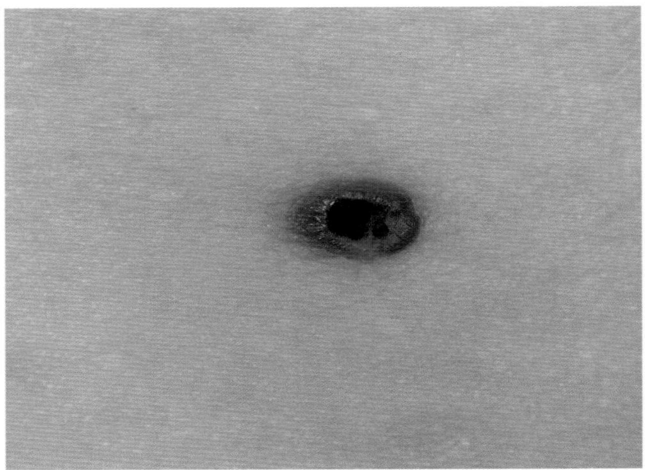

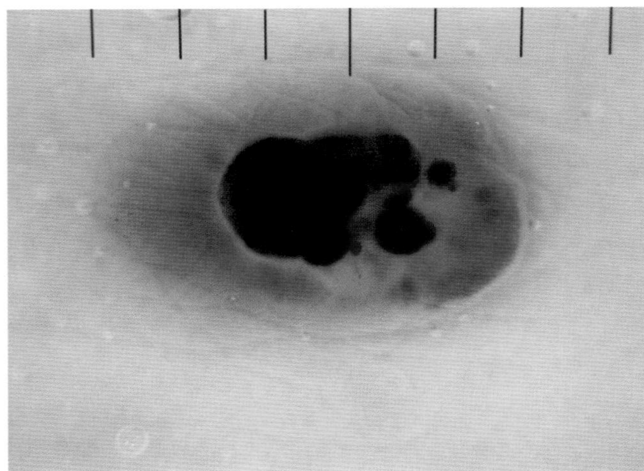

A new solitary hyperpigmented plaque on the upper thigh of a 30-year-old woman: dermoscopy shows a central black/purple blotch with a surrounding whitish veil and peripheral erythema in keeping with an angiokeratoma.

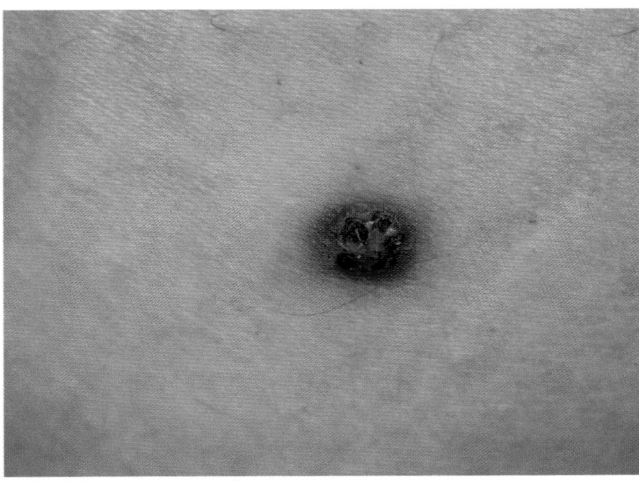

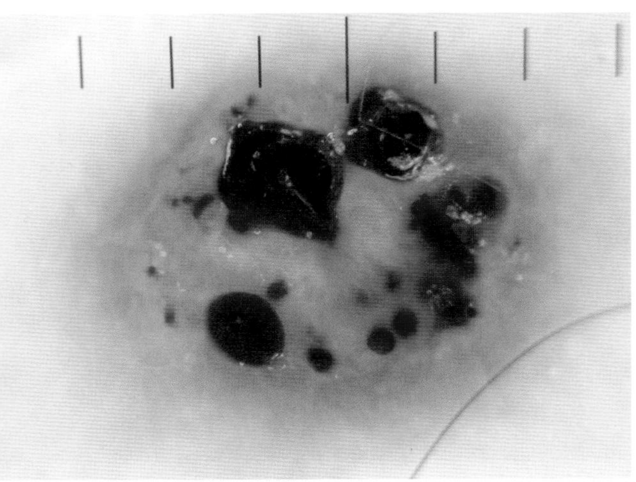

A new hyperpigmented papule on the calf of a 40-year-old woman: dermoscopy shows discrete black/purple lacunae with a whitish veil and peripheral ill-defined erythema in this histopathologically confirmed angiokeratoma.

Zaballos, P. et al. Dermoscopy of solitary angiokeratomas: a morphological study. *Arch Dermatol*. 2007;143(3):318–325.

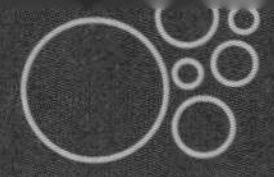

Lymphangiomas

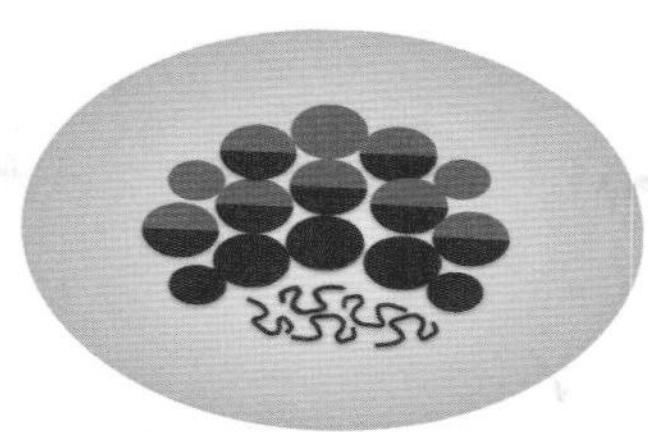

Lymphangiomas are localised proliferations of lymphatic vessels that present as flesh-coloured papules. With trauma they may increase in size and develop purple haemorrhagic foci. Dermoscopic features include orange, pink colours and two-tone lacunae with a fluid level with varying volumes of purple blood. With gravity, the purple component of the two-tone lacune should be at the inferior aspect and the orange component located superiorly.

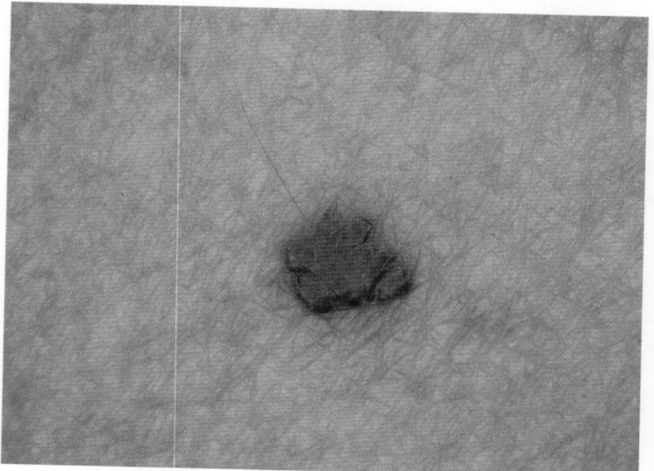

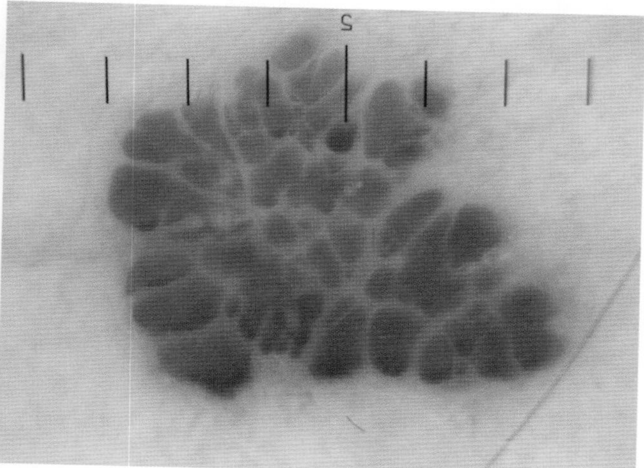

An orange-pink plaque on the lateral thigh of a 60-year-old man: dermoscopy shows multiple lacunae with orange colouration superiorly and purple inferiorly in keeping with a lymphangioma.

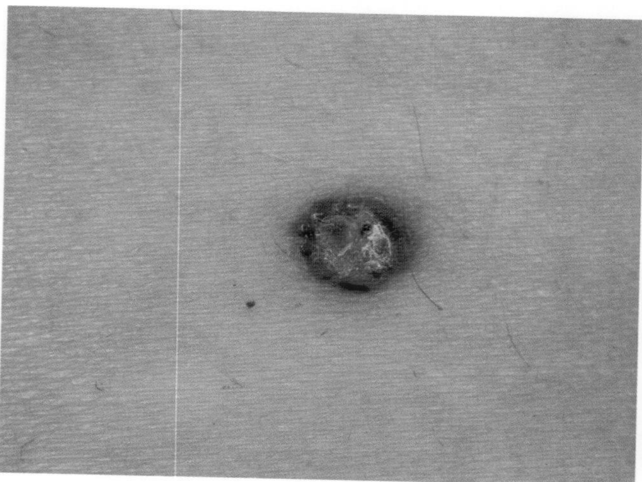

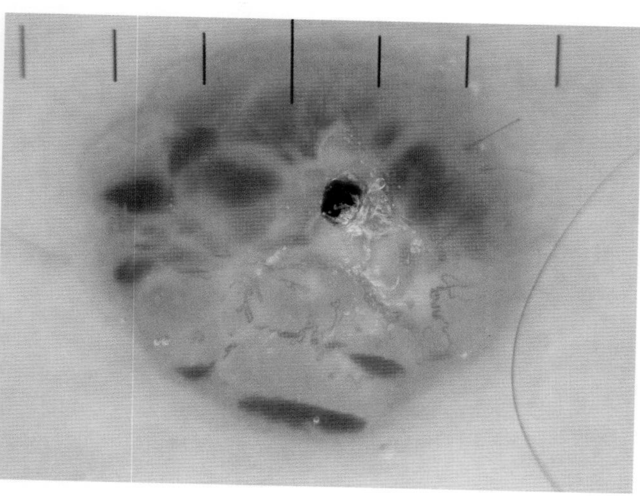

A purple-orange papule on the flank of a 50-year-old man: dermoscopy shows two-tone (half-and-half) lacunae of orange and purple as well as sharply in-focus anastomosing vessels in this histopathologically confirmed lymphangioma.

Jha, A.K. et al. Dermoscopy of cutaneous lymphangioma circumscriptum. *Dermatol Pract Concept*. 2017;7(2):37–38.

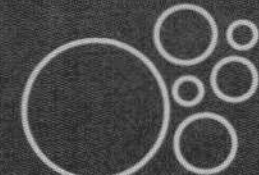

Pyogenic granulomas

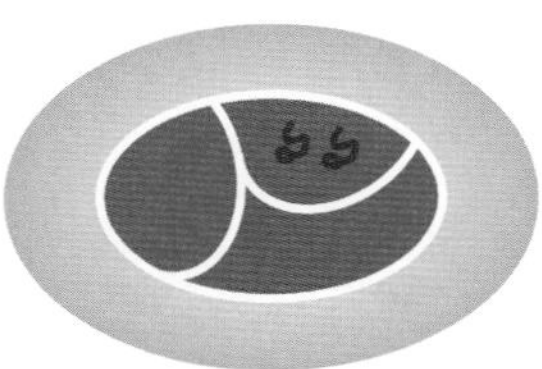

Lobular capillary haemangiomas, also known as pyogenic granulomas, are localised vascular proliferations that typically occur following trauma. They commonly occur on acral skin though they may also be found on lips, trunk and limbs. Pyogenic granulomas bleed easily. Dermoscopically, they present with red homogeneous areas (with or without irregular vessels) separated by white lines/septae and/or surrounded by a white collarette. Vessels may also be present.

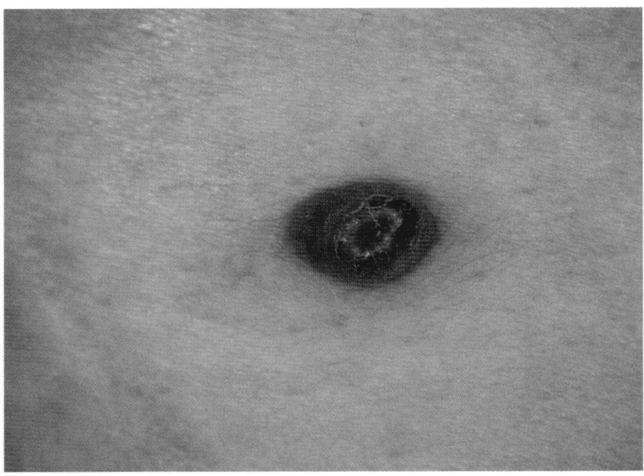

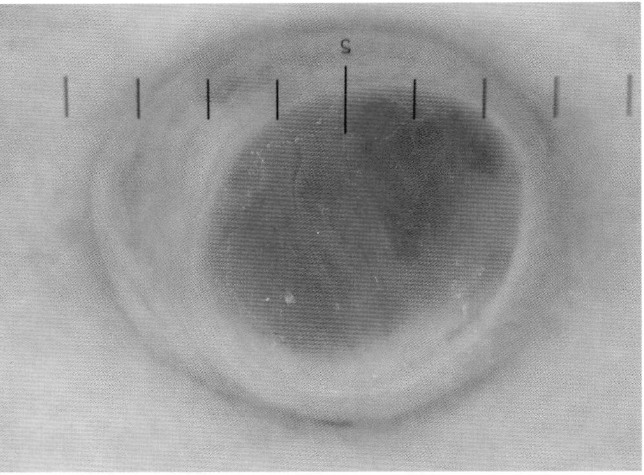

A vascular papule on the thigh of a 40-year old female: dermoscopy shows a peripheral collarette with central homogeneous red colouration with histopathology confirming pyogenic granuloma.

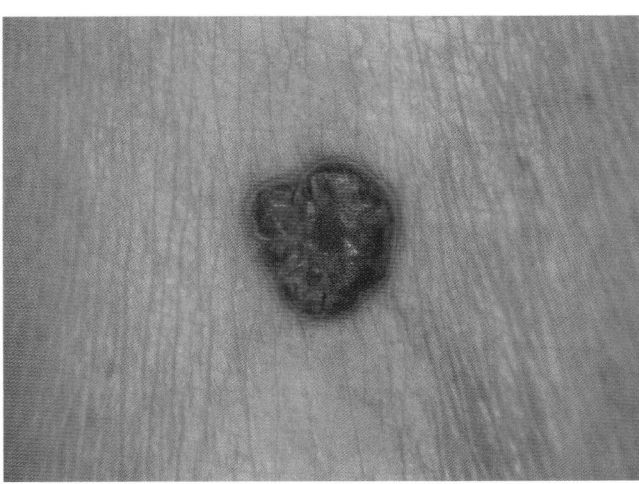

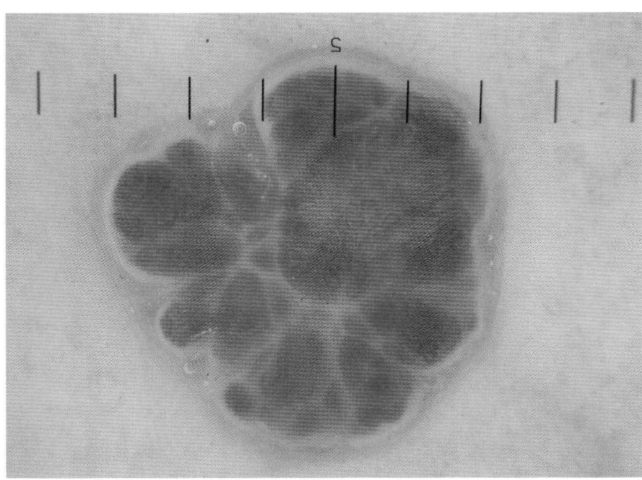

A vascular plaque on the lower leg of a 30-year-old female: dermoscopy shows a peripheral collarette, white septae/lines, irregular vessels and uniform cherry red colouration in this histopathologically confirmed pyogenic granuloma.

Zaballos, P. et al. Dermoscopic findings in pyogenic granuloma. *Br J Dermatol*. 2006;154(6):1108–1111.

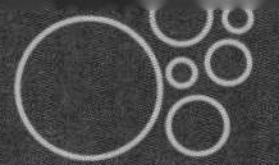

Pyogenic granulomas – acral cases

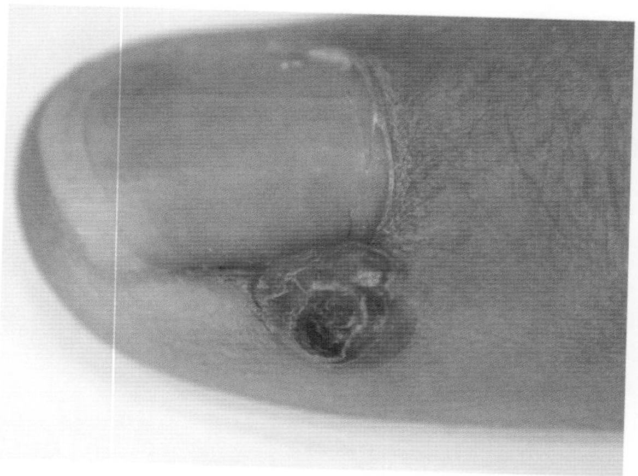

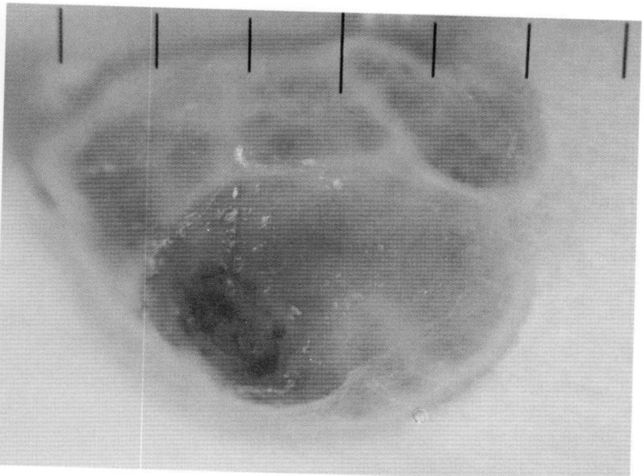

A vascular papule on the index finger lateral nail fold: dermoscopy shows a peripheral collarette, red homogeneous areas separated by white lines and a focus of erosion.

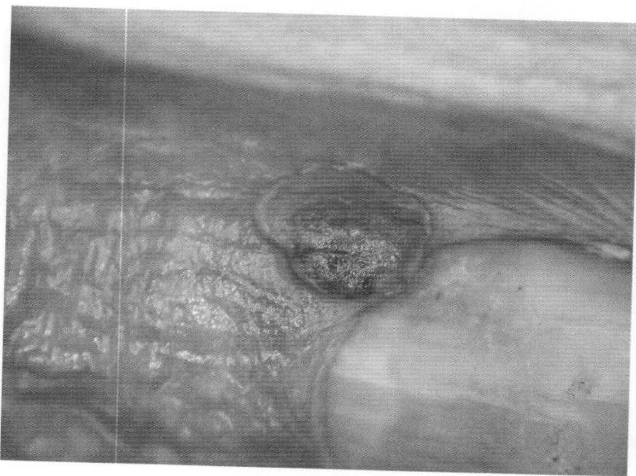

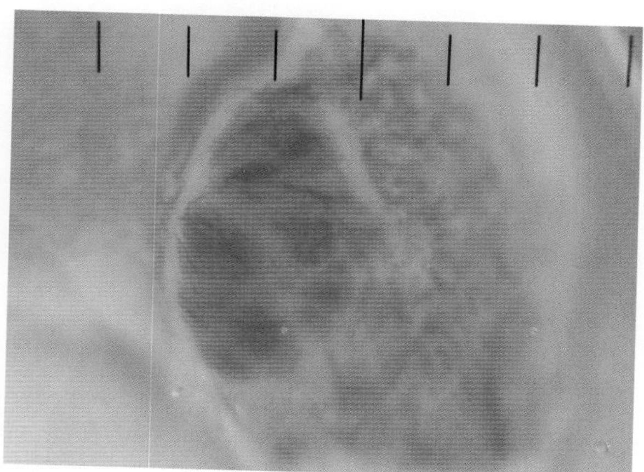

A vascular papule on the index finger proximal nail fold following minimal trauma: dermoscopy shows peripheral white collarette, erythema and dilated vessels.

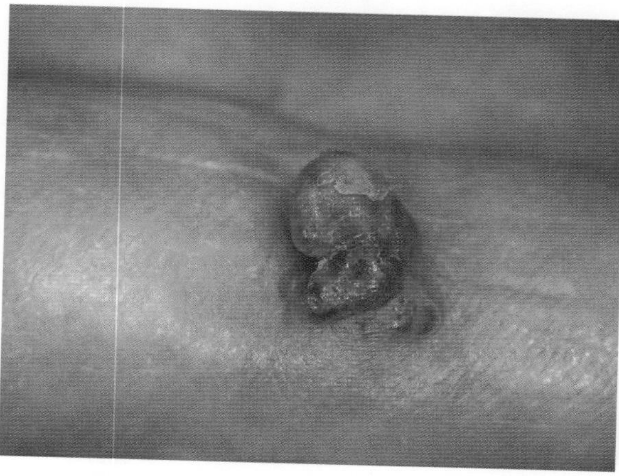

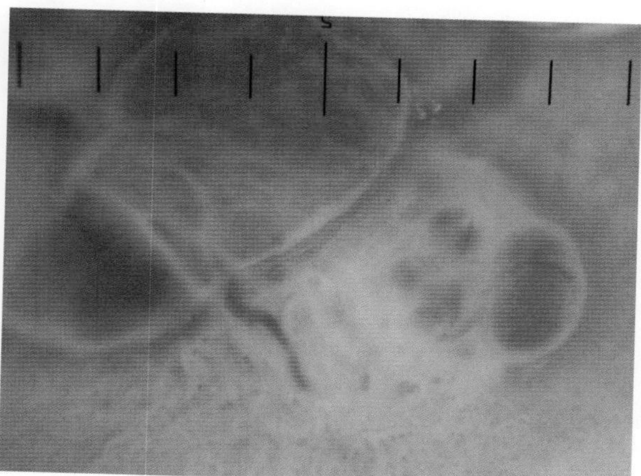

An exophytic vascular papule on the palmar surface of the left middle finger: dermoscopy shows peripheral white collarette and white lines surrounding the erythematous areas and dilated vessels.

Always send the surgical sample for histopathologic confirmation to exclude amelanotic melanoma or other malignant tumours.

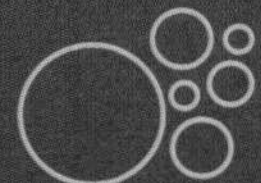

Vascular tumours

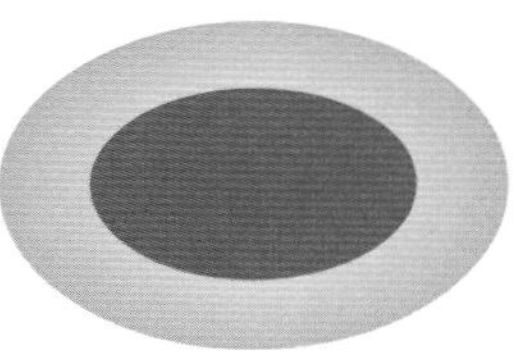

Vascular tumours, with small vessel proliferation on histopathology, will tend to show similar clinical and dermoscopic features. These include tumours such as microvenular haemangioma, hobnail haemangiomas and Kaposi sarcoma.
Note: consider diagnostic biopsy for any long-standing pink macule where there is diagnostic uncertainty.

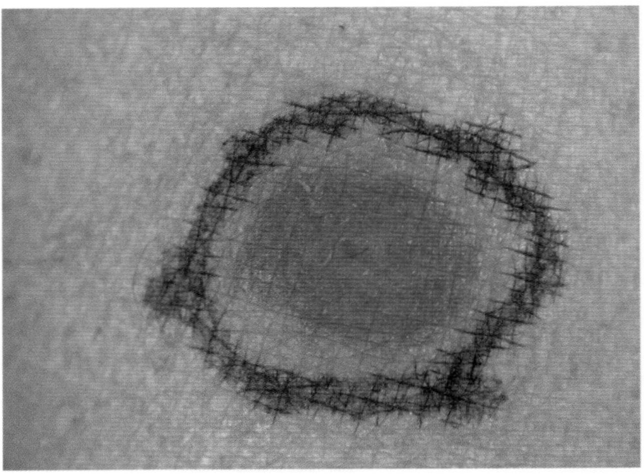

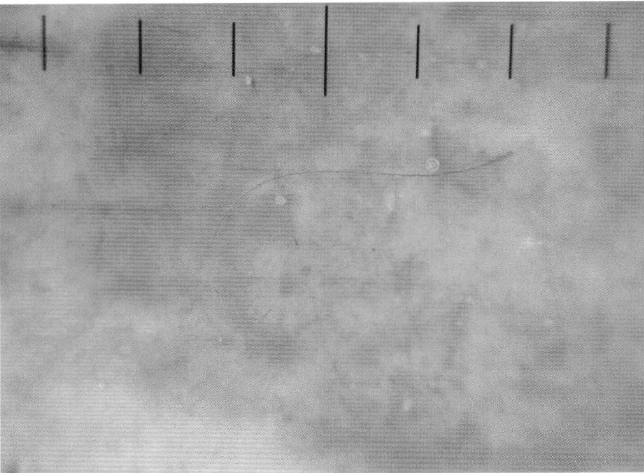

A long-standing pink macule, unresponsive to topical steroids, on the thigh of a 40-year-old woman: dermoscopy shows patchy erythema with no other diagnostic features; histopathology confirmed a microvenular haemangioma.

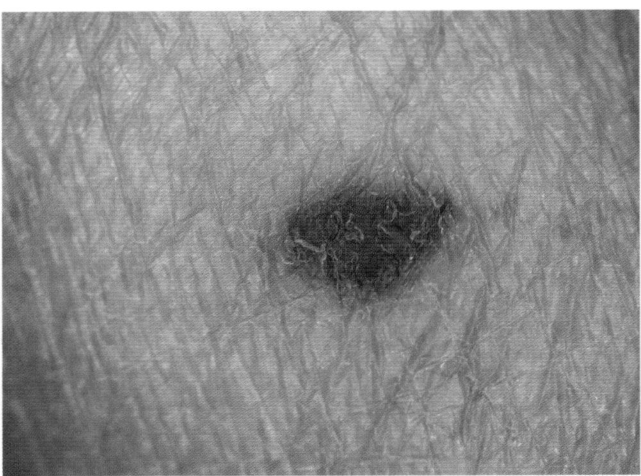

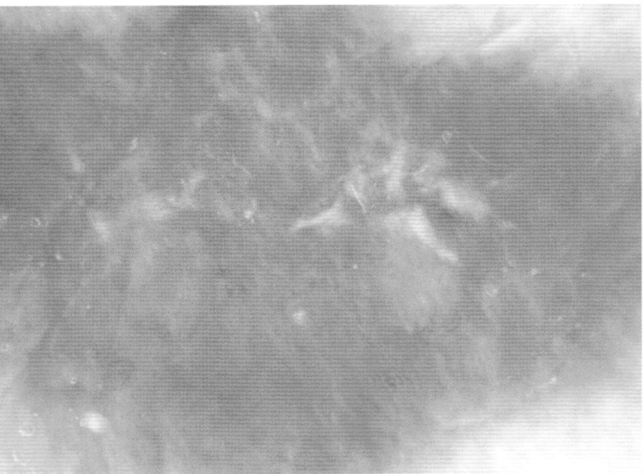

An 85-year-old man with multiple purple plaques on the lower limb: dermoscopy shows milky erythema and shiny white blotches and strands; histopathology confirmed a Kaposi sarcoma of classical type. Diagnosis here relies on good clinical correlation.

Coates, D. and Bowling, J. Dermoscopy is not always helpful in the diagnosis of vascular lesions. *Australas J Dermatol.* 2010;51(4):292–294.

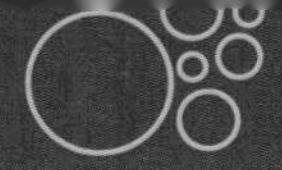

Purpura – traumatic

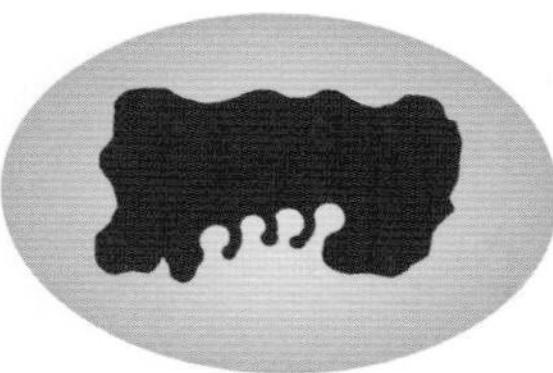

Traumatic purpura (also known as Bateman's purpura, senile purpura and actinic purpura) is a common, benign condition in the elderly characterised by recurrent, often multiple, purple ecchymoses typically on the extensor surfaces of the hands, forearms or legs. They arise following minor trauma and are self-limiting. Dermoscopy shows well-demarcated purple blotches with a well-defined peripheral margin, often with perifollicular sparing.

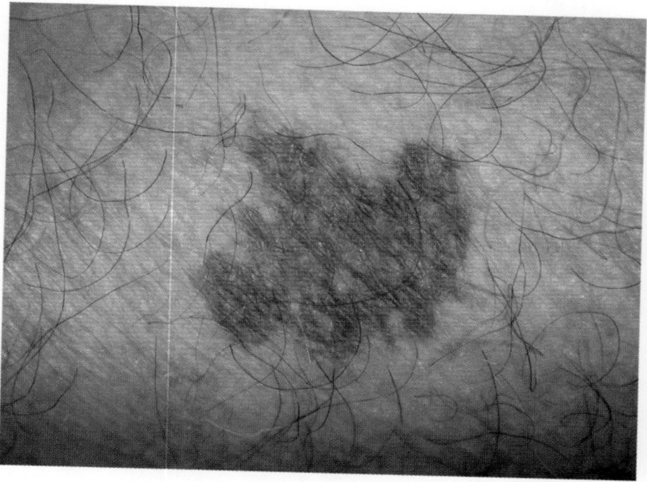

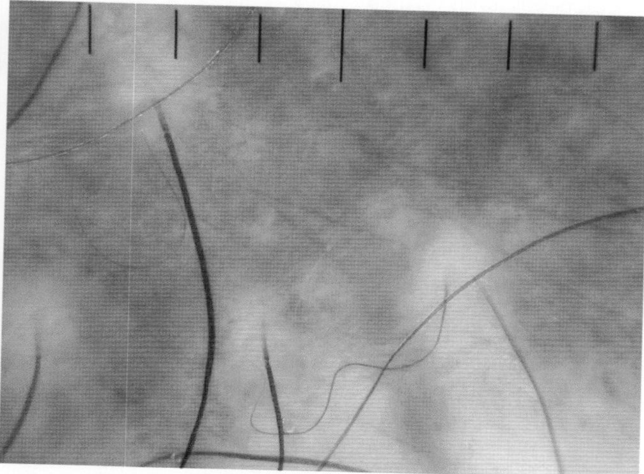

A new purple macule on the forearm of a 75-year-old man with no overt history of trauma: dermoscopy shows a large well-demarcated homogeneous purple colour with perifollicular sparing at the margin in this benign purpuric macule.

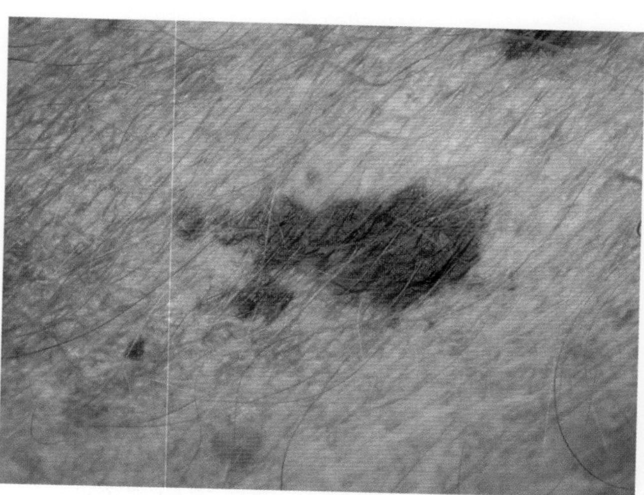

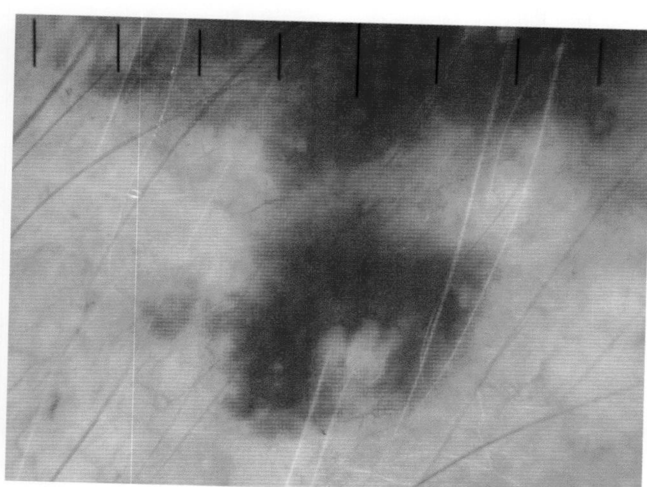

Multiple purple macules on the forearm of an 80-year-old man: polarised dermoscopy shows well-demarcated homogeneous purple colour with perifollicular sparing at the margin in this benign purpuric macule.

Consider further investigations if spontaneous purpuric macules occur in young adults to exclude haematological causes.

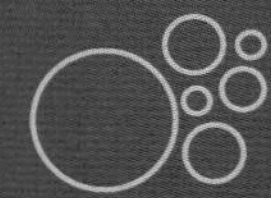

9 Inflammoscopy

Mastocytosis 275
Acne 276
Rosacea 277
Eczema 278
Psoriasis 279
Lichen planus 280
Lichen planus pigmentosus 281
Capillaritis 282
Vasculitis 283
Granulomatous conditions 284
Granuloma annulare 285
Tinea corporis 286
Pityriasis rosea 287
Cutaneous lupus erythematosus 288

Diagnostic Dermoscopy: The Illustrated Guide, Second Edition. Jonathan Bowling.

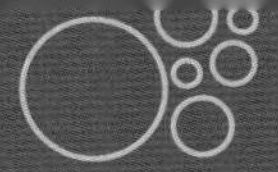

Mastocytosis

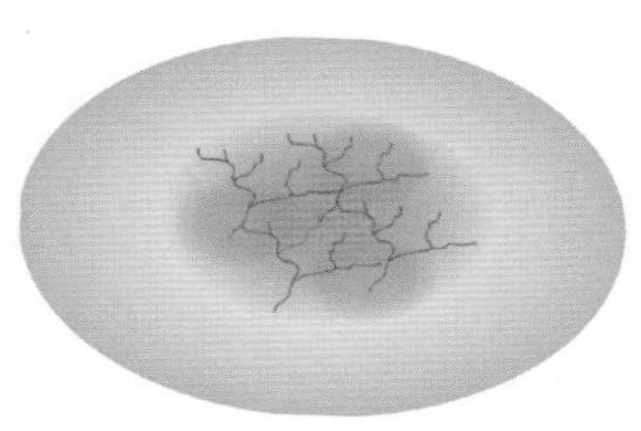

Cutaneous mastocytoses are a group of rare disorders characterised by an increase in mast cells in the skin. Clinically, they may present in a number of ways, either as a solitary plaque or multiple macules. Rarely, cutaneous mastocytosis can progress to systemic mastocytosis. Dermoscopic features are subtle and include erythema, vascular network and brown reticular pigmentation.

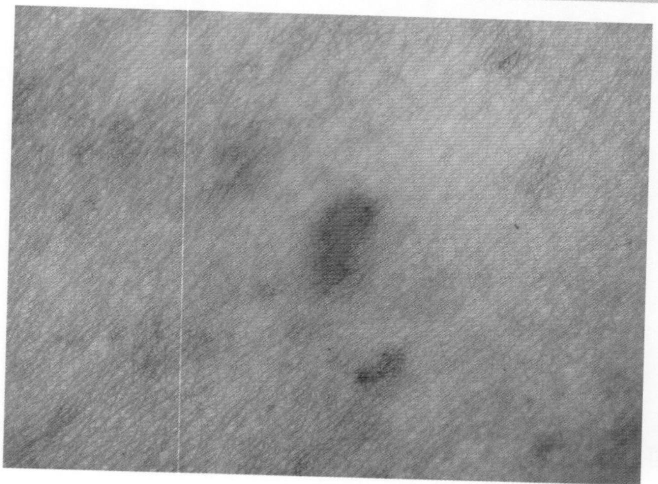

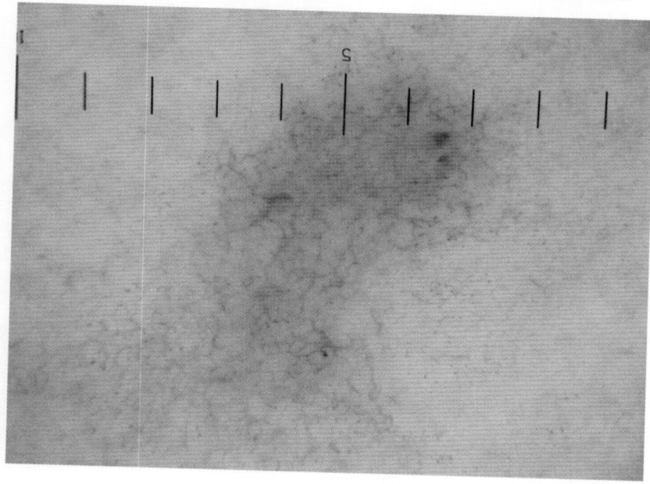

Multiple asymptomatic erythematous macules on the thighs of a 20-year-old woman: dermoscopy shows erythema, a reticular vascular network and foci of faint pigmentation in this case of histopathologically confirmed urticaria pigmentosa.

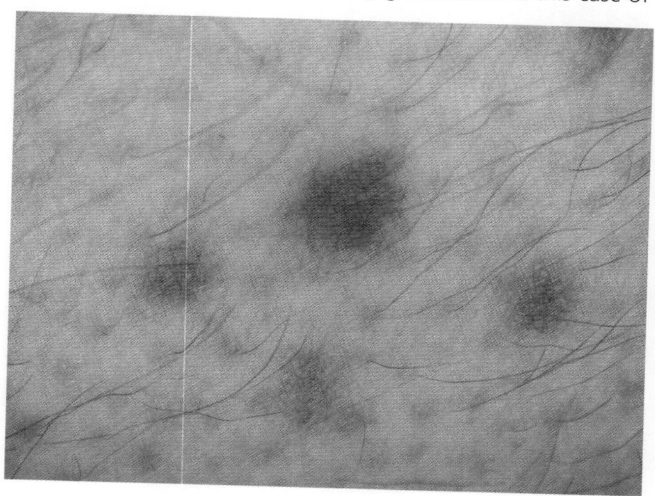

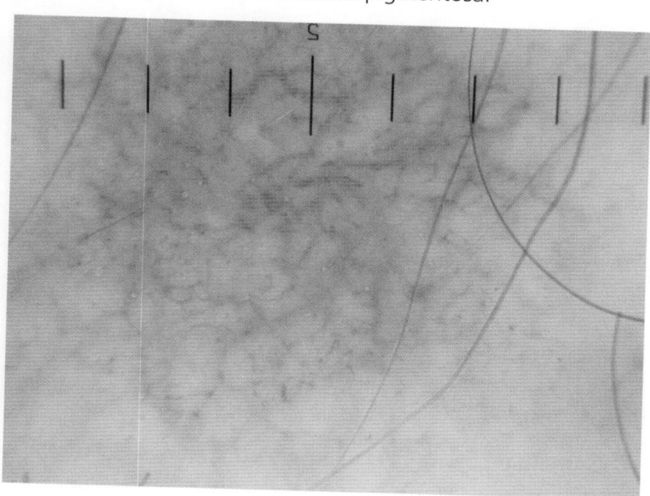

Multiple asymptomatic erythematous macules on the thighs and abdomen of a 40-year-old man: dermoscopy shows a blurry vascular network on an erythematous background in this histopathologically confirmed telangiectasia macularis eruptiva perstans.

Vano-Galvan, S. et al. Dermoscopic features of skin lesions in patients with mastocytosis. *Arch Dermatol*. 2011;147(8):932–940.

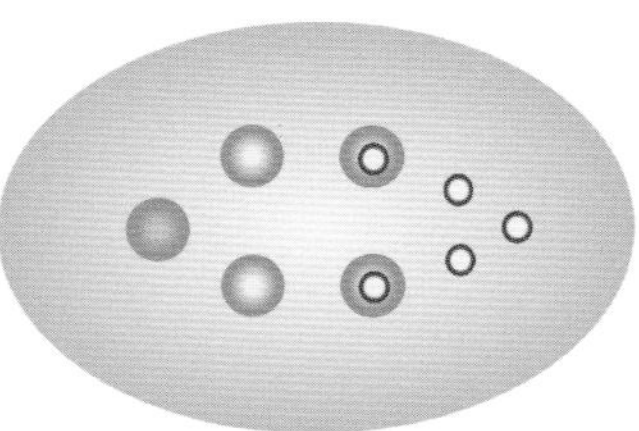

The severity of acne will influence treatment decisions. Dermal granulomatous inflammation can be associated with scar formation, which on dermoscopy appears as well-defined foci of orange and erythematous perifollicular blotches.

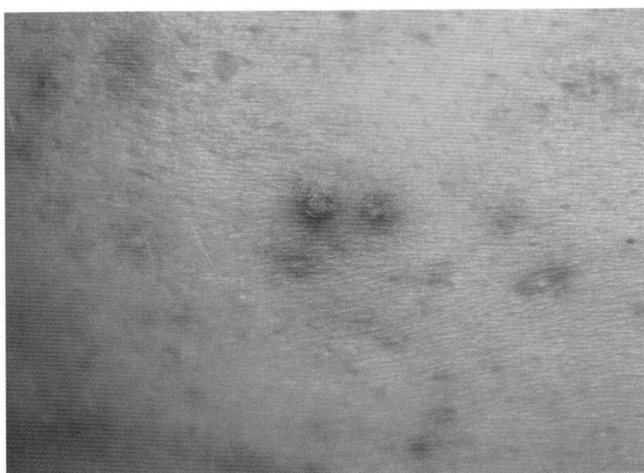

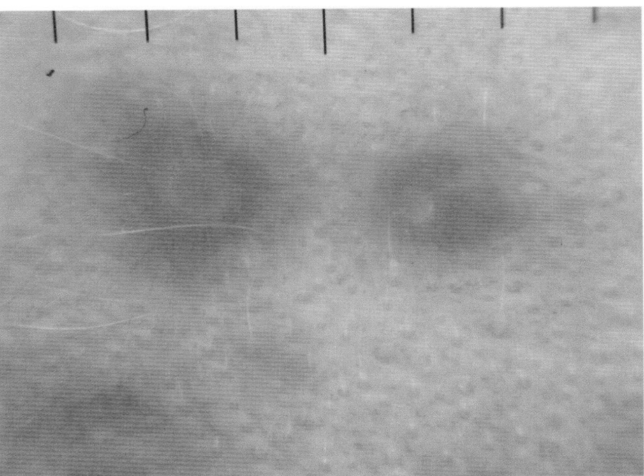

A 20-year-old woman with acne: dermoscopy shows foci of orange and erythematous perifollicular inflammation in keeping with ongoing acne activity.

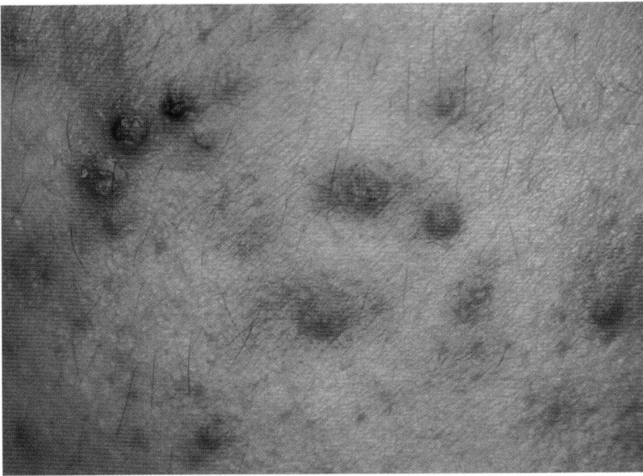

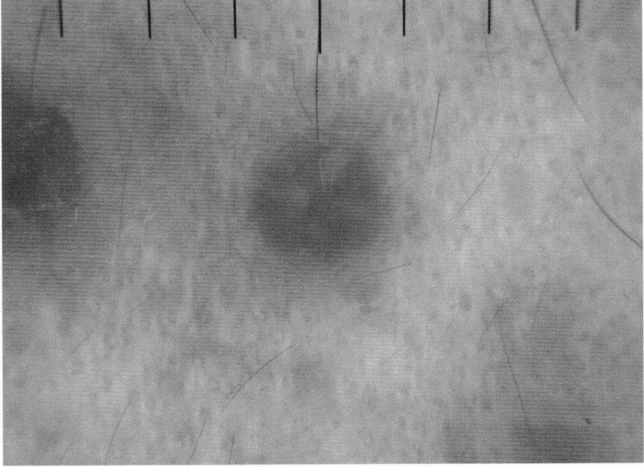

A 15-year-old boy with acne: dermoscopy shows foci of orange and erythematous perifollicular inflammation in keeping with ongoing acne activity.

Documentation of granulomatous inflammation can be useful when monitoring treatment in acne patients. Ongoing presence of dermal granulomatous inflammation can indicate whether escalation or prolongation of treatment may be required.

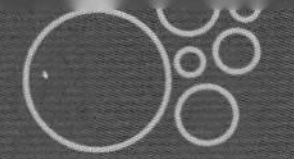

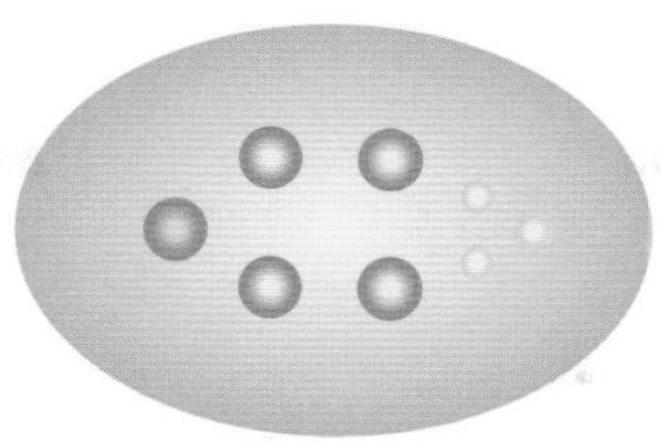

The severity of rosacea will influence clinical presentation and treatment decisions. Dermal granulomatous inflammation, which on dermoscopy appears as well-defined foci of orange or erythematous perifollicular blotches, may indicate that escalation to systemic treatment over topical alone may be required for a complete response.

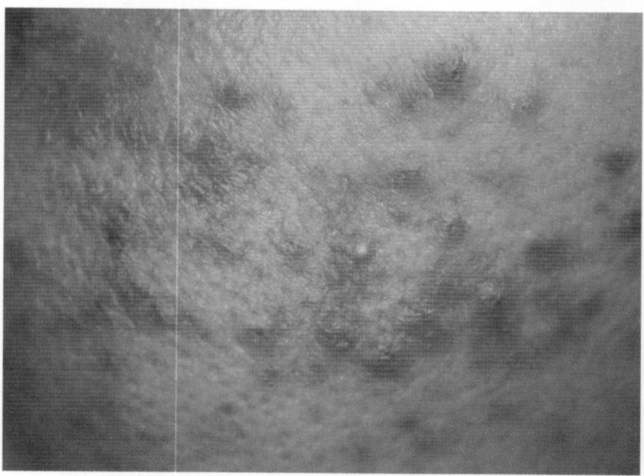

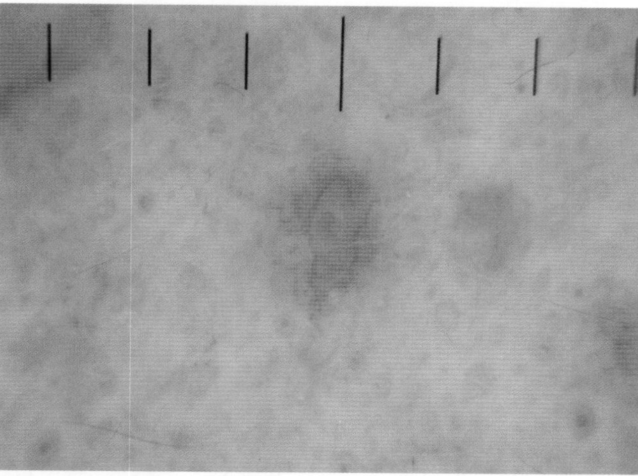

A 40-year-old woman with multiple papules and pustules on both cheeks without comedones in keeping with granulomatous rosacea: dermoscopy shows orange-erythematous perifollicular inflammation and linear vessels.

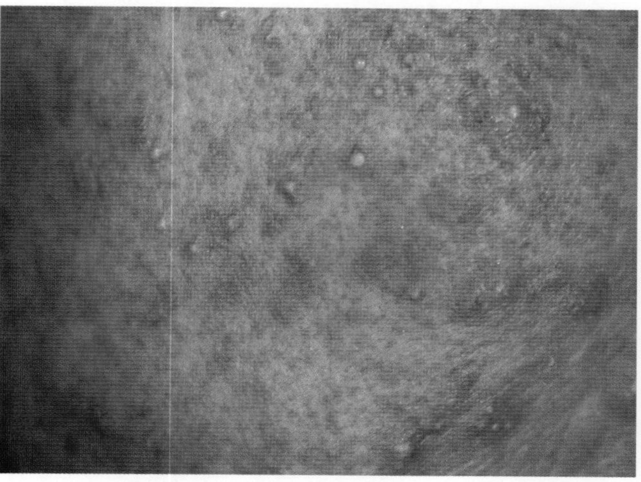

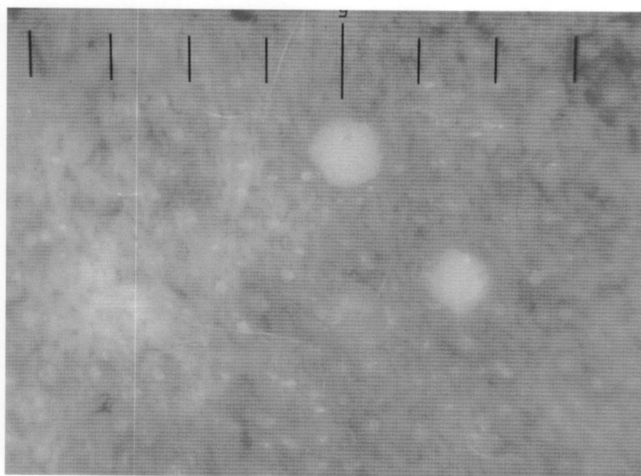

A 65-year-old man with widespread facial telangiectasia and erythema with multiple pustules: dermoscopy shows foci of orange-yellow well-circumscribed globules corresponding to pustules in this case of granulomatous rosacea.

Errichetti, E. et al. Standardization of dermoscopic terminology and basic dermoscopic parameters to evaluate in general dermatology (non-neoplastic dermatoses): an expert consensus on behalf of the International Dermoscopy Society. *Br J Dermatol* 2020;182(2):454–467.

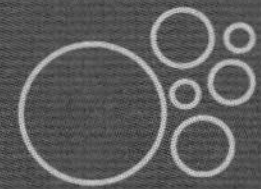

Eczema

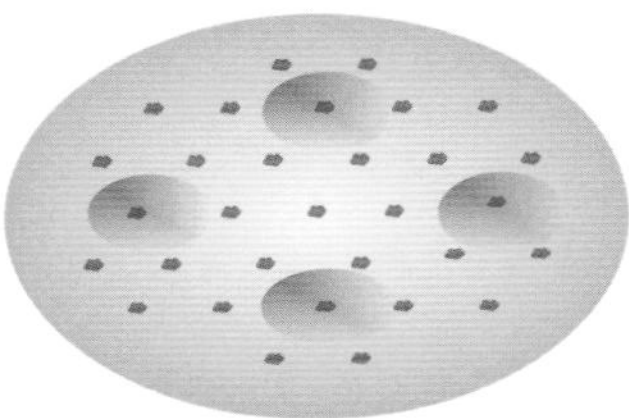

Eczema is characterised as an ill-defined inflammatory dermatosis with itch and exudation. It has many presentations depending upon aetiology; hence a detailed history is essential. Nummular eczema may initially present as a solitary well-defined erythematous plaque in which case it may cause diagnostic concern. Dermoscopy shows dotted, multifocal erosions and exudative yellow crusts corresponding histopathologically to underlying spongiosis.

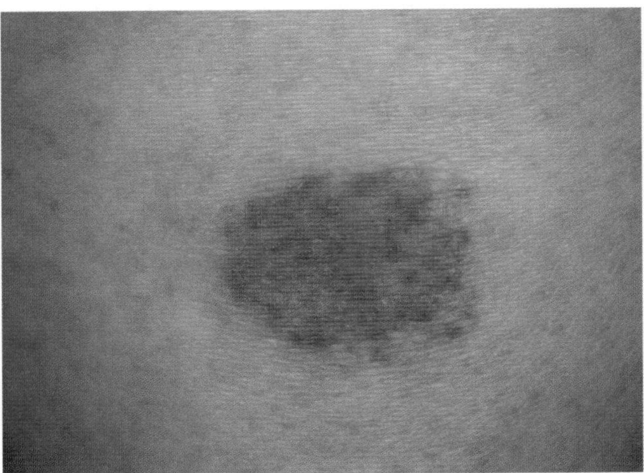

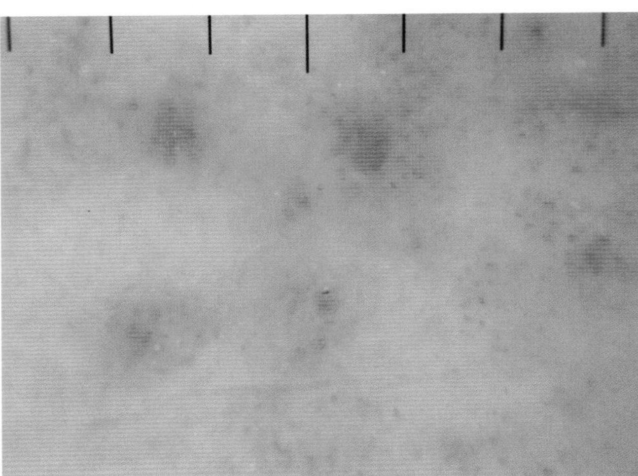

A solitary itchy plaque on the posterior thigh of a 70-year-old man: dermoscopy shows multifocal clusters of dotted vessels with multiple erosions and erythema in this case of nummular eczema, which responded to topical treatment.

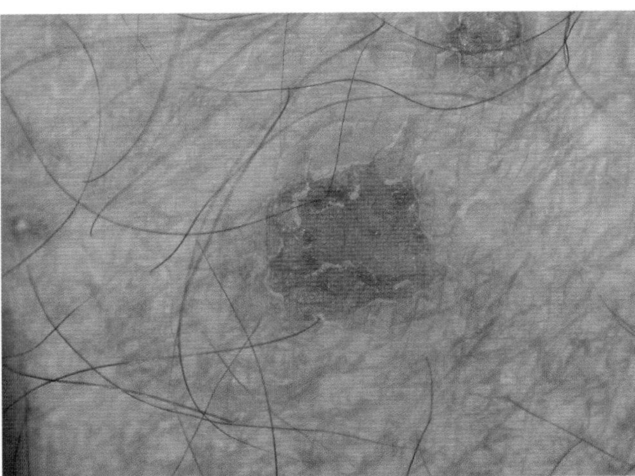

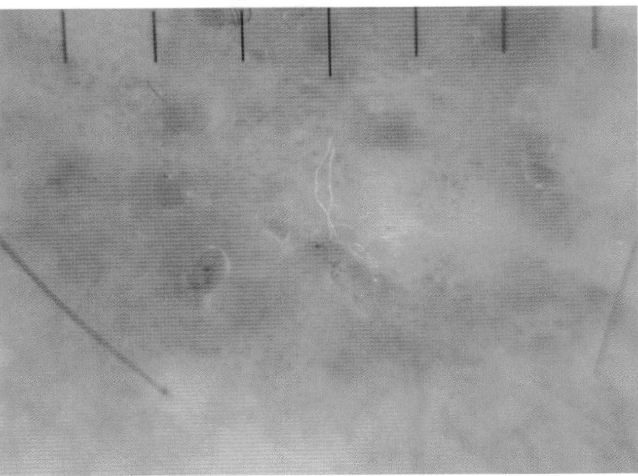

Multiple itchy exudative plaques on the lower leg of a 60-year-old man: dermoscopy shows multifocal clusters of dotted vessels, erosions, fibre from clothing, milky erythema and yellow crusts in this case of nummular eczema.

If an initial trial of topical steroid fails to clear a patch/plaque of presumed eczema, then one should consider either increasing the strength of steroid or, importantly, an alternative diagnosis.

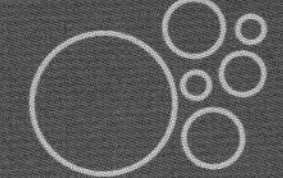

Psoriasis

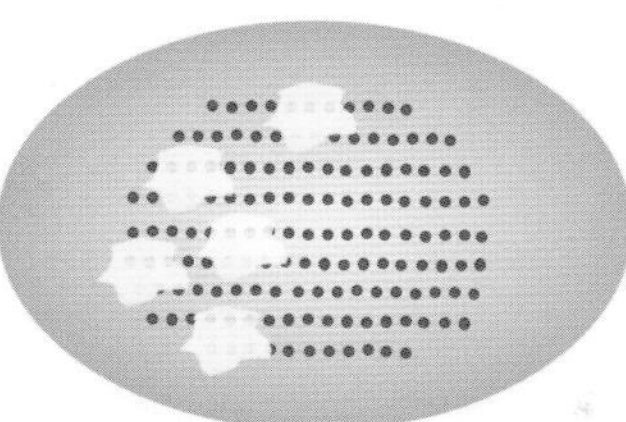

Psoriasis is characterised as an inflammatory dermatosis with well-defined erythrosquamous plaques. It has many presentations; hence a detailed history is essential. Dermoscopy shows parallel lines of dotted vessels, which, if traumatised by scale removal, may illustrate Auspitz sign (pin-point bleeding). When chronic plaque psoriasis develops there may only be a few plaques at initial presentation, thus the differential diagnosis is broad.

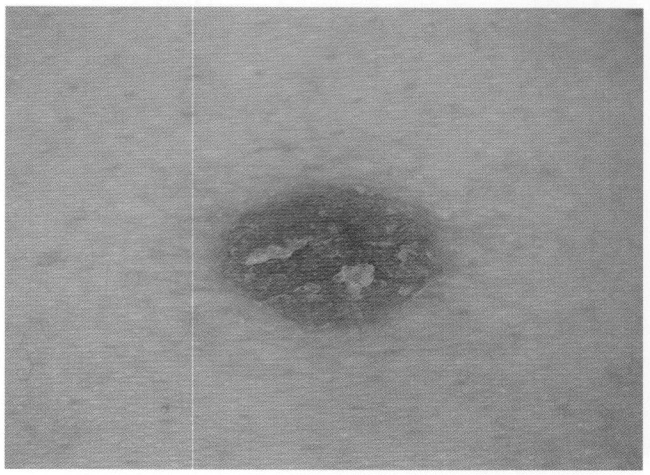

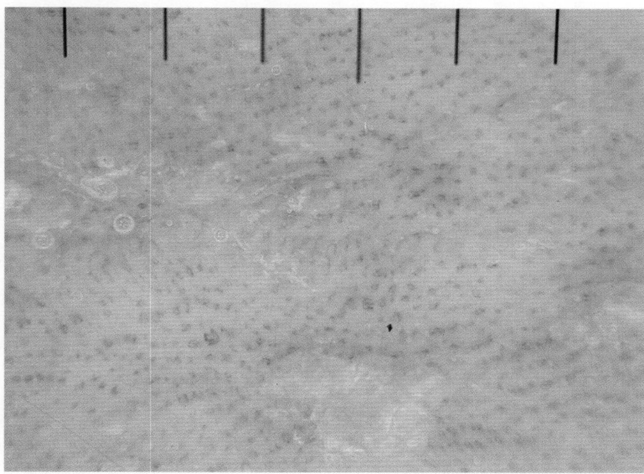

A solitary plaque on the flank of a 40-year-old man: dermoscopy shows multiple lines of dotted and small coiled or glomerular vessels in parallel in this case of plaque psoriasis.

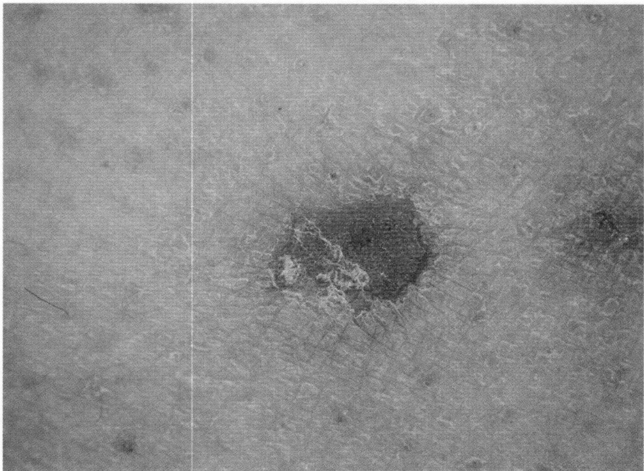

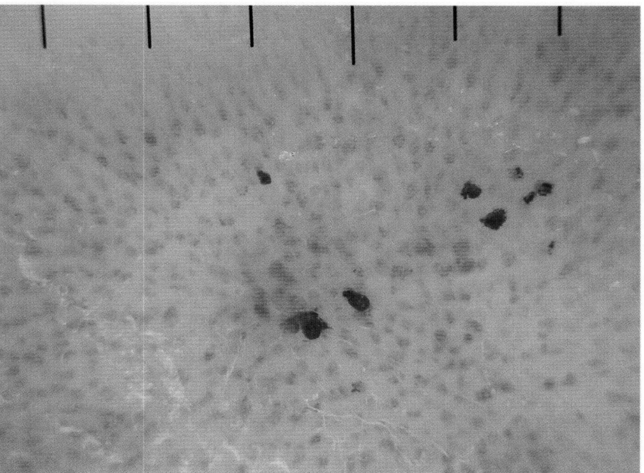

Multiple erythematous scaly psoriatic plaques on the trunk and limbs of a 50-year-old man with known psoriasis: dermoscopy shows multiple, small coiled or glomerular vessels with small foci of haemorrhage.

Unlike Bowen's disease where the dotted/glomerular or coiled vessels are clustered, in psoriasis the vessels all appear to be heading in the same direction like a school of fish.

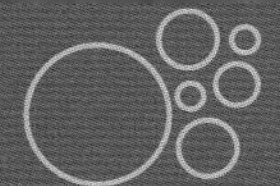

Lichen planus

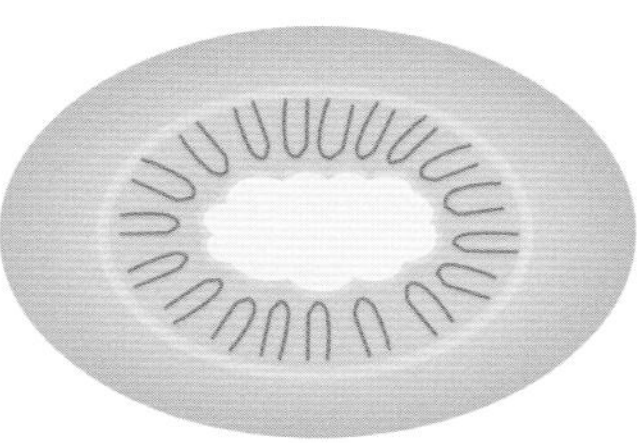

Lichen planus is an inflammatory dermatosis characterised clinically by multiple itchy flat-topped violaceous macules and plaques. In individuals with darker skin, prominent pigmentation may develop. Dermoscopy shows peripheral linear looped vessels and central pink structureless areas corresponding to Wickham's striae clinically.

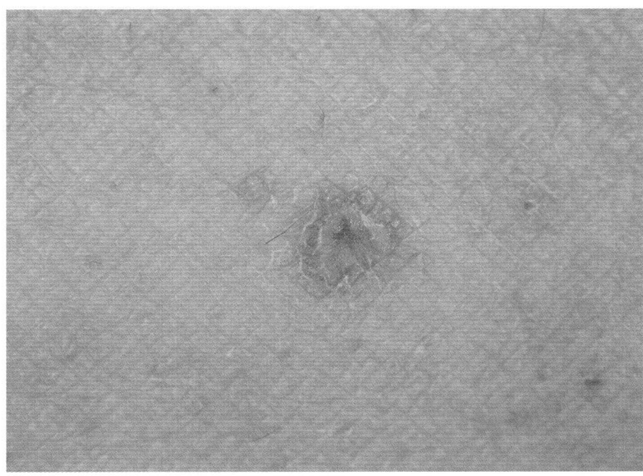

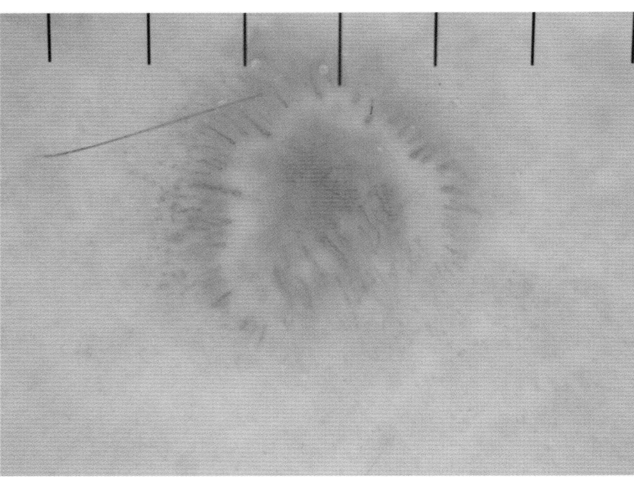

Multiple itchy discrete pink flat-topped macules on the forearms of a 30-year-old woman: dermoscopy shows multiple peripheral linear looped vessels, central erythema and pink structureless areas in this case of lichen planus.

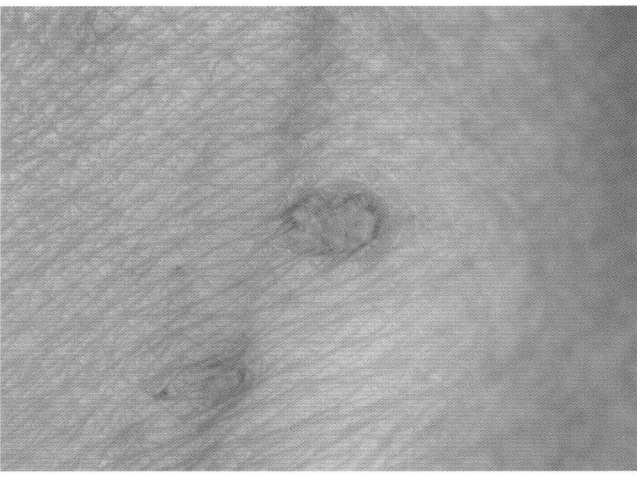

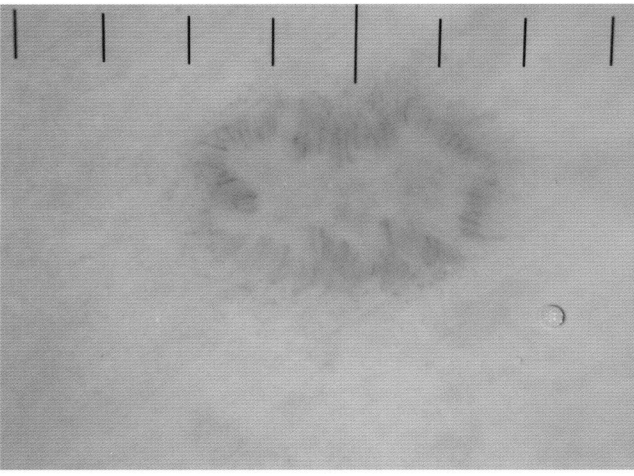

Multiple itchy discrete pink flat-topped macules on the limbs of a 30-year-old man: dermoscopy shows multiple peripheral linear looped vessels and pink structureless areas in this case of lichen planus.

Friedman, P. et al. Dermoscopic findings in different clinical variants of lichen planus. Is dermoscopy useful? *Dermatol Pract Concept.* 2015;5(4):51–55.

Lichen planus pigmentosus

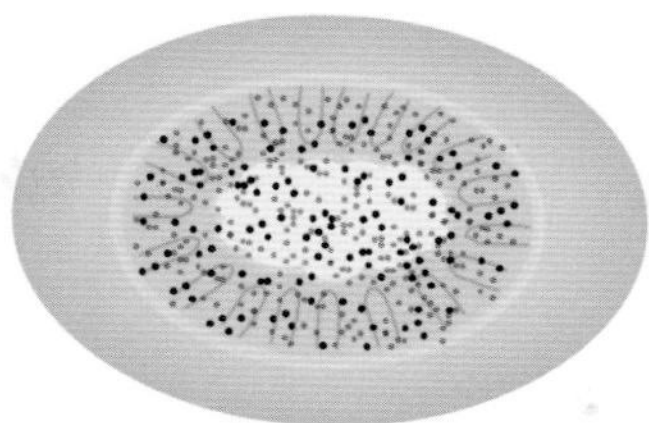

Lichen planus pigmentosus is a clinical variant of lichen planus characterised by multiple lichenoid pigmented macules with prominent pigment incontinence, commonly found in individuals with darker skin phototypes. Dermoscopy shows widespread brown-grey granular pigmentation and pink structureless areas.

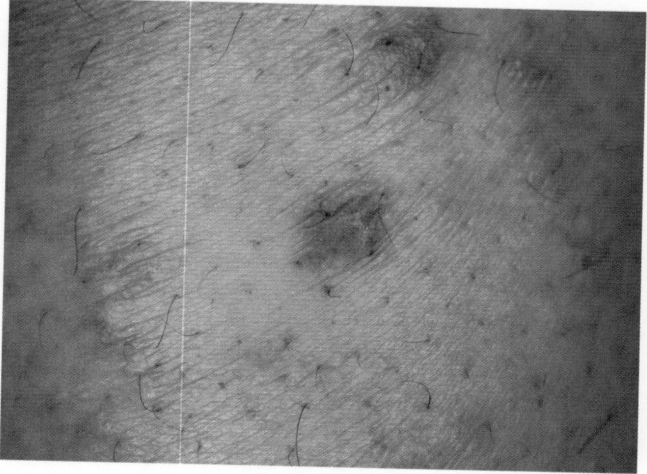

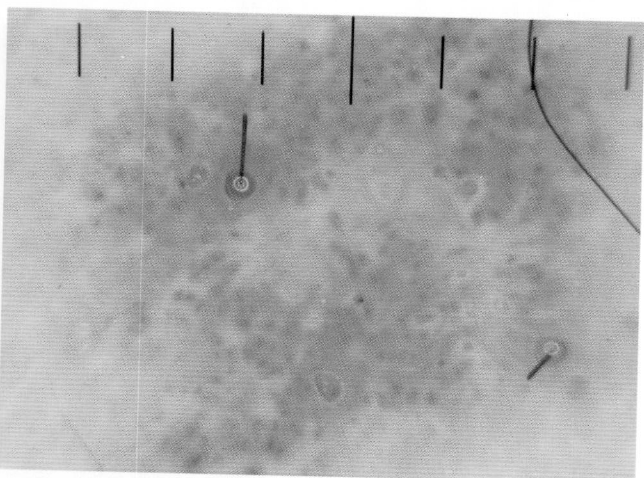

Multiple itchy violaceous pink macules in a 50-year-old man with dark skin: dermoscopy shows granular grey-brown pigmentation with central pink structureless areas in this case of lichen planus pigmentosus.

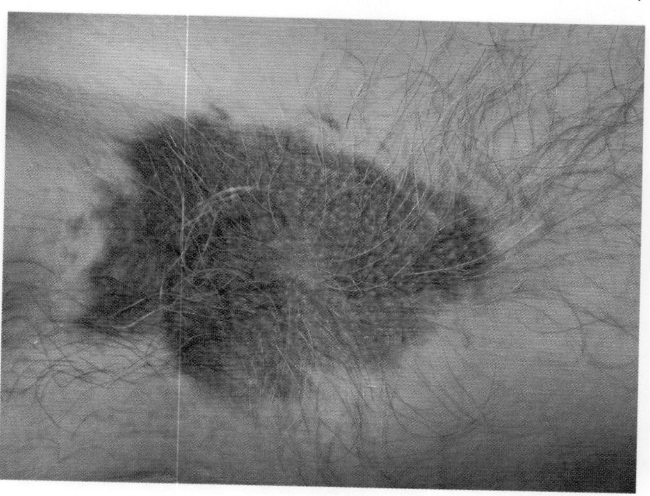

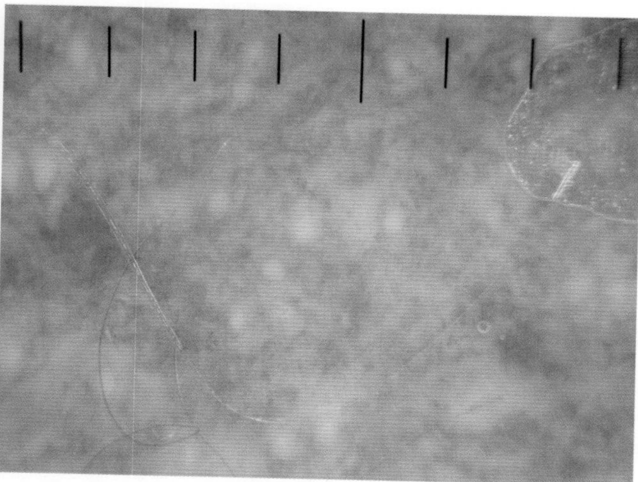

A hyperpigmented axillary patch in a 50-year-old man: dermoscopy shows brown-grey granular pigmentation and milky erythema in this case of lichen planus pigmentosus.

Murzaku, E.C. et al. Axillary lichen planus pigmentosus-inversus: dermoscopic clues of a rare entity. Diagnosis: lichen planus pigmentosus (LPP). *J Am Acad Dermatol*. 2014;71(4):e119–120.

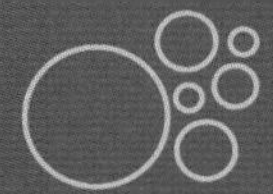

Capillaritis

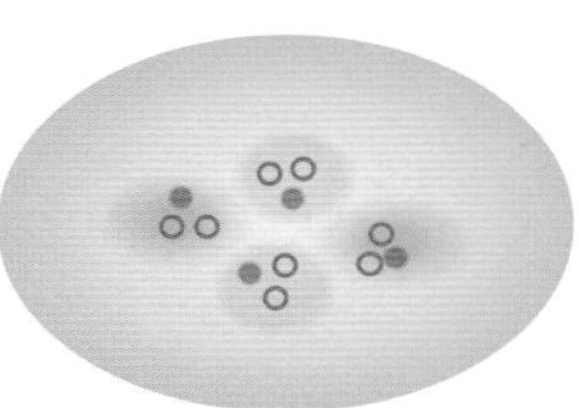

Capillaritis, also known as pigmented purpuric dermatosis, is a harmless inflammatory dermatosis affecting the small skin capillaries. Capillary leakage and extravasation of red blood cells causes petechial 'cayenne pepper'-like pigmentation, which gradually fades, depositing haemosiderin in the upper dermis. On dermoscopy the extravasation can outline dermal papillae as globules or red ring-like annular structures in addition to rust brown-orange background colouration.

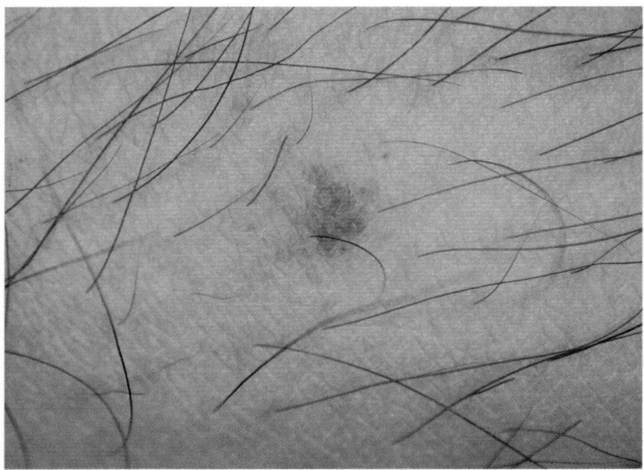

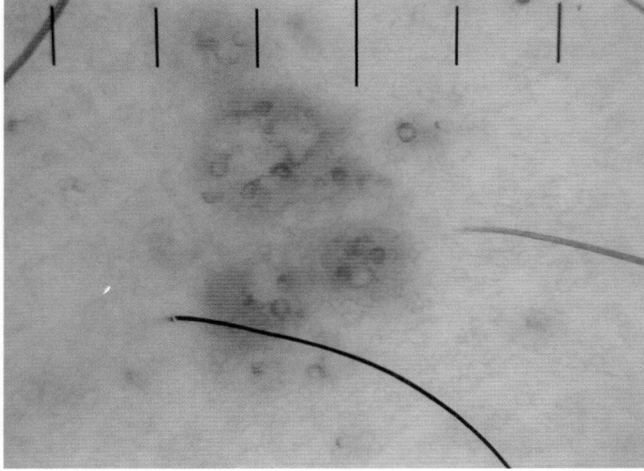

Multiple asymptomatic petechial macules on the lower legs of a 20-year-old man: dermoscopy shows erythematous ring-like vascular structures and orange-brown background in this histopathologically confirmed case of capillaritis.

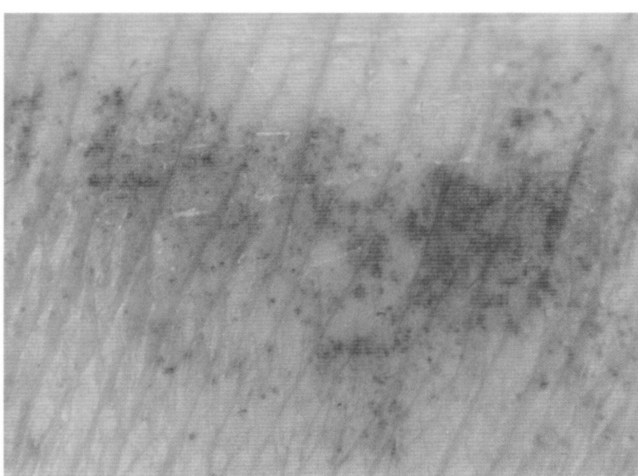

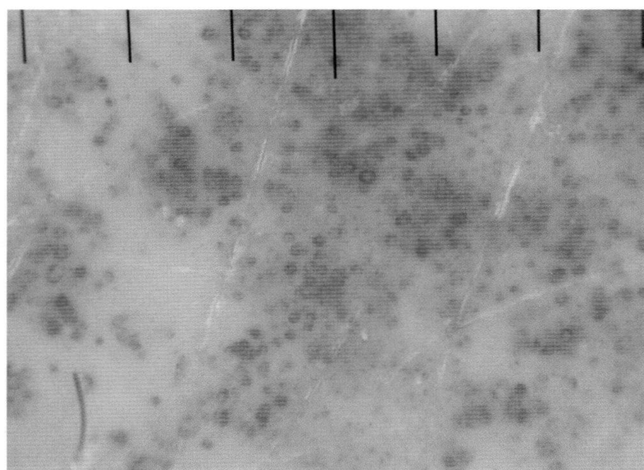

Multiple petechial patches on the lower legs of a 30-year-old man: dermoscopy shows widespread erythematous ring-like vascular structures and orange-brown background in this histopathologically confirmed case of capillaritis.

Zaballos, P. et al. Dermoscopy of pigmented purpuric dermatoses (lichen aureus): a useful tool for clinical diagnosis. *Arch Dermatol.* 2004;140(10):1290–1291.

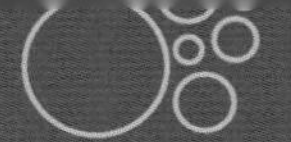

Vasculitis

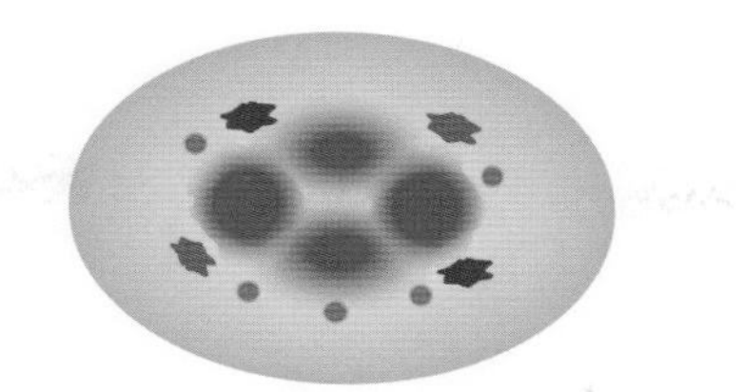

In contrast to capillaritis, small vessel vasculitis needs investigating to confirm the severity and subtype of vasculitis in addition to identification of systemic complications. Clinically it presents with multiple purpuric blotches and, if severe, skin necrosis and ulceration. Dermoscopy typically shows different features despending upon the timing of presentation and the severity, which includes purple, blue-grey and erythematous blotches, erythematous dots or globules and crusts if ulceration is present.

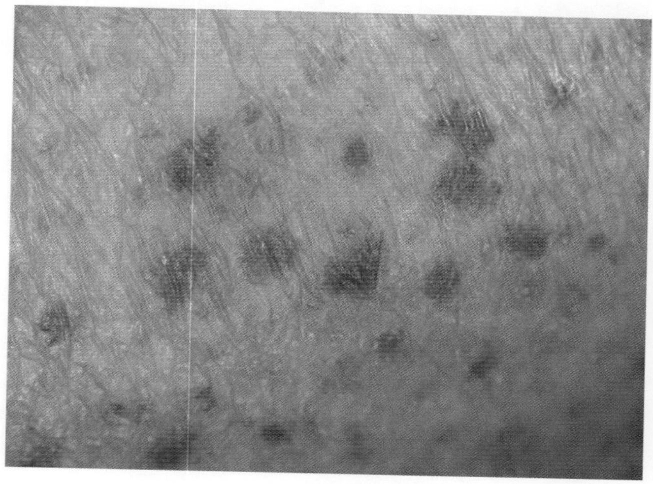

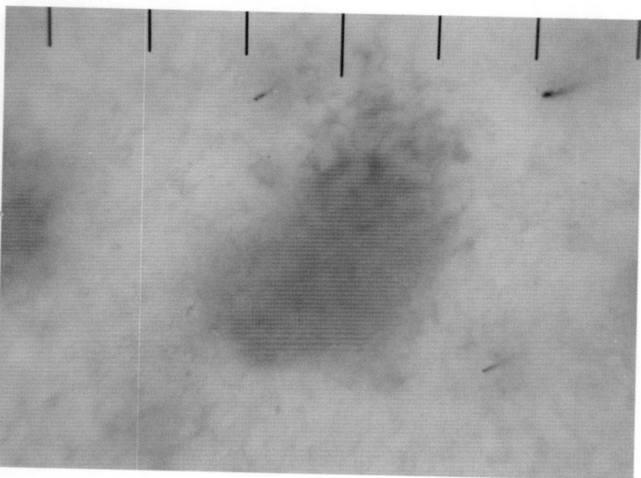

Multiple purpuric macules on the lower legs of a 20-year-old man: dermoscopy shows blurred erythematous/purple blotches in this histopathologically confirmed case of vasculitis.

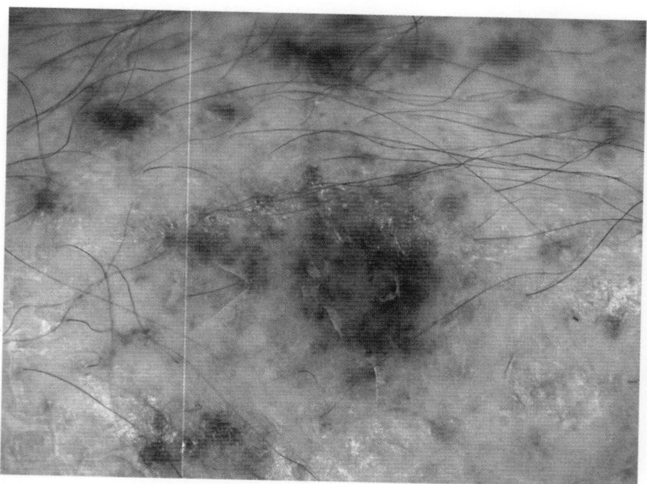

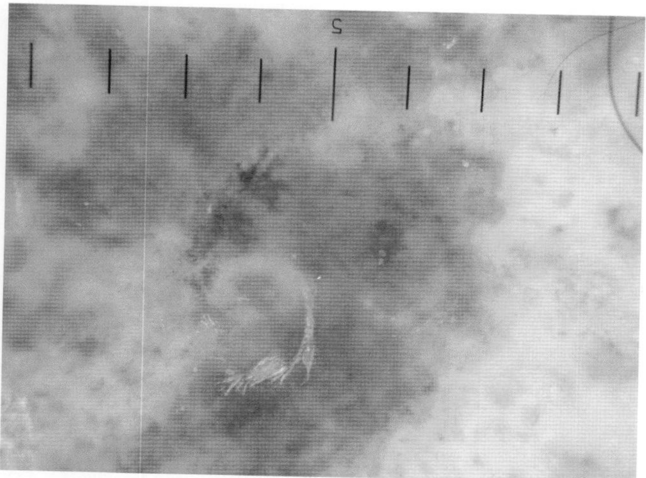

Multiple petechial macules on the lower legs of a 60-year-old man: dermoscopy shows irregular erythematous and haemorrhagic blotches in this histopathologically confirmed case of polyarteritis nodosa.

Choo, J.Y. et al. Blue-gray blotch: A helpful dermoscopic finding in optimal biopsy site selection for true vasculitis. *J Am Acad Dermatol*. 2016;75(4):836–838.

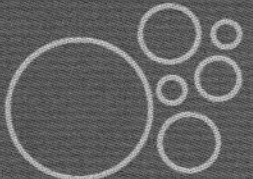

Granulomatous conditions

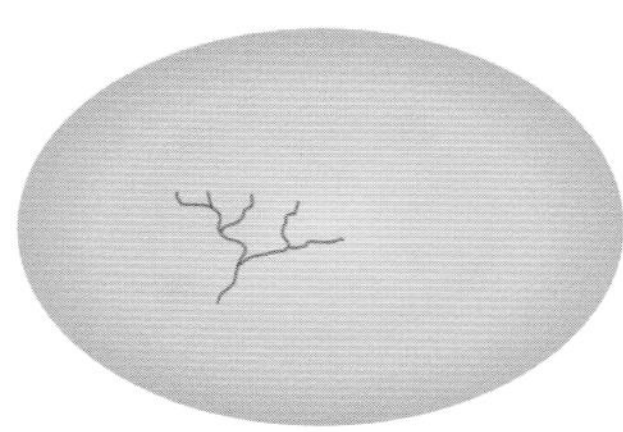

Non-infectious granulomatous skin conditions may share clinical and dermoscopic features. Dermoscopy features include linear vessels and orange structureless areas and background colour. Histopathology is therefore recommended to reliably confirm the diagnosis.

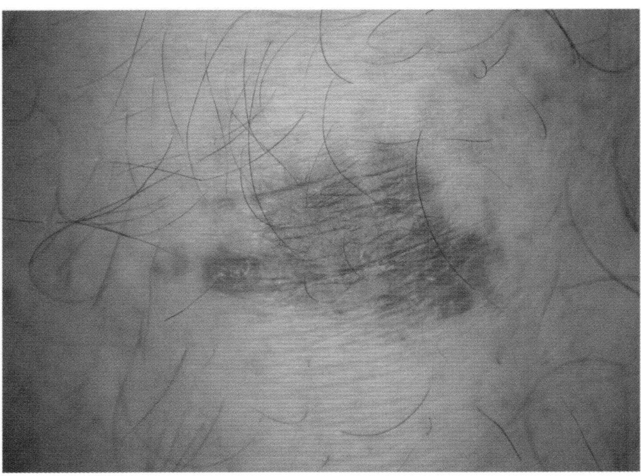

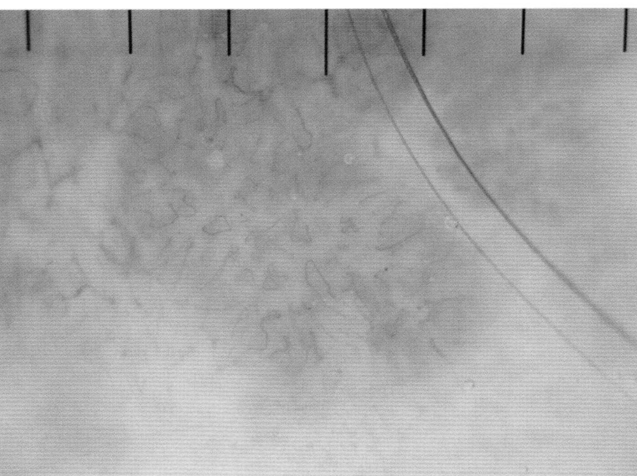

A solitary orange and erythematous granulomatous plaque on the knee of a 40-year-old man: dermoscopy shows multiple linear vessels upon an orange background colour in this histopathologically confirmed case of cutaneous sarcoidosis.

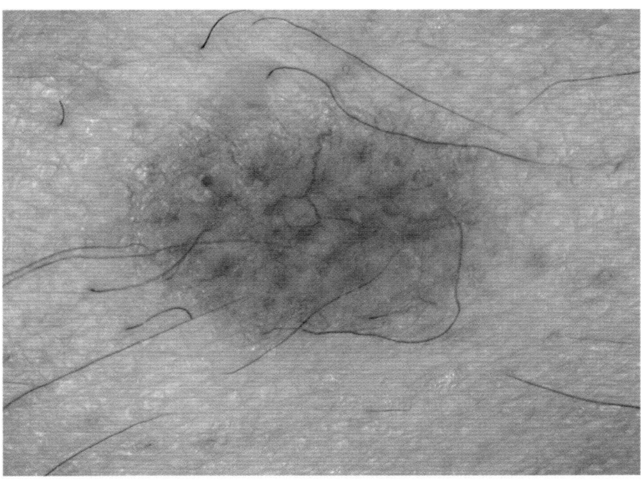

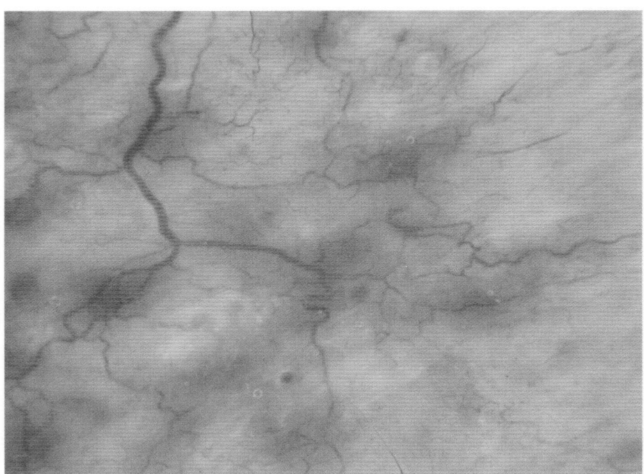

A solitary orange and erythematous granulomatous plaque on the shin of a 60-year-old woman: dermoscopy shows linear vessels and yellowish background in this histopathologically confirmed case of necrobiosis lipoidica.

Errichetti, E. and Stinco, G. Dermatoscopy of granulomatous disorders. *Dermatol Clin*. 2018;36(4):369–375.

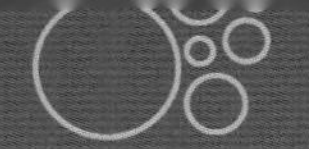

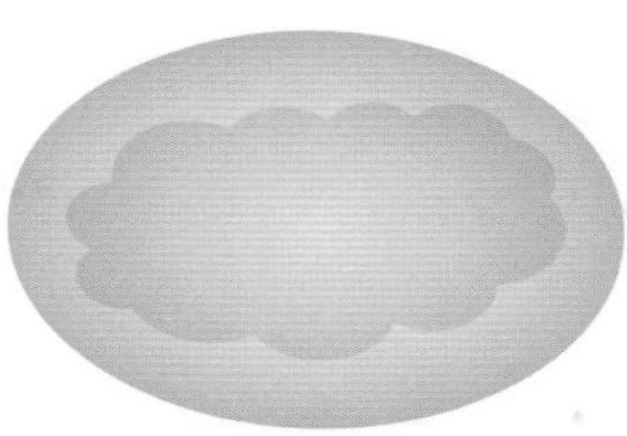

Granuloma annulare is a non-infectious granulomatous skin condition that typically presents in a variety of morphologies including skin-coloured or lightly erythematous papules and annular plaques. The diagnosis is usually made clinically as the dermoscopic features are very subtle, which include a pinkish-reddish and orange background and blurry dotted and linear vessels.

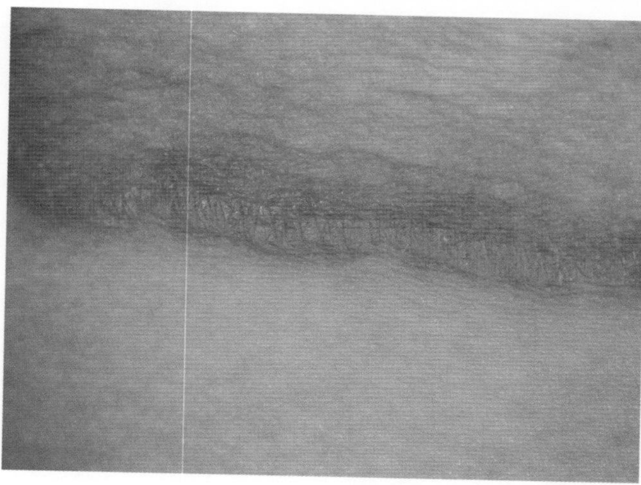

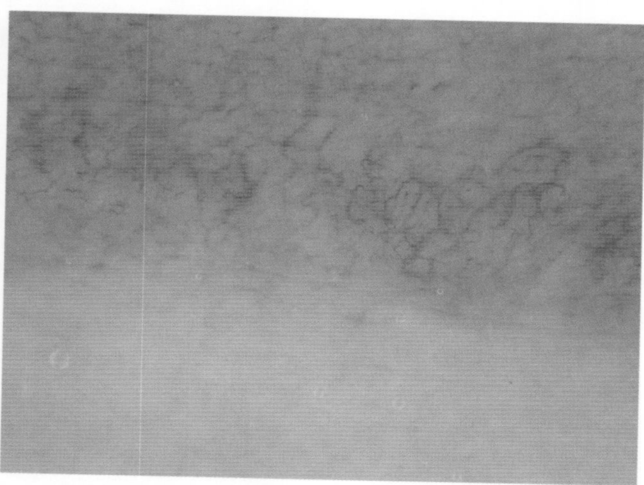

A solitary granulomatous violaceous plaque on the ankle of a 40-year-old woman: dermoscopy shows blurred dotted vessels and an orange-reddish background in this histopathologically confirmed case of granuloma annulare.

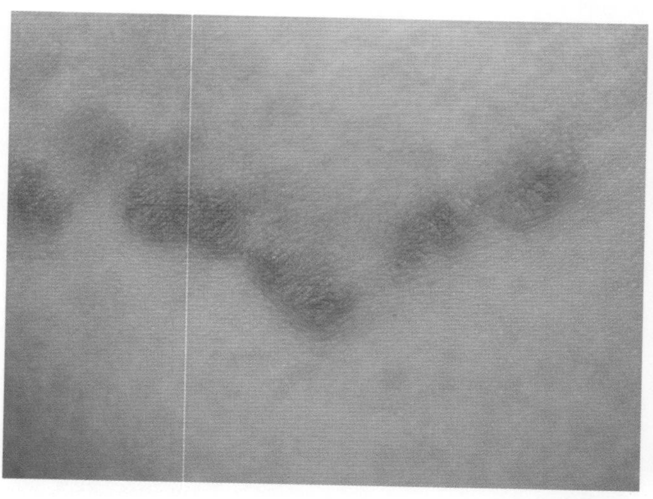

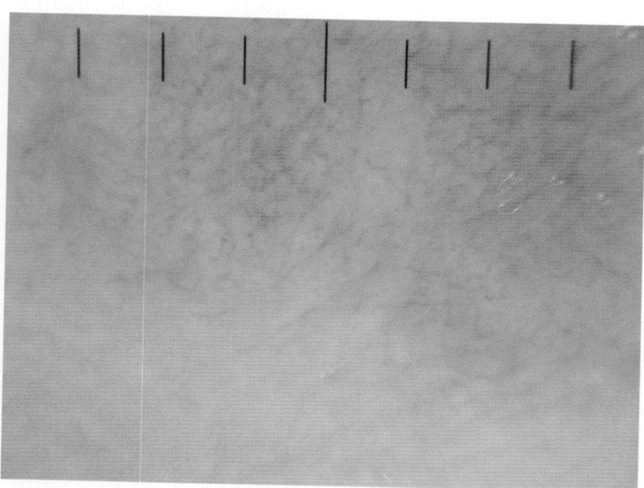

Multiple granulomatous papules coalescing to form a linear plaque on the arm of a 60-year-old woman: dermoscopy shows blurry linear vessels and a pinkish-reddish background in this histopathologically confirmed case of granuloma annulare.

Errichetti, E. et al. Dermoscopy of granuloma annulare: a clinical and histological correlation study. *Dermatology*. 2017;233(1):74–79.

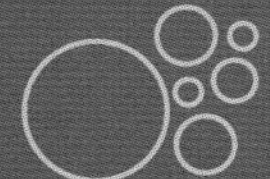

Tinea corporis

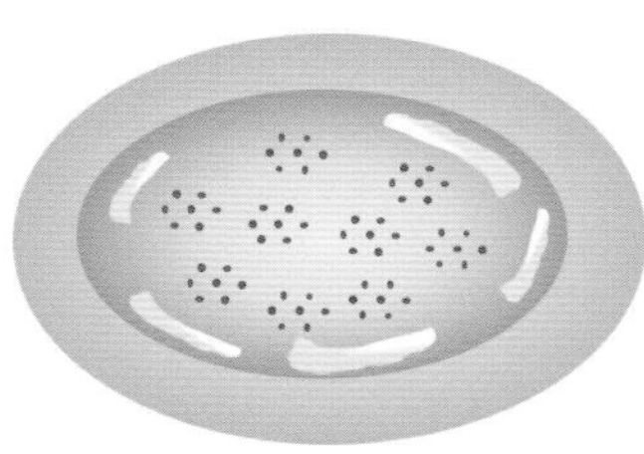

The clinical presentation of dermatophyte infection of the skin or tinea is influenced by many factors including the site of infection and the causative infective organism. Clinically, tinea corporis typically presents as an erythematous scaly plaque with a peripheral erythematous margin with desquamation medially. Dermoscopy shows peripheral erythema, dotted vessels, and on dry dermoscopy peripheral desquamation. Diagnosis is based on a combination of clinical features and mycology.

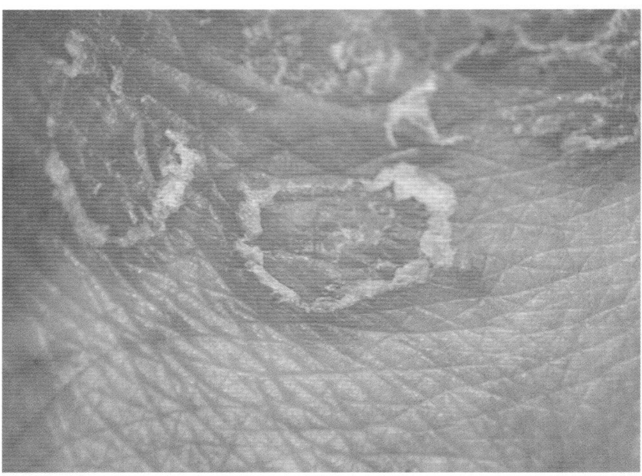

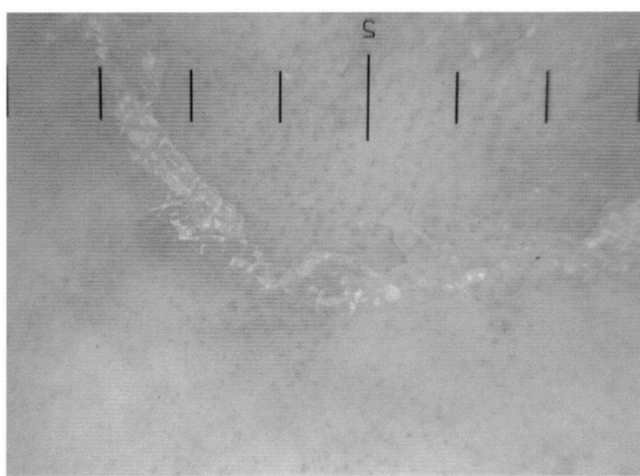

A scaly plaque on the ankle of a 40-year-old man: dermoscopy shows erythema with dotted vessels and peripheral desquamation in this case of mycologically confirmed *Trichophyton rubrum* tinea corporis.

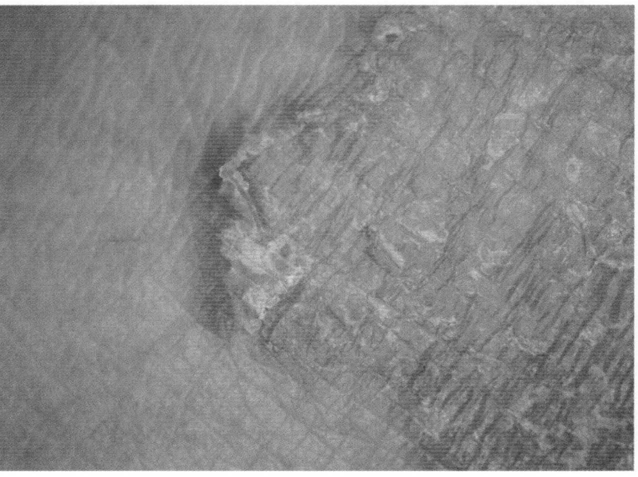

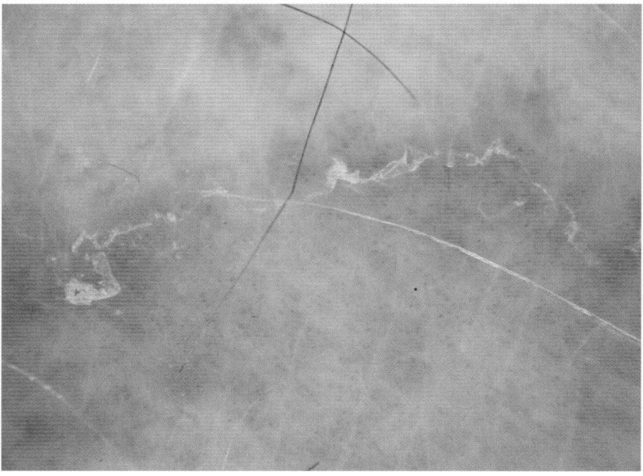

A solitary scaly plaque on the wrist of a 50-year-old man: dermoscopy shows erythema with dotted vessels and peripheral desquamation in this case of mycologically confirmed *Trichophyton rubrum* tinea corporis.

Leung, A.K. et al. Tinea corporis: an updated review. *Drugs Context*. 2020;9:2020-5-6.

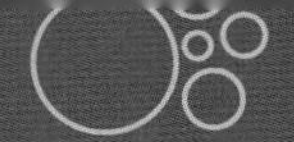

Pityriasis rosea

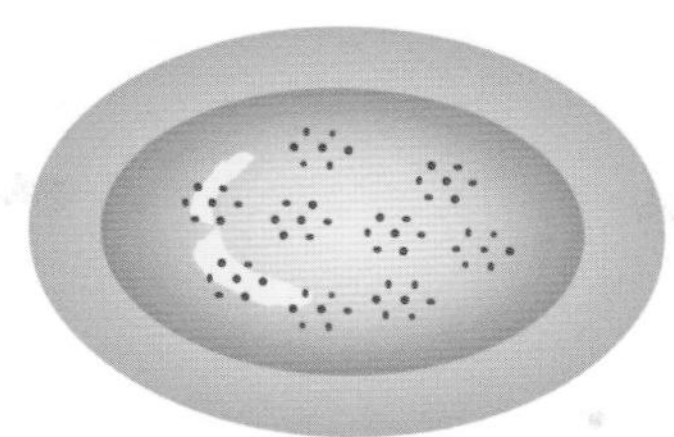

Pityriasis rosea is an inflammatory dermatosis associated with HHV-6 and HHV-7 infection. Clinically it is characterised by an in initial erythematous 'herald' patch followed by the development of multiple scaly patches and plaques mainly on the trunk and proximal extremities. Dermoscopy shows erythema and dotted vessels centrally with peripheral desquamation.

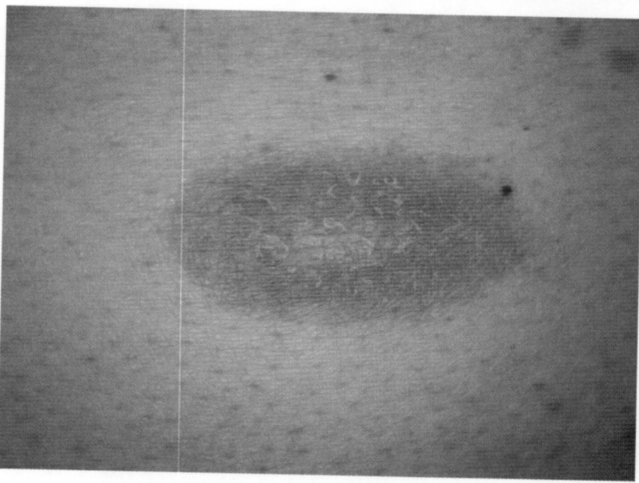

An indurated erythematous herald patch on the chest of a 50-year-old man with widespread erythematous macules on the trunk and limbs: dermoscopy shows erythema with dotted vessels in this case of pityriasis rosea.

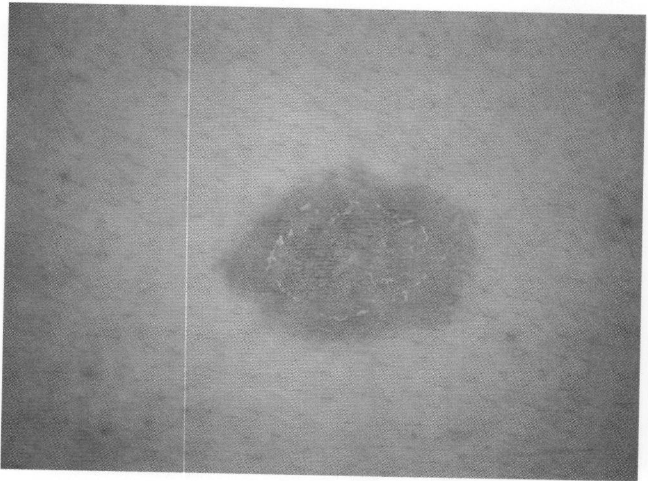

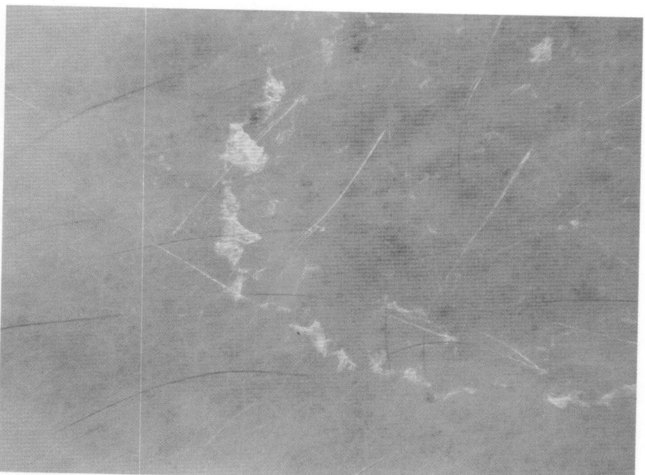

A herald patch on the back of a 30-year-old woman: dry dermoscopy shows erythema and dotted vessels with inward facing peripheral desquamation in this case of pityriasis rosea.

Lallas, A. et al. Accuracy of dermoscopic criteria for the diagnosis of psoriasis, dermatitis, lichen planus and pityriasis rosea. *Br J Dermatol.* 2012;166:1198–205.

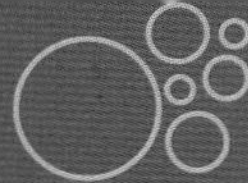

Cutaneous lupus erythematosus

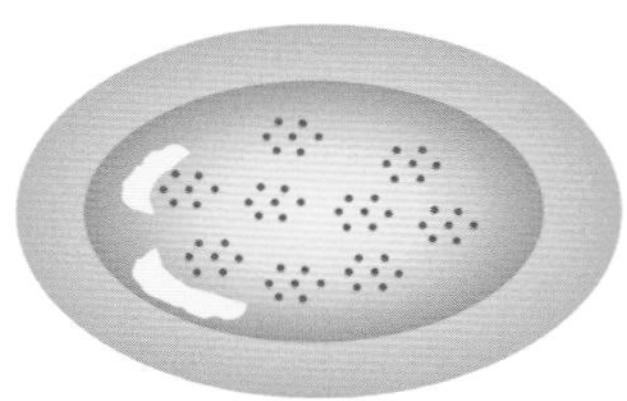

Cutaneous lupus erythematosus is an autoimmune disease with many clinical manifestations, including an acute, subacute or chronic form. The typical histopathological feature is an interface dermatitis. Dermoscopic features include perifollicular white halos, erythema, linear and dotted vessels, and rosettes on polarised dermoscopy. Diagnosis is typically based upon the clinical history, examination and histopathology.

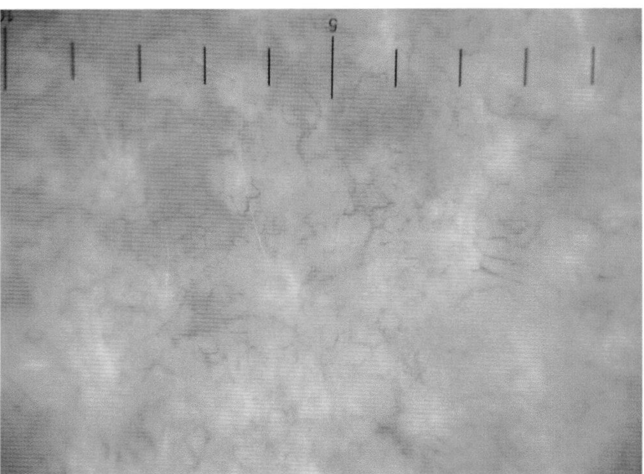

A solitary erythematous indurated plaque on the upper arm of a 60-year-old woman: dermoscopy shows erythema with a perifollicular whitish halo and linear vessels in this histopathologically confirmed case of cutaneous lupus erythematosus.

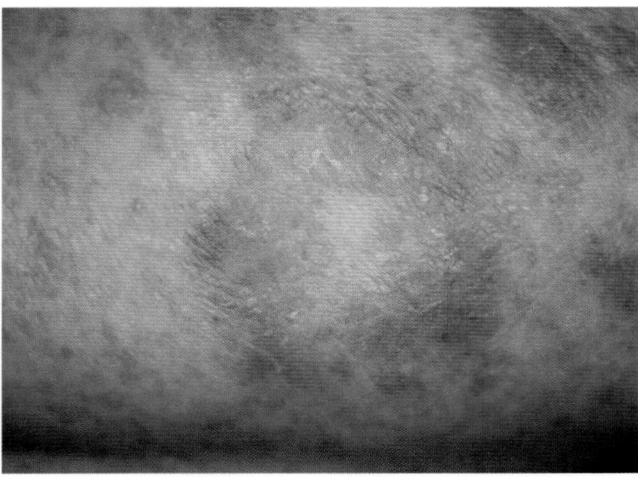

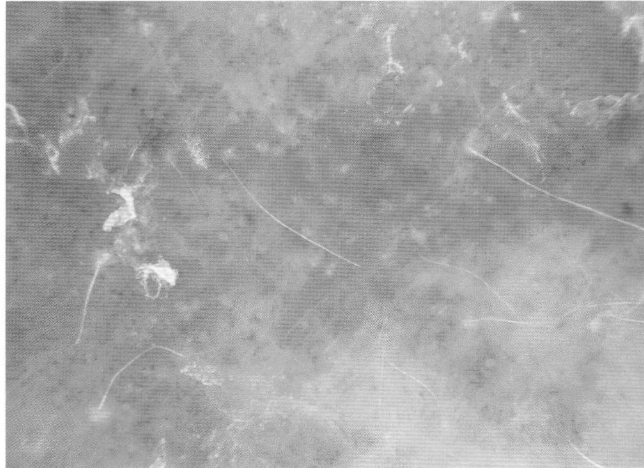

Multiple polycyclic annular erythematous plaques on the forearms of a 60-year-old woman: dermoscopy shows dotted vessels, erythema, rosettes and hyperkeratosis in this confirmed case of subacute cutaneous lupus erythematosus.

Errichetti, E. et al. Dermoscopy of subacute cutaneous lupus erythematosus. *Int J Dermatol.* 2016;55(11):e605–e607.

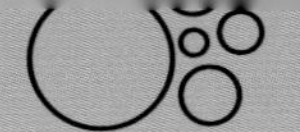

10 Genodermatoses

Gorlin syndrome 290
Cowden syndrome 291
Birt-Hogg-Dubé syndrome 292
Familial cylindromatosis syndrome 293
Muir-Torre syndrome 294
Reed syndrome 295
Familial melanoma 296
Carney complex 297

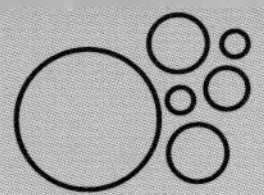

Gorlin syndrome

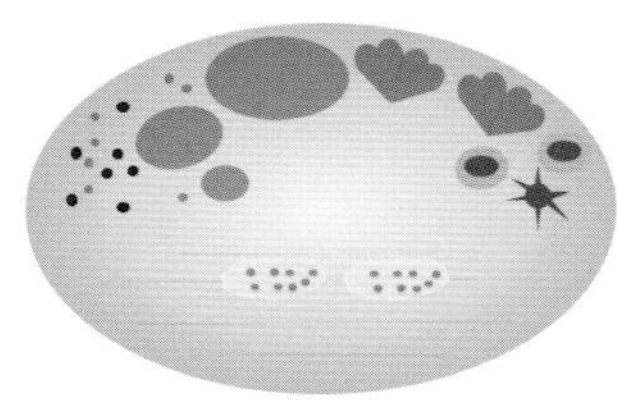

Gorlin syndrome or naevoid basal cell carcinoma syndrome is an autosomal dominant genodermatosis caused by mutations in the PTCH1 gene. Cutaneous features include multiple basal cell carcinomas (BCCs), which may develop in childhood/adolescence in addition to palmoplantar pits. Dermoscopy is helpful in differentiating pigmented BCCs from naevi in affected individuals.

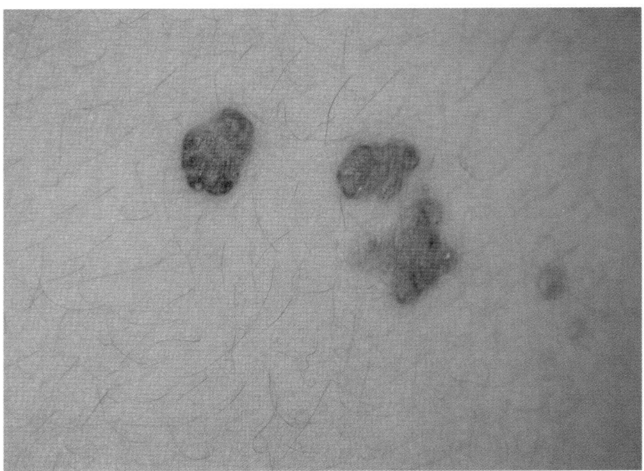

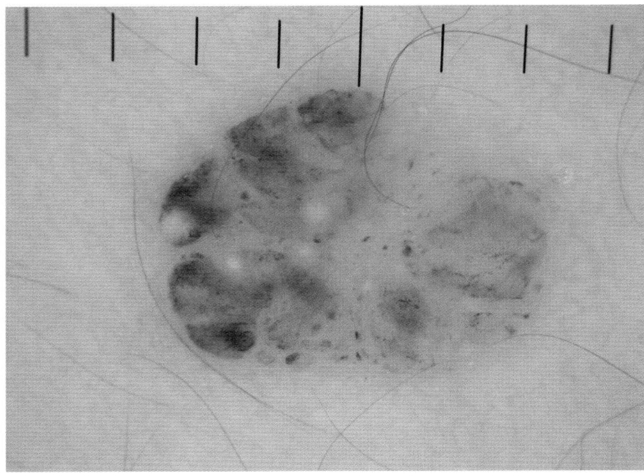

Multiple pigmented macules and plaques on the trunk of an 11-year-old girl with known Gorlin syndrome: dermoscopy shows short telangiectatic vessels with multiple irregular brown/grey dots and granules in this pigmented BCC.

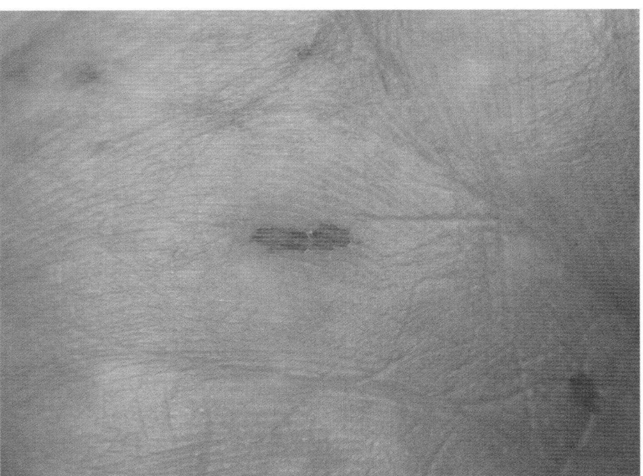

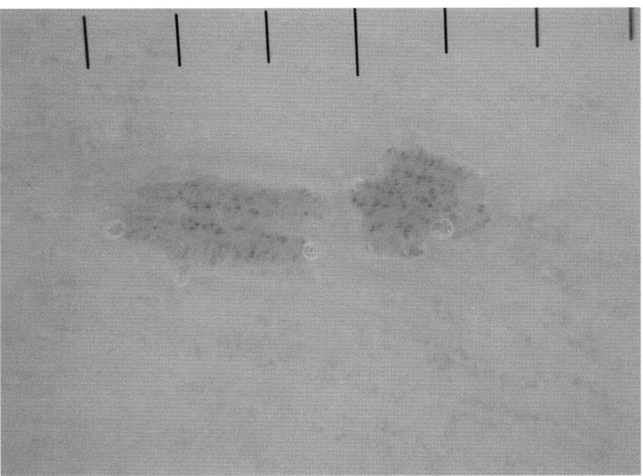

Multiple asymptomatic palmar pits in a 50-year-old woman with Gorlin syndrome: dermoscopy shows focal hypokeratosis with a clear view of the underlying dotted vessels of the acral dermatoglyphics.

Jarrett, R. et al. The dermoscopy of Gorlin syndrome: pursuit of the pits revisited. *Arch Dermatol.* 2010;146(5):582.

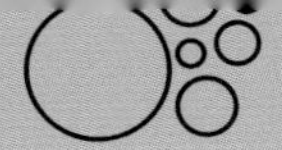

Cowden syndrome

Cowden syndrome (CS) is an autosomal dominant genodermatosis is caused by mutations in the PTEN (tumour suppressor) gene. Cutaneous features include trichilemmomas and acral keratoses, which have a characteristic orthokeratotic plate of keratin on histopathology. The acral keratoses show classical dermoscopy with yellow structureless areas with a prominent collarette. People with CS are at an increased risk of developing internal malignancies.

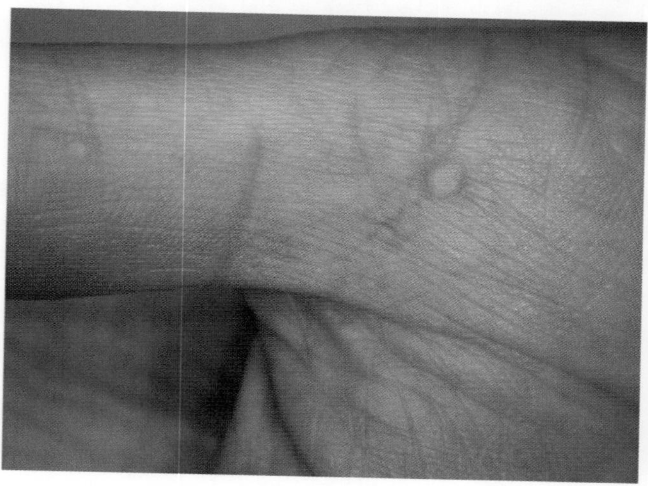

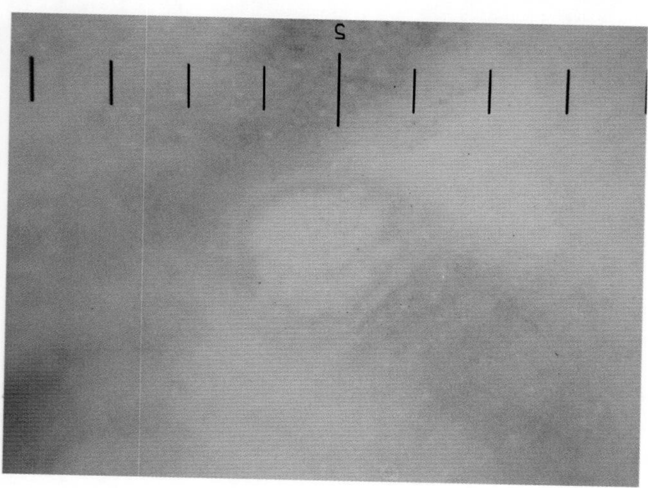

Multiple acral keratoses on the palm of a 50-year-old woman with known CS: dermoscopy shows a characteristic yellow structureless focus of keratin with a well-defined collarette.

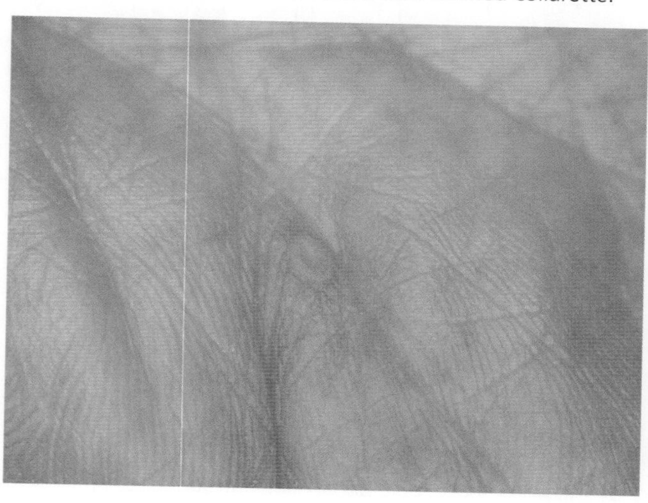

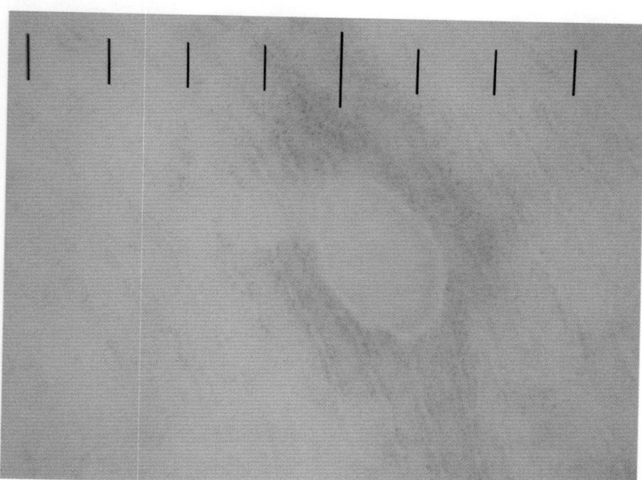

Multiple acral keratoses on the palm and thumb of a 30-year-old woman with known CS: dermoscopy of a keratosis shows the characteristic keratin plate with a prominent peripheral yellow collarette.

Images with permission from: Jarrett, R. et al. Dermoscopy of Cowden syndrome. *Arch. Dermatol.* 2009;145(4):508–509.

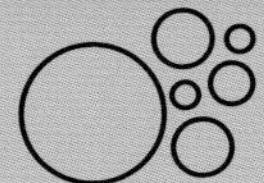

Birt-Hogg-Dubé syndrome

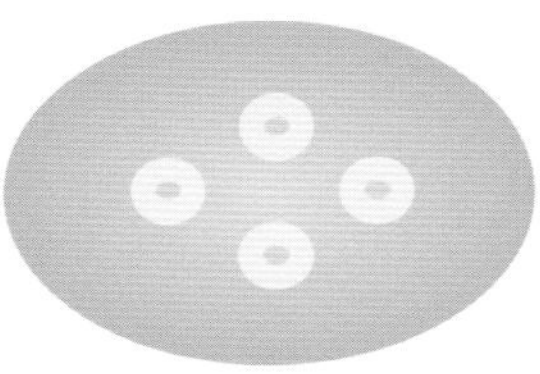

Birt-Hogg-Dubé syndrome is an autosomal dominant genodermatosis caused by mutations in the folliculin (FLCN) gene, which causes skin lesions and in up to 30% of patients renal tumours including renal cell cancer. The clinical features include multiple firm sclerotic fibrofolliculomas which occur on the head and neck and upper trunk. These typically appear in the third and fourth decade. Lung cysts are also common, which may lead to spontaneous pneumothorax.

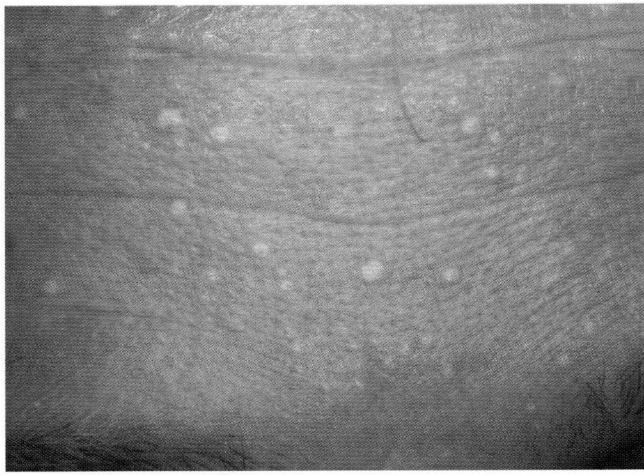

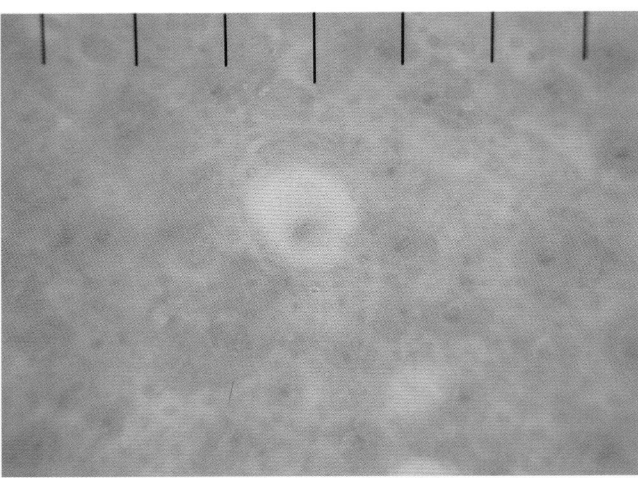

Multiple skin-coloured papules on the forehead of a 40-year-old man: dermoscopy shows multiple perifollicular pale structureless areas confirmed as fibrofolliculomas on histopathology in a patient with Birt-Hogg-Dubé syndrome.

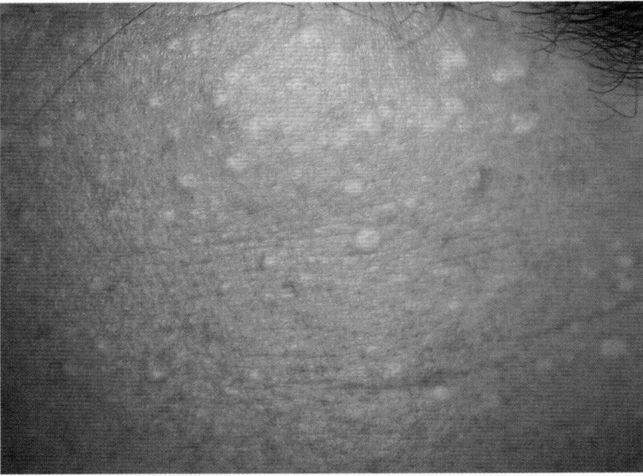

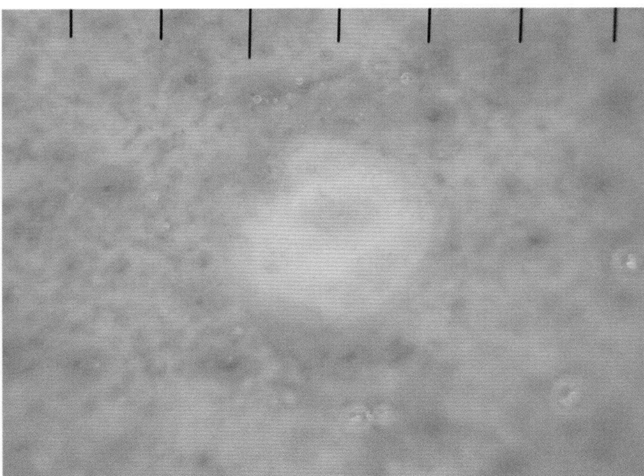

Multiple skin-coloured papules on the face of a 50-year-old woman: dermoscopy shows pale perifollicular structureless areas with central yellow keratin mass, confirmed as fibrofolliculomas in a patient with Birt-Hogg-Dubé syndrome.

Jarrett, R. et al. Dermoscopic features of Birt-Hogg-Dubé syndrome. *Arch Dermatol.* 2009;145(10):1208.

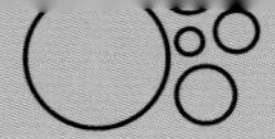

Familial cylindromatosis syndrome

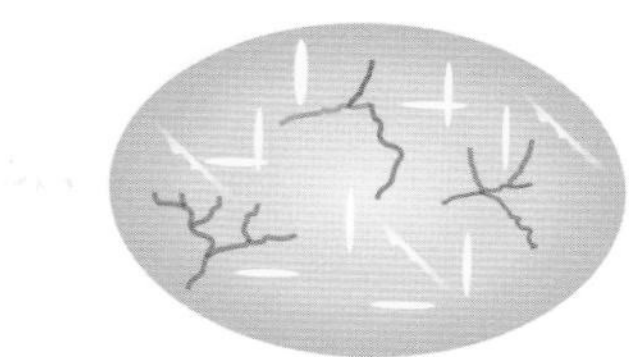

Familial cylindromatosis is caused by mutations in the CYLD gene. Cylindromas manifest as multiple firm pink telangiectatic papules and nodules arising on the scalp and hairline. Dermoscopy shows branching linear vessels, structureless areas and shiny white structures on polarisation mimicking BCC. Cylindromatosis is on a phenotypic spectrum with Brooke-Spiegler syndrome which is also characterised by eccrine spiradenoms and facial trichoepitheliomas.

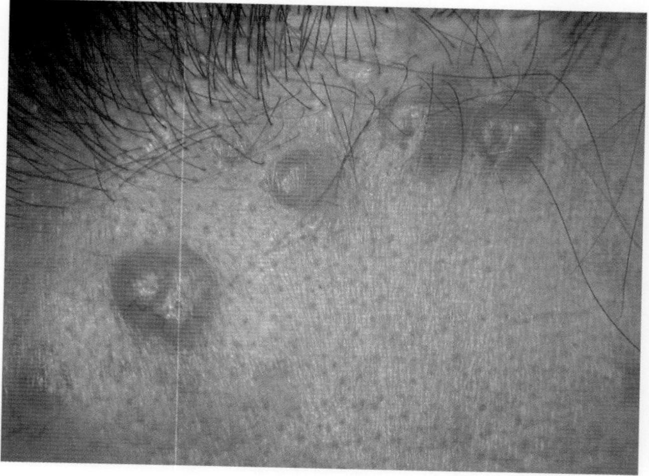

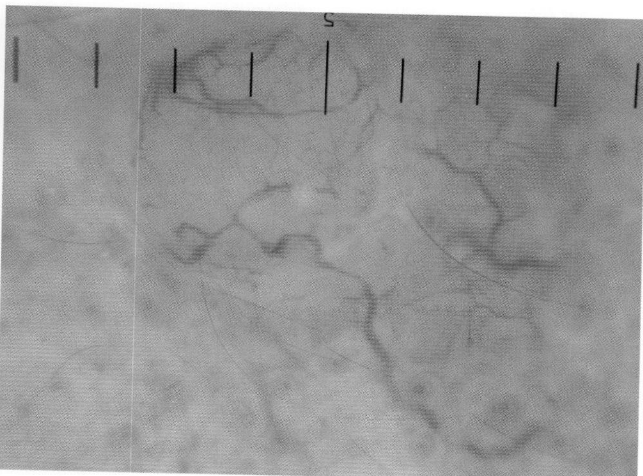

Multiple pink papules and nodules along the frontal scalp in a 40-year-old woman: dermoscopy shows pink structureless areas with poorly focused linear branching vessels in this woman with known cylindromatosis.

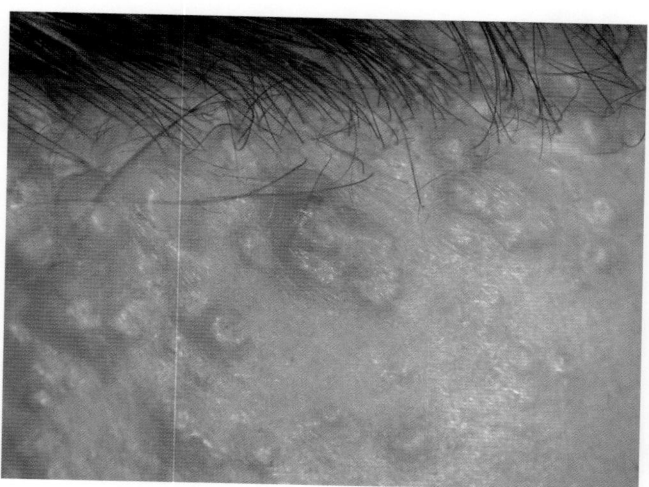

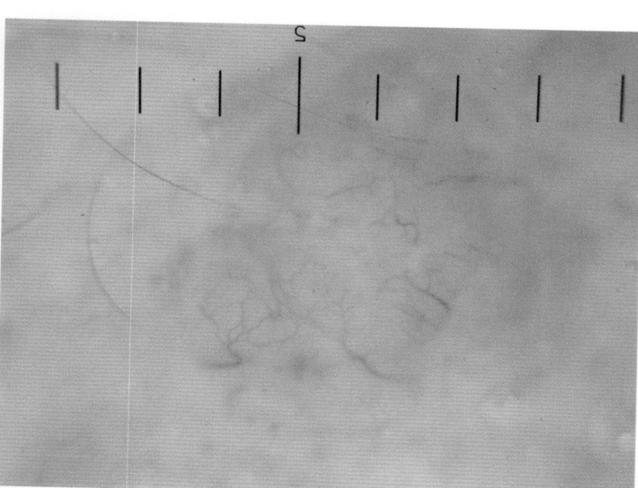

Multiple firm pink papules and nodules on the scalp and forehead in a 60-year-old woman with known CYLD mutation: dermoscopy shows poorly focused branching linear vessels with pink structureless areas in this cylindroma.

Jarrett, R. et al. Dermoscopy of Brooke-Spiegler Syndrome. *Arch Dermatol*. 2009;145(7):854.

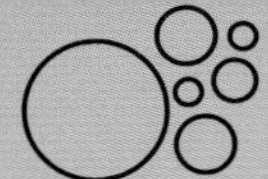

Muir-Torre syndrome

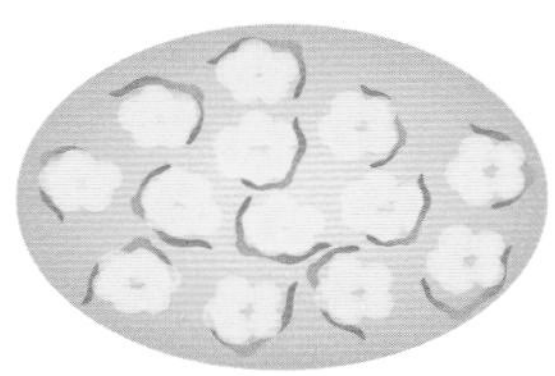

Muir-Torre syndrome (MTS), a subset of Lynch syndrome, is an autosomal dominant genetic disorder that is associated with the development of colonic or genito-urinary malignancy. It is caused by mutations in the mismatch repair genes including MLH1, MSH2 and MSH6. Cutaneous features include sebaceous tumours and keratoacanthomas. Immunohistochemistry can identify changes in expression of mismatch repair genes.

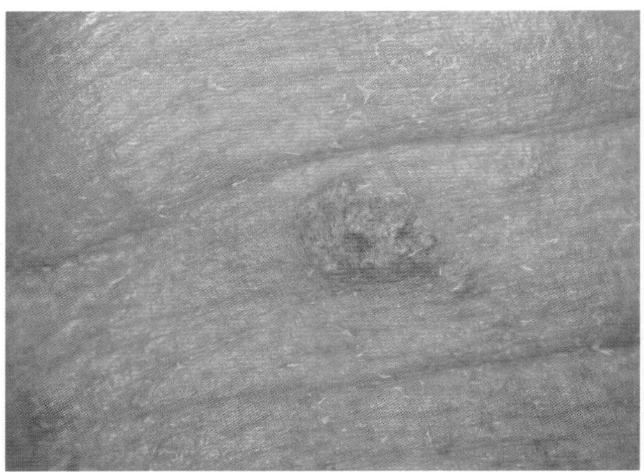

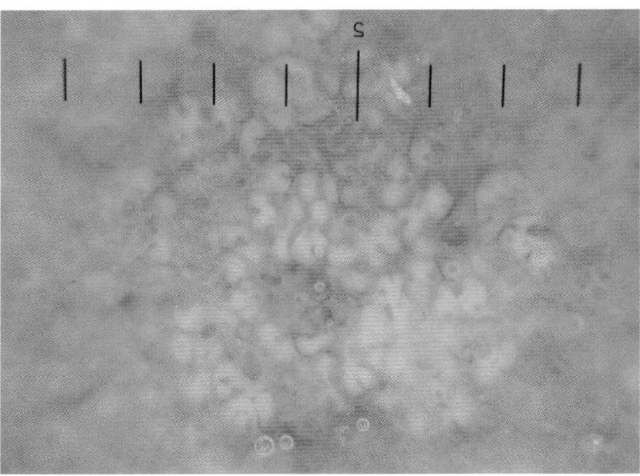

An 8 mm waxy plaque on the forehead of a 70-year-old man with Lynch syndrome: dermoscopy shows sebaceous gland aggregates, comedo-like openings and curvilinear branching vessels in this sebaceous adenoma.

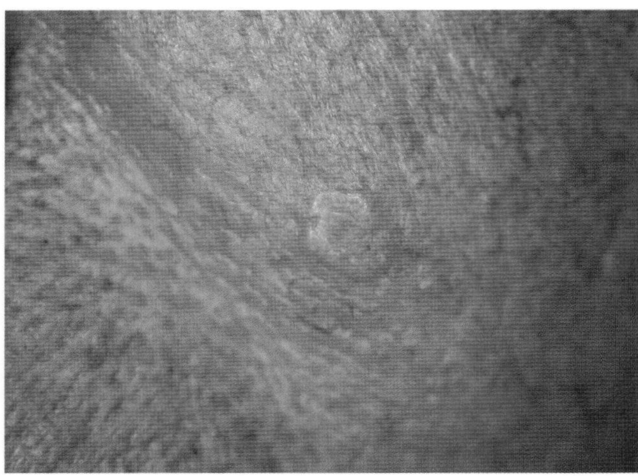

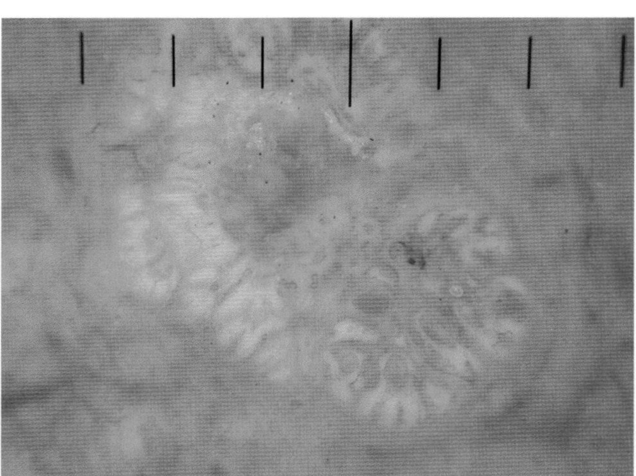

A large waxy yellow plaque on the medial cheek of a 70-year-old man with Lynch syndrome: dermoscopy shows yellow aggregates and small linear vessels in this sebaceous adenoma.

Be aware of the significant associations of sebaceous adenomas in younger patients.

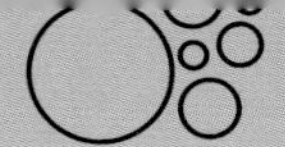

Reed syndrome

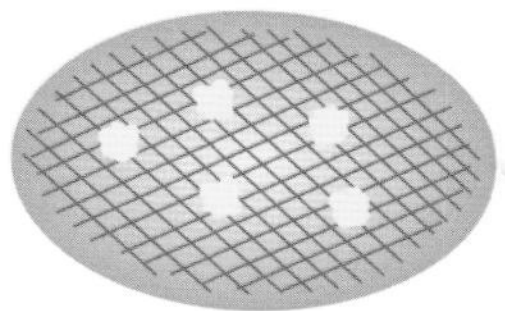

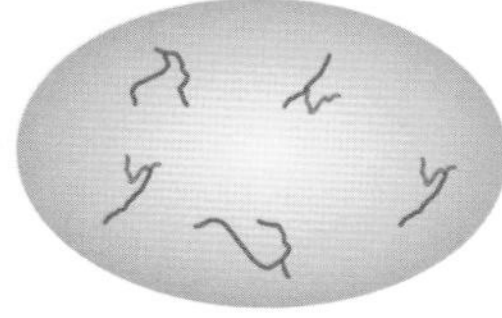

Reed syndrome is an autosomal dominant genodermatosis that causes smooth muscle tumours (leiomyomas) in the skin and in the uterus, and an increased risk of renal cell cancer (hereditary leiomyomatosis and renal cell carcinoma, HLRCC). It is caused by a mutation in the fumarate hydratase gene. Cutaneous leiomyomas may present as scattered lesions or in a zosteriform pattern. They may mimic dermatofibromas or other pink skin tumours clinically and on dermoscopy.

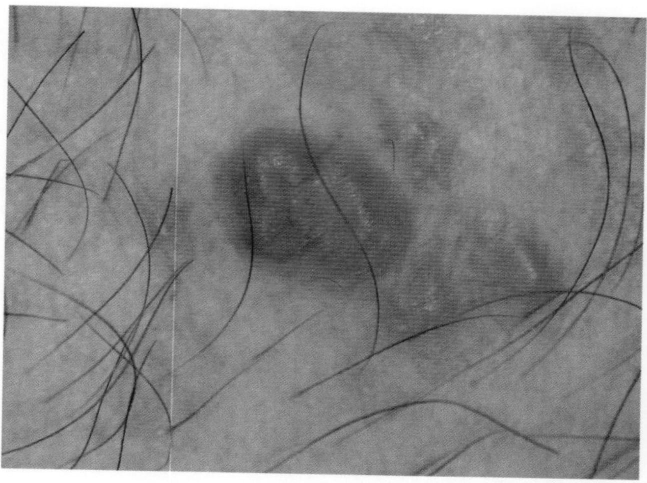

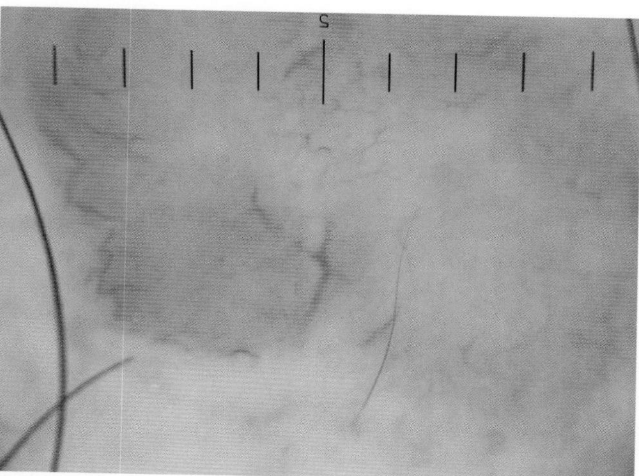

Multiple pink dermal plaques, plaques and nodules on the chest of a 20-year-old man with HLRCC: dermoscopy shows linear branching vessels with a pink structureless background confirmed as cutaneous leiomyomas on histopathology.

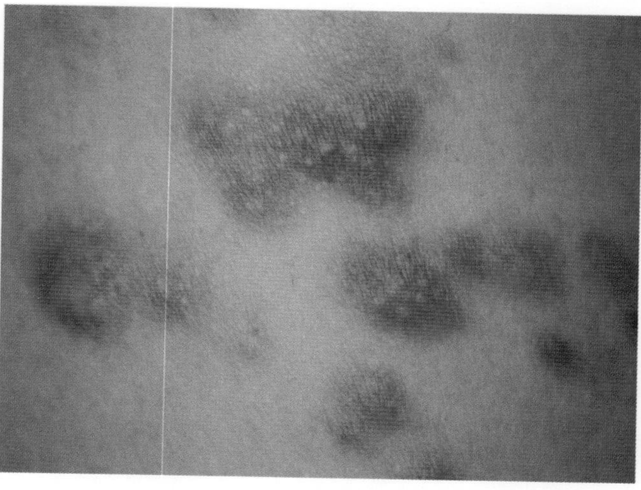

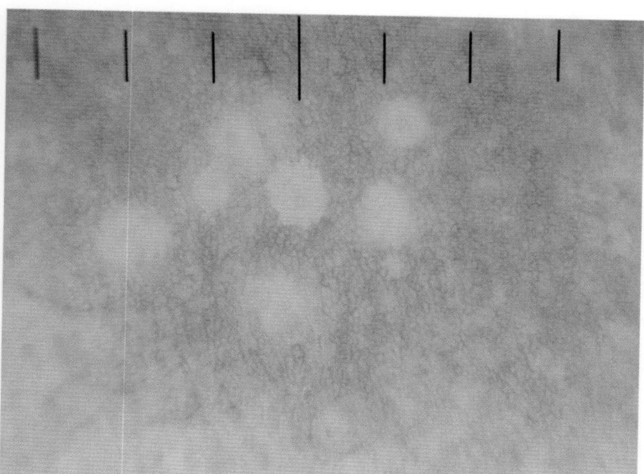

Multiple tender pale brown dermal plaques and nodules in a zosteriform pattern on the leg of a 40-year-old woman with HLRCC: dermoscopy shows reticular pigmentation with focal structureless areas confirmed as cutaneous leiomyomas on histopathology.

Consider a biopsy for any symptomatic dermal nodule or any nodules in a zosteriform distribution. Leiomyomas can be painful with exposure to cold or pressure, a key symptom.

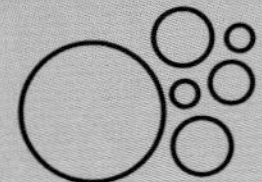

Familial melanoma

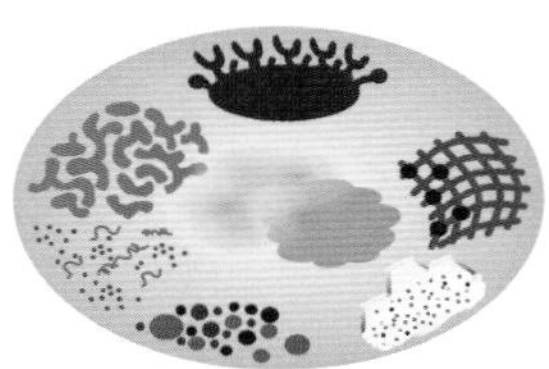

Familial melanoma is an inherited condition characterised by a high risk for developing melanoma and commonly multiple naevi that may be clinically atypical. It can be caused by mutations in the CDKN2A gene or rarely the CDK4 gene. Typically, multiple family members will be affected. Patients with familial melanoma should be closely monitored with total body photography and sequential digital dermoscopy as well as educated on self-surveillance.

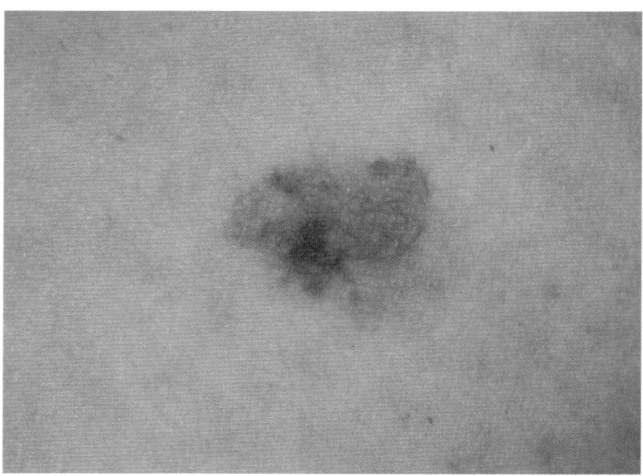

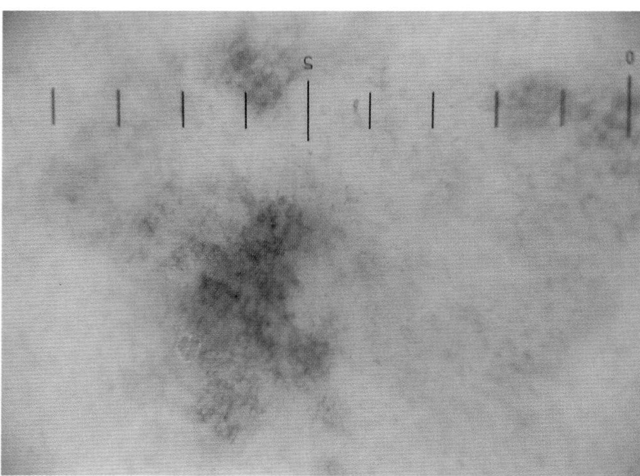

An irregular melanocytic lesion on the arm of a 30-year-old woman with a CDKN2A gene mutation: dermoscopy shows eccentric brown granular pigmentation, dotted and curved vessels in this 0.6 mm superficial spreading melanoma.

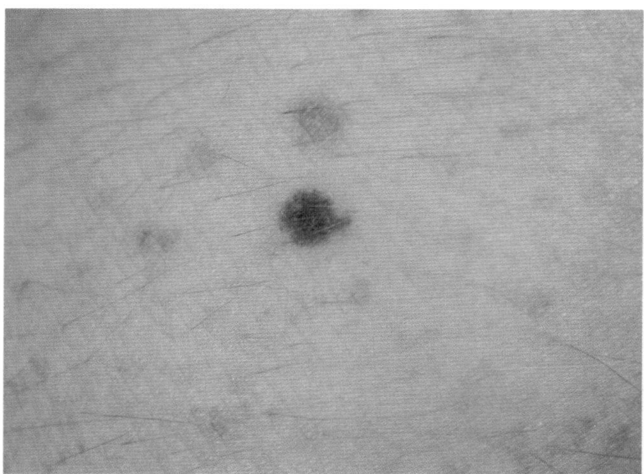

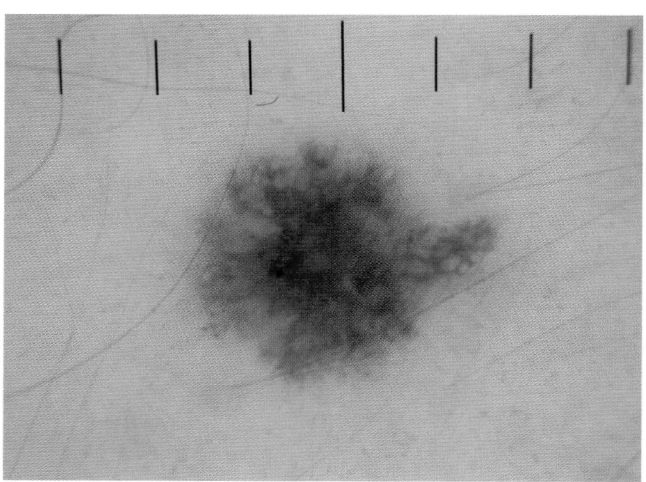

New eccentric pigment arising in a melanocytic lesion noticed by the same patient with CDKN2A gene mutation five years after the original diagnosis: dermoscopy shows atypical network in this melanoma in situ.

The aim of close follow-up and patient education on self-surveillance is to ensure whenever possible that patients with familial melanoma, who develop a subsequent second melanoma, present at an earlier stage than their original melanoma.

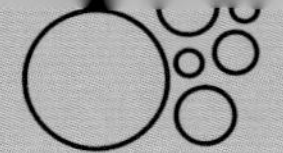

Carney complex

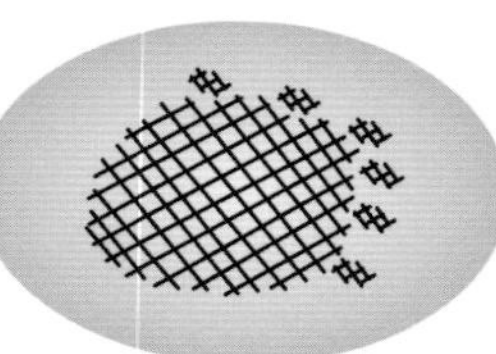

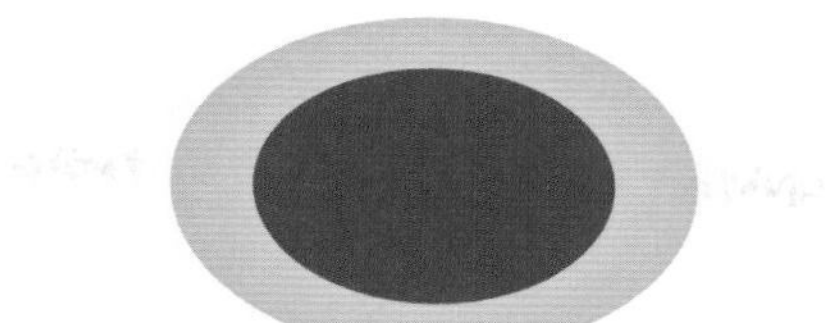

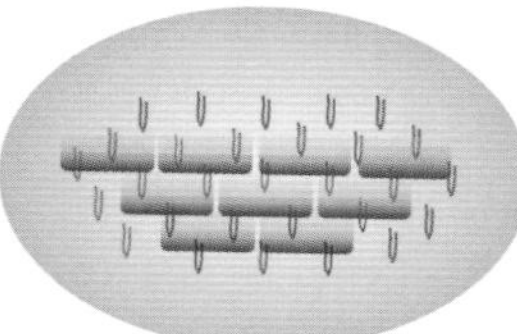

Carney complex is an autosomal dominant genetic disorder caused by mutations in the PRKAR1A gene, causing uncontrolled cellular proliferation. Multiple benign myxomas develop in tissues including the skin and the four chambers of the heart, where they can be multiple and fatal. Endocrine tumours may also develop. Cutaneous clues to diagnosis include cutaneous myxomas, multiple ink spot lentigines, blue naevi and mucosal melanotic macules.

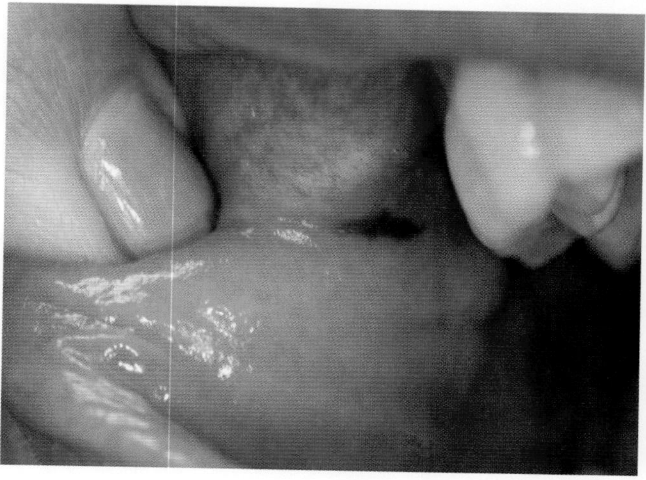

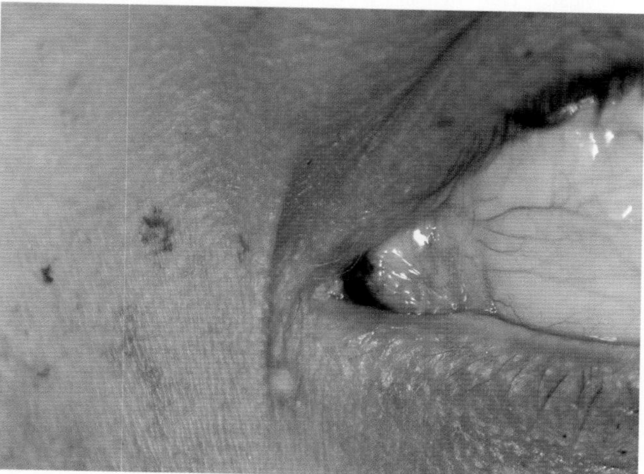

Multiple pigmented macules on the buccal mucosae and conjunctival caruncle, along with widespread solar lentigines in a 20-year-old woman with known Carney complex caused by PRKAR1A gene mutation.

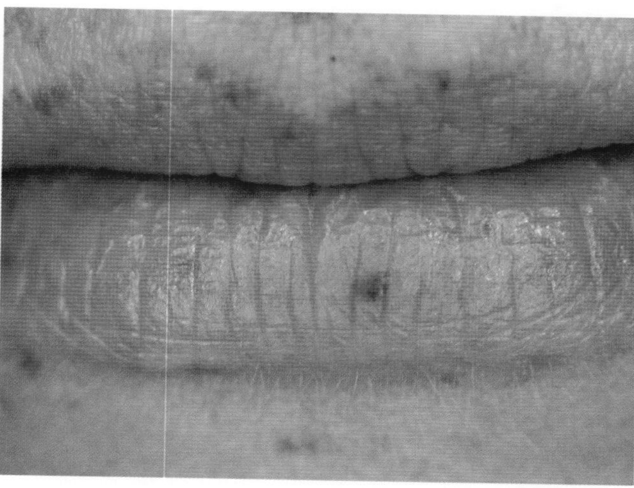

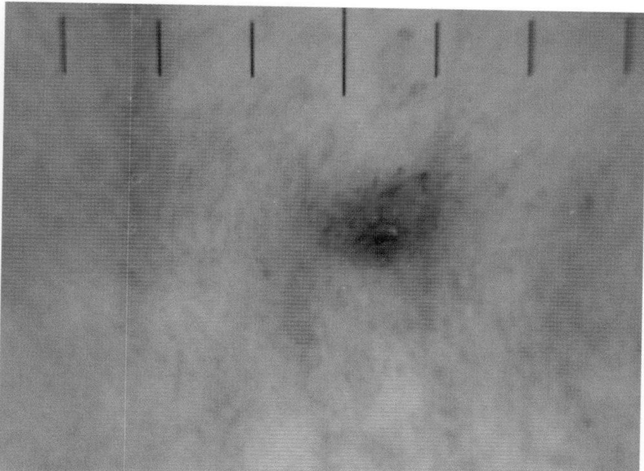

Mucosal melanosis on the lower lip in a woman with known Carney complex: dermoscopy of the lower lip shows regular grey-brown pigmentation typical for mucosal melanosis.

Consider further investigations to exclude Carney complex in patients with an unusual presentation or a high number of ink spot lentigines, melanotic macules and blue naevi.

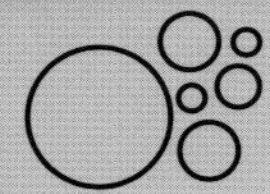

11 Entomodermoscopy

Delusional parasitosis	299
Scabies – *Sarcoptes scabiei*	300
Scabies cases	301
Head lice – *Pediculosis capitis*	302
Bed bugs – *Cimex lectularius*	303
Tick bites – Ixodidae	304
Leishmaniasis	305
Molluscum contagiosum	306
Viral warts – Verrucae vulgaris	307
Sea urchin – Echinoidea	308
Jellyfish – Cnidaria	309
Tungiasis – *Tunga penetrans*	310
Myiasis – *Dermatobia hominis*	311

Diagnostic Dermoscopy: The Illustrated Guide, Second Edition. Jonathan Bowling.

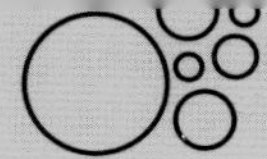

Delusional parasitosis

Delusional Parasitosis, the false perception of infestation by invertebrates, hexapoda, arachnids, etc., sometimes presents to the clinician. Commonly, material from the presumed infestation is presented by the patient. Dermoscopy imaging of the material presented can help confirm the origin of the material presented. Clarification of diagnosis is particularly important when the potential for infectious sequelae exists, e.g. a *Borrelia* infection from tick bites.

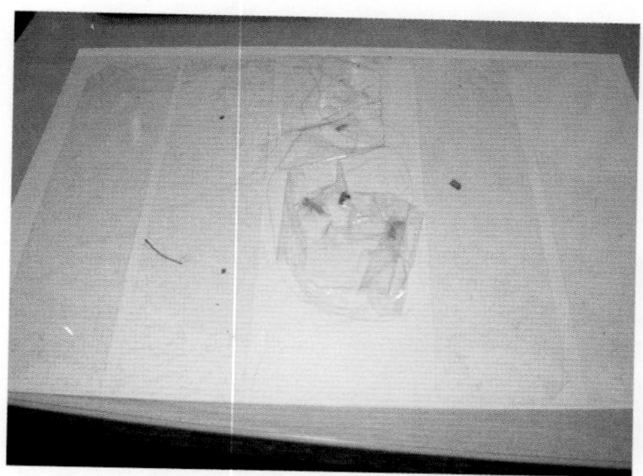

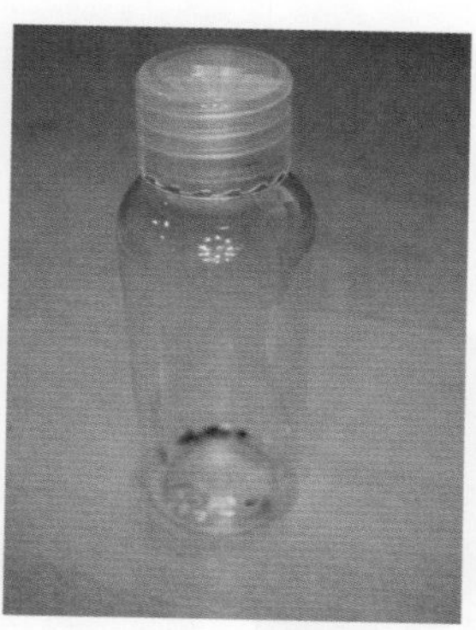

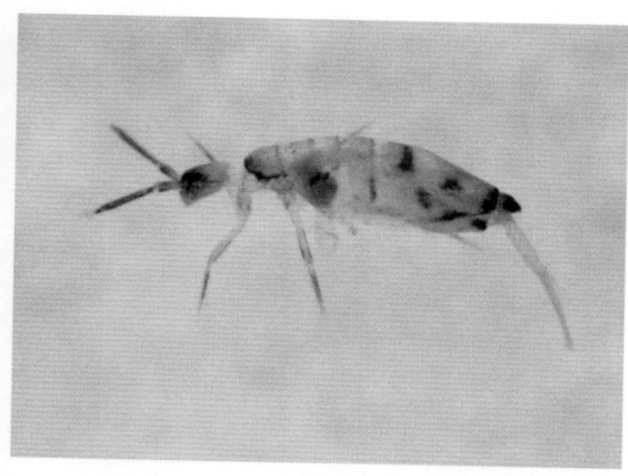

A 50-year-old woman with a 12-month history of 'infestation' with jumping insects presented a collection of samples for examination: dermoscopy showed crushed invertebrates and a live sample, confirming collembola, 'springtails', as the cause for her concern (although unlikely a true infestation). As springtails do not bite humans the patient could be reassured. Occasionally an expert entomologist will be required to identify species accurately.

Zalaudek, I. et al. Entodermoscopy: a new tool for diagnosing skin infections and infestations. *Dermatol*. 2008;216:14–23.

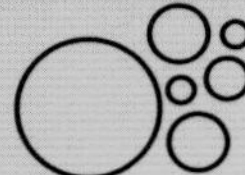

Scabies – *Sarcoptes scabiei*

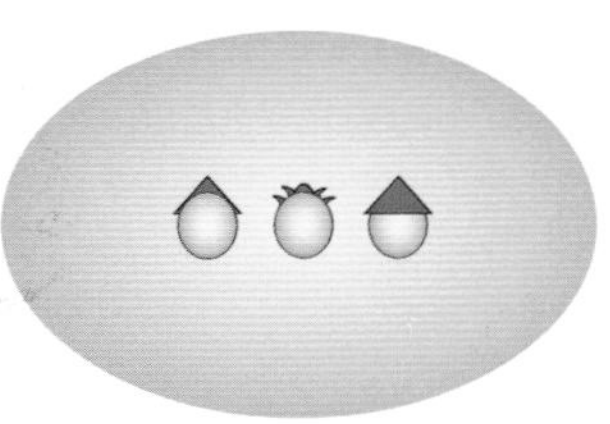

Scabies is confirmed by identification of the mite, which range in size up to 0.5 mm. Dermoscopy can easily identify a pigmented triangle, representing the forelimbs and mouth of the mite, at the end of a keratotic burrow. The mite's orientation will reveal a full triangle (ventral view) or a partial one (dorsal view). Eggs and faeces may also be seen within the burrow. The mite and burrow have been likened to a delta wing jet with contrail.

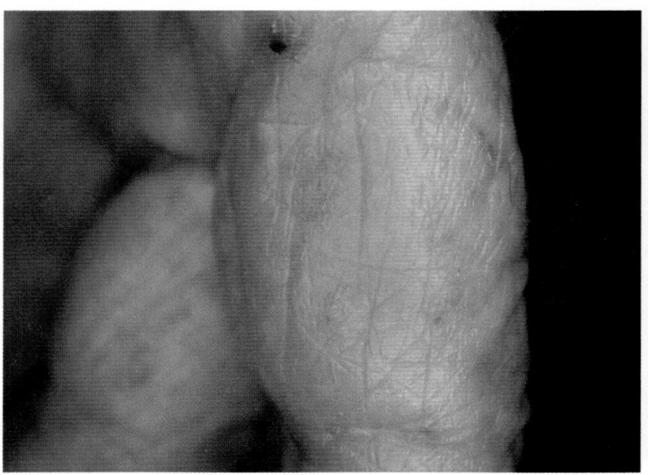

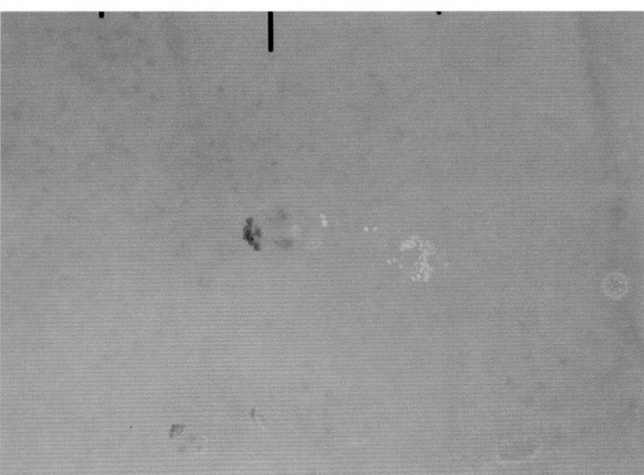

Multiple burrows on the hand of an elderly female nursing home resident: dermoscopy show multiple mites, with eggs visible within the burrow delineated by white faeces.

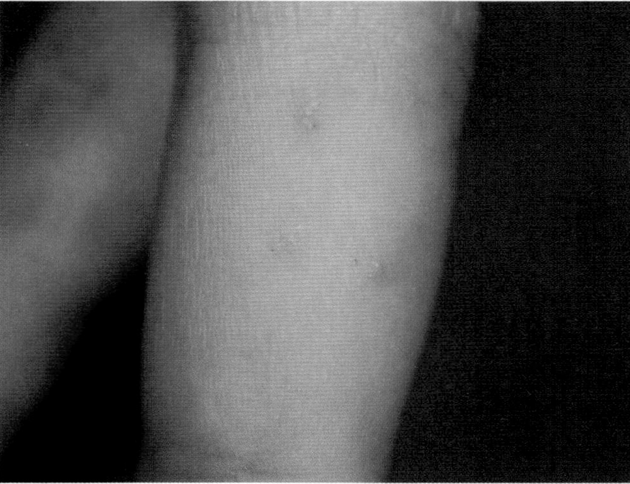

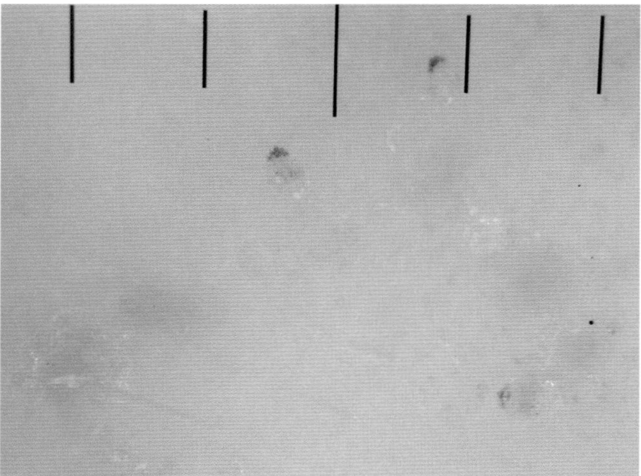

Multiple burrows seen on the hand of a 20-year-old university student: dermoscopy shows the pigmented triangles of the scabies mites in varying degrees of orientation.

Prins, C. et al. Dermoscopy for the detection of sarcoptes scabiei. *Dermatology* 2004;208(3):241–243.

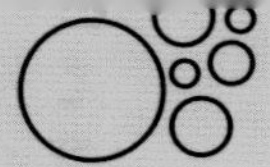

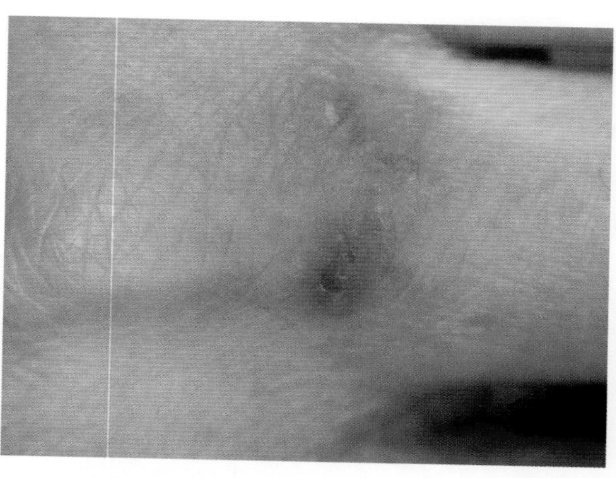

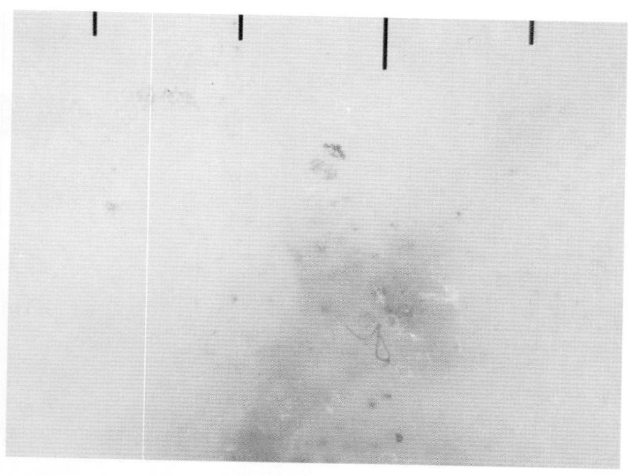

An inflamed scabies burrow on the dorsum of the index finger: dermoscopy shows inflammation and erosion with a small triangular pigmented structure confirming the presence of a scabies mite.

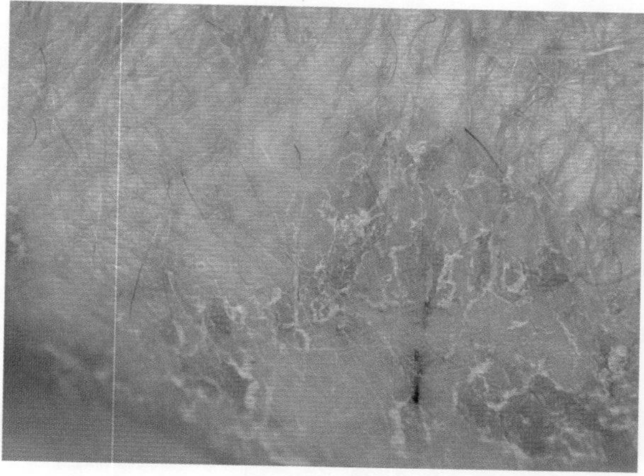

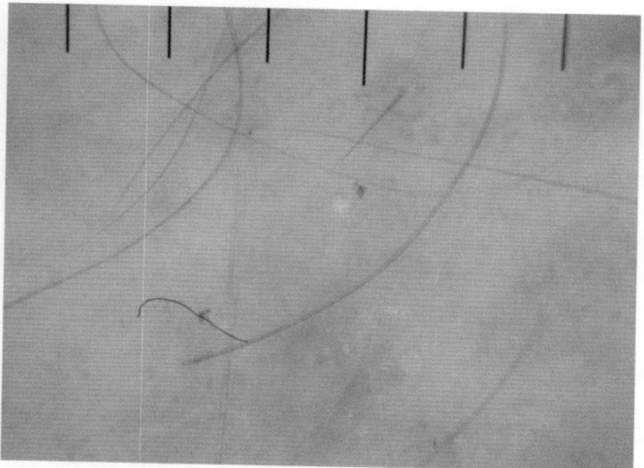

A 60-year-old builder with long-standing hand dermatitis unresponsive to topical steroids: dermoscopy shows multiple small triangular pigmented structures, confirming a scabies infestation.

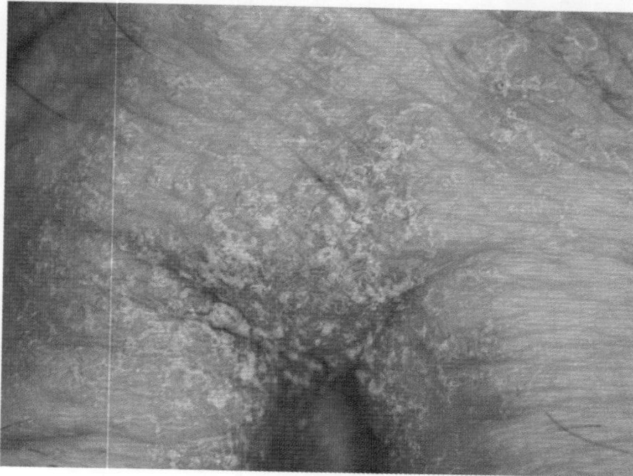

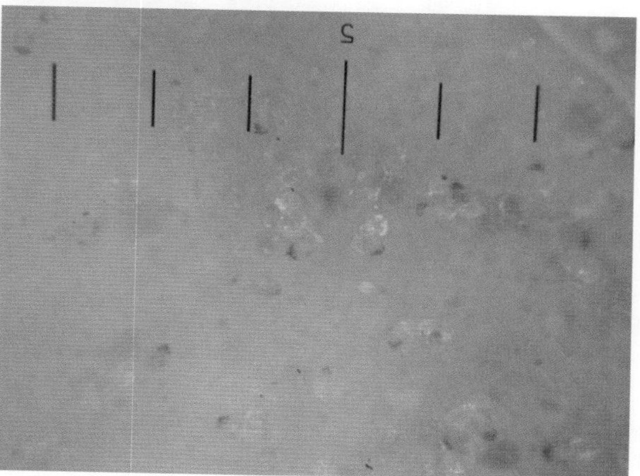

A 70-year-old man with a five-year history of hand dermatitis unresponsive to treatment: dermoscopy shows extensive crusting and multiple ill-defined triangular pigmented structures in keeping with a heavy infestation of crusted scabies.

In a heavy infestation of scabies with pronounced crusting the clear-cut image of the mite can be obscured. Videodermoscopy using higher magnification up to x 50 is superior to conventional x10 dermoscopy.

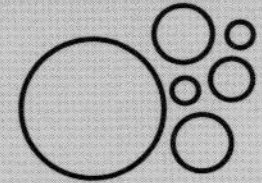

Head lice – *Pediculosis capitis*

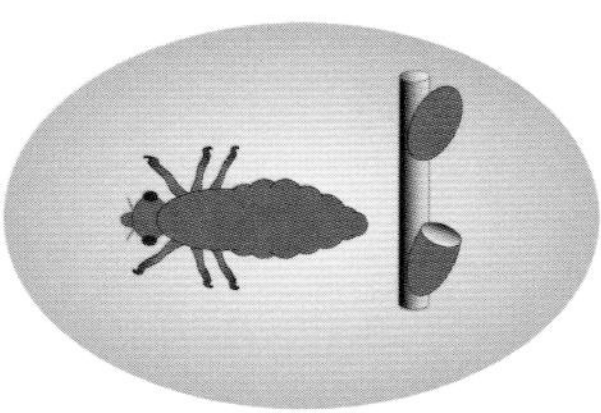

Head lice is a common and easy condition to diagnose. Dermoscopy allows for not only accurate diagnosis of this condition, but also to monitor therapeutic response to treatment.

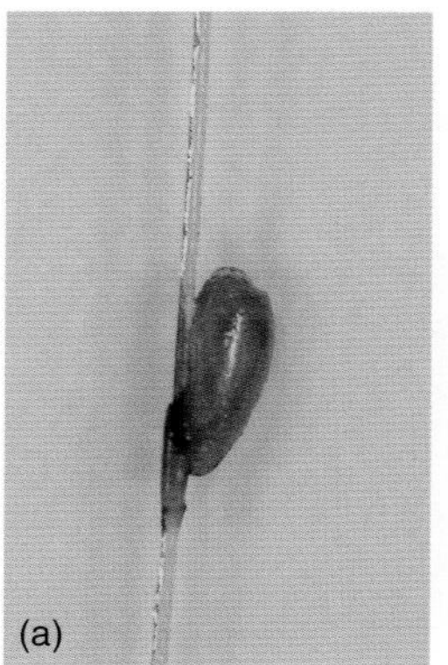

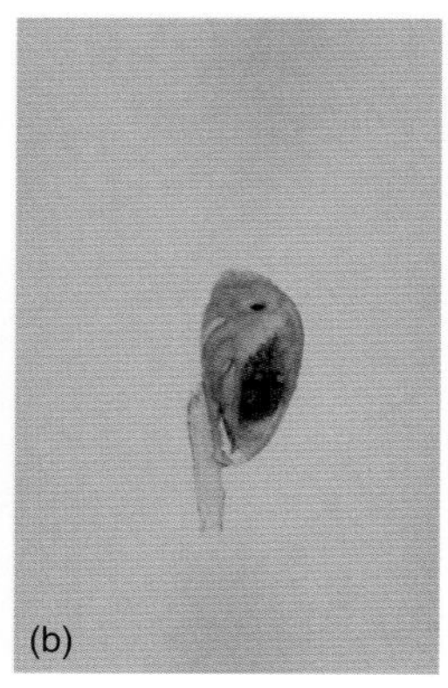

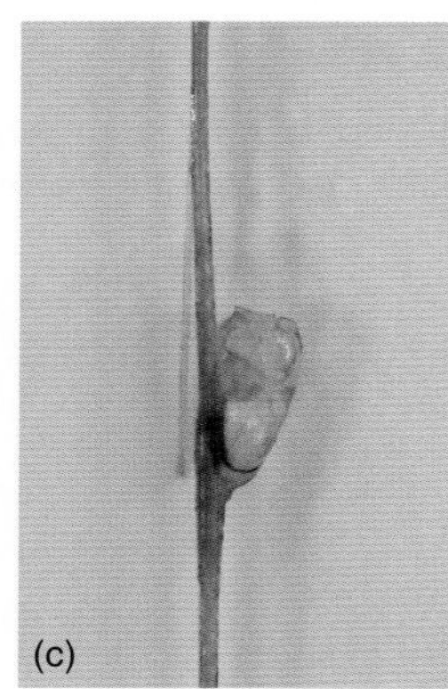

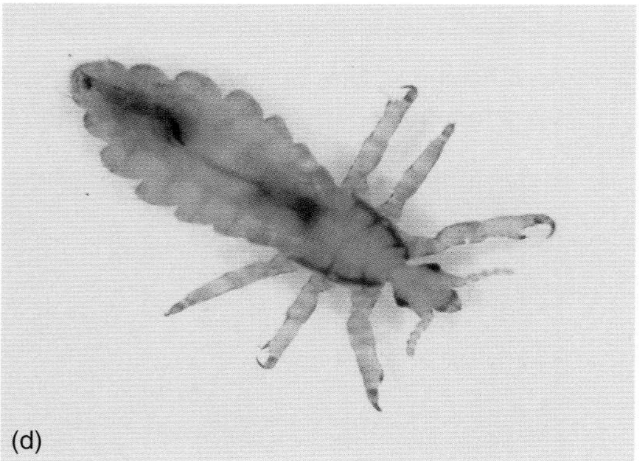

A nit attached to the hair shaft (a); the developing nymph can be seen about to emerge from the egg (b); the empty nit cast is clearly seen (c) and the anatomy of an adult louse (d).

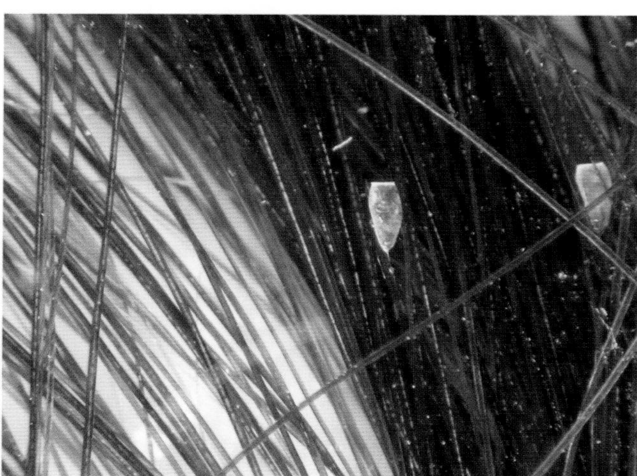
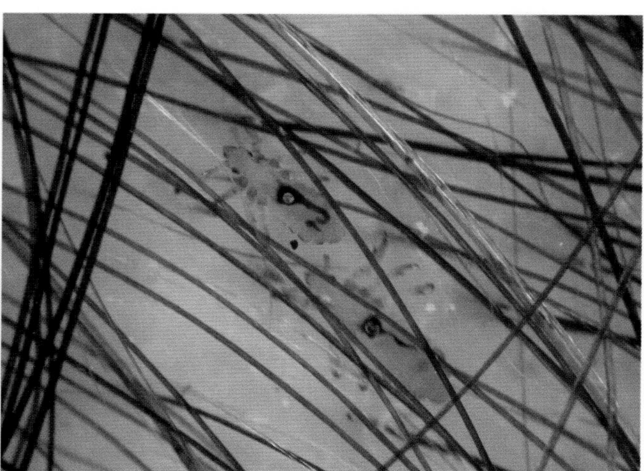

Polarised dermoscopy of hair shafts show the firmly attached empty nit casts; nearby the adult lice can be seen post-prandial with a blood meal in their stomachs.

Zalaudek, I. and Argenziano, G. Images in clinical medicine. Dermoscopy of nits and pseudonits. *N Engl J Med.* 2012;367(18):1741.

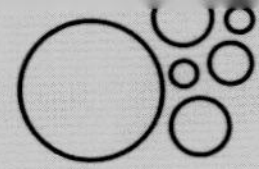

Bed bug – *Cimex lectularius*

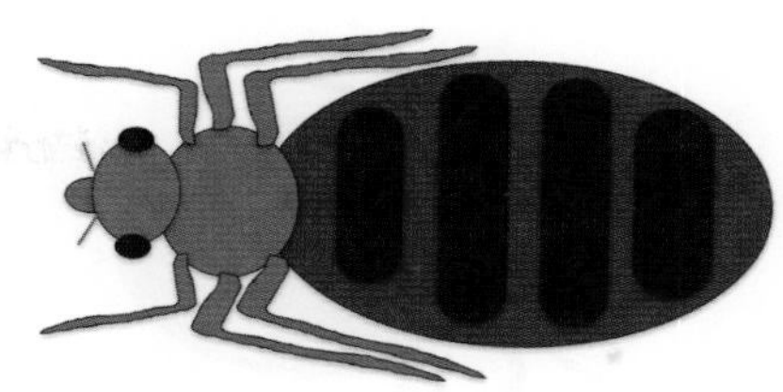

Insect bites can create inflammatory papules and nodules with or without vesiculation, bullae, haemorrhage and ulceration. For patients with recurrent insect bites, attempts to identify the causative insect should be undertaken. Common features of insect bites on dermoscopy include erythema, dotted vessels haemorrhage, erosions and vesiculation. Bed bugs (*Cimex lectularius*) and their eggs are easily identified on dermoscopy.

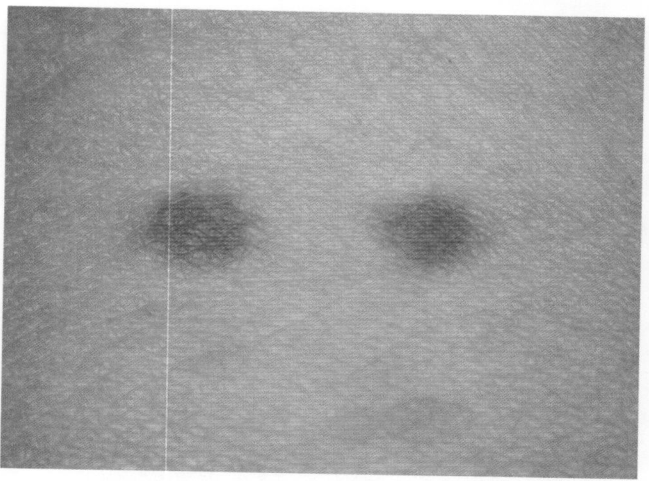

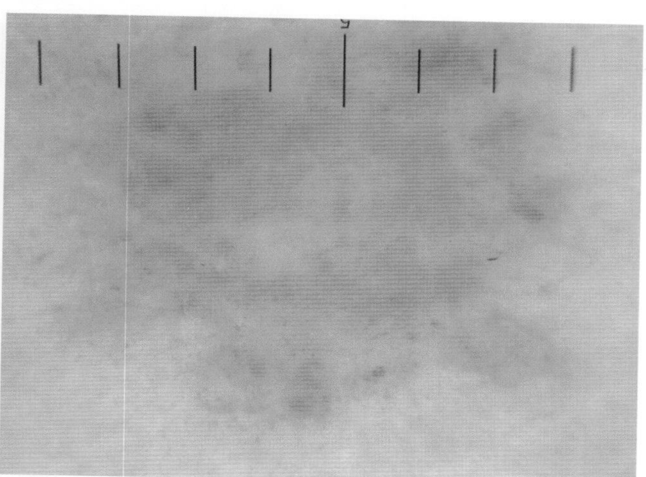

A series of insect bites across the trunk and limbs in a 14-year-old boy: dermoscopy shows erythema and dotted vessels.

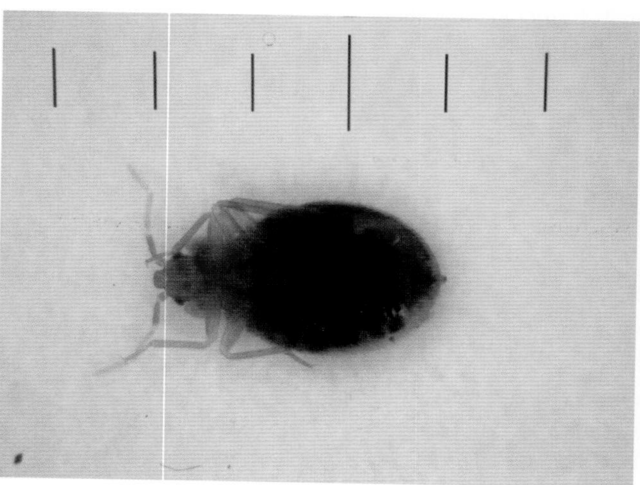

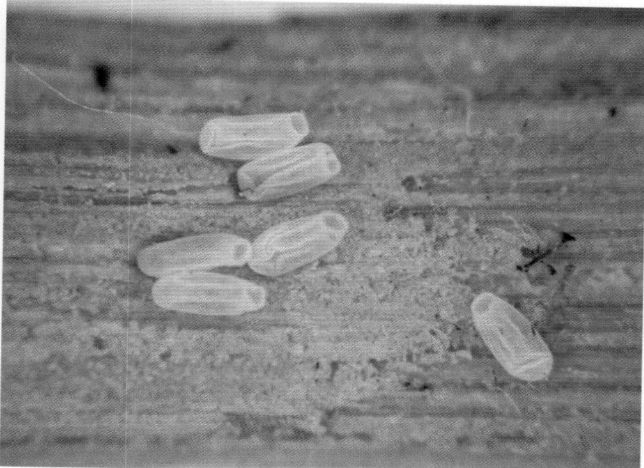

Dermoscopy of a retrieved bed bug from a wooden bed frame identifying *Cimex lectularius* and of a fragment of the bed frame with empty egg casts.

Shirato, T. et al. Dermoscopy is useful for bug (*Cimex lectularius*) bites. *J Eur Acad Dermatol Venereol*. 2016;(3):539–540.

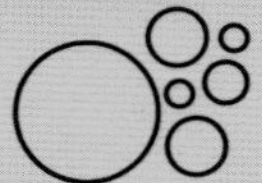

Tick bites – Ixodidae

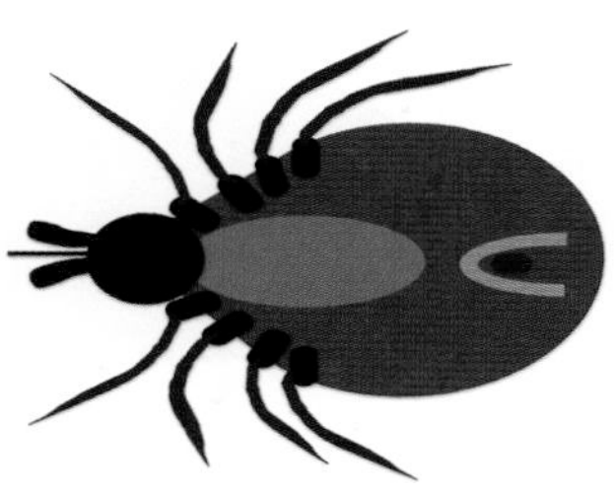

Ticks are a common cause of cutaneous reactions, particularly erythema chronicum migrans caused by the transmission of *Borrelia burgdorferi* causing Lyme disease. The species of ticks responsible for Lyme disease are numerous and belong to the genus *Ixodes*, family Ixodidae and include *I. scapularis, I. ricinus* and *I. pacificus*. It is possible to simply identify ticks from the *Ixodes* genus by the presence on dermoscopic examination of a small groove that wraps around the anus in an anterior direction.

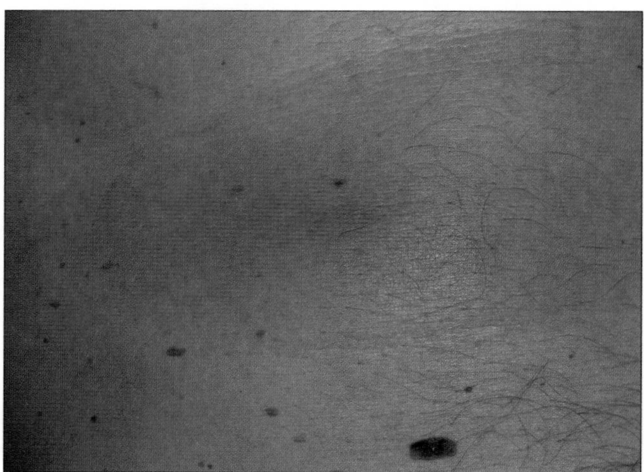

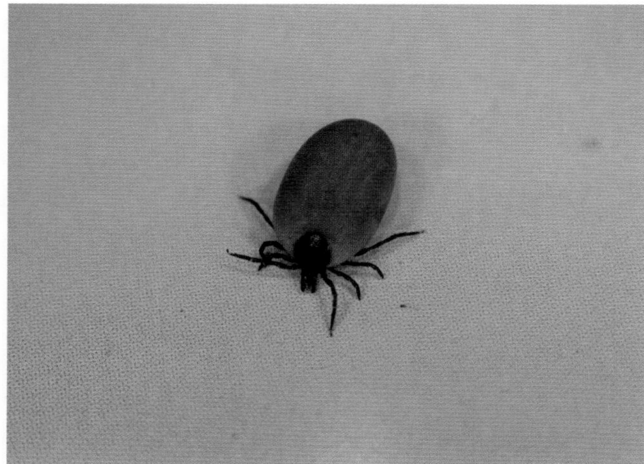

An evolving erythematous patch on the right abdomen in keeping with erythema chronicum migrans caused by a tick bite in a confirmed case of Lyme disease. The dorsal view of the 'hard tick' limits further identification.

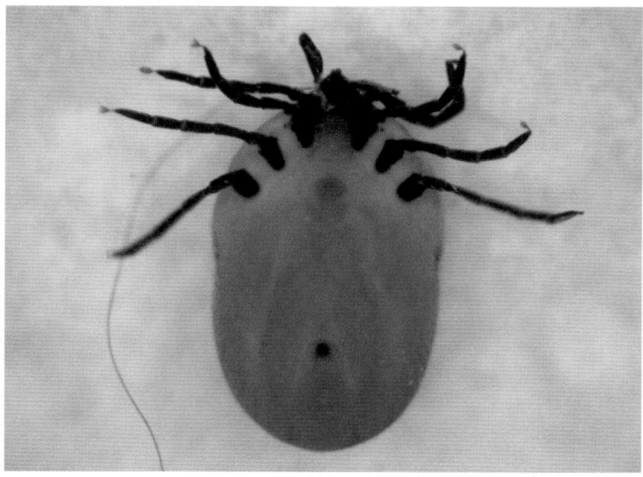

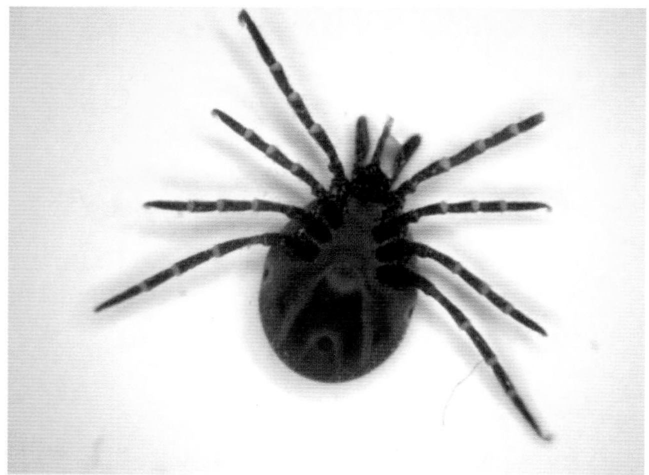

Dermoscopy of the ventral aspect of these ticks, in various stages of engorgement, shows a groove running anteriorly around the anus and confirming the presence of ticks belonging to the *Ixodes* genus.

Connoly, M. and Lee, J. The anal groove sign: the use of dermatoscopy for identification of Ixodes ticks. *J Am Acad Dermatol* 2017;76(2):S64–S65

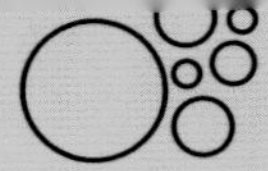

Leishmaniasis

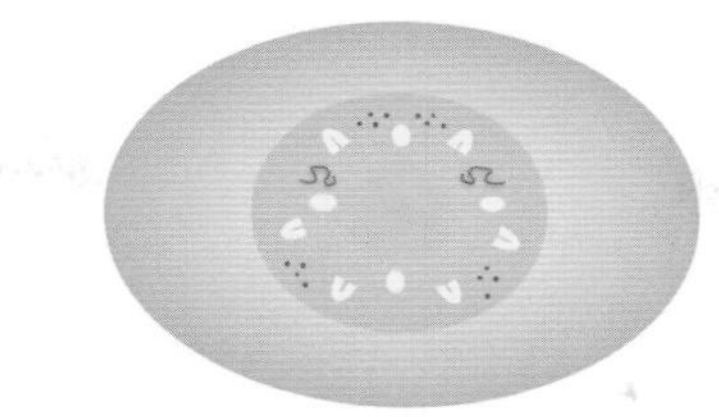

Cutaneous leishmaniasis may present as a solitary inflammatory papulo-nodule, plaque, with or without ulceration, typically appearing a few weeks after a traveller returns from an area where leishmaniasis is endemic. Clinical presentations are variable and may reflect the strain of infection. Dermoscopic features include comma, linear irregular and polymorphous vessels, erythema, multiple yellow-whitish blurred ovoid/teardrop-shaped globules creating a 'white starburst-like' pattern due to follicular ostia occlusion.

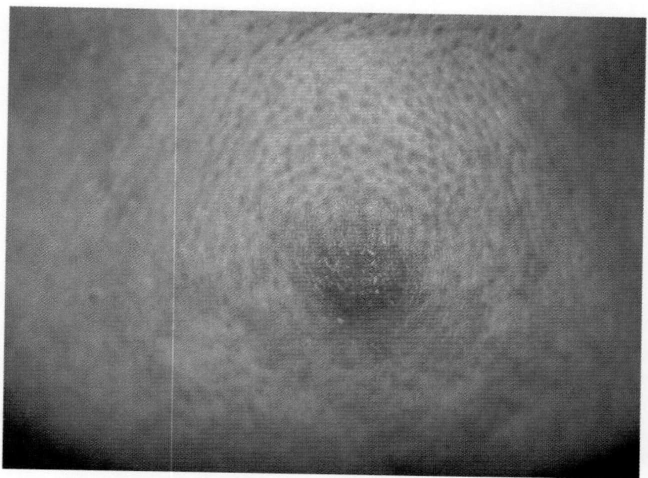

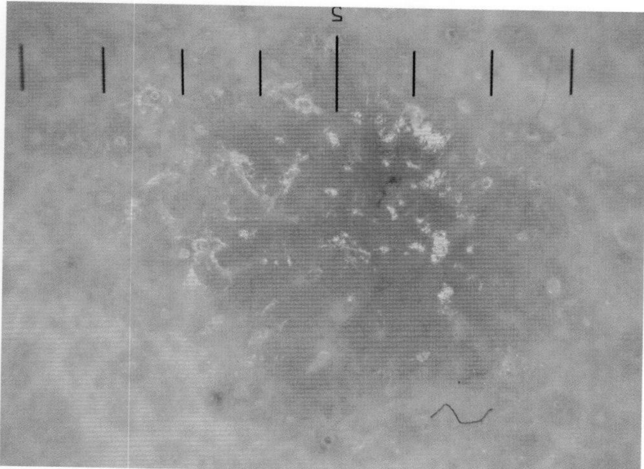

A painless firm papule on the chin, appearing six weeks after a trip to Italy: dermoscopy shows erythema, a 'white starburst-like' pattern, linear irregular vessels and hyperkeratosis in this case of leishmaniasis.

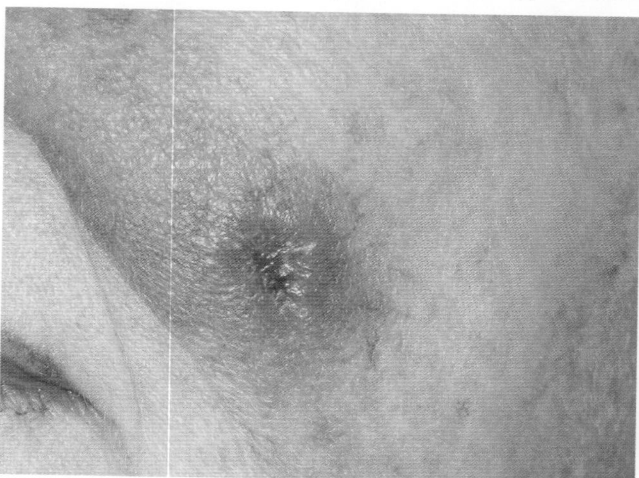

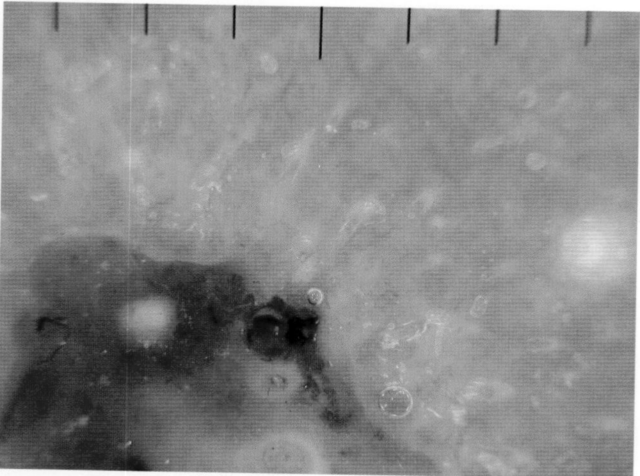

An inflamed ulcerated nodule on the left cheek in a traveller six weeks after returning from Cyprus: dermoscopy shows ulceration, erythema, a radial 'white starburst-like' pattern and irregular vessels (*L. infantum* was confirmed with PCR).

Llambrich, A. et al. Dermoscopy of cutaneous leishmaniasis. *Br J Dermatol.* 2009;160(4):756–761

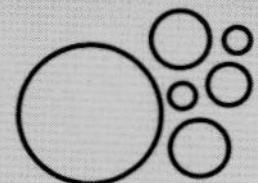

Molluscum contagiosum

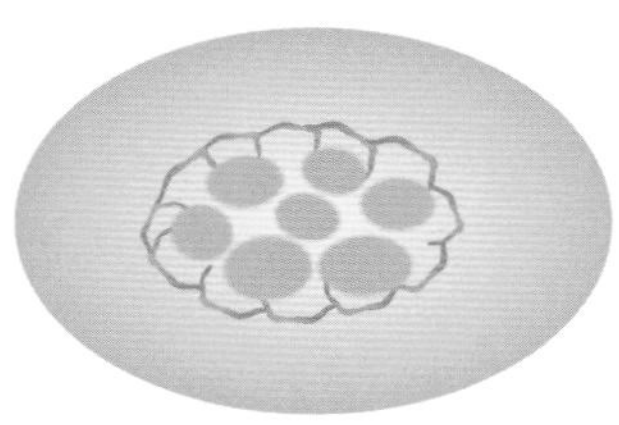

Molluscum contagiosum is a common childhood skin infection characterised by multiple crops of umbilicated flesh-coloured papules. When adults are affected, the individual lesions may be solitary and larger and are more common in those with an impaired immune system. Dermoscopy shows large central pink homogeneous globules with peripheral/marginal curvilinear (crown) vessels which do not cross the midline. Prominent vessels are more common in inflamed lesions.

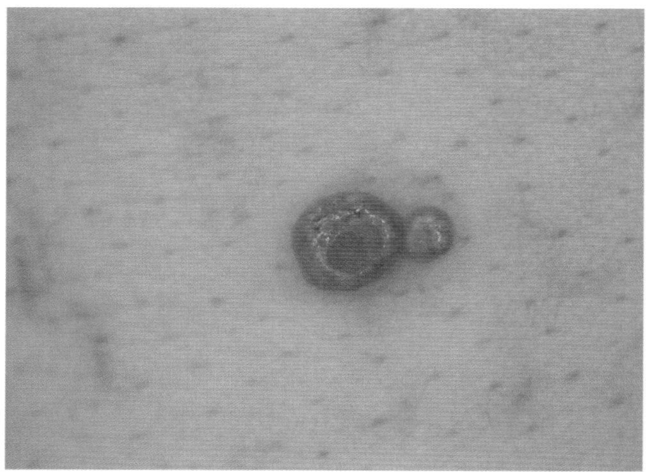

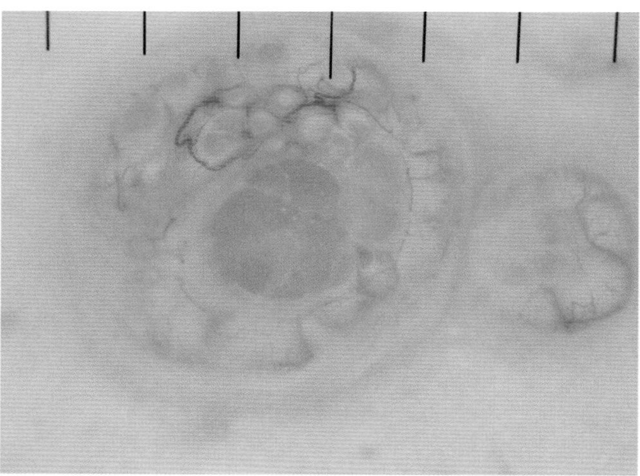

Umbilicated papules on the arm of a Caucasian male whose daughter has active mollusca: dermoscopy shows erythema and curvilinear crown vessels surrounding multiple, central, homogeneous yellow-orange globules.

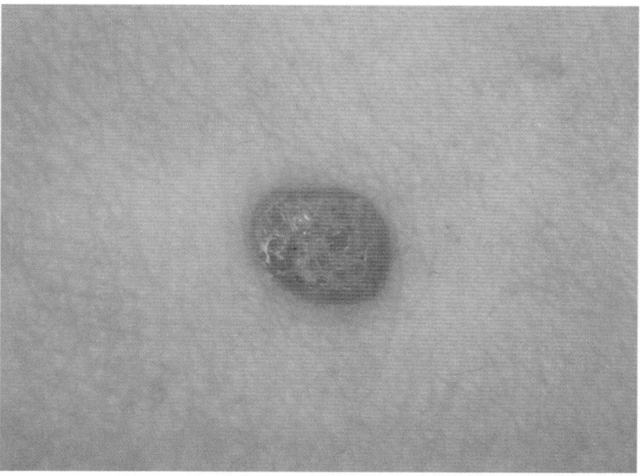

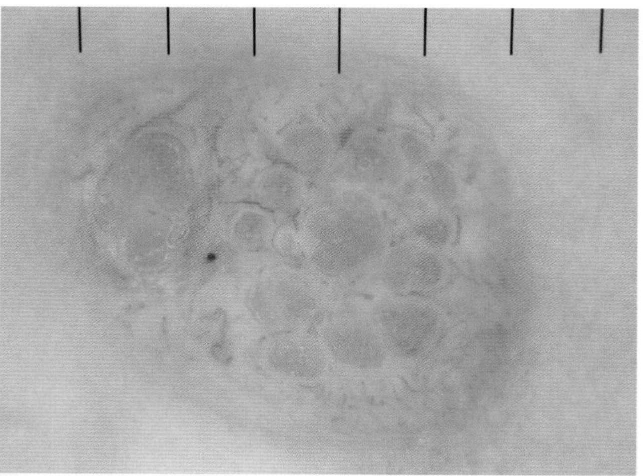

A solitary inflamed well-circumscribed papule on the thigh of a 50-year-old woman: dermoscopy shows multiple yellow homogeneous central globules with curvilinear crown vessels in this inflamed lesion of *Molluscum contagiosum*.

Morales, A. et al. Dermoscopy of *Molluscum contagiosum*. *Arch Dermatol*. 2005;141(12):1644.

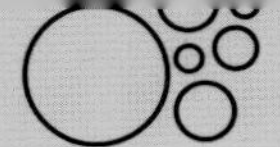

Viral warts – Verrucae vulgaris

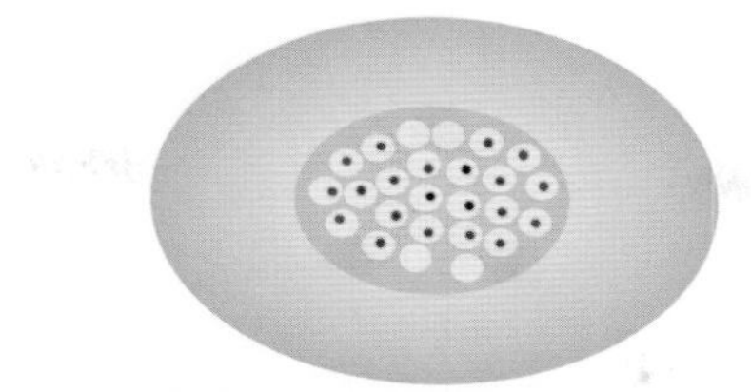

Viral warts can be easily distinguished from a callus on dermoscopy by the presence of multiple whitish keratotic halos, often with a central red/purple dot. The red dots are often associated with micro-haemorrhages, particularly if the wart has been irritated. Yellow colouration reflects hyperkeratosis. Confident diagnosis of viral warts from keratinocyte cancers and their precursors is particularly helpful in the transplant population.

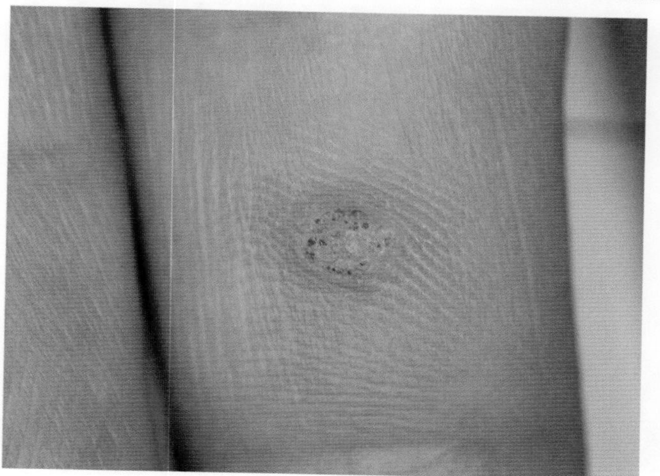

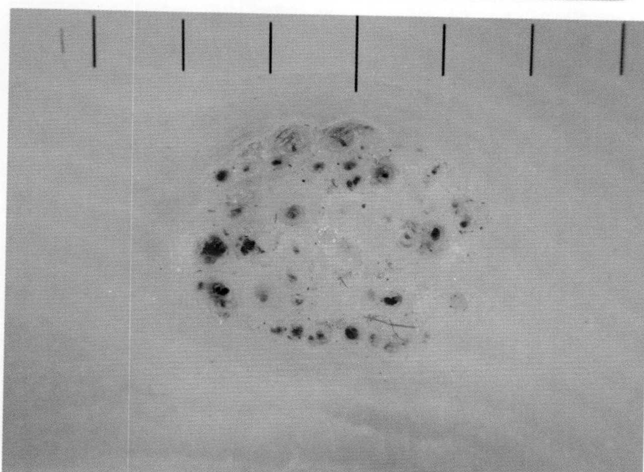

A viral wart with a keratotic plaque on the index finger: dermoscopy shows multiple whitish halos with central red/purple dots in this viral wart.

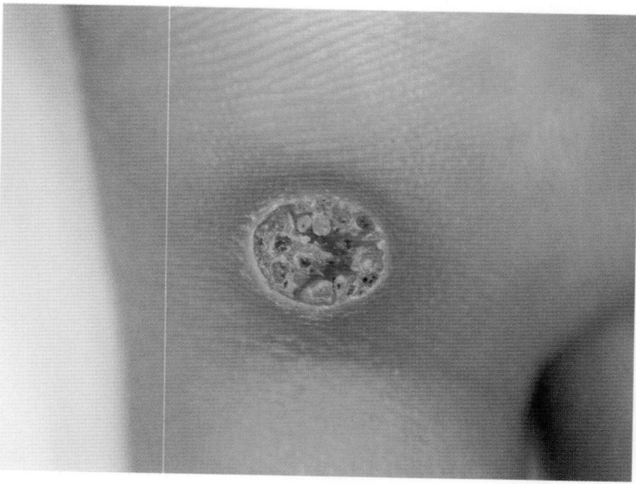

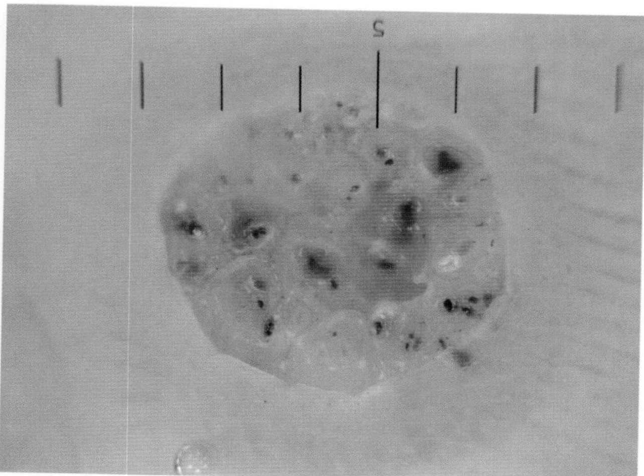

A painful keratotic crateriform, endophytic plaque on the palm: dermoscopy shows orange homogeneous areas with multiple focal red dots with whitish keratotic halos (micro-haemorrhages) in this myrmecia (deep plantar wart).

Bae, J.M. et al. Differential diagnosis of a plantar wart from corn and a healed wart with the aid of dermoscopy. *Br J Dermatol.* 2009;160(1);509–515.

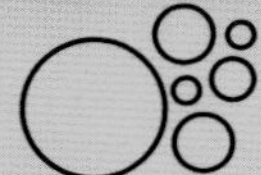

Sea urchins – Echinoidea

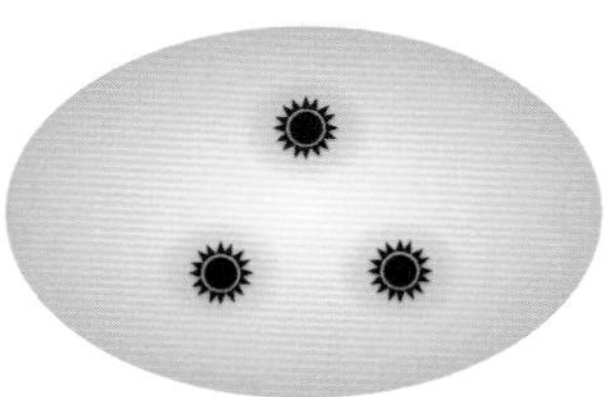

Sea urchin injury is not uncommon in the barefoot holiday maker, whereby the spines are implanted into the sole of the foot when the sea urchin is trodden upon. The cross-section of the spines shows a crenulated disc, which can be seen on dermoscopy. If the spines are not removed, secondary infection can develop.

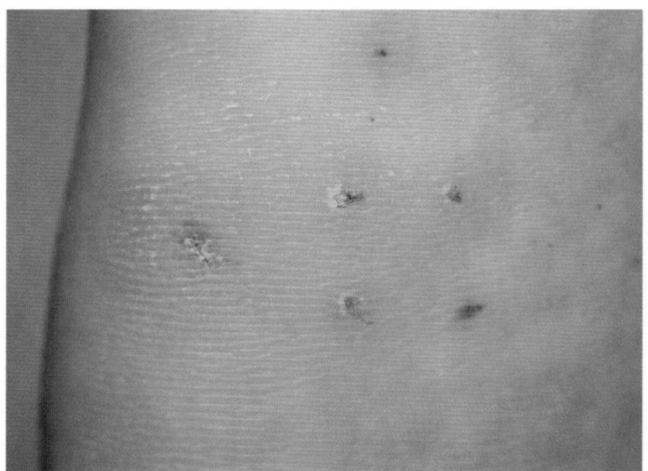

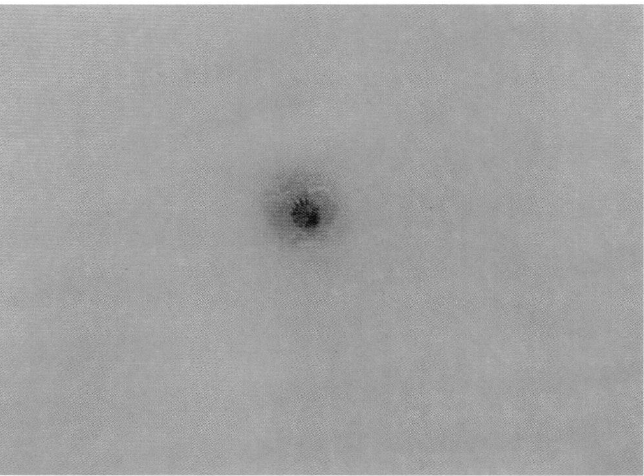

A 40-year-old returning from France with multiple tender puncture points on the sole following a sea urchin injury: dermoscopy of a puncture point shows a crenulated disc corresponding to the cross-section of a sea urchin spine.

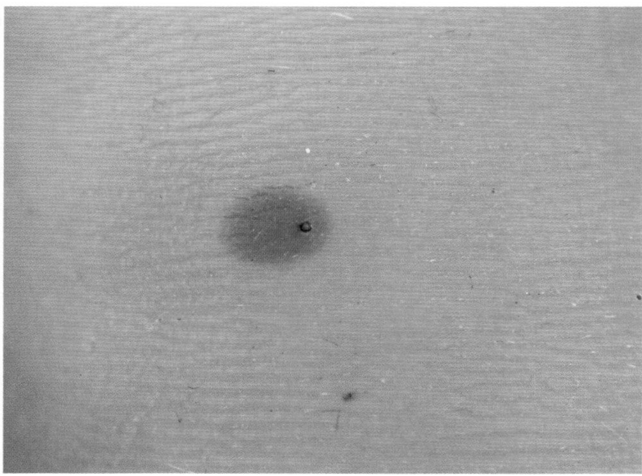

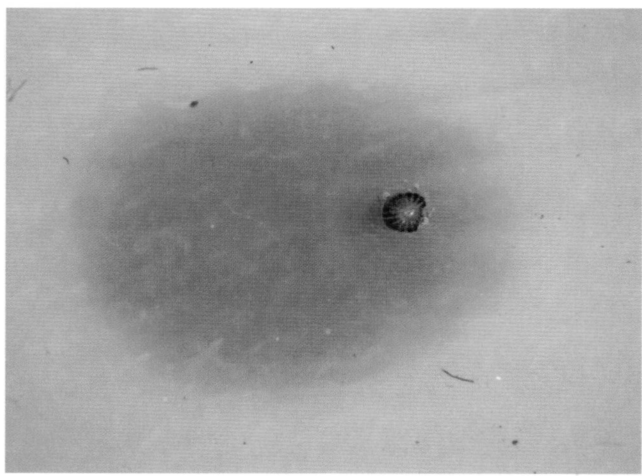

A 30-year-old with inflammation and discomfort around the site of a sea urchin injury two weeks earlier: dermoscopy shows a homogeneous greenish yellow area (pseudomonas infection) with a crenulated disc corresponding to the sea urchin spine.

Ex vivo dermoscopy of the material causing a foreign body injury can be a useful addition to the clinical record.

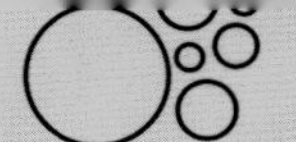

Jellyfish – Cnidaria

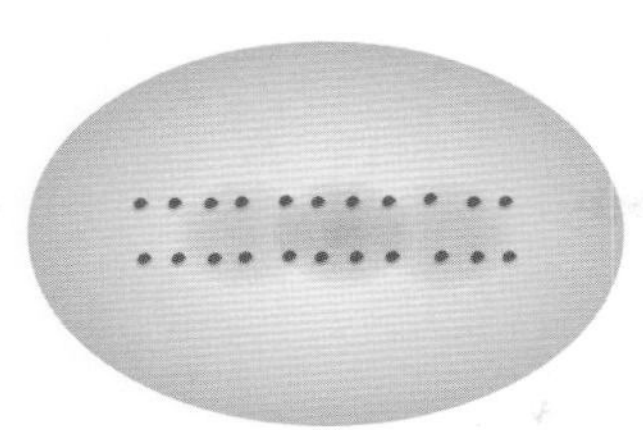

Jellyfish stings are usually accompanied by a reliable history with visual identification of the offending jellyfish. The cutaneous features are typical in keeping with contact with the stinging tentacles, causing parallel lines of erythema, haemorrhage and vesiculation. Other marine organisms can also cause envenomation; therefore, close inspection of the resulting cutaneous signs may be helpful in identifying the cause.

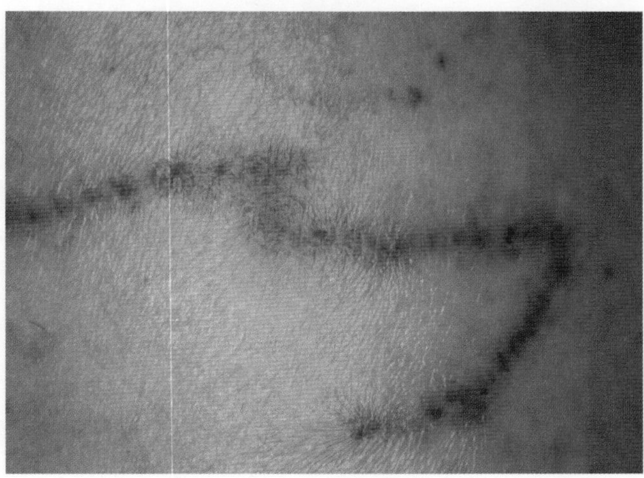

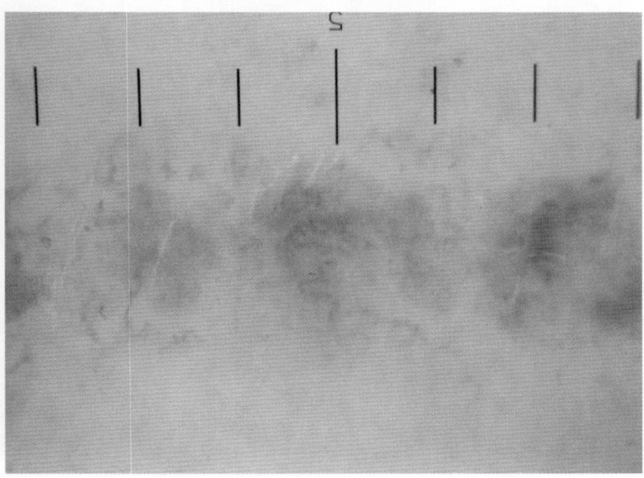

A 40-year-old woman returning from the Mediterranean two weeks after contact from an unidentified species of jellyfish: dermoscopy shows a linear arrangement of regularly spaced telangiectasia, purpura and hyperpigmentation.

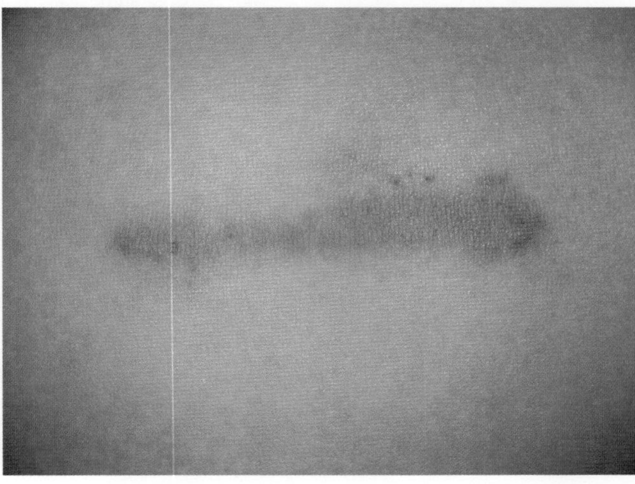

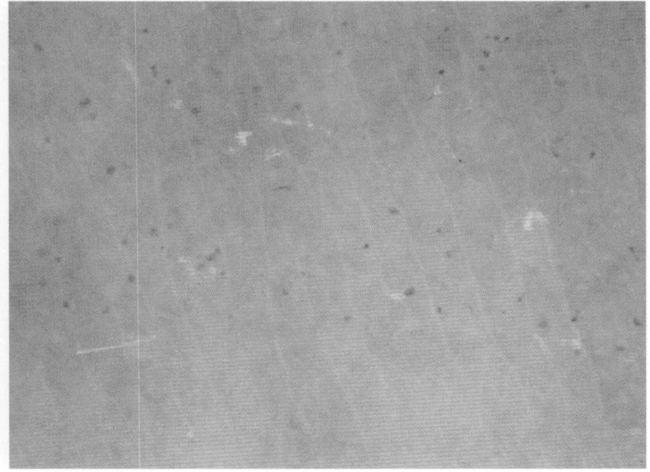

Reactivation of a jellyfish sting caused by *Pelagia noctiluca*, one week after exposure: dermoscopy shows erythema and multiple pinpoint dots in parallel lines corresponding to sites of nematocyst discharge and envenomation.

Del Pozo, L.J. et al. Dermoscopic findings of jellyfish stings caused by *Pelagia noctiluca*. *Actas Dermosifiliogr*. 2016;107(6):509–515.

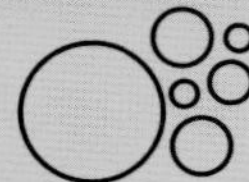

Tungiasis – *Tunga penetrans*

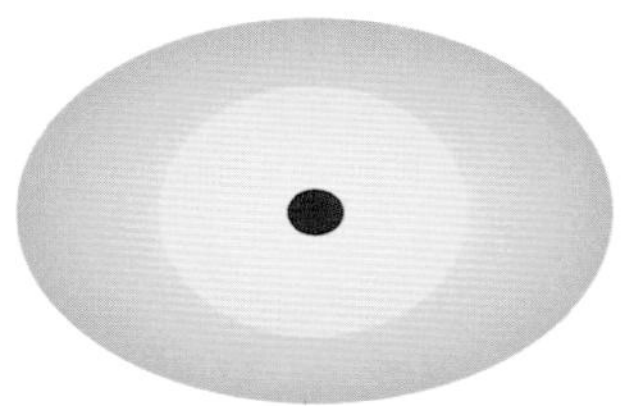

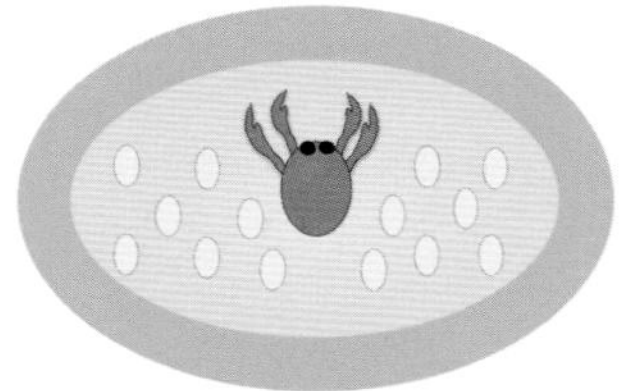

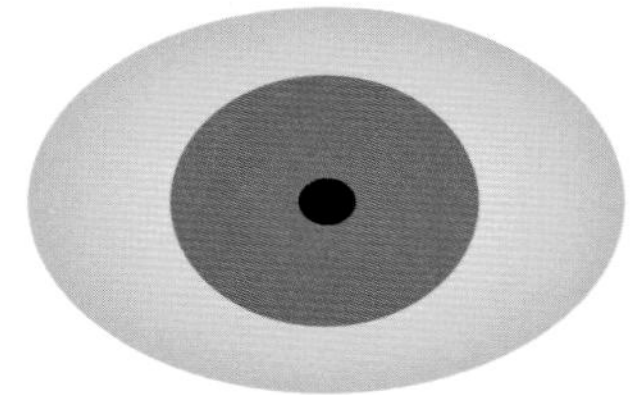

Tunga penetrans infection presents as single or multiple acral papules with a visible central pore. The skin surrounding the pore may become pale as the pregnant flea enlarges or purple if infection or haemorrhage occurs. A clinico-dermoscopic diagnosis allows the flea to be removed intact for *ex vivo* dermoscopic confirmation.

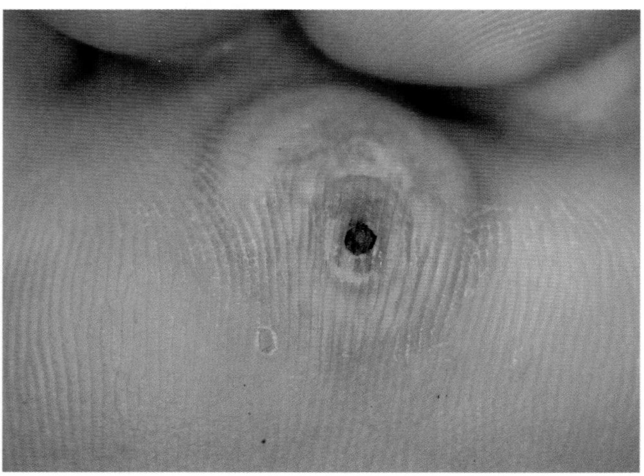

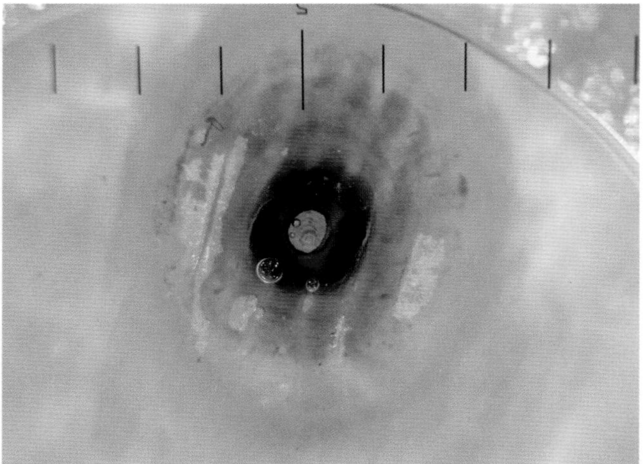

A tender acral papule on the forefoot of a traveller returning from Mozambique: dermoscopy shows a dilated central haemorrhagic pore with surrounding pale yellow discoloration.

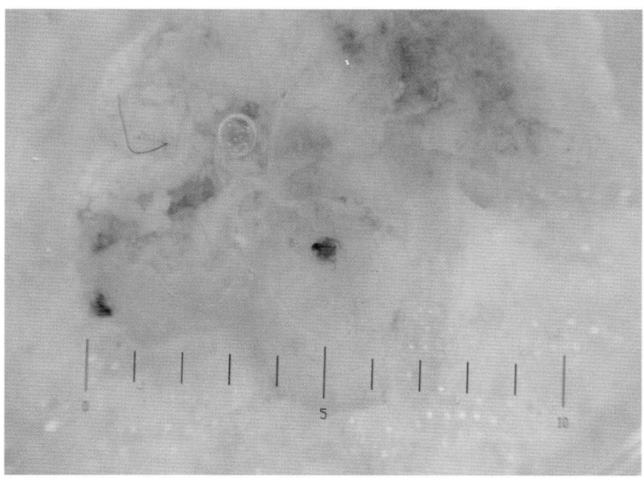

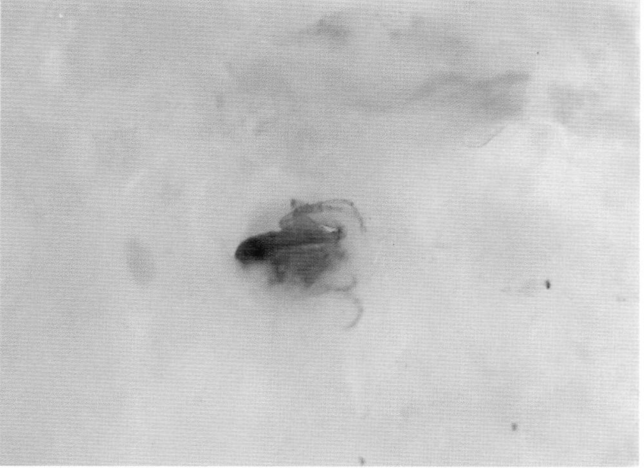

Ex vivo examination of the flea shows the head and thorax of the flea on top of a massively distended abdomen full of eggs: dermoscopy of the head and thorax confirms the diagnosis.

Dunn, R. et al. Dermoscopy: Ex-vivo visualization of flea's head and bag of eggs confirms the diagnosis of tungiasis. *Austral J Dermatol*. 2012;53(2):120–122.

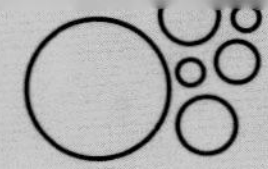

Myiasis – *Dermatobia hominis*

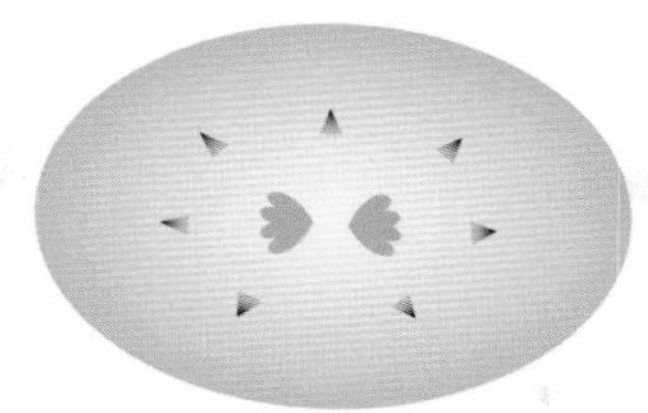

Myiasis is a not uncommon cutaneous infection affecting humans in tropical climates. The condition is caused by the larva of dual-winged flies (Diptera) burrowing into the skin. It commonly presents as a solitary (although may be multiple) boil-like inflammatory papule, often accompanied with sensations of movement within. Dermoscopy of the larva *in vivo* may show 'bird's feet' structures corresponding to the breathing spiracles of the larva.

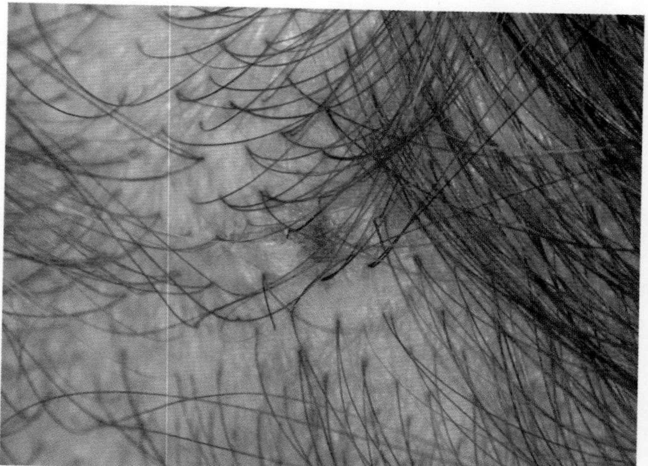

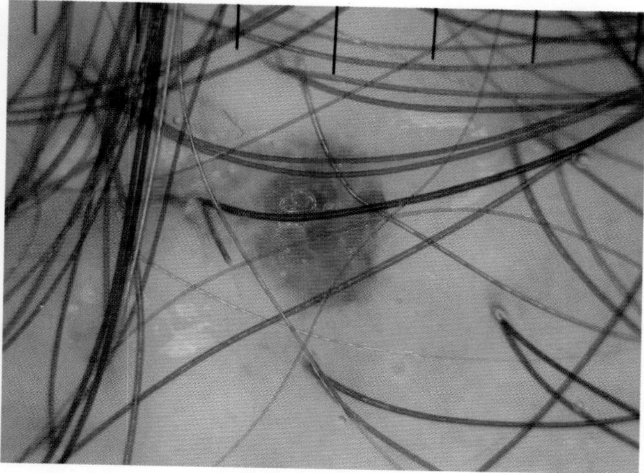

A tender inflammatory furuncle on the left temple of a traveller returning from Belize, with a history of the sensation of movement within the furuncle: dermoscopy showed a central erosion only and no overt diagnostic features.

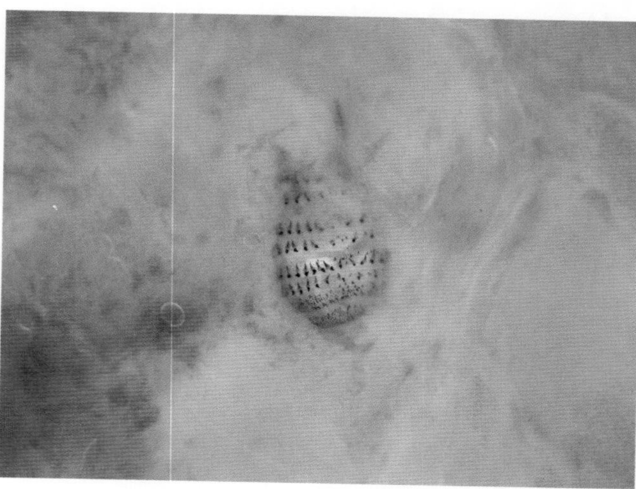

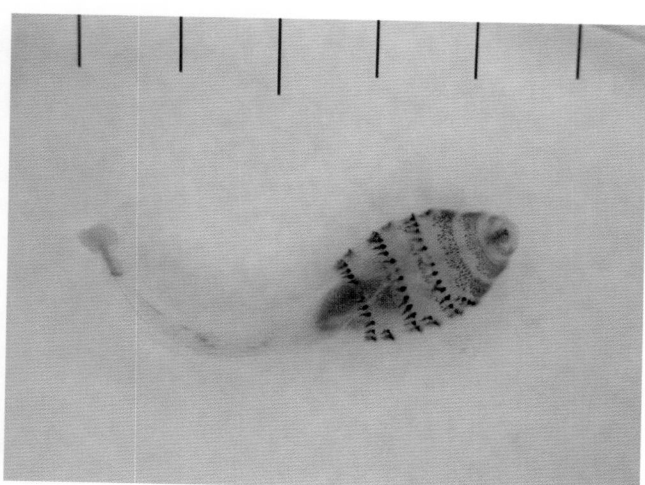

Excision and *ex vivo* examination of the tissue showed an embedded barbed larva: dermoscopy confirmed infection with *Dermatobia hominis* causing furuncular myiasis. (Reproduced from Esdaile et al. with permission from John Wiley.)

Esdaile, B.A. et al. Residents' corner July 2013. Clues in DeRmosCopy: Entodermoscopy. *Eur J Dermatol*. 2013;23(4):574–575.

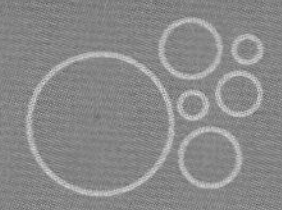

12 Miscellaneous

Keloids and hypertrophic scars 313
Foreign body 314
Foreign body cases 315
Exogenous pigmentation 316
Exogenous pigmentation cases 317
Laser 318
Cryotherapy 319
Radiotherapy 320

Diagnostic Dermoscopy: The Illustrated Guide, Second Edition. Jonathan Bowling.

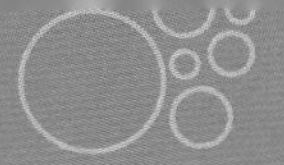

Keloids and hypertrophic scars

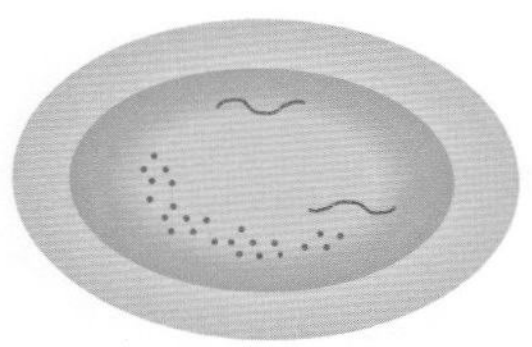

Keloids and hypertrophic scars are not uncommon following surgical episodes or trauma to the skin and do not cause diagnostic concern in this scenario. However, they may also develop spontaneously in patients with inflammatory or infective conditions. If solitary, they may cause diagnostic concern, particularly if features of a coexistent inflammatory process are subtle or have cleared. They may mimic skin tumours and therefore a careful examination and history should be taken.

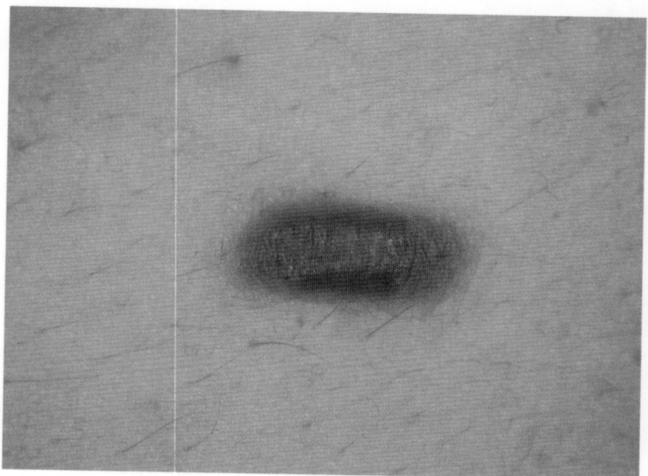

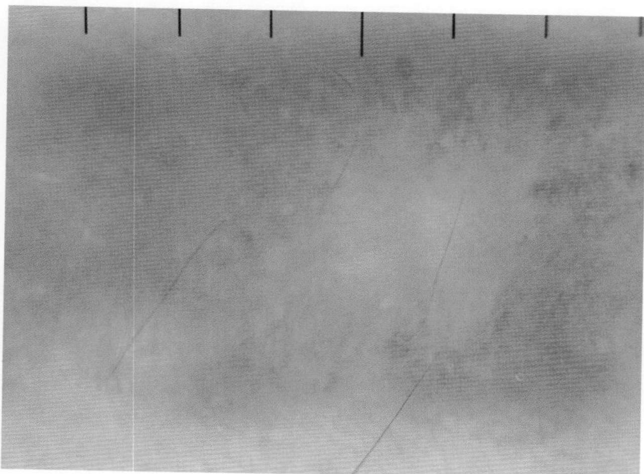

A spontaneous linear scarred plaque on the shoulder of a 25-year-old woman with acne: dermoscopy shows peripheral erythema and central structureless light brown pigmentation in this hypertrophic scar.

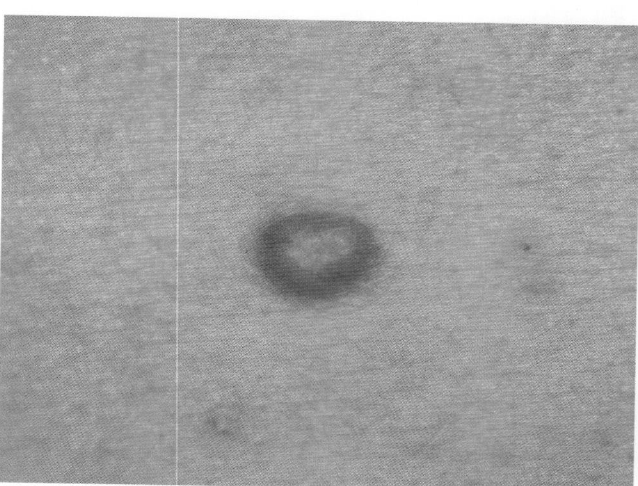

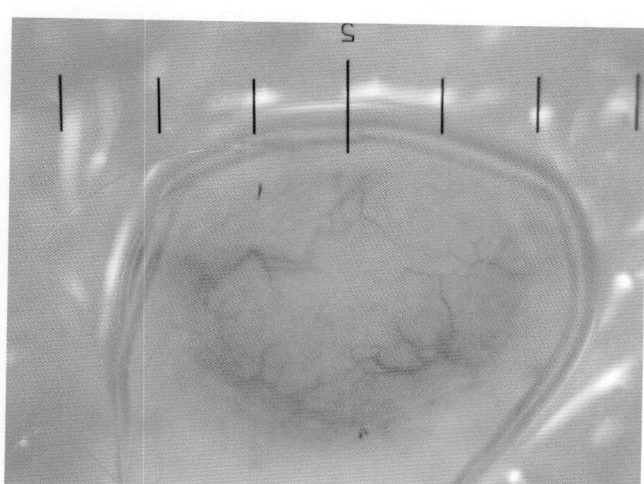

A well-circumscribed firm nodule on the back of a 30-year-old woman with known acne: dermoscopy shows poorly focused linear branching vessels and a pink homogeneous, structureless background in this hypertrophic scar.

Consider a keloid or hypertrophic scar in the differential of a solitary pink plaque in patients with a history of acne.

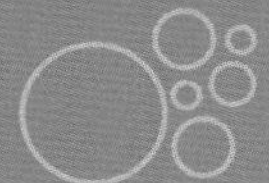

Foreign body

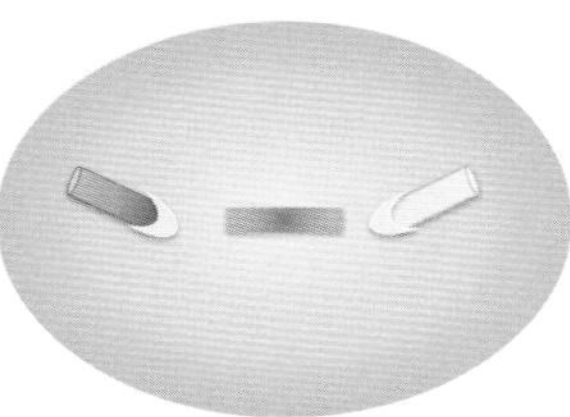

Dermoscopy examination allows identification of not only inflammatory, infective and neoplastic skin conditions but can also aid in diagnosis when foreign materials lodge in the skin. Foreign material can be from traumatic, surgical or accidental events.

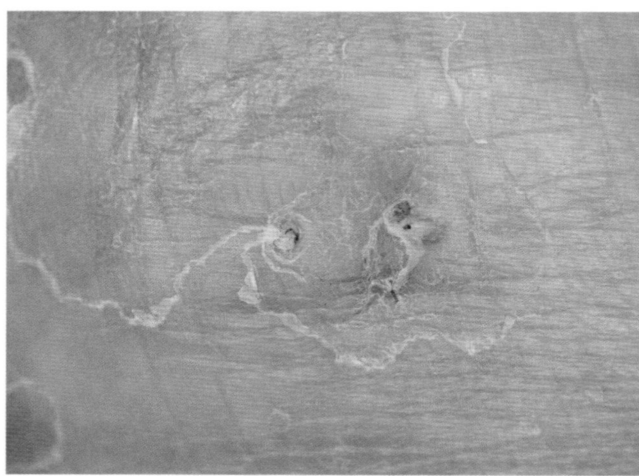

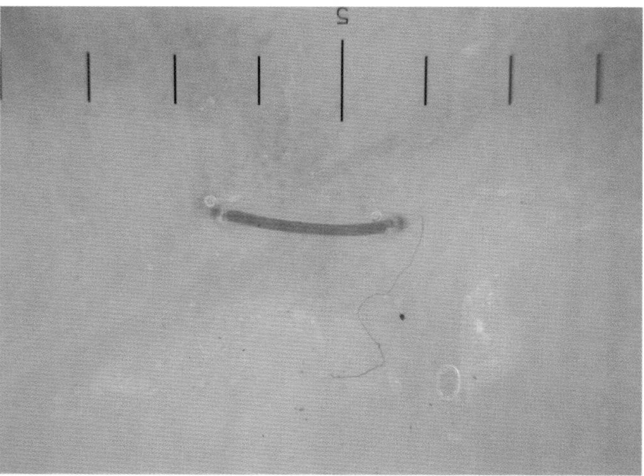

Ongoing pain and hyperkeratosis following a lacerated hand after a bicycle accident eight weeks earlier: dermoscopy shows residual polypropylene suture protruding through the skin.

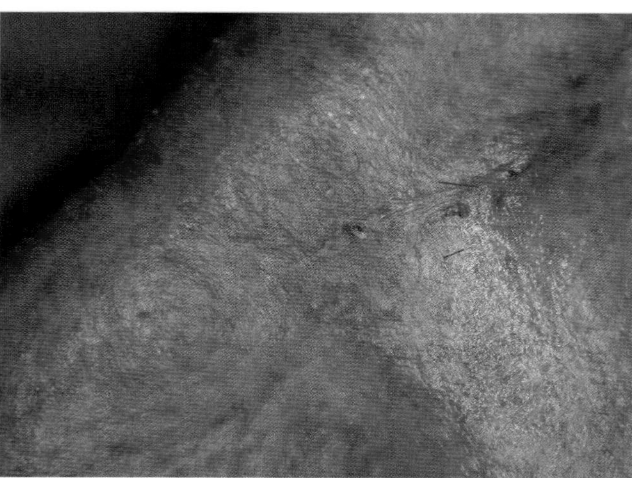

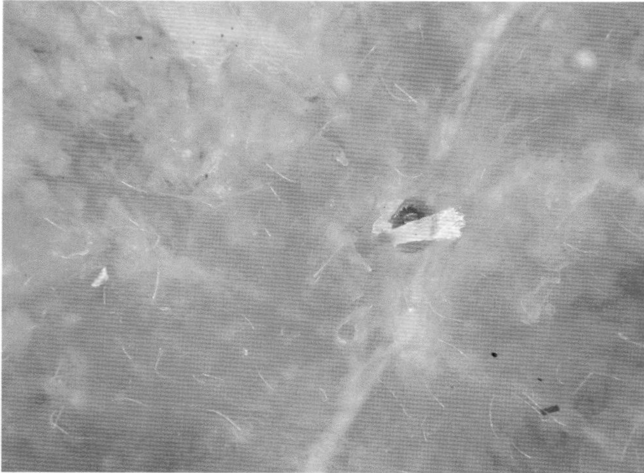

Transepidermal elimination of a dermal polyglactin suture six weeks post-excision of a well-differentiated squamous cell carcinoma on the left nasal side wall: polarised dermoscopy confirms suture material and facilitates easy removal.

Naimer, S.A. Dermoscopic prevention and improved detection of retained sutures. *J Am Acad Dermatol*. 2014;70(3):e57–58.

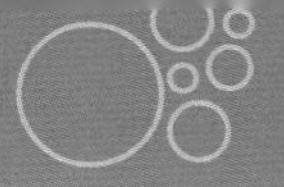

Foreign body cases

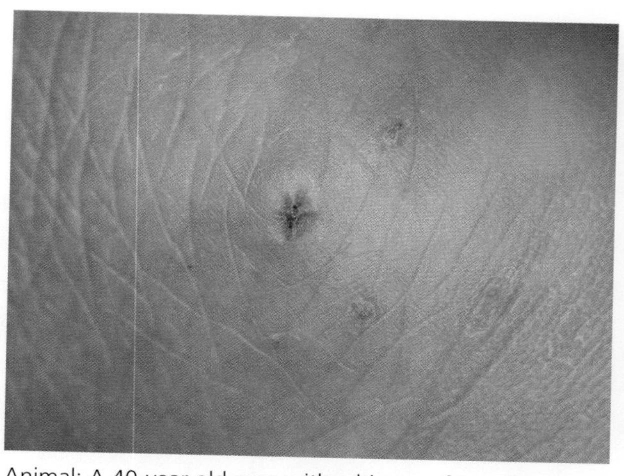

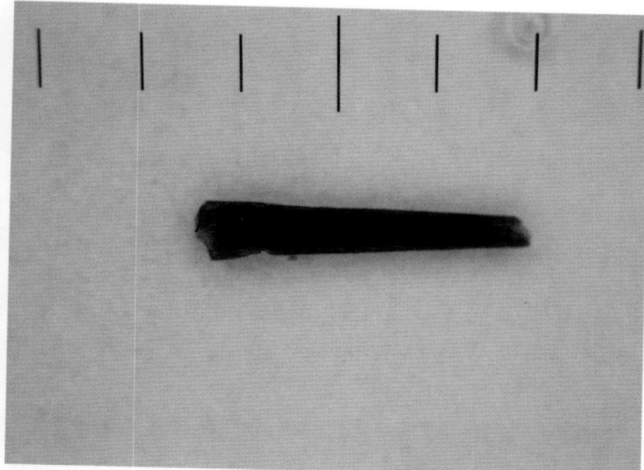

Animal: A 40-year-old man with a history of treading on a sea urchin presented with persistent pain on the heel. A foreign body was removed and confirmed on dermoscopy as a fractured tip of a sea urchin spine.

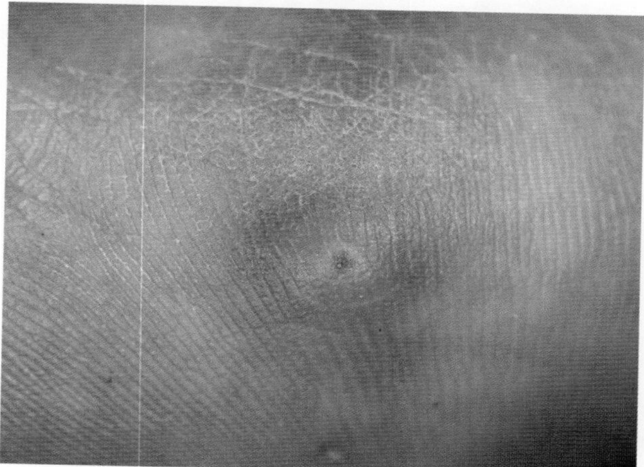

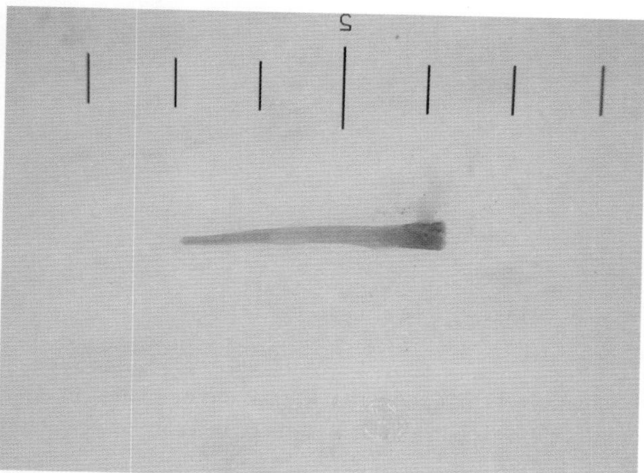

Vegetable: A tender abscess on the instep of a keen gardener; dermoscopy confirmed a penetrating thorn as the cause.

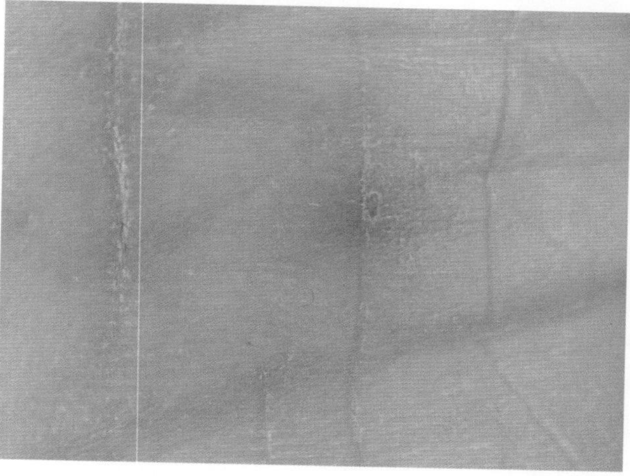

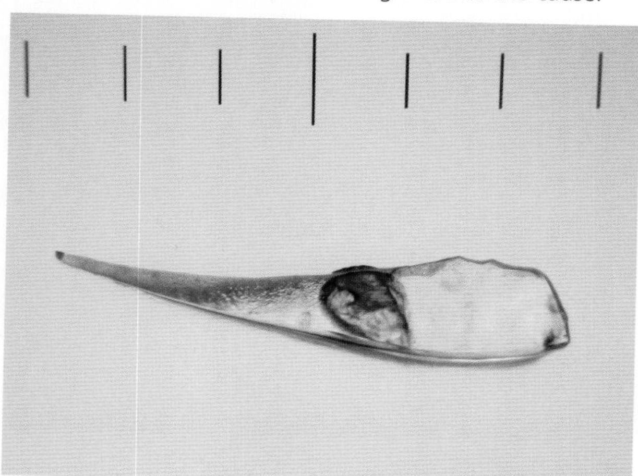

Mineral: A 45-year-old woman with a history of persistent pain on the instep four months after sustaining a penetrating glass injury to the sole of the foot. A shard of glass was removed under local anaesthetic and confirmed on dermoscopy.

Dermoscopic confirmation and digital imaging of any foreign body material removed should be considered. Confirmation of the foreign body may not only help guide medical management but also act as an accurate addition to the medical record.

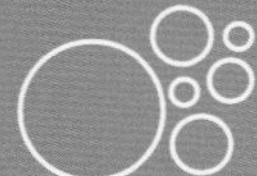

Exogenous pigmentation

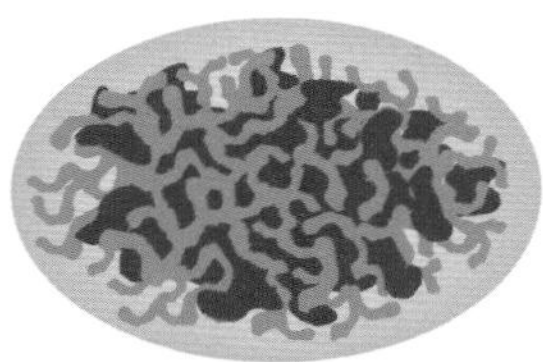

When pigment is applied to the skin either intentionally or accidentally it has the opportunity to collect in the surface contours of any skin lesion with a prominent epidermal component. The pigment accumulates on the skin surface, exaggerating the topographical features of the underlying lesions and often leading to bizzare patterns. Common epidermal lesions that can be affected include seborrhoeic keratoses, dermal naevi, actinic keratoses and porokeratoses.

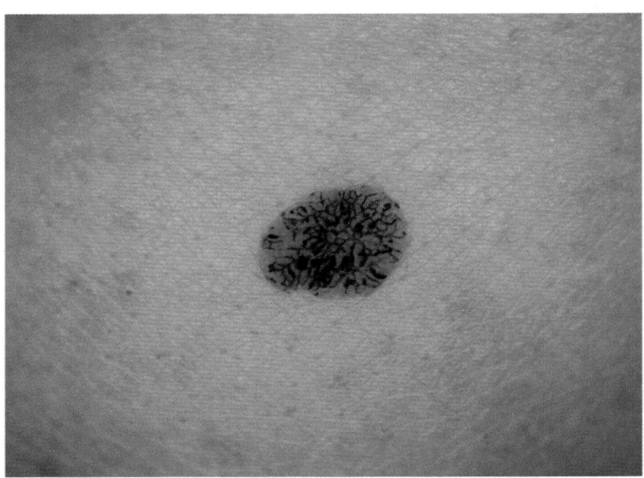

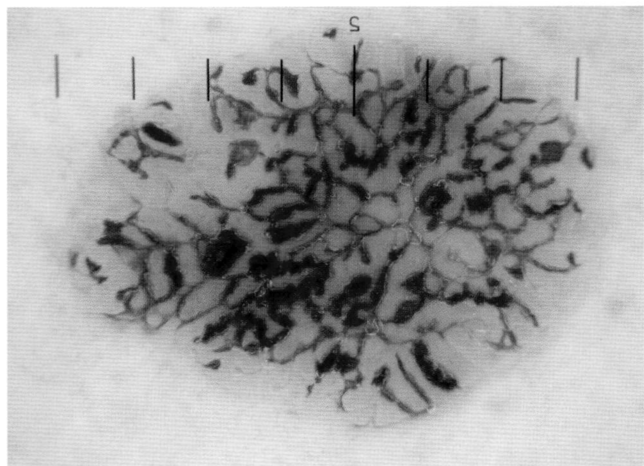

Fake tan applied to the skin in a 40-year-old woman with a past history of melanoma: dermoscopy shows accentuated pigmentation within the surface clefts of this seborrhoeic keratosis.

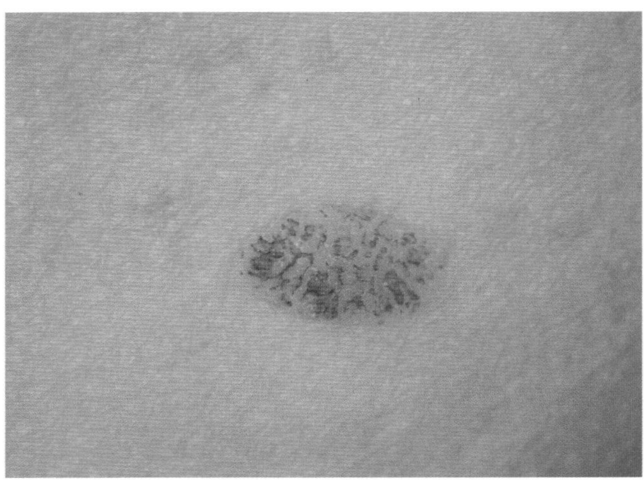

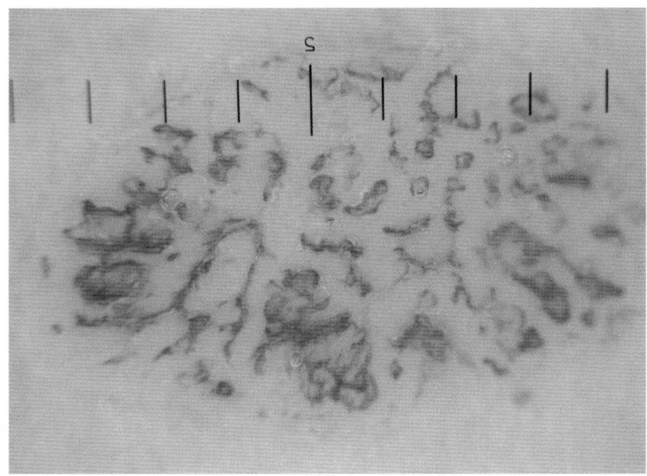

An unusual new pink macule appearing following abdominal surgery to a 30-year-old woman: dermoscopy shows pink tinting (skin surgical marker) of the surface clefts of this seborrhoeic keratosis.

Orpin, S.D. et al. The 'St. Tropez' sign; a new dermoscopic feature of seborrhoeic keratoses? *Clin Exp Dermatol*. 2006;31(5): 707–709.

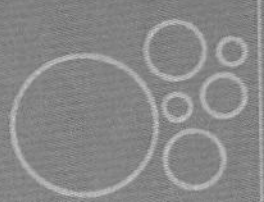

Exogenous pigmentation cases

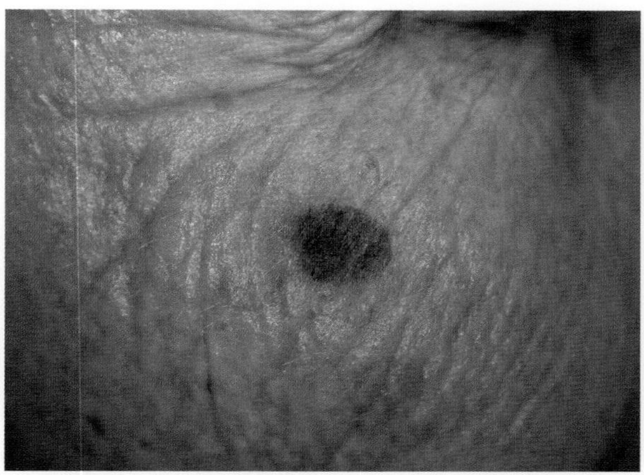

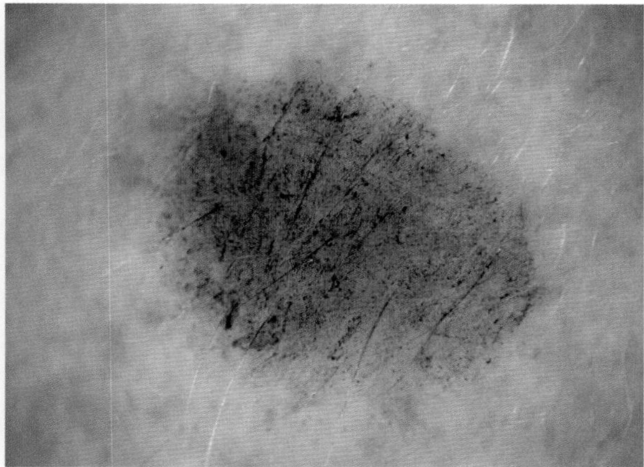

Daily self-application of make-up to create a 'beauty spot' on the cheek of an 87-year-old lady: dermoscopy shows pigment outlining the skin surface markings, hairs and follicular openings, illustrating an exogenous pigment.

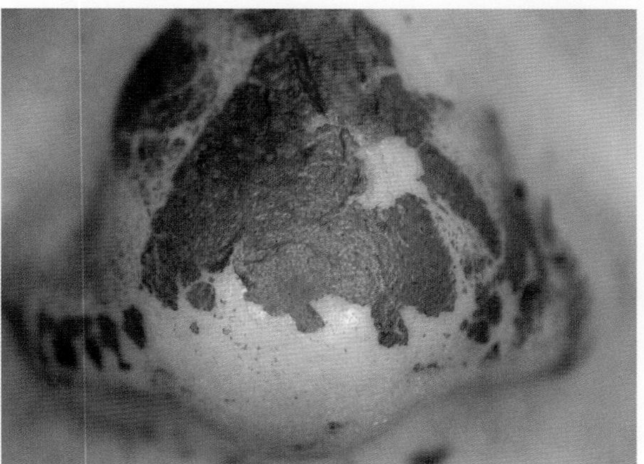

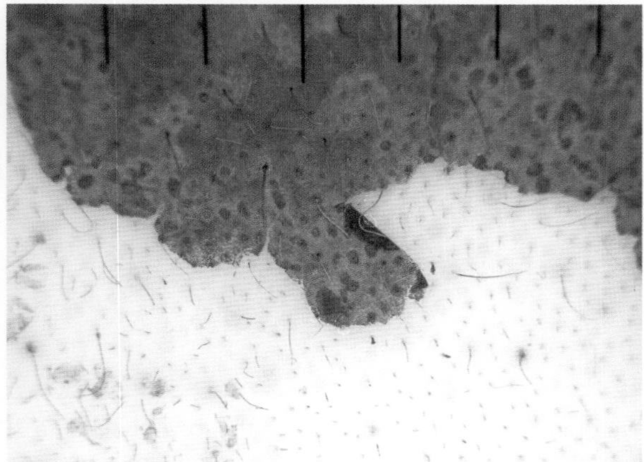

A 14-year-old girl with sudden staining across the central face following application of out-of-date 'aftersun cream': dermoscopy shows the demarcation of external pigmentation with oxidation of a component of the product.

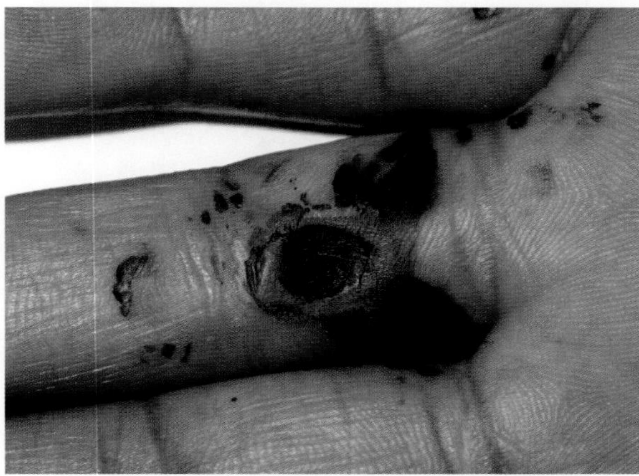

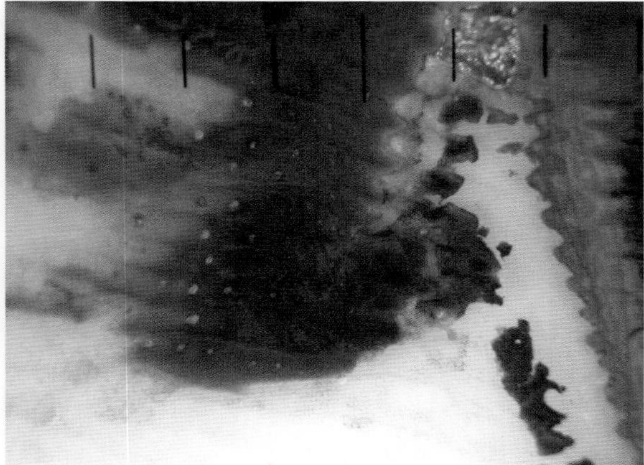

Self-application of silver nitrate to treat a viral wart on the hand of a 55-year-old woman: dermoscopy shows the clear demarcation and multiple colours of oxidised silver nitrate effectively tattooing the skin.

Although rarely causing diagnostic concern, digital documentation of exogenous pigmentation can be a helpful addition to the clinical record.

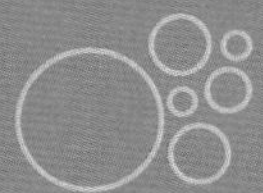

Laser

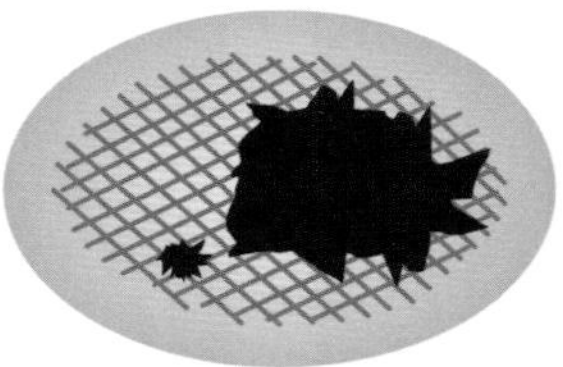

Laser depilation therapy is an increasingly popular treatment for removing excess pigmented body hair. If a melanocytic naevus is also included in the treatment field hyperpigmentation may occur within it. This iatrogenic hyperpigmentation may develop at variable time points post-procedure, leading to bizarre hyperpigmented blotches and diagnostic uncertainty. The history will confirm the diagnosis as the changes are relatively short-lived.

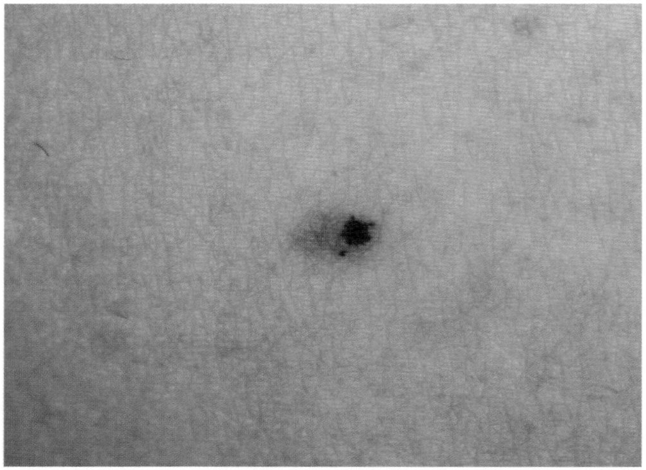

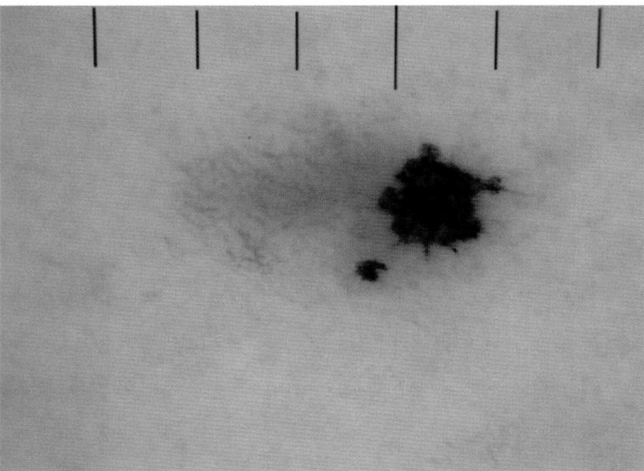

Focal hyperpigmentation in a naevus on the lower back of a 20-year-old woman with a history of recent laser depilation treatment: dermoscopy shows hyperpigmented blotches superimposed on a background reticular naevus.

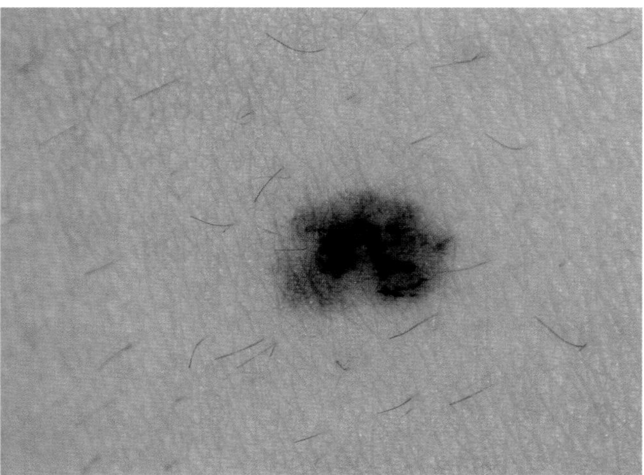

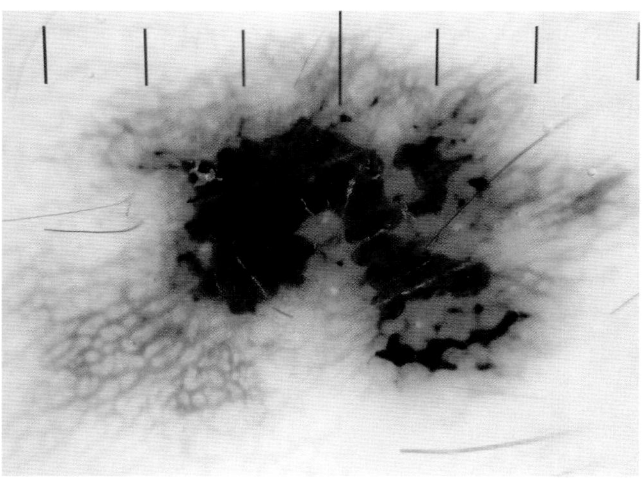

Multiple foci of hyperpigmentation on a naevus in another 20-year-old woman with a history of recent laser depilation treatment: dermoscopy shows hyperpigmented blotches on a background reticular naevus.

If the laser treatment episode was a few weeks earlier and diagnostic uncertainty persists, consider an initial trial of tape stripping, which, if it clears the pigmentation, may prevent an unnecessary biopsy.

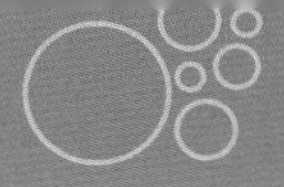

Cryotherapy

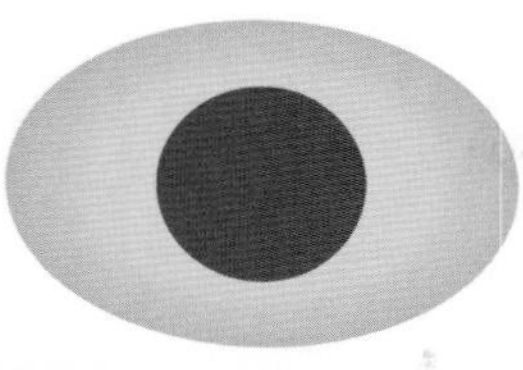

Following cryotherapy to the skin, an iatrogenic subcorneal haematoma may develop. This is not an uncommon finding following treatment for acral viral warts. The area of purple discolouration tends to be circular, corresponding to the area treated with cryotherapy. Additionally, the peripheral margin is well-demarcated and uniform and does not tend to show separate distinct peripheral globules, which are present when a subcorneal haematoma arises from a traumatic episode.

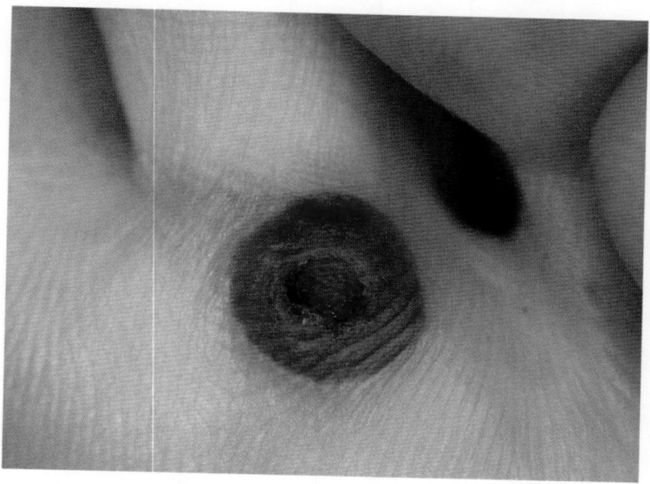

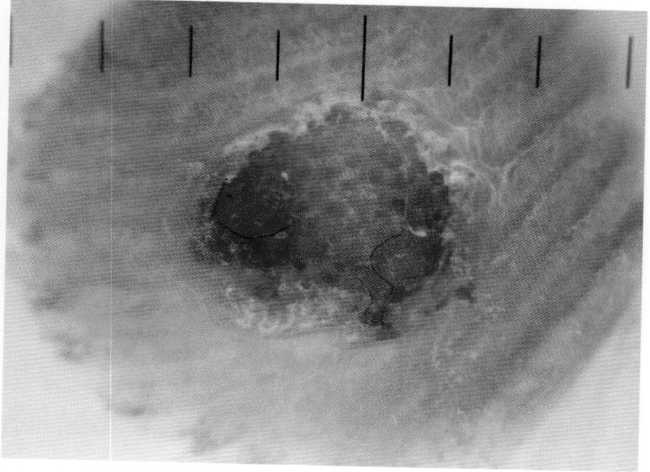

Post-cryotherapy iatrogenic subcorneal haematoma on the forefoot of a 14-year-old girl: dermoscopy shows a uniform purple circular blotch with a distinct peripheral margin surrounding the ulcerated central area.

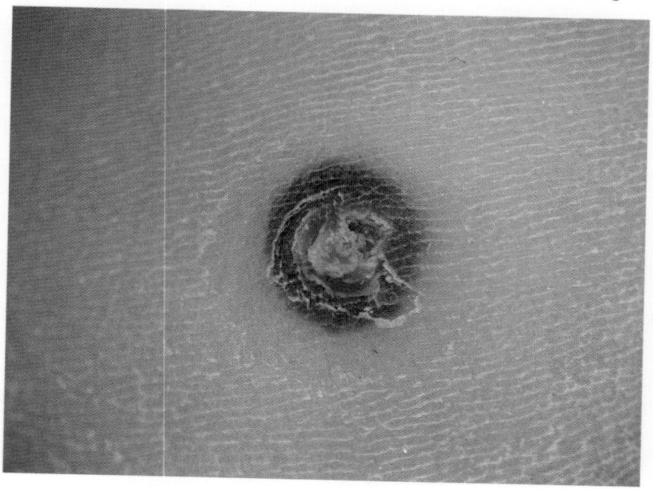

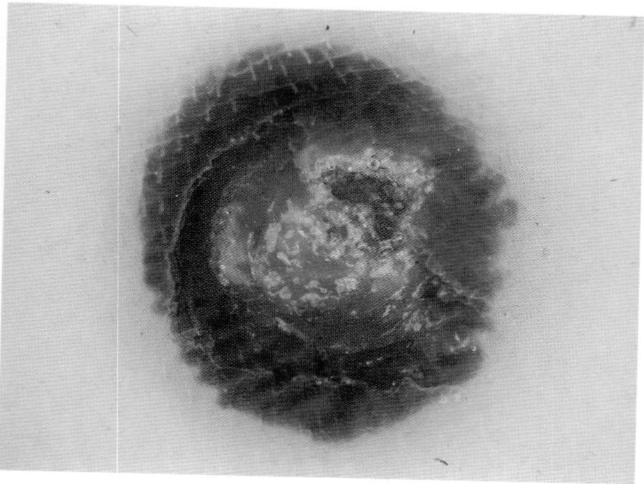

Post-cryotherapy iatrogenic subcorneal haematoma on the heel of a 30-year-old woman: dermoscopy shows a solitary purple circular blotch with central hyperkeratosis with a distinct peripheral margin.

Although a subtle feature, the absence of marginal/peripheral globules of blood may be a good discriminator to distinguish subcorneal haematomas caused by thermal injury rather than those caused from impact causes.

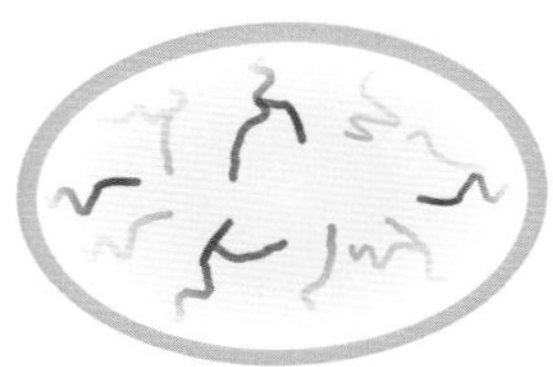

Radiotherapy scars can in themselves mimic infiltrative basal cell carcinomas (BCCs) due to the vascular structures and scarring that develop over time. Unlike BCCs, the vessels within radiotherapy scars are of variable thickness, tortuous, and course a path of variable depth and focus through the skin.

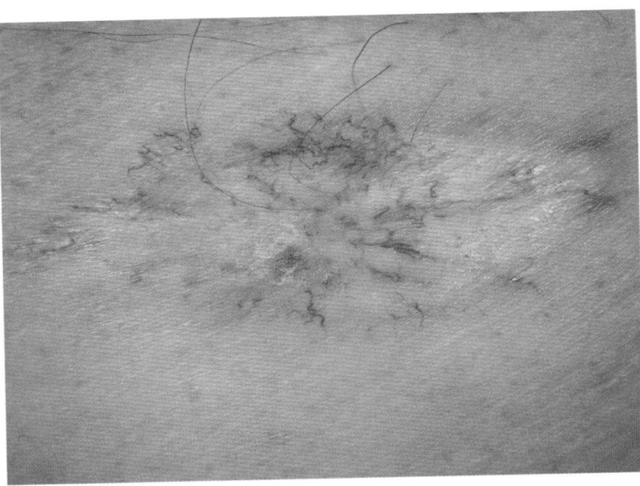

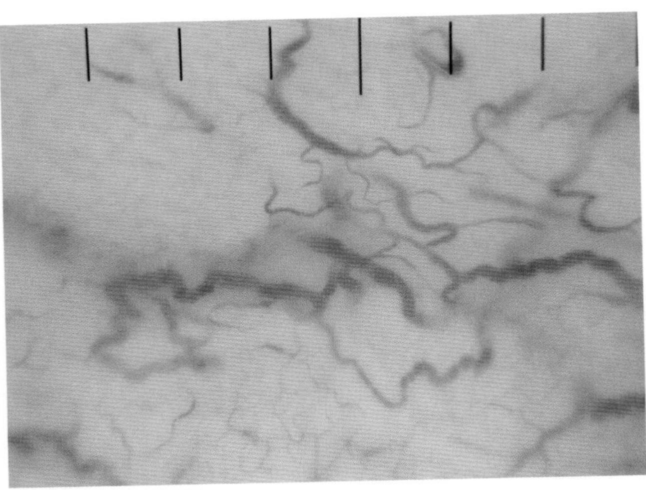

A radiotherapy scar 10 years following treatment to a BCC on the shoulder of a 55-year-old man: dermoscopy shows thick linear vessels with a tortuous path coming in and out of focus.

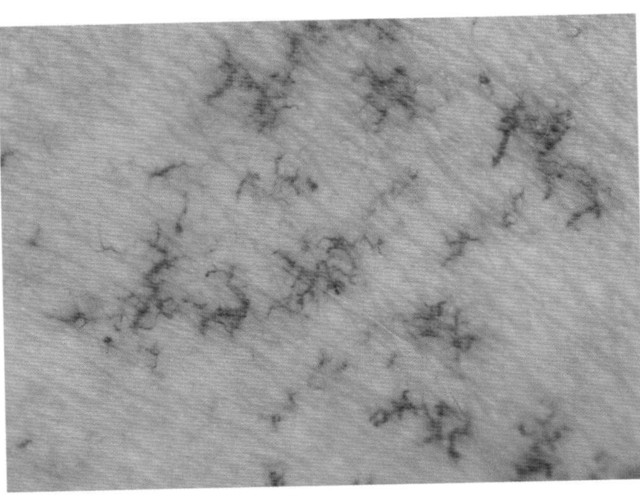

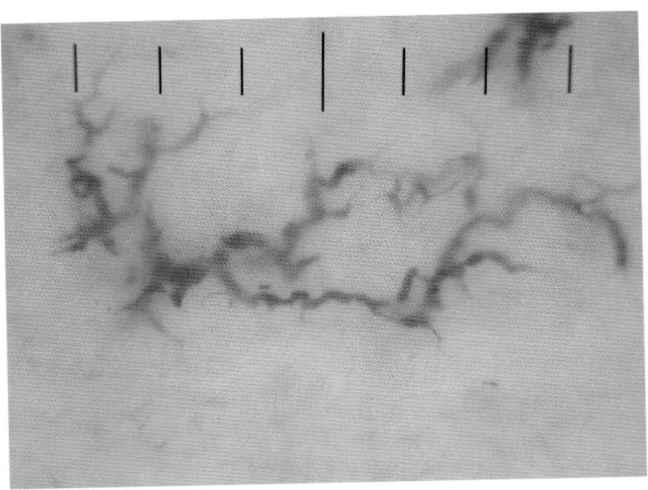

A patch of telangiectatic vessels on the chest wall of a 50-year-old woman treated for breast cancer with adjuvant radiotherapy five years earlier: dermoscopy shows linear tortuous vessels of variable diameter and focus, in keeping with radiotherapy scarring.

Secondary dermatoses and tumours may rarely develop within radiotherapy fields.
Soilleux, E.J. et al. Cutaneous mastocytosis localized to a radiotherapy field. *Clin Exp Dermatol*. 2009;34(1):111–112.

Index

acne, 276, 313
acral melanocytic lesions
acquired acral naevi, 173
acral lentiginous melanoma, 178–182, 186
acral parallel furrow pattern, 174
advanced acral lentiginous melanoma, 182
congenital acral naevi, 177
fibrillar pattern, 176
lattice pattern, 175
acral skin, 10, 262, 264, 270
acrosyringia, 174, 175
actinic keratosis
follicular, 159, 160, 162
grade 1, 159
grade 2, 160
grade 3, 161
hyperkeratotic, 159–162
agminated naevus, *see* naevus
alopecia, *see* trichoscopy
angulated lines, 73, 82, 83, 87, 99, 193, 222, 223, 227, 228, 237
annular granular pigmentation, 222, 223, 228
anonychia, 188
atypical beaded network, 72–73, 97, 109
atypical melanocytic lesions, 22, 23, 124, 155
atypical network, 23, 43, 47, 49, 53, 68–71, 73, 75, 86, 97, 99, 102, 104, 296
Auspitz sign, 279

barcode sign, 185
basal cell carcinoma
hyperpigmented, 155
hypopigmented, 154
morphoeic/infiltrative, 152, 153
nodular, 146–151
pigmented, 6, 148
scalp, 240, 241
seborrhoeic keratosis-like, 156
superficial, 142–145, 164
bed bug, 303
benign lichenoid keratosis, 126, 127, 220–221
Birt-Hogg-Dubé syndrome, 212, 292
blotch
eccentric black, 78, 79
eccentric brown, 76, 77
eccentric grey, 80, 81
blue-grey ovoid nests, 145, 148, 151, 155
blue-gray dots/globules, 144, 149, 151, 154, 157
blue naevus, *see* naevu
blue-whitish veil, 41, 44, 50, 52, 53, 55, 56, 57, 67, 90–93, 99, 102, 103, 107, 238
Bowen's disease
classical, 163
digital, 166
hypertrophic, 164
pigmented, 165
BRAAFF checklist, 179
branched vessels. *see* vessels
broken hairs, 256, 257
Brooke-Spiegler syndrome, 243, 293

callus, 194, 307
Campbell de Morgan spots, 266
candy cane sign, 190
capillaritis, 282, 283
capillaroscopy, 198
capillary effect, 193
Carney complex, 219, 297
cayenne pepper, 282
cerebriform pattern, 116–118, 121, 234, 235
'cherry' angiomas, 266
chloronychia, 196
chromophores, 6, 7, 121
Cimex lectularius. see bed bug
clear cell acanthoma, 125
Cnidaria. *see* jellyfish
cobblestone pattern, 22, 24–27, 31, 32, 48, 177, 214, 215, 230, 267
coiled vessels. *see* vessels
collagen, 7, 14, 89, 128
collarette, 140, 270, 271, 291
comedo-like openings, 74, 118–121, 206, 207, 234, 235, 294
comma vessels, *see* vessels
congenital naevus, *see* naevus
corkscrew vessels, *see* vessels
cornoid lamella, 134
Cowden syndrome, 213, 291
crenulated disc, 308
crown vessels, *see* vessels
cryotherapy, 319
curved vessels. *see* vessels
curvilinear vessels. *see* vessels
cutaneous lupus erythematosus, 288

Diagnostic Dermoscopy: The Illustrated Guide, Second Edition. Jonathan Bowling.

cutaneous T-cell lymphoma
  anaplastic large cell lymphoma, 138
  mycosis fungoides, 138
cylindroma, 243, 293

Darier's disease, 190, 191
dark skin, 10, 26, 120, 130, 281
delusional parasitosis, 299
dermal naevus, *see* naevus
Dermatobia hominis. *see* myiasis
dermatofibroma
  aneurysmal, 131
  cellular, 131
  non-typical, 131
dermatofibrosarcoma protuberans, 132
dermatoglyphics, 10, 174–176, 180, 263, 265, 290
dermatomyositis, 198
dermoscopy
  nail plate, 184, 185, 187, 188, 191, 192, 195, 197
  non-polarised, 4, 8, 9, 119
  polarised, 4, 8, 9, 14, 89, 118, 119, 143, 150, 151, 273, 288, 302, 314
digital dermoscopy, 22, 296
discoid lupus erythematosus, 250
dissecting cellulitis, 251
dots
  black, 42, 44, 45, 48, 55, 56, 57, 67, 72, 74, 75, 79, 91, 97, 130, 136, 179, 182, 187, 238, 246, 257 6–8, 28, 29, 34, 36, 41, 42, 47, 52, 53, 54, 67, 79, 103, 118, 126, 131, 144, 151, 179, 185, 192, 193, 196, 201, 204, 209, 211, 216, 223, 241, 244, 262, 264, 267, 269, 273, 284, 317
  blue-grey dots, 36, 57, 74, 144, 149, 154, 157
  and globules, 36, 40, 41, 44, 45, 47, 50, 56, 57, 59, 67, 71–75, 79, 97, 130, 149, 179, 238, 283
dotted vessels. *see* vessels
dysplastic naevus, *see* naevus
dystrophic hairs, 246

eccrine gland openings, 174
eccrine poroma, 140
eccrine spiradenomas, 293
Echinoidea. *see* sea urchins
eczema
  lichen simplex chronicus, 256
  nummular, 278
egg casts, 303
entomodermoscopy
  bed bug, 303
  delusional parasitosis, 299
  head lice, 302
  jellyfish, 309
  leishmaniasis, 305
  Molluscum contagiosum, 306
  myiasis, 311
  scabies, 300, 301
  sea urchins, 308
  tick bites, 304
  tungiasis, 310
  viral warts, 307
epidermal naevus, 136, 137
epidermoid cysts, 202, 204
erythronychia, 190, 191
erythroxanthonychia, 188
eumelanin, 6
exclamation hairs, 246
exogenous pigmentation, 316, 317

facial lesions
  benign lichenoid keratosis, 220–221
  dermal naevus, 214, 215
  epidermoid cysts, 204
  fibrous papules, 212
  granulomatous folliculitis, 211
  hidrocystomas, 203
  ink spot lentigo, 219
  juvenile xanthogranuloma, 210
  lentigo maligna, 222–226
  lentigo maligna melanoma, 227–228
  malignant adnexal carcinomas, 209
  milium/keratin cysts, 202
  mucosal melanosis, 201, 297
  pilomatricomas, 205
  sebaceous adenomas, 207, 294
  sebaceous hyperplasia, 206, 207
  sebaceous naevus, 208
  solar lentigo, 216–218
  trichilemmomas, 213
  venous lake, 200
facial skin, 10
familial cylindromatosis syndrome, 293
fibroepithelioma of Pinkus, 157
fibrofolliculomas, 212, 292
fibrous papules, 212
follicular density, 10, 224, 244
follicular destruction, 212, 222, 227, 228
follicular plugging, 250
folliculitis decalvans, 251
foreign body, 308, 314, 315
frictional alopecia, 257

genodermatoses
  Birt-Hogg-Dubé syndrome, 292
  Carney complex, 297
  Cowden syndrome, 291
  familial cylindromatosis, 293
  familial melanoma, 296
  Gorlin syndrome, 290
  Muir-Torre syndrome, 294
  Reed syndrome, 295
globules
  black, 34, 44, 45, 56, 57, 67, 74, 75, 79, 94, 130, 178, 179
  blue-grey globules, 36, 57, 74, 86, 149, 151, 154
  cobblestone, 22, 24–27, 31, 32, 48, 177, 214, 215, 230, 267
  multiple aggregated yellow-white globules, 154
  splatter, 192, 264
glomerular vessels. *see* vessels
glomus tumour, 190, 191
Gorlin syndrome, 290
granuloma annulare, 285
granulomatous folliculitis, 211

haemangioma
  lobular capillary, 270
  microvenular, 272
haemoglobin, 7
hair
  broken, 256, 257
  circle, 254
  coiled, 246, 254
  dystrophic, 246
  exclamation, 246, 257
  peripilar casts, 248, 249

vellus, 247, 248, 255
hairpin vessels, *see* vessels
halo naevus, *see* naevus
head lice, 258, 302
helical vessels. *see* vessels
herald patch, 287
hereditary leiomyomatosis and renal cell carcinoma (HLRCC), 295
hidrocystomas, 203
histopathological correlation, 2, 136
Hutchinson's sign, 185–187
hypertrophic scars, 313
hypokeratosis, 290

illumination, 2, 4
ILVEN, 136
imaging modes, 2, 4, 8, 9
inflammatory linear verrucous epidermal naevus, 136
inflammoscopy
acne, 276
capillaritis, 282
cutaneous lupus erythematosus, 288
eczema, 278
granuloma annulare, 285
granulomatous conditions, 284
lichen planus, 280
lichen planus pigmentosus, 281
mastocytosis, 275
pityriasis rosea, 287
psoriasis, 279
rosacea, 277
tinea corporis, 286
vasculitis, 283
Insect bite reaction, 139
inverse network, *see* negative network
Ixodidae. *see* tick bites

jellyfish, 309
junctional naevus, *see* naevus
juvenile xanthogranuloma (JXG), 210

Kaposi sarcoma, 272
keloids, 313
keratin, 7, 9, 25, 74, 117, 119, 159, 161, 165, 189, 200, 202, 204, 211, 213, 258, 291, 292
aggregates, 124, 137, 258
collarette, 140, 291
concentric, 111
crust, 161
debris, 182, 189
laminated, 111
plugs, 119
rim, 134, 135
spires, 136
keratinocyte dysplasia
actinic keratosis, 159–162
Bowen's disease, 163–166
squamous cell carcinoma, 167–171
keratoacanthoma, 168, 170, 294

labial melanotic macule, 200, 201
laser, 318
leaf-like structures, *see* structures
leiomyomas, 295
leishmaniasis, 305
lentigo
ink spot, 115, 219
solar, 112–116, 126, 127, 216–218, 220, 223
lentigo maligna, 82, 114–116, 216–218, 221–227, 222–226, 237
lentigo maligna melanoma, 225, 227, 228, 237, 238
leukoxanthonychia, 189
lichen planopilaris, 249, 250, 252
lichen planus, 191, 220, 280, 281, 287
lichen-planus like keratosis, 220
lichen planus pigmentosus, 281
lichen simplex chronicus, 256
light skin, 10, 20, 58, 59, 62, 63, 64, 109, 121, 129, 233
linear irregular vessels. *see* vessels
linear vessels. *see* vessels
lipids, 7
'Little Red Riding Hood' sign, 41
looped vessels. *see* vessels
lunula, 184, 191
Lyme disease, 304
lymphangioma, 269
lymphoma
B-cell lymphoma scalp, 242
primary cutaneous follicle centre lymphoma, 242
Lynch syndrome, 207, 294

macrocomedone, 111
magnification, 4, 5, 301
medium-toned skin, 21
melanoma
amelanotic, 58–61, 129, 187
amelanotic nodular, 104, 105
congenital melanocytic naevus-associated, 50
dermal pigmentation, 92, 93
desmoplastic melanoma, 129
disordered polarity, 46–47
familial, 296
feature-poor, 100, 101
geographic border, 44–45
geometric border, 42–43
high-risk scenarios, 98–109
hypermelanotic, 56–57
hypomelanotic, 62–65
in situ, 185
late features, 99
metastatic, 106, 107
multicoloured, 52–53
multicomponent, 54–55
naevus-associated, 48–49
nail apparatus, 185–188
nail matrix, 184, 186, 188
nodular melanoma, 155
rare subtypes, 108
scalp, 236
small diameter, 40–41
synchronous, 109
verrucous melanoma, 120
melanoma in situ, 5, 22, 42, 43, 45–49, 58, 62, 67, 69, 70, 72–75, 77, 78, 80, 82–87, 89, 96, 97, 100, 178, 185, 236, 296
melanoma-specific features, 67, 99
melanonychia
broad band, 185
fungal, 187, 195
longitudinal, 186
metastases, 107, 239
microcystic adnexal carcinoma, 209
micro-haemorrhages, 194, 307
micro-Hutchinson's sign, 186

microvenular haemangioma, 272
milia-like cyst, 118–121, 123, 157, 235
milium/keratin cysts, 202
Mohs surgery, 153
Molluscum contagiosum, 306
moth-eaten border, 113, 116, 216, 218
mucosal melanosis, 201, 297
Muir-Torre syndrome (MTS), 294
myiasis, 311
myrmecia, 307

naevus
  acral, 174
  agminated, 33
  blue, 27, 28, 232, 263
  blue scalp, 232
  blue sclerotic, 29
  combined, 27
  congenital, 32, 33, 48, 177, 263
  dermal, 16, 24–27, 48, 154, 214, 215, 230, 255, 316
  dermal scalp, 230
  dysplastic, 22, 23, 46, 48
  eclipse, 233
  halo, 31
  junctional, 17, 19, 27, 174–176, 214
  junctional scalp, 231
  nail matrix, 184
  pigmented Spitz, 36
  recurrent, 30
  Reed, 34–36
  spilus, 33
  Spitz, 6, 34, 36-38, 59, 84
naevus spilus, *see* naevus
nail bed capillaries, *see* vessels
nail matrix
  biopsy, 188
  melanoma, 184, 186, 188
  naevus, 184
nail plate
  dystrophy, 185–188, 195
  erosion, 188
  fissure, 186
  fragility, 186
  loss/anonychia, 187, 188
nail unit/apparatus
  fungus, 187, 195
  melanoma, 185–188
  naevus, 184
  squamous cell carcinoma, 189
necrobiosis lipoidica, 284
negative network, 5, 22, 36, 37, 44, 46, 47, 49, 50, 58, 59, 62, 64, 65, 67, 84, 85, 88, 91, 94, 100–102, 104, 124, 131, 179
neurofibromas, 133
neurofibromatosis, segmental, 133
nit cast, 302
nodular melanoma (NM), 37, 44, 91, 95, 102–105, 131, 155, 240
non-eumelanin, 7
non-melanocytic lesions
  benign lichenoid keratosis, 126–127
  clear cell acanthoma, 125
  dermatofibroma, 128–131
  dermatofibrosarcoma protuberans, 132
  macrocomedone, 111
  neurofibroma, 133
  seborrhoeic keratosis, 117–124
  solar lentigo, 112–116
non-polarised dermoscopy, *see* dermoscopy
normal skin, 10, 33, 56, 130, 152, 260

onycholysis, 188, 189, 195, 196
onychomycosis, *Trichophyton rubrum,* 195, 286
onychopapilloma, 191
onychoscopy
  capillaroscopy, 192, 198
  chloronychia, 196
  erythronychia, 190
  nail apparatus melanoma, 186–188
  nail apparatus melanoma in situ, 185
  nail apparatus squamous cell carcinoma, 189
  nail matrix naevus, 184
  nail pigmentation, 197
  onychomycosis, 195
  onychopapilloma, 191
  periungual warts, 194
  subungual haematoma, 193
orthogonal lines, *see* shiny white lines

palmoplantar pits, 290
pattern
  atypical fibrillar, 176
  cerebriform, 116–118, 121, 234, 235
  circles, 112, 216, 224
  cobblestone, 22, 24–27, 31, 32, 48, 177, 214, 215, 230, 267
  double-edged line, 114, 134
  evolving, 19, 117
  fat fingers, 117
  fibrillar/filamentous pattern, 173, 176
  fingerprint, 112, 216, 218
  globular, 16, 18, 19, 32, 34, 44, 78, 80, 81, 84, 89, 99, 103
  homogeneous, 18, 19, 22, 34, 35, 47, 55, 63, 65, 78, 103, 105, 113, 118, 125, 155, 192, 193, 196, 202, 203, 206, 213, 217, 218, 220, 231, 233, 262, 264–267, 270, 271, 273, 306, 307, 308, 313
  keratotic halos, 194, 307
  lattice pattern, 173, 175, 177
  mosaic, 194
  multicomponent, 44, 49, 54–55, 70, 79, 97, 132
  non-typical acral pattern, 178
  parallel furrow, 173, 174, 175, 177
  parallel lines, 112, 176, 184, 216, 262, 279, 309
  parallel ridge, 180, 181, 185, 263, 264
  reticular, 10, 11, 17–21, 27, 31–34, 46, 48–50, 55, 68, 71, 72, 74, 80, 82, 89, 112, 114–116, 178, 216, 231, 233, 260, 275, 295, 318
  scar-like area, 88, 128, 130
  starburst, 35, 79, 305
  strawberry, 160
  string of pearls, 125
  structureless, 72, 81, 87, 89, 99–101, 103, 105, 129, 132, 133, 138, 142, 146, 147, 177, 242, 291, 295, 313
  structureless area, 47, 49, 53, 71, 75, 77, 82, 83, 86, 89, 102, 104, 106, 108, 129, 132, 133, 143, 145, 147, 151, 153, 156, 177, 179, 182, 200, 206, 228, 233, 239, 242, 243, 280, 281, 284, 291, 292, 293, 295
  vascular, 7, 11–13, 25, 28, 52, 59, 60, 63, 94, 100, 103, 104, 107, 121, 122, 125, 126, 130, 148, 164, 169, 170, 190, 200, 214, 215, 221, 232, 252, 266, 268, 270–272, 275, 282, 320
  white circles, 159, 167, 169, 170
  white halos, 136, 160, 288
Pediculosis capitis. see head lice
peppering, 54, 81, 86, 88, 89, 123, 127

perifollicular pigmentation, 217, 221–226, 228
peripilar casts, 248, 249
phaeomelanin, 6, 7, 62
photodamaged skin, 11, 260
picker's nodule, 256
pigmentation
brown granular pigmentation, 148, 151, 156, 159, 179, 223, 296
brown-grey, 180, 181, 237, 281
exogenous nail, 197
fibrillar, 176
follicular, 130, 212, 217, 221–226, 228, 237
granular, 30, 45, 55, 57, 80, 81, 86–89, 102, 106, 107, 123, 127, 130, 144, 148, 151, 156, 159, 179–181, 192, 221–223, 226, 228, 236, 237, 281, 296
lattice, 173, 175
nail band, 184
parallel furrow, 174, 175, 177
polychromasia, 186
tar staining, 197
white granular, 192
pigmented purpuric dermatosis, 282
pilomatricomas, 205
pityriasis amiantacea, 258
pityriasis rosea, 287
polarisation structures, *see* shiny white structures
polarised dermoscopy, 4, 8, 9, 14, 89, 118, 119, 143, 150, 151, 273, 288, 302, 314
polyarteritis nodosa, 283
polygonal structures, *see* angulated lines
porokeratosis
disseminated superficial actinic porokeratosis, 134
porokeratosis of Mibelli, 134, 135
pseudolymphoma, 139
Pseudomonas aeruginosa, 196
pseudopelade, 253
psoriasis, 258, 279, 287
purpura
actinic, 273
Bateman's, 273
traumatic, 273
pyocyanin, 196
pyoverdin, 196

radiotherapy, 320
recurrent naevus, *see* naevus
red pseudonetwork, 160
Reed naevus, *see* naevus
Reed syndrome, 295
regression
extensive, 54, 86, 87
focal, 88, 89
rhomboidal structures, *see* angulated lines
rosacea, 277
rosettes, *see* shiny white structures
ruptured follicle, 211

sarcoidosis, 284
scalp, 244
Sarcoptes scabiei. see scabies
scabies, 300, 301
crusted, 301
jet with contrail, 300
scalp lesions
basal cell carcinoma, 240–241
B-cell lymphoma, 242
cylindromas/spiradenomas, 243
melanoma, 236–238
metastases, 239
naevus, 230–233
sarcoidosis, 244
seborrhoeic keratosis, 234–235
scar-like areas, 88, 128, 130
scarring alopecia, 248–251, 253
scleroderma, 198
sea urchins, 308, 315
sebaceous adenomas, 207, 294
sebaceous carcinoma, 209
sebaceous hyperplasia, 206, 207
sebaceous naevus, 208
seborrhoeic keratosis
clonal, 124
evolving, 116, 117
hyperkeratotic, 119
hyperpigmented, 120
hypopigmented, 121
irritated, 122
scalp, 234
traumatised, 123
serpentine vessels. *see* vessels
shiny white structures
blotches and strands, 14, 142, 143, 148, 150, 154, 272
lines, 14, 89, 102, 157, 193, 203, 270, 271
rosettes, 14, 203, 288
site-specific features, 10
skin surface markings, 83, 96, 97, 113, 317
solar lentigo, 126, 127, 220, 223
evolving seborrhoeic keratosis, 116
fingerprint pattern, 112, 216
homogeneous pattern, 113, 217
hyperpigmented 'ink spot,' 115
moth-eaten border, 218
reticular pattern, 114
spider telangiectasia, 261
spiradenomas, 243
Spitz naevus, *see* naevus
splinter haemorrhages, 191
squamous cell carcinoma
in situ, *see* Bowen's disease
moderately differentiated, 167, 169, 170, 189
nail apparatus, 189
poorly differentiated, 169–171, 240
subungual, 189
well-differentiated, 168, 170, 314
steroid-induced telangiectasia, *see* trichoscopy
structures, 9
blue pigmented, 52, 92, 146
keratinising, 7, 118, 159, 168–171, 254
leaf-like, 144, 145, 149
shiny white, *see* shiny white structures
structureless areas/background, 47, 49, 53, 71, 75, 77, 82, 83, 86, 89, 102, 104, 106, 108, 129, 132, 133, 143, 145, 147, 151, 153, 156, 177, 179, 182, 200, 206, 228, 233, 239, 242, 243, 280, 281, 284, 291–293, 295
'St. Tropez' sign, 316
subungual haematoma, 192, 193
suture material, 314

tape stripping, 318
tattoo reaction, 139
telangiectasia, *see* vessels
steroid-induced, 252

telangiectasia macularis eruptiva perstans, 275
teledermoscopy, 2
telogen bulbs, 258
tick bites, 299, 304
tinea corporis, 286
total body photography, 22, 296
traction alopecia, 257
transgredal zone, 178
triangle sign, 186
trichilemmomas, 213, 291
trichoepitheliomas, 208, 293
Trichophyton rubrum, 195, 286
trichoptilosis, *see* trichoscopy
trichoscopy
  alopecia areata, 246, 257
  androgenetic alopecia, 247
  circle hairs, 254
  discoid lupus erythematosus, 250
  frontal fibrosing alopecia, 248, 249
  lichen planopliaris, 249
  non-scarring, 246, 247
  picker's nodule, 256
  pseudonits, 258
  pseudopelade, 253
  scarring, 248–251, 253
  steroid-induced telangiectasia, 252
  traction/frictional alopecia, 257
  trichotillosis, 257
  trichoptilosis, 256
  trichostasis spinulosa, 255
  tufted folliculitis, 251
trichostasis spinulosa, *see* trichoscopy
trichotillomania, *see* trichoscopy
trichotillosis, *see* trichoscopy
tufted folliculitis, *see* trichoscopy
Tunga penetrans. see tungiasis
tungiasis, 310

urticaria pigmentosa, 275

vascular lesions
  angiokeratomas, 268
  haemangiomas, 266–267
  lymphangiomas, 269
  purpura, 273
  pyogenic granulomas, 270–271
  spider telangiectasia, 261
  subcorneal haematoma, homogeneous pattern, 264–265
  subcorneal haematoma, parallel pattern, 262–263
  telangiectasia, 260
  vascular tumours, 272
vascular morphologies, 12
vascular patterns, 13, 59, 60, 100, 103, 104, 121, 122, 214, 232
vasculitis, 283
vellus (miniaturised) hairs, 247, 248, 255
venous lake, 200
verrucae vulgaris. *see* viral warts
vessels
  arborising/branched, 11, 12, 142, 143, 146–157, 203, 204, 206–209, 211, 215, 216, 232, 240, 241–244, 260, 293, 294, 295, 313
  atypical, 50, 52, 61, 84, 94, 104, 106, 169, 179, 189, 232, 267
  clustered, 163, 166, 279
  comma/curvilinear, 12, 25, 32, 49, 117, 212, 214, 215, 230, 294, 305, 306
  corkscrew/helical, 12, 60, 94
  crown, 206, 208, 209, 306
  curved, 12, 207, 296
  dotted, 12, 36, 37, 40, 41, 46, 47, 49, 50, 52, 58, 59, 60, 62, 63, 64, 65, 71, 92, 94, 109, 125, 126, 128, 129, 134, 135, 163, 165, 194, 278, 279, 285, 286, 287, 288, 290, 296, 303
  glomerular/coiled, 12, 37, 50, 60, 108, 124, 125, 135, 137, 140, 163, 164, 166, 171, 279
  hairpin/looped, 12, 63, 65, 107, 121, 122, 125, 131, 135, 136, 140, 167, 168, 169, 170, 201, 230, 234, 280
  interfollicular, 160, 251
  irregular, 55, 58, 60, 62, 63, 64, 101–106, 109, 124, 132, 167, 169, 170, 171, 205, 239, 241, 250, 270, 305
  linear, 12, 41, 49, 67, 106, 108, 133, 135, 137–139, 138, 139, 201, 204, 207, 208, 210–214, 242, 249–252, 260, 261, 277, 284, 285, 288, 293, 294, 320
  linear-irregular, 94, 167, 169, 170, 171, 305
  nail bed capillaries, 192
  nail fold capillaries, 198
  polymorphous, 40, 53, 55, 60, 61, 63, 65, 77, 93, 94, 95, 99, 102, 104, 107, 119, 124, 157, 171, 188, 209, 305
  serpentine, 12, 242
  short fine telangiectasias, 142, 143, 145, 156
  telangiectasia, 11, 139, 142, 143, 145, 155, 156, 204, 211, 244, 245, 252, 260, 261, 275, 277, 309
viral warts, 136, 194, 307, 317, 319

Wallace's line, 178
warts
  plantar, 194, 307
  viral, 136, 194, 307, 317, 319
white starburst-like pattern, 305
Wickham's striae, 280

yellow dots, 246, 257

zig-zag lines, *see* angulated lines